Atlas of
Correlative Surgical Neuropathology and Imaging

DEDICATION
To the memory of

BETTY BROWNELL, FRCPath, 1925–1989

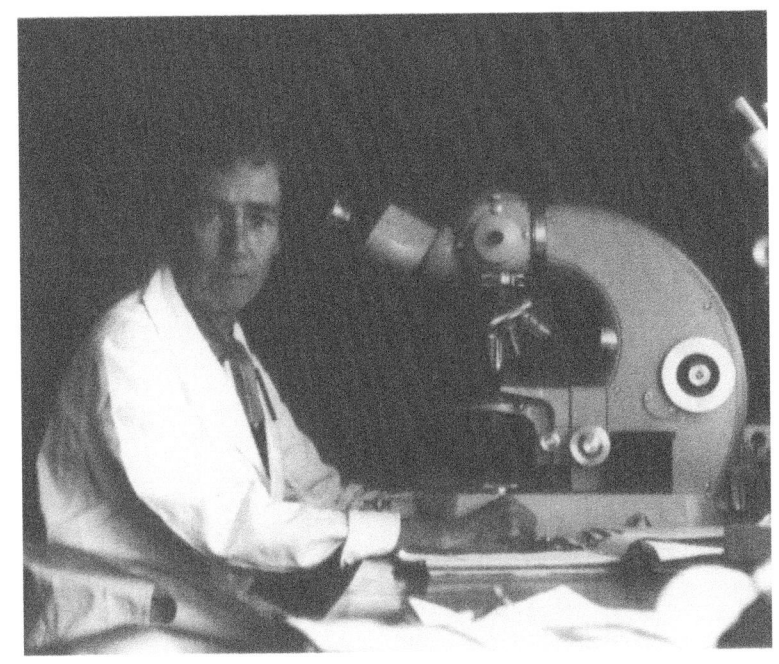

Current Histopathology

Consultant Editor
Professor G. Austin Gresham, TD, ScD, MD, FRCPath.
Emeritus Professor of Morbid Anatomy and Histopathology,
University of Cambridge

Volume Twenty-four

ATLAS OF CORRELATIVE SURGICAL NEUROPATHOLOGY AND IMAGING

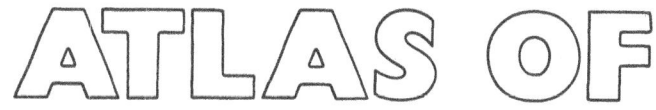

G. STUART RUTHERFOORD
Head, Neuropathology Unit
Department of Anatomical Pathology
Tygerberg Hospital
and Senior Lecturer
University of Stellenbosch
Cape Town, South Africa

and

R. H. HEWLETT
Consultant Neuropathologist
MRI Unit, City Park Hospital and
Department of Radiology (Neuroimaging)
Tygerberg Hospital
and Senior Lecturer
University of Stellenbosch
Cape Town, South Africa

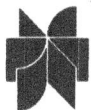
SPRINGER-SCIENCE+BUSINESS MEDIA, B.V.

A catalogue record for this book is available from the British Library.

ISBN 978-0-7923-8951-4

Library of Congress Cataloging-in-Publication Data

Rutherfoord, G. Stuart.
  Atlas of correlative surgical neuropathology and
imaging / G. Stuart Rutherfoord and R.H. Hewlett.
     p.   cm. — (Current histopathology ; v. 24)
  Includes index.
  ISBN 978-0-7923-8951-4   ISBN 978-94-011-1434-9 (eBook)
  DOI 10.1007/978-94-011-1434-9

    1. Nervous system—Histopathology—Atlases.
2. Nervous system—Imaging—Atlases. 3. Nervous
system—Surgery—Atlases. I. Hewlett, R. H.
II. Title III. Series.
    [DNLM: 1. Nervous System Diseases—
pathology—atlases. 2. Nervous System Diseases—
surgery—atlases. 3. Diagnostic Imaging—atlases.
W1 CU788JBA v. 24 1994 / WL 17 R975a 1994]
RC358.5.R88   1994
616.8'047—dc20
DNLM/DLC
for Library of Congress   94-11237
                                                      CIP

Typeset and originated by Speedlith Photo Litho Ltd., Stretford, Manchester M32 0JT

Contents

Consultant Editor's Note

At the present time books on morbid anatomy and histopathology can be divided into two broad groups: extensive textbooks often written primarily for students and monographs on research topics.

This takes no account of the fact that the vast majority of pathologists are involved in an essentially practical field of general diagnostic pathology providing an important service to their clinical colleagues. Many of these pathologists are expected to cover a broad range of disciplines and even those who remain solely within the field of histopathology usually have single and sole responsibility within the hospital for all this work. They may often have no colleagues in the same department. In the field of histopathology, no less than in other medical fields, there have been extensive and recent advances, not only in new histochemical techniques but also in the type of specimen provided by new surgical procedures.

There is a great need for the provision of appropriate information for this group. This need has been defined in the following terms:

1. It should be aimed at the general clinical pathologist or histopathologist with existing practical training, but should have value for the trainee pathologist.

2. It should concentrate on the practical aspects of histopathology taking account of the new techniques which should be within the compass of the worker in a unit with reasonable facilities.

3. New types of material, e.g. those derived from endoscopic biopsy should be covered fully.

4. There should be an adequate number of illustrations on each subject to demonstrate the variation in appearance that is encountered.

5. Colour illustrations should be used wherever they aid recognition.

The use of computerized tomography (CT) and magnetic resonance imaging (MRI) has revolutionized the diagnosis of neurological disorders. Details of normal anatomy and the precise location of lesions in the brain and spinal cord are clearly shown by the new methods. Histopathologists should be familiar with the results of CT and MRI scanning in order to make an accurate diagnosis of smears and sections of such lesions. The aim of this atlas is to achieve this familiarity. It will be most useful to neuropathologists and will be a valuable addition to the library of pathologists in training.

G.A. Gresham

Preface

Of the many factors which have combined to persuade us of the need to prepare this text, a historical association of neuroimaging and neuropathology in our professional lives has been the most influential. Beginning with the installation of the United Kingdom's second CT scanner at Frenchay Hospital, Bristol, in 1974, to the first private MR unit in Cape Town in 1989, we have never ceased to be intimately involved with clinical neuroimaging. Moreover, we have with increasing confidence found ourselves employing the standard terminology of anatomical pathology in the interpretation of images, and therefore of having to explain and justify the use of such terms to our colleagues in radiology.

Of course, the direct contribution of imaging to neuropathology has been as immense as Raymond Clasen predicted in 1982, when he wrote that 'the CT scan is, if anything, more important than electron microscopy to the neuropathologist, and [that] no description of a disease process is complete without reference to its CT characteristics'[1]. MR, with its exquisite and extraordinary depiction of the normal and abnormal neural parenchyma, has proved the ultimate reinforcement of the synthesis of optical and molecular-computed morphology, and has additionally placed neuropathology at the very centre of clinical neuroscience (even if only for the time being). This inescapable fact of present-day morbid anatomical life is the motivation for the book, and although it has, in the first place been written for pathologists, it is our hope that neuroradiologists and neurosurgeons will also find it of use.

The literature notwithstanding, our views and interpretations are based mainly on our personal experience with material in the archives of the Neuropathology Unit at Stellenbosch University Medical School, and the City Park Hospital MRI Unit. This, in turn has been accumulated from the clinical departments of Radiology and Neurosurgery at Tygerberg Hospital, and the Medical Research Council MR Unit. In addition, many invaluable cases have been made available to us from the university departments at Groote Schuur Hospital and the Red Cross Children's Hospital, as well as the Constantiaberg and Panorama private hospitals, all in greater Cape Town. Throughout we have taken care to use the images and tissue from the same individual patient; however, when the biopsy has proven unexceptional, a set of images may have been correlatively illustrated with a routine micrograph of the typical lesion, or we have simply referred to an appropriate example elsewhere in the text.

The topographic organization of subject-matter reflects the condition of contemporary surgical neuropathology: because of the images, the pathologist is not only made aware of the precise anatomical location of the tissue sample, but is also frequently presented with a reasonable differential diagnosis, whilst with stereotaxis, even specific parts of a lesion may be sampled. The immediate disadvantage of such an approach is that of repetition and fragmentation, and we have attempted to alleviate this problem by means of brief topical discussions in which particular emphasis is placed on clinical and technical factors influencing the biopsy material, together with detailed cross-referencing and careful indexing.

It is as a direct result of the gross or macroscopic morphology now supplied by the images, MR especially, that the neuropathologist is so frequently called upon to make intraoperative diagnoses on very small, or even minute, tissue samples. Smear preparations are the most effective (and often the only) way to examine these specimens, and it is for this reason that so much emphasis has been placed on this cytological technique. Without for a moment denying the essentiality of detailed histological investigation, the fact is that in a significant number of cases the final anatomical diagnosis will be a composite one, derived as much from the images and clinical data as from the histomorphology, even including nosological aspects and grades of malignancy in glial neoplasms.

Thus, the aim of the atlas is to illustrate and correlate those morphological features affecting CT and MR images, to formulate precepts where possible and, in turn, to show the influence that neuroimaging modalities have on the microscopic interpretation of smear preparations and paraffin sections. Whilst the majority of commonly biopsied lesions are presented, sometimes in a fair amount of detail, we have not attempted to cover the range of surgical neuropathology. Occasional rare conditions have been included, chiefly in order to illustrate certain principles or to draw attention to diagnostic difficulties.

ACKNOWLEDGEMENTS

In the academic environment one is expected to write; in the private hospital, however, maintaining a viable balance sheet is the primary concern. It is all the more remarkable, therefore, that one of us (R.H.H.) should have been able to devote a great deal of time to the preparation of this book, whilst employed by the Magnetic Resonance Imaging Unit of City Park Hospital. This extraordinary concession to academic neuroscience, which includes every aspect of support from contrast material to computer software, is not fortuitous, but instead the result of the calculated efforts of Dr Jan Lotz, together with the generosity of Mr Barney Hurwitz and Mr Allan Matthews. We are principally indebted to them, as well as to Prof. Hannes van der Walt, Head of Anatomical Pathology; Prof. Alan Scher, Clinical Radiology, University Stellenbosch; and Sinclair Wynchank, Head of Medical Biophysics, Medical Research Council.

Prof. A. Beyers initiated the full-time participation of a neuropathologist in the neuroradiology service and Dr Roger Smith, besides setting the standards of neuroimaging in Cape Town, has given us advice and encouragement.

W. Pieterse, Annemarie Beukes, D. Geiger, S. van Dyk, Paulette du Plessis, Ingrid Vogel, Giselle Rouillard, Enver Ebrahim, Neville Hans, Ingrid Cloete and Lesley Harley provided technical, darkroom and graphics expertise. Mrs Aniel Allen has borne the secretarial burdens without in any way giving in.

Drs Pat Kirby and S. Wynchank read and criticized the manuscript, and Dr Freddie Kieck, neurosurgeon at City Park Hospital, made his magnificent library freely available to us.

Material in the form of scans, blocks and slides has come from all the major hospitals in the greater Cape Town area, as well as from many other centres in the South African Republic, and we are particularly grateful to those colleagues and friends who have been unstinting

Abbreviations

Ab	antibody
AB	Alcian blue stain for acid mucins
Ag	antigen
AOCVM	angiographically occult cerebrovascular malformation
APAS	combined Alcian blue/PAS stain
AVM	arteriovenous malformation
BB	Bismark Brown stain for mast cells
BBB	blood–brain barrier
CP	cerebello-pontine
CR	Congo red stain for amyloid
CT	computerized tomography
CT+C	CT scan with contrast
CTBW	CT bone window
CV	cresyl fast violet (Nissl) stain
EM	electron microscopy
EMA	epithelial membrane antigen
EVG	Verhoeff's elastic stain, VG counterstain
FF	frozen fat stain
GFAP	glial fibrillary acidic protein
Giemsa	Giemsa stain
Gram	Gram stain for micro-organisms
HE	haematoxylin and eosin stain
Holmes/LB	combined Holmes/Luxol blue stain
Holmes	Holmes method for neuritic processes
IAM	internal auditory meatus
ITC	individual tumour cells
JPA	juvenile pilocytic astrocytoma
LB	Luxol blue stain for myelin
LBCV	combined Luxol blue/cresyl violet stain
LBHE	combined Luxol blue/haematoxylin and eosin stain
MAB	monoclonal antibody
MFH	malignant fibrous histiocytoma
MGP	methyl green-pyronin stain for RNA
MS	Grocott-Gomori methenamine silver stain for fungi
MT	Masson's trichrome stain for connective tissue
NF	neurofilament
NOS	not otherwise specified
OFG	orange fuchsin green for anterior pituitary cells
PAP	peroxidase–anti-peroxidase method to localize Ag
PAS	periodic acid–Schiff reaction for glycogen
PAS/OG	combined PAS/orange G for anterior pituitary cells
PCNSL	primary central nervous system lymphoma
PD	proton density
PDWI	proton density weighted image
Perls'	Perls' prussian blue reaction for ferric iron

PNET	primitive neuroectodermal tumour
PTAH	Mallory's phosphotungstic acid haematoxylin stain
Retic	Gordon and Sweets' silver stain for reticular fibres
RNA	ribonucleic acid
SEGC, SEGCA	subependymal giant cell (astrocytoma)
T1WI	T1 weighted image
T1WI+C	T1WI with contrast
T2WI	T2 weighted image
TBH	Tygerberg Hospital
TBM	tuberculous meningitis
Tol blue	toluidine blue stain
TR	repetition time
UCHL1	University College Hospital, antibody L1 (T-cell marker)
VG	van Gieson's stain for collagen
VK	von Kossa stain for calcium
Zn	Ziehl-Neelsen stain for tubercle bacilli

Introduction to neuroimaging, diagnostic approach, smear technique and principles

1.1. INTRODUCTION TO THE PRINCIPLES OF NEUROIMAGING

The advent of magnetic resonance imaging (MRI) has had the same profound effect on medical and surgical neurology that computerized tomography (CT) had, when that modality first appeared. Compared with CT, however, MR images are both more detailed and more specific, whilst views in any axis are possible, the so-called multiplanar facility. That MRI has superseded CT in aspects of neurology is beyond doubt: yet CT continues to be a cost-effective investigation in many circumstances, and in most institutions the two modalities thrive side by side. Many patients, therefore, have undergone both types of imaging, and the diagnostic process oscillates between the terminologies of each. This assumption of parallel interpretation is made throughout the text.

The reader, by default, will be a pathologist who has accepted the necessity for some imaging competence[1], the level of which is determined by a number of technical questions, such as why do the pictures vary in grain and greyness; in relation to what is density determined on the CT; what is meant by spin echo and by TR/TE; what is enhancement? For most clinicians a non-mathematical approach to these technicalities is essential, and the extent to which this can be achieved by language and picture is very well exemplified in the remarkable booklet by Hans Schild[2]. However, in our opinion there is no satisfactory account of MRI for those individuals whose mental capabilities and clinical needs do not permit fluency with nuclear and atomic physics, even allowing for admirable, current texts[3]. In the brief following account the aim has been to emphasize the jargon of imaging within concepts, since it is over the use of technical terms that ways invariably part.

1.2. COMPUTERIZED TOMOGRAPHY OR CT SCANNING

It is worth recalling that the introduction of CT scanning in the early 1970s was the single biggest advance in radiology since the discovery of X-rays. The principle of CT, elaborated by the English and South African physicists, Hounsfield and Cormack, involves the delivery, from several angles, of a gated X-ray beam through an object as depicted in Figure 1.1. Sensors detect and measure the photons which pass through the object, and comparison with their initial intensity allows a determination of what is called *attenuation* – that is, their diminution in number. At the same time, the number of *volume elements* (voxels) of tissue generated by the composite slice angles is calculated, and each voxel is represented in two dimensions, as a point of photon intensity or *picture element* (pixel) in the final image. Pixels are arranged in rows and columns, referred to as a *matrix*, a minimum number for acceptable resolution being a square of 256 by 256 pixels (Figure 1.1). It follows that computation of pixel intensity will be a reflection of X-ray intensity and slice width, both factors having now been optimized and standardized by convention.

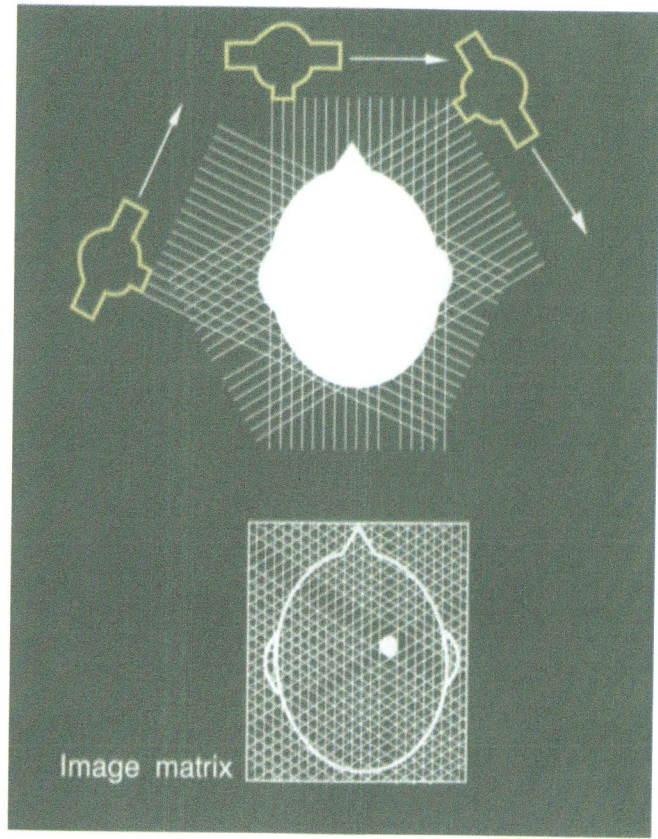

Figure 1.1 Mathematical image construction: by means of a convolutional algorithm the calculated attenuation values are converted into shades of grey and displayed as an image. Every punctiform picture element (pixel) corresponds to a volume element (voxel), and the grey value of the pixel represents the attenuation value of the voxel

Pixel counts, representing as they do, the passage of X-rays through the volume elements (*voxels*) of various tissues, also reflect the attenuation of these same rays, and therefore the 'density-value' of the tissue(s); conversely, the tissues themselves have their own absorption properties or density coefficients, which have been graded as *Hounsfield Units* (HU). The measurement and pixel-conversion of photons is achieved by means of a convolution algorithm and forms the basis of the computed tomogram.

It will be immediately apparent that for a noticeable difference to occur between an object and its surroundings the voxel must bear an appropriate proportion to the X-ray slice width. In a slice of 8 mm thickness, a mean density difference of about 5 HU (under optimal conditions) is enough to permit a recognizable alteration of tissue detail. A homogeneous object larger than the slice width can be seen with density differences even smaller than 5 HU. Any abnormal substance or structure which only partially occupies the volume element will be read as the so-called *partial volume average*, and the resultant image may be unrecognizable or spurious. A

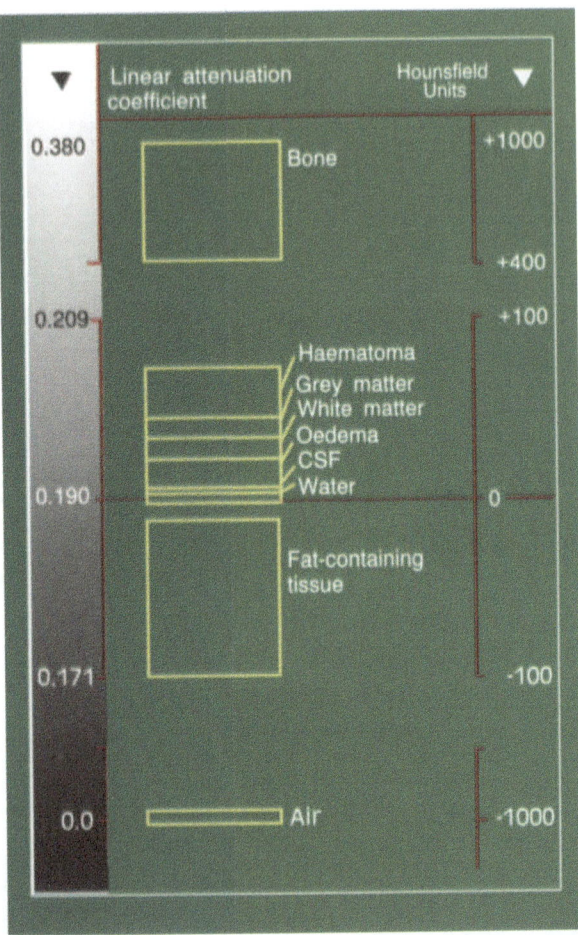

Figure 1.2 **Grey scale**: attenuation values of the structures occurring in a cranial slice at a tube voltage of 120 kV

common example of morphologic 'artefact' resulting from partial volume averaging is when a cerebral sulcus and portion of adjacent cortex lie horizontally within the same slice, so that CSF and brain are measured together.

In the representation of Hounsfield Units in terms of grey (the so-called grey scale), water has been arbitrarily set as 0, with dense mineral and air making the extremes of hyperdensity (1000) and hypodensity (−1000) respectively (Figure 1.2). For practical purposes the pathologist needs to be aware of the average densities of CSF, white matter, grey matter and mixtures of the latter two, as seen in the pontine basis. The visual perception of normal brain and other tissue densities on the CT scan is subject to the *window settings* of the display unit or console: these are *width*, in which the grey-scale bands are widened or compressed, with resulting alteration of grain; and *level*, where the image is set at any point of the grey scale, with appropriate alteration of tissue density (Figure 1.3). Contemporary scanners have certain pre-selected image parameters or protocols, in which the window settings are chosen for specific tissue studies, e.g. brain, bone and abdomen. The effects of these different programmes on a standard axial slice of the brain are shown in Figures 1.3 and 1.4.

The *density* of normal and abnormal tissues can be altered in the direction of increased brightness (or increased attenuation – a double-negative demanded by the fact that the usual CT pictures are themselves negatives!) by the administration of *contrast agents*. These contain iodine, and are injected intravenously, as rapidly as possible. The composition, dose, injection rate and circulation time of contrast determine the degree of brightness or *enhancement*, which is then described as normal or abnormal with regard to a specific tissue or structure. Because of their very large molecular weights, contrast media do not cross the intact blood–brain barrier; thus in the normal state transient enhancement is seen

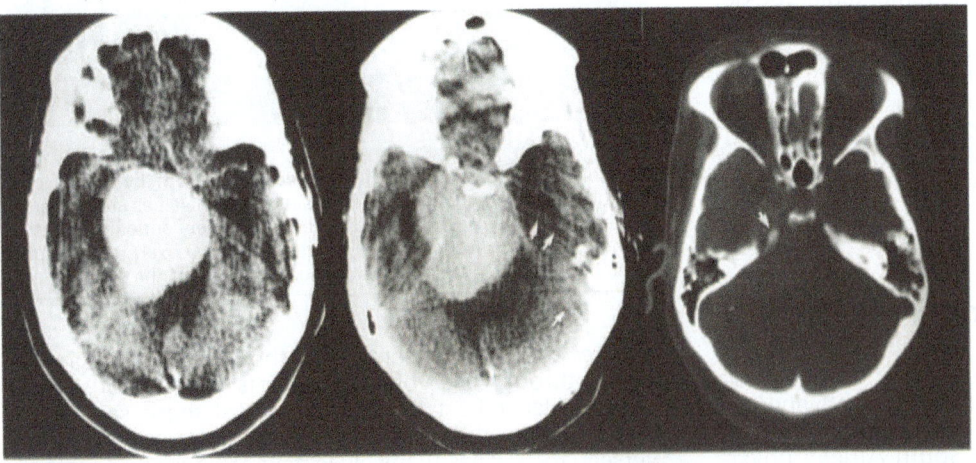

Figure 1.3 **Window settings** (clivus meningioma): (**a–c**) CT + C; standard protocol for cerebral hemispheres (**a**), posterior fossa (**b**) and bone window (**c**). Bony artefacts (**b**, arrows) of posterior fossa necessitate the use of a protocol resulting in a finer grain and contrast reduction. With bone window setting, soft tissue detail is lost; note erosion of petrous apex (**c**, arrow), only visible with this protocol

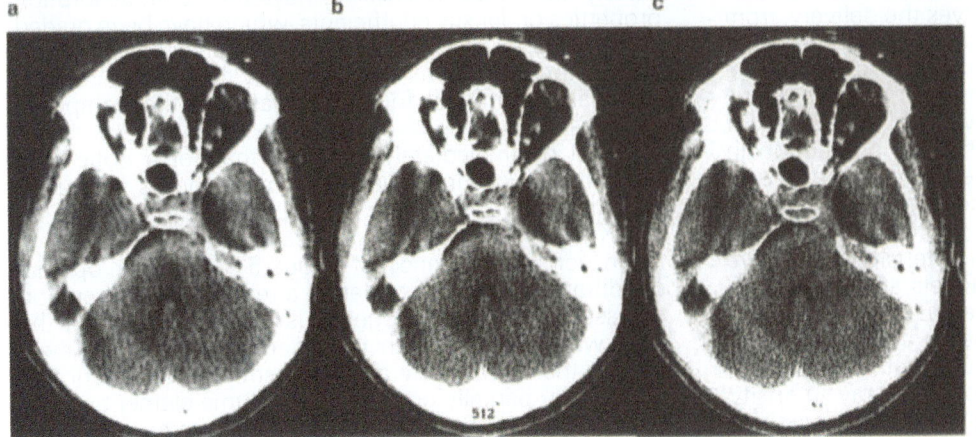

Figure 1.4 **Technical factors**: (**a**) CT matrix 256 × 256, (**b**) CT matrix 512 × 512 (**c**) CT bone-edge enhancement filter: technically imposed variations in density and grain, on an identical posterior fossa slice

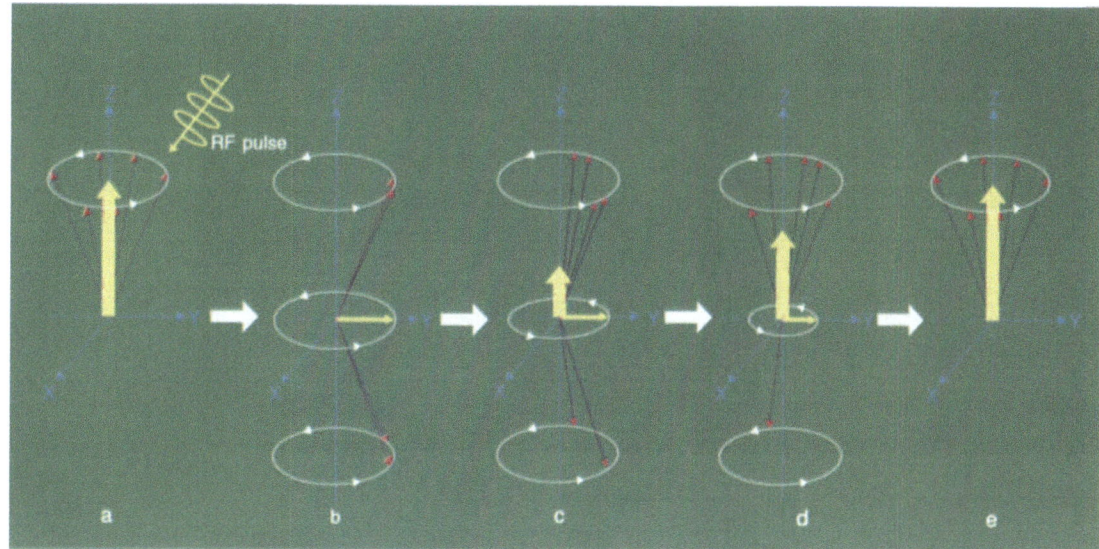

Figure 1.5 (**a**) Depicts aligned hydrogen protons within the applied magnetic field, and the consequent net longitudinal magnetization. (**b**) Following application of RF pulse, precession is synchronized (phase coherence), with resultant net transverse magnetization (*x–y* axis). (**c,d**) Cessation of RF pulse results in dephasing of protons, decay of transverse magnetization (spin-spin relaxation/T2 signal) and progressive resumption of longitudinal magnetization (spin-lattice relaxation/T1 signal). (**e**) Return to steady state within the applied magnetic field. (Broad arrows represent magnetic vectors; individual precessing protons are shown by red arrows)

macroscopically within the larger intracranial vessels, both arterial and venous, whilst tissues with a rich microvasculature, such as grey matter, choroid plexus and pituitary infundibulum, also brighten appreciably. In the neuropathological context, immediate enhancement seen in abnormal tissues is probably mainly on the basis of vascular density[4], whilst leakage from structurally defective capillaries, combined with the presence of a suitable perivascular interstitial space, constitute the other necessary conditions.

1.3. MAGNETIC RESONANCE IMAGING (MRI)

1.3a. The basis of the signal

MR imaging makes use of three aspects of atomic physics in particular; the predominance of magnetic *hydrogen protons* in biological tissues; the ability of protons to *resonate* in response to a radiofrequency (RF) pulse after more or less uniform alignment has been induced by means of a static, external magnetic field; and the capture of resonant signals or *echoes* after the orchestrated protons have been made to perform uniform changes of alignment within the magnetic field by means of pulsed radio waves. The frequency of the radio pulse, referred to as the *Larmor frequency*, is a function of the intrinsic resonating frequency of hydrogen protons at any specified magnetic field strength, and at 1 Tesla this happens to be about 43 MHz. The intervals which separate the RF pulses and echoes are called *repetition time* (*TR*) and *time to echo* (*TE*) respectively.

In brief, within the bore of the magnet, the patient's precessing protons and their magnetic fields become aligned parallel (lower energy state) or anti-parallel (higher energy state), to the external magnetic field, with the establishment of a new *longitudinal magnetic vector* (in the *z* axis). Protons, precessing (or wobbling) at a specific frequency, have the 'ability' to absorb energy from a radio wave of the same frequency (a phenomenon called resonance); thus the application of a RF pulse of specific angle and duration alters the ratio of parallel to anti-parallel protons and at the same time stimulates 'in-phase' or synchronous precession. The net effect is the disappearance of the longitudinal vector, and the development of a *rotating transverse* (x–y *axis*) *magnetic vector*, moving at the same frequency as the in-phase, precessing protons (Figure 1.5).

The most commonly-used MR imaging technique is referred to as *spin echo*, short for *saturation recovery– spin echo*. Although this term strictly refers to the MR signal (echo) derived from the transverse, rotational movement and dephasing of protons (*T2 relaxation*), by convention it is also applied to that part of the sequence when the ensemble of magnetized protons (actually their summed magnetic moments), after having been tipped out of the north–south axis of the magnet, return to their former position, that is the return to longitudinal magnetization (*T1 relaxation*).

Thus, the T1 time is associated with the rate at which the protons 'relax' by disseminating energy to their surroundings, or lattice; hence the term *spin-lattice* relaxation, and from it is derived the *T1 signal* (Figure 1.5). Protons within complex biological tissues have a mix of T1 relaxation properties, and by keeping the TR short (*T1 weighting*), the signal (energy release) from molecules with short (rapid) relaxation (e.g. lipids) will be captured as image hyperintensity, whilst those with long relaxation times, especially water, are excluded, thereby providing the component of image hypointensity (Figure 1.6).

As already described, the other principal component of the MR technique, is concerned with the induced, synchronized precession or *phase coherence* of hydrogen protons and their subsequent *dephasing*, or loss of phase coherence, due to cancelling-out of the magnetic moments of the hydrogen protons, mainly by nearby molecules with their own magnetic fields, a process denoted by the term *spin-spin* relaxation. In this synchronized but unstable state the transversely rotating (resonating), magnetic vector induces an electrical current in an appropriately positioned receiving antenna, producing a transient echo. However, the rate of decay of this vector is so rapid that, in order to accurately determine the so-called *T2 relaxation*, the protons require to be repeatedly rephased as they continue to spiral (or flip back) toward the north–south axis, thus generating multiple diminishing echoes which collectively represent the *T2 signal* (and hence the term *multi-echo sequence* (Figure 1.5). The

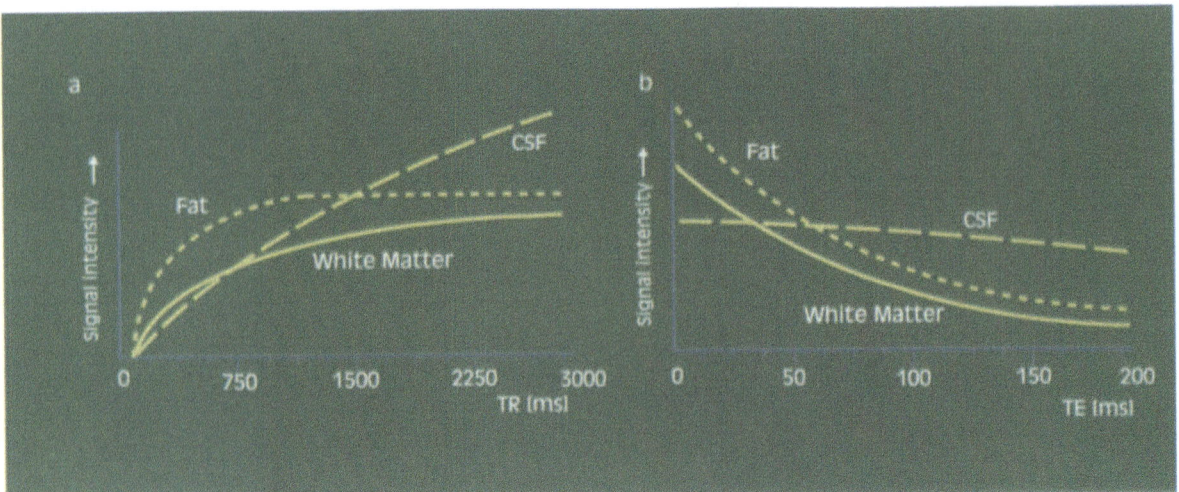

Figure 1.6 Spin-echo technique: graphic representation illustrating dependence on TR and TE

innate length of the multi-echo acquisition requires a long TR (*T2 weighting*), and thus favours signals from protons within tissues and substances with long relaxation times (ultimately free water in bulk), whilst excluding, or rendering hypointense, those of short relaxation properties (Figure 1.6).

Another important effect of the repeated late (long TR) rephasing of protons is that the rotating transverse vector has an initial magnitude roughly equal to that of the original static *z* axis vector, both being proportional to the density of proton nuclei in the tissue. Thus, very early (short TE) recording of the signal produced by this rotating vector, before T2 effects have had time to really show up, results in an image (Figure 1.8) where differences in tissue contrast are dependent on *proton density* (also called spin density).

1.3b. Construction of the image

The spatial localization of ensembles of protons within the *slice* of excited tissues, requires the use of suitably placed coils inside the main magnet, so providing *field gradients* along the three principal axes. In this way each volume element will possess a population of protons whose frequency and phase coherence differs slightly from that of its neighbour. The computation of these differences, called *phase and frequency encoding*, forms the basis of the image, and it is easy to see how the slightest movement of protons between adjacent voxels will give rise to artefacts (Figure 1.7).

1.3c. Paramagnetism and contrast enhancement

Paramagnetic substances with unpaired electrons, such as *gadolinium*, have small local magnetic fields which enhance or shorten the relaxation of surrounding protons (but only in the presence of an external magnetic field). Effectively, this is most easily demonstrated with short TR, producing signal hyperintensity in the T1 image and forms the basis of *contrast enhancement* in MRI. Because gadolinium exerts its effect only when in close proximity to protons, and does not cross the intact blood–brain barrier, enhancement occurs only with barrier deficiency or disruption, together with an extravascular space to permit pooling. *Ferromagnetism*, by inducing *fixed inhomogeneities*, accelerates spin–spin relaxation, and is most apparent as hypointensity with long TR/TE.

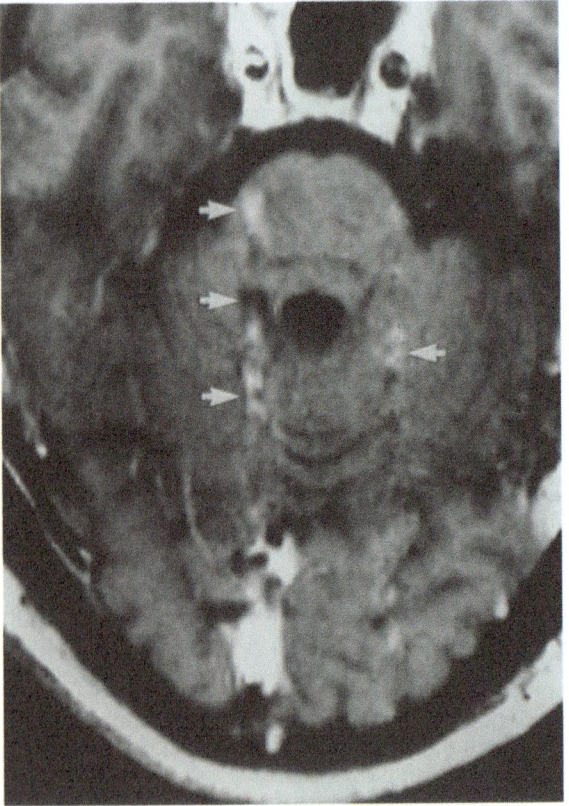

Figure 1.7 Phase encoding artefact (due to carotid pulsation); characteristic bands of alternating signal intensity are aligned with the carotid vessels (arrows); this type of artefact[a] may seriously affect the normal signal intensity composition of the brainstem
[a]Clark JA, Kelly WM. Common artefacts encountered in magnetic resonance imaging. Radiol Clin N Am. 1988;26:893–920.

1.3d. The grey scale in MRI

By now the reader will be aware that, compared with CT, the physical basis of the grey scale in MRI is totally different, being a composite of individually differing pulse sequences, in turn reflecting proton density, molecular composition, etc., and all being subject to the strength of, and variations in, the ambient magnetic field. The fact is that no *single combination* of TR/TE can capture the necessary range of normal or abnormal tissue signal intensities, and at the same time express these in terms

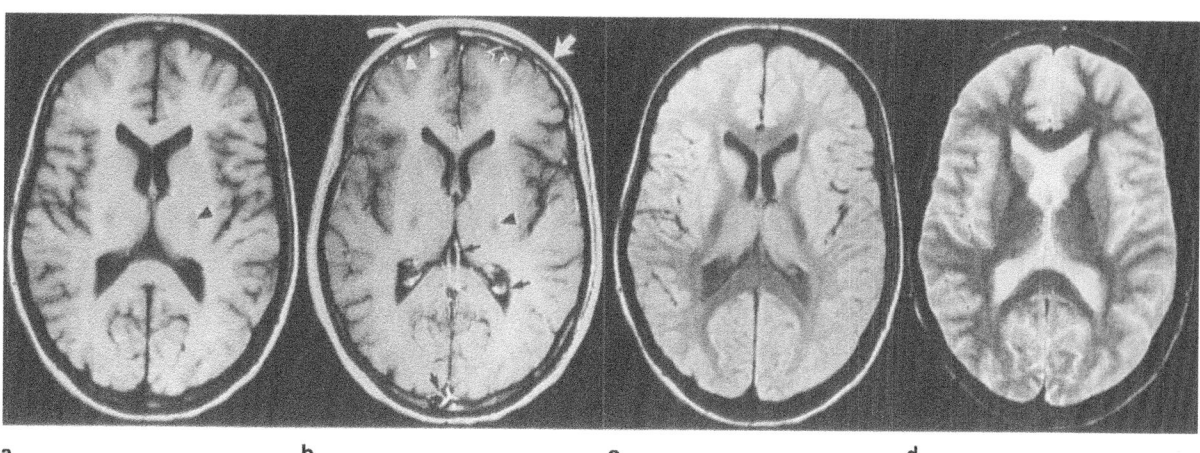

a   b   c   d

Figure 1.8 Normal brain, spin-echo sequence: (a) T1WI (TR560/TE15 ms), (b) T1WI + C, (c) PDWI (TR2800/TE15 ms), (d) T2WI (TR2800/TE90 ms); grey matter has intermediate signal intensity at short TR, whilst white matter is relatively bright (a,b). Signals become reversed at long TR (c,d). CSF remains hypointense on PDWI (c), becoming hyperintense at full T2 weighting (d). Variation in frontal and occipital white-matter hypointensity (d) is technical. Note prominent hyperintensity of scalp (b, closed arrow) and marrow (b, open arrow) adipose tissue; signal is greatly reduced at long TR/TE (d). Outer hypointense rim (b, curved arrows) is cortical bone, whilst inner rim is composite of inner table bone and CSF (b, arrow-heads). Enhancement is occurring in choroid plexus, cerebral veins and sagittal sinus (b, dark arrows – compare with a). Focal internal capsule hypointensities (a,b, arrow-heads) are normal

of *contrast* sufficient to provide meaningful anatomical or gross pathological detail. For each series of images the description of signal intensities always has to be made in terms of relationships, these being the norms of grey and white matter, CSF and adipose tissue respectively.

Where tissues are concerned, these comparisons can often be restricted to the short TR (T1 weighted) and long TR/TE (T2 weighted) images, but because of its dependence on protein concentration, long TR/short TE (proton density weighted) images are needed in any assessment of water, including CSF and cyst fluid. Bony and dense fibrous tissue (Figure 4.68), having little or no water, will not appear at all in the images, nor will blood which is moving sufficiently fast for protons to have escaped from the slice where their echoes cannot be captured – the *flow (signal) void*.

1.4. INTERPRETATION OF THE IMAGE
1.4a. The normal neural parenchyma

The crisp profile of the brain provided by the surrounding CSF space, and the structured inhomogeneity of grey and white matter, respectively, comprise the features of *morphology* and *signal intensity*, the latter being the pathoanatomical equivalent of colour and consistency. At short TR (T1 weighted image) white matter is relatively bright (hyperintense) compared with grey, a manifestation of the short relaxation time of myelin lipids, the cause of which is not entirely explained at present, but might be the effect of cholesterol[5] (Figure 1.8). Lengthening the TR but not the TE (proton density weighted image) starts to include less tightly bound tissue hydrogen protons and some forms of water (hydration water), but not that which is 'free' in the CSF; the signal intensity of grey and white matter is reversed as tissue with short relaxivity is excluded (Figure 1.8). With long TR/TE (T2 weighted image), progressive brightening of all grey matter occurs, as a result increasing the signal from tissue water, with real T2 hyperintensity of bulk water in the CSF; coincidentally, the myelin and other short-relaxation tissues become hypointense as the combination of long TR/TE excludes their signal (Figure 1.8).

As a working principle, T1 weighted images are used for the assessment of *anatomical* detail and those pathological processes exhibiting signal shortening or hyperintensity (notably haemorrhage, lipids and contrast agents), whilst T2 weighted images are used for the assessment of any *pathological* alteration of normal brain water, manifested as signal prolongation or hyperintensity, as well as those substances which shorten the signal (notably iron and mucin). Besides the specified deviations of hyper- or hypointensity in each sequence, signal abnormalities are also defined in terms of *homogeneity* or its reverse.

The concept of relative signal intensities of soft tissues in spin-echo images, is the result of the obvious need for the viewer to assess the diagnostic significance of grey-scale differences. Relaxation-time maps generated from such studies[6,7] show the difference between most soft tissue, muscle and fat, for which purpose, having a homogeneous structure such as the liver as a reference point is a great advantage. The distinct signal intensity differences of grey and white matter, however, necessitate specific reference to cortex or white matter at least, and sometimes to brainstem parenchyma and CSF as well, and is the cause of descriptive prolixity in neuroimaging. That aside, it can never be too strongly emphasized that all assessments of grey scale variation have to be translated into alterations of signal within the context of the imaging parameters.

1.4b. Adipose tissue

The protons in adipose cell non-polar lipids exhibit exceptionally short T1 (spin-lattice) and moderate T2 (spin-spin) relaxation, thus constituting the most commonly encountered form of T1 tissue hyperintensity (Figure 1.8). Although fat cells are also the principal source of marrow hyperintensity at short TR, assessment of signal, especially the vertebral bodies, requires consideration of the normal, age-related conversion of red to yellow type[8], as well as the pathological alterations secondary to discogenic disease[9].

1.4c. Tissue water, cerebral oedema and spongiosis

Tissue water exists in three principal physical states, namely, *bound* (i.e. bonded to a macromolecule or ion); *structured* (i.e. having its motion restricted or 'perturbed' by the macromolecule or membrane); *bulk* (i.e. relatively freely mobile), with respective T1 or spin-lattice relaxation times varying from short to long[5]. Regardless of the

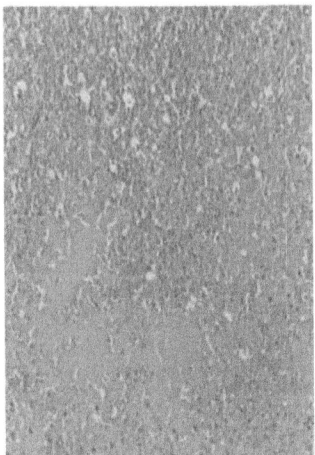
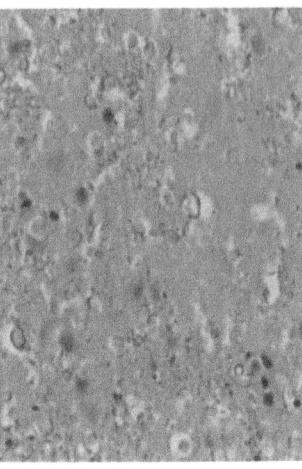

Figure 1.9 Oedema, vasogenic: parenchyma is disrupted by lakes of eosinophilic, proteinaceous fluid; interspersed fibres exhibit axonal spheroids, myelin ballooning and fragmentation; necrotic oligodendroglial nuclei stain indistinctly. Images at this stage are characteristically CT hypodense, T2 hyperintense, with volumetric expansion; T1 signal may be unaltered. LBHE × 40/ × 400

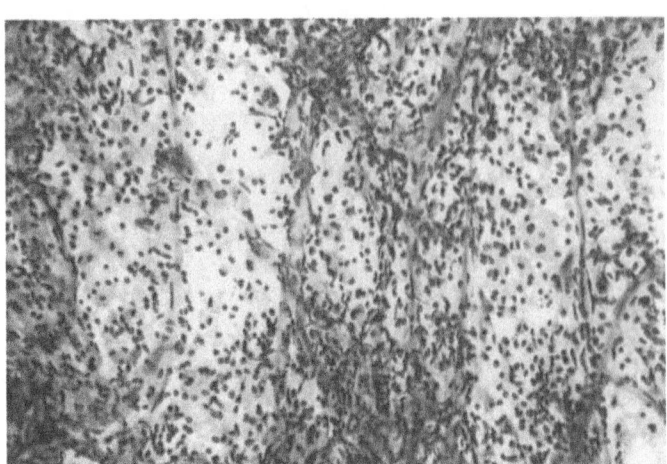

Figure 1.10 Infarct, early subacute: smear preparation, illustrating vascular leashes with intervening macrophages. Giemsa × 100

mechanism, any water expansion of the parenchymal interstitial space is readily apparent as abnormal hyperintensity on T2W images (CT hypodense), with maximal contrast afforded by the relatively hypointense myelin. By the same token, T1 hypointensity tends to be unobtrusive until bulk water is present in sufficient amount. The macromolecular-associated or structured water, also known as hydration water[10], is of great importance in neuroimaging, since it exhibits selective T1 shortening on the proton density images (long TR/short TE) and therefore distinguishes hyperintense pathological parenchyma adjacent to the hypointense ventricle (Figure 4.20). For practical purposes the signal alterations of oedema and spongiosis are identical, the former being identified by the presence of volumetric expansion and fibre tract-associated bulk flow[11] (Figure 1.9).

1.4d. Cyst fluids and protein content

In the neuropil and subarachnoid space the fluid content of many degenerative and congenital cysts follows the signal intensity of CSF on all sequences (see also section 3.1). However, in some cysts increasing protein concentration (whether secretory, transudative or exudative) produces T1 shortening, so that accumulated fluid is often isointense with brain and therefore invisible at short TR, although still T2 hyperintense. With macromolecular protein concentrations in excess of 20%, mucocele and Rathke's cleft cyst being good examples (Figures 2.3 and 5.4), the T1 signal is shortest, even resembling that of adipose tissue in hyperintensity, whilst the T2 hyperintensity declines; such accumulations have been noted to have gel viscosity. However, with progressive inspissation, bulk proteins become hypointense at both short and long TR[12]. In addition to the factor of concentration, glycoproteins, including mucin, have the capacity to bind free water, effectively shortening spin-spin relaxation time, and thus constituting an important mechanism of selective T2 hypointensity[13].

1.4e. Necrosis

Necrosis is generally identified as water-dependent T2 hyperintensity and T1 hypointensity, but is modified by the underlying tissue substrate, as well as the degree

and blend of coagulation and liquefaction. Subacute ischaemic necrosis of neural parenchyma (i.e. prior to cavitation) presents a uniform inhomogeneity, resulting from the mix of debris, macrophages and vascular relics, the last presenting as characteristic strings on smearing (Figure 1.10). Similar morphological factors must account for a comparable picture in glioma necrosis (Figure 4.29). Pure coagulative necrosis, as exemplified in the tuberculous gumma, must contain mainly structured water (or else free radicals), since it is relatively T2 hypointense (white matter isointense), T1 isointense and also CT isodense (see section 3.2). The liquefied necrotic contents of a pyogenic abscess are diffusely T2 hyperintense/T1 hypointense, CT hypodense (see section 4.4a.), and may be indistinguishable from necrotic metastasis (see section 4.12).

1.4f. Gliosis, gliomesodermal response and granulation tissue

These glial-vasoproliferative reactions are brain isodense and isointense, and are identified passively because of T2 highlighting (i.e. surrounding oedema) and actively with contrast administration (Figure 4.8). No distinction can be made between inflammatory granulation tissue of pyogenic (abscess wall) (Figure 4.9) or granulomatous (epithelioid cell-associated) aetiopathogenesis (Figure 4.17), and usually neither type displays water-dependent T2 hyperintensity. The reason(s) for this are uncertain, but are currently thought to be associated with the effects of free radicals. While collagen and reticulin are almost invariably found in the inflammatory response, making smear preparation difficult, the even spread of abnormally plentiful vessels, together with reactive glia and myelinophages typifying ischaemic granulation tissue, provides no obstruction in the preparation of cytological specimens. Pure gliosis is characterized by T2 hyperintensity because of the inevitable accompanying spongiotic interstitium (Figure 1.11).

When the reparative process is associated with significant haemorrhage, haemosiderin induces paramagnetic T2 signal shortening or hypointensity which is even more pronounced than the normally hypointense myelin. The basis of contrast enhancement in granulation tissue includes increased vascular density together with leakage which, because of its transience, is assumed to be maturational[14].

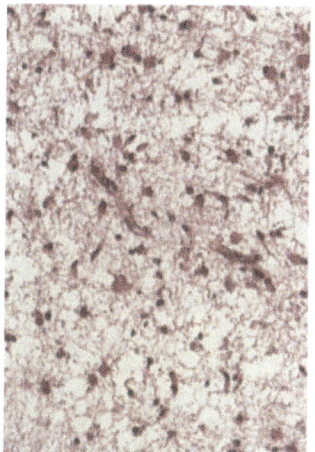 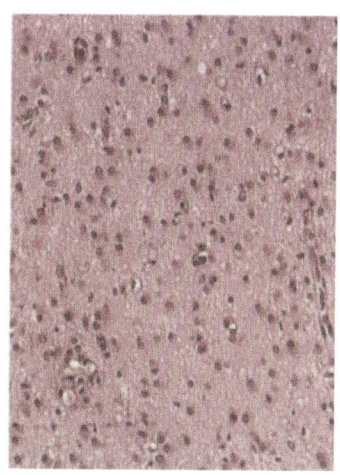

Figure 1.11 Spongiosis/gliosis: illustrates marked (left), and mild (right) spongiosis, in association with gliosis; former probably determines hyperintensity on T2 weighted images, and if sufficiently extensive, T1 hypointensity. HE ×100

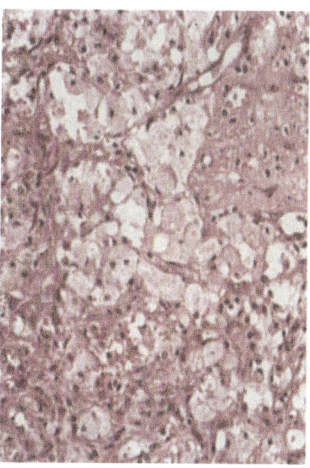 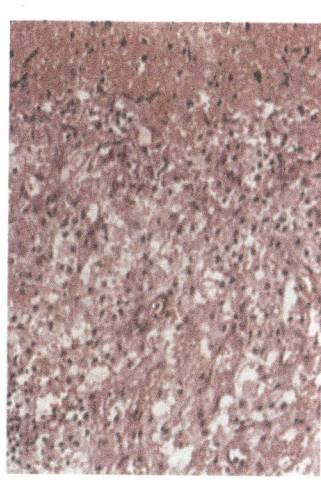

Figure 1.12 Gliomesodermal response: stages in the gliomesodermal response illustrating vascular proliferation and progressive engorgement of macrophages; criteria for enhancement are apparent, including vascular density and widened interstitial space; immature vessels are known to be leaking mainly on account of deficient junctional complexes. HE ×100

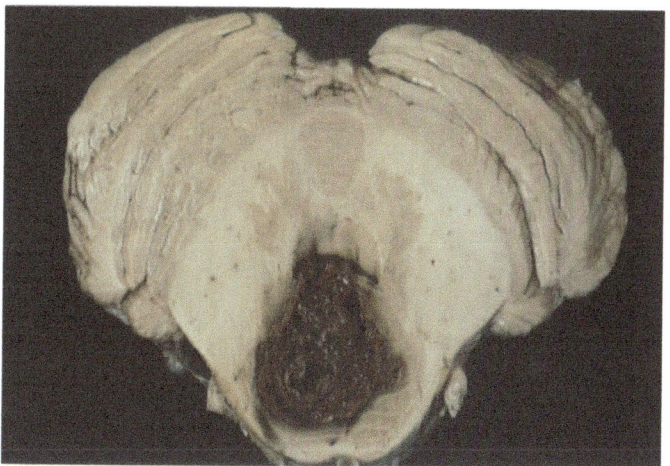

Figure 1.13 Haematoma, resolving (late subacute), brainstem: peripheral part of lesion is brick-red due to blood breakdown products, mainly haemosiderin (CT hypodense, T1 hyperintense/T2 hypointense), whilst central part is still gelatinous, consisting of serum, lysed red cells and fibrin (CT hyperdense, T1/T2 hyperintense). (Dark pigmentation of surrounding parenchyma is due to the formation of acid haematin, consequent to formalin fixation)

1.4g. Haemorrhage

With CT, acute haemorrhage confined to the brain parenchyma is hyperdense, usually homogeneous, with a sharply circumscribed border (Figure 4.1); after a week, contrast injection shows a thin rim of enhancement separated from the shrinking hyperdensity by a progressively widening zone of isodensity (Figure 4.1); this enhancement represents the gliomesodermal reaction (Figure 1.12), whilst the isodense tissue is composed of hordes of haemosiderophages with interspersed degenerate fibrin and red blood cells (Figure 4.1). By the third or fourth week all hyperdensity disappears and, apart from anatomical distortion, the enhancing ring lesion, usually perceptibly smaller, may be all that can be demonstrated; at this stage macroscopic examination shows the haematoma to be brick red and gelatinous throughout (Figure 1.13). The organized, resorbing clot is then replaced by fluid, with progressive loss of density and, depending on the degree of infarction accompanying the original haemorrhage, an angular CSF-isodense cavity, often less

than a quarter of the volume of the original haematoma, is the residuum. These events are summarized diagrammatically in Figure 1.14.

By comparison with this simple and pathogenetically satisfactory series of events, MR of parenchymal haemorrhage is complex in the extreme, being a reflection of the differing magnetic susceptibilities of blood and its degradation products, as well as the effects of intervening tissue fluid. It is also one area of imaging where pathologists need to be particularly aware of the signal variations generated with different magnetic field strengths and data acquisition techniques (i.e. spin echo versus gradient echo)[15,16]. The events in spin echo sequences at 1 Tesla may be summarized as follows: (1) Fresh or hyperacute haematoma resembles the CT image, being strongly hyperintense on the T2 and PD weighted images and slightly T1 hyperintense, (2) At 12–24 hours later, intracellular deoxyhaemoglobin initiates T2 shortening (hypointensity) but has little effect on the T1 signal; contrast on the T2W image is provided by the surrounding hyperintensity of vasogenic oedema, (3) Over the next few days the accumulation of intracellular methaemoglobin initiates T1 shortening (hyperintensity), and maintains T2 shortening (hypointensity), (4) At about 10–14 days the lysis of red cells allows methaemoglobin to go into solution, initiating T2 signal prolongation (hyperintensity) whilst maintaining T1 signal hyperintensity. These four phases of signal alteration also correspond, generally, to the stages of hyperacute, acute, subacute and chronic haematoma, respectively. Studied with this information, the diagram reproduced after Chaney et al.[17] (Figure 1.15) displays the temporal profile to advantage. A feature unique to MR is the presence of a T2 hypointense rim to the resorbing haematoma (Figure 4.1), caused by haemosiderin (see also below), whilst the decline of T1 hyperintensity and maintenance of T2 hyperintensity reflect the gradual conversion of the clot to interstitial fluid, copying the density fall on CT.

Apart from neoplastic haemorrhages, biopsy samples from haematomas are encountered only in the treatment of occult angioma and the rare chronic expanding haematoma (section 4.1a). Autopsy material will therefore remain crucial in correlating these lesions with the images, and it is also worth remarking that, in our opinion, of the many current accounts of brain haemorrhage on MR, that of Thulborn and Atlas is the most satisfactory[17].

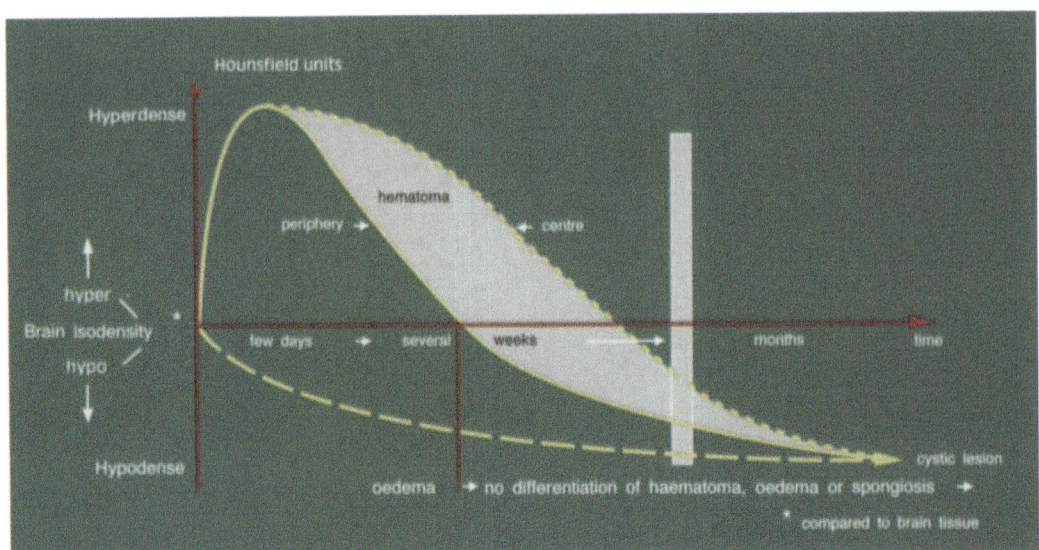

Figure 1.14 Haematoma: CT features (see text for explanation)

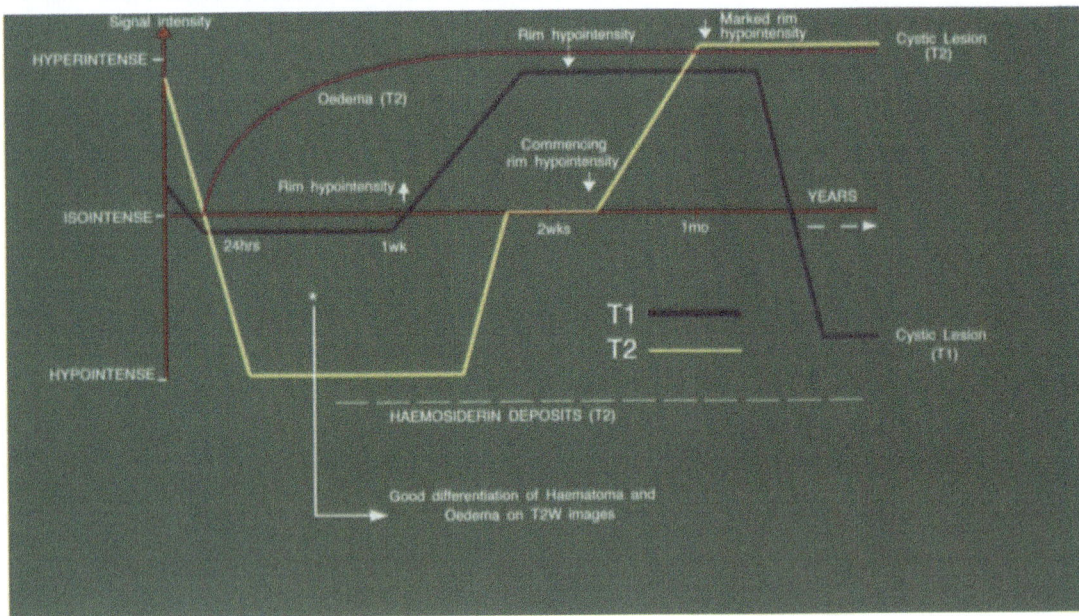

Figure 1.15 Haematoma: MRI features (see text for explanation)

1.4h. Calcification and mineralization

The demonstration of various elements, besides calcium, in tissues conventionally regarded as calcified[18], has prompted the use of the term 'mineralization' by most pathologists, without clarifying the role or nomenclature for iron, which can often be determined coincidentally[19].

Calcification, even when presenting as obvious hyperdensity on CT, is non-specific in spin-echo images, including signal void or damping, or no alteration of signal intensity[20]. Gradient echo hypointensity of calcification is not clearly explained.

Brain iron deposition, whether as submicroscopic ferritin or in the form of haemosiderin pigment granules, is generally accepted as inducing T2 hypointensity (long TR/TE signal shortening), although tissue concentration and signal alteration are mysteriously equivocal[21].

The routine finding of a band of T2 signal hypointensity (surrounding a subacute haematoma) (Figure 4.1), much wider than the corresponding T1 hyperintensity band (when present), appears to correlate pathologically with the demonstration of ferritin (PAP method) and iron (Perl's) respectively[22]. It must, however, be emphasized that Perl's method identifies only loosely bound ferric iron, and thus will only ever reveal a fraction of the true amount of tissue iron. This fact, applied to ferrocalcinosis, might explain the paradoxical T1 hyperintensity (signal shortening) reported from neural tissue in which mineral deposits stain strongly for calcium but weakly for iron[23]

1.4i. Neoplasia and dysplasia

With the exception of those neoplasms containing or producing large amounts of melanin, mucin or osteoid, neoplastic cells have intermediate signal intensities through the ranges of TR/TE, and cannot, *per se*, be easily distinguished from the neural parenchyma. Signal abnormalities from neoplastic aggregates are therefore a reflection of an abnormal interstitial space, with or without an abnormal vasculature.

Epithelial tumours having the attributes of low cytoplasmic spin density, intracytoplasmic filaments and desmosomes, do not possess an interstitial space significantly different from the neuropil, and can be detected only on account of disturbance of the blood–brain barrier, i.e. surrounding oedema (T2 hyperintensity) and enhancement of tumour vessels (section 4.12). By contrast,

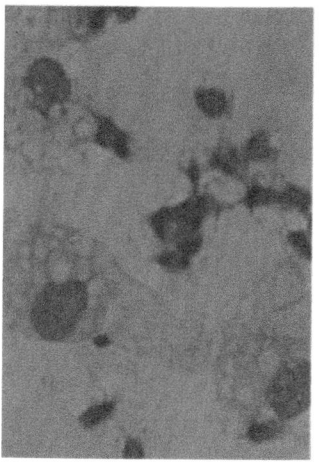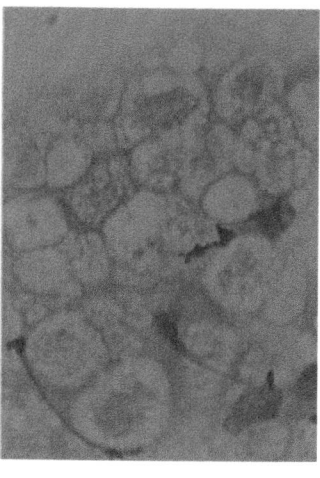

a

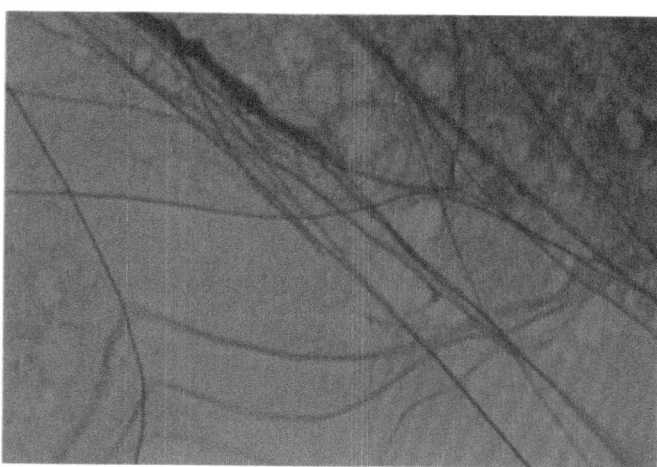

b

Figure 1.16 Focal demyelinating myelopathy: (a) HE/LBHE ×1000, (b) HE ×1000; vacuolated macrophages (a, left), contain blue staining myelin debris (a, right); field also contains numerous axonal processes (b), which should not be confused with astrocytic processes

neoplastic glia are characteristically non-adherent, and are almost invariably associated with a widened intercellular space, even when infiltrating the parenchyma diffusely (section 4.6). Collections of dysplastic glia also exhibit these features. Tumours composed of neuronal (or precursor) cells tend to possess packing akin to the neuropil itself, and are thus brain isodense and isointense, as are germ cell neoplasms. It need hardly be added that, in any neoplasm, the profoundest changes in density and signal intensity follow the occurrence of degeneration, necrosis and haemorrhage.

1.5. THE DIAGNOSTIC APPROACH, SMEAR TECHNIQUE AND PRINCIPLES

The vital role of neuroimaging in pathological diagnosis being self-evident, and the fact (difficult for some to recognize) that a level of indivisibility of these two branches of neurology exists, necessitates an approach. That is the message of this book, and we conceptualize the *anschluss* in the form of an *ideal diagnosis*, which includes patient data, imaging features, pathomorphology and, where appropriate, previous treatment. Such a concept has, of course, for many years formed the basis of *SNOMED* coding[24], which, despite its irrefutable logic and usefulness, is nonetheless constantly resisted by innumerable clinicians of all disciplines.

1.5a. Consultation

A clinical summary should always be sought, and we have found that information crucial to the neuropathology includes patient age, race and geographic origin, chest X-ray, serology, and the temporal profile of symptomatology. In many instances, particularly in spinal disease, the CSF biochemistry and plain films are also essential. The era has closed when the pathologist relied principally on his own acumen in the examination of intraoperative biopsy material, and it is now quite usual for the clinician to request tissue confirmation of a firm diagnosis obtained from the images (surprises notwithstanding). Study of the scans should be done systematically in the same way that a brain-cut is conducted, with identical objectives in terms of anatomical diagnosis: that is, the topography and macroscopic morphology of the lesion, deduced from alterations of density, signal intensity and enhancement. Cursory assessment of topographic anatomy on the operating theatre viewing box should be avoided; for if radiologists are able to affirm their dependence on histology[25], the opposite holds equally, and every imaging

examination requires the opinion of a radiologist. We have found the clinical-neuroradiology meeting to be the best forum for this, as well as for the follow-up discussion. However, it seems to be a fact of present clinical life that the effort required for preoperative imaging consultation has to come from the pathologist.

1.5b. Tissue examination

The diagnostic bias provided by CT and MR almost always determines the surgical approach and method of tissue examination. In any practice a number of cases are treated by means of primary excision, and some of these can be sent off to the laboratory, in fixative. Meningiomas are the usual lesions in this category, but attendance in theatre by the pathologist remains the rule, particularly in teaching institutions where even common lesions may require to be properly photographed or re-examined. Sclerosing conditions such as hypertrophic pachymeningitis require careful excision samples under the eye of the pathologist (which usually means the observer microscope eyepiece), and orientation for paraffin processing alone. In the majority of cases lesions are biopsied by rongeur or needle instrumentation, and it is gratifying that the usually tiny samples obtained are entirely suitable for cytological examination using the smear technique[26,27]. It is also smear cytology which has made stereotactic biopsy possible and, in our experience, these preparations have no substitute, and even fibrous neoplasms will yield adequate tissue with scraping or squashing. Thus frozen sections have no part in intraoperative diagnosis.

Smears are made by placing a tissue sample 1–2 mm in diameter on one end of a clean glass slide; pressure, appropriate to the consistency of the tissue, is then applied with a second glass slide and, with the tissue squashed between the two slides, the sample is spread out as evenly as possible and then fixed immediately (while still moist) by immersion in a 50:50 ether/alcohol solution. After rinsing in water, the fixed preparation is stained, dehydrated, cleared and mounted in DPX. It is our policy to prepare and examine at least two smears, stained separately in 1% aqueous toluidine blue or Giemsa, and with haematoxylin and eosin (HE). If adequate material is available, extra slides should always be made for staining at a later stage. We have found that a variety of stain techniques are possible (Figure 1.16), including immunohistochemistry (Figure 1.17). Tissue is also routinely fixed for paraffin processing and ultrastructure.

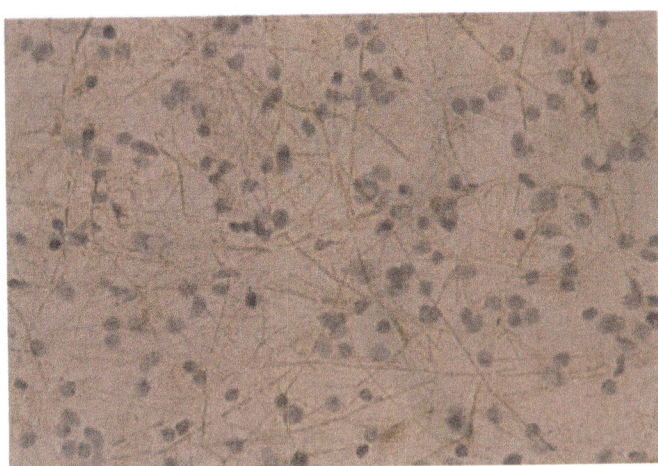

Figure 1.17 Astrocytoma: immunohistochemistry performed on intra-operative smear preparation; astrocytic processes are easily seen. GFAP ×400

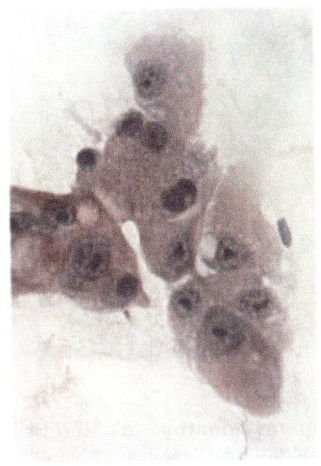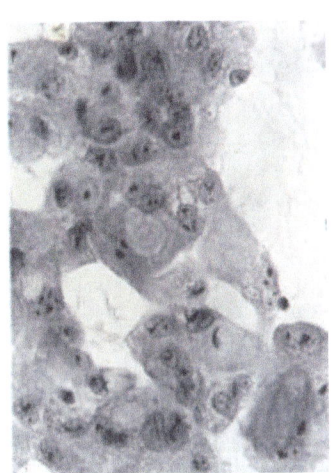

Figure 1.18 Metastatic adenocarcinoma: characteristic clumping of epithelial cells during smear preparation. HE/Tol blue ×400

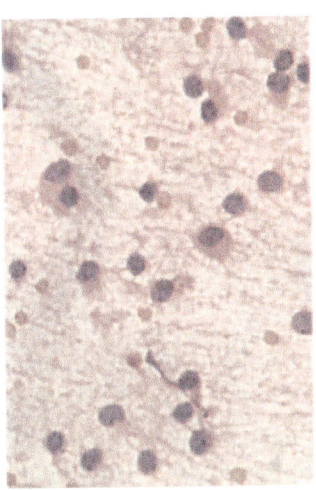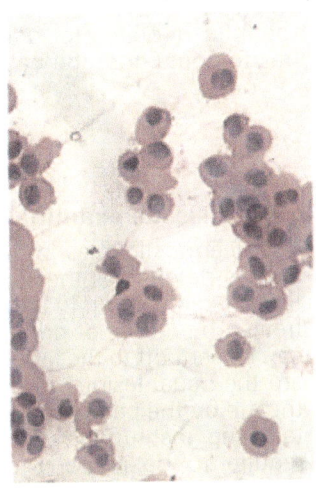

Figure 1.19 Adenoma, pituitary: illustrates disruption of adenoma cells during smearing process (left), but cytoplasmic preservation if 'dabbed' (right). HE ×400

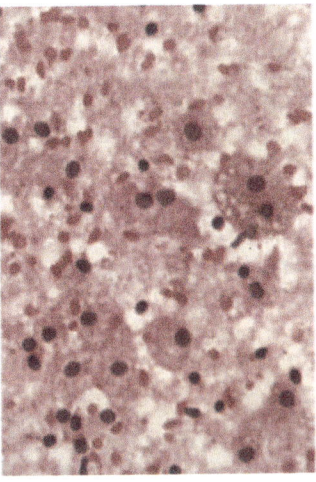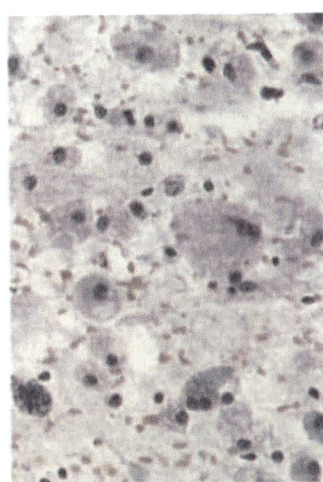

Figure 1.20 Liquefactive necrosis (subacute infarct): sheets of compound granular corpuscles; note lipid vacuoles and myelin debris. HE/Giemsa ×400

1.5c. Biopsy cytology

It is to be expected that a number of the factors influencing the imaging features of normal and abnormal brain, inflammatory and neoplastic tissue are also responsible for the physical characteristics of smear cytology. Thus, the propensity of a tissue to smear out evenly into a monolayer of intact cells is related to: (1) intercellular fibrous support; (2) angio-architecture and relationship of cells to vessels; (3) intercellular contact and presence or absence of cell junctions; (4) cytoskeleton and concentration of intracytoplasmic organelles. Based on these principles, certain generalizations can be made. Normal brain tissue, devoid of collagen-reticulin, and having a predominantly capillary vasculature, tends to smear rather like blood, in a thin, even film. The processes of reactive and well-differentiated neoplastic astrocytes, whose forms are maintained on account of intermediate filament aggregates, result in some cytological clustering (Figure 4.24), but not to the same degree as occurs in more malignant gliomas, where clumping of cells is greatly accentuated by the associated stromal reaction, proliferation of glioma vessels and presence or absence of tumour necrosis. Epithelial cells with strong desmosomal attachments and a filamentous cytoskeleton, e.g. meta-

static carcinoma, craniopharyngioma and epidermoidoma, form cohesive groups with visible intercellular junctions (Figure 1.18). On the other hand, cells with junctions but no cytoskeleton (e.g. pituitary adenoma), show some tendency to adhere to each other (at a microscopic level), but are easily disrupted, with loss of cytoplasmic detail (Figure 1.19), this artefact being maximal in tissues lacking junctions and filaments, such as lymphoma, medulloblastoma and oligodendroglioma. Tumours and proliferative inflammatory processes which are highly vascular and/or contain abundant reticulin, smear with great difficulty; examples include haemangioblastoma, some meningeal sarcomas, certain cerebromeningeal gliomas, desmoplastic medulloblastoma, gliofibroma, hypertrophic pachymeningitis and proliferative granulomatous disease. However, liquefactive necrosis, in which the necrotic tissue consists predominantly of macrophages (Figure 1.20), with dead and viable vessels (Figure 1.10), smears easily. Perivascular orientation and attachment, as occurs in ependymoma and metastatic papillary carcinoma, yields a distinct papillary pattern (Figure 1.21), whilst the tearing apart of cells joined by complex interdigitations, e.g. meningioma, causes the formation of characteristic stumpy cytoplasmic process (Figure 4.88).

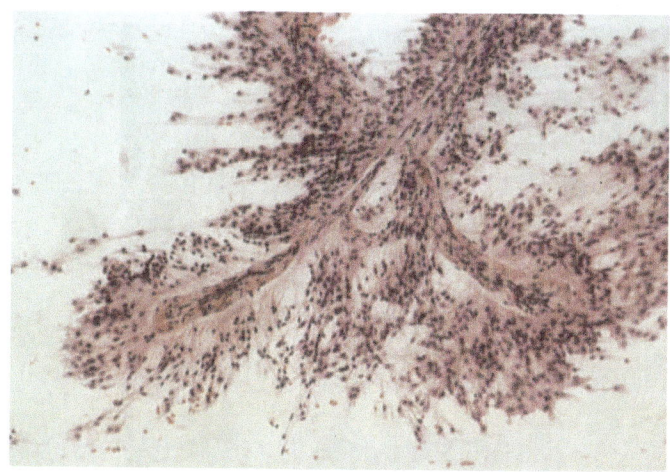

Figure 1.21   Ependymoma: smear illustrating characteristic papillary arrangement and perivascular nuclear-free zones. HE × 100

The case discussed below and shown in Figure 1.22 illustrates the application of the correlative approach in arriving at an 'ideal diagnosis'. The patient, a male of 53 years, had received 66 Gy to the region of the L trigeminal ganglion for a malignant nerve sheath tumour. Three months after completing the course of therapy he presented to the neurologist with headaches and cognitive disturbance. The MR scan at that stage revealed T1 hypointense, T2 hyperintense expansion of the L temporal lobe white matter, with a focal, linear-ring enhancing component. Radiation encephalopathy was diagnosed, and treatment with steroids commenced. Follow-up scan a month later (not shown), showed reduction in the temporal lobe swelling, with clinical improvement. Two months later the patient's condition again worsened, and after consultation with the surgeon and neuropathologist, needle biopsy of the temporal lobe was undertaken on the assumption that cytology alone would be adequate for the purpose of distinguishing radiation necrosis from a glial neoplasm which, on account of the pattern of enhancement, would in all probability be malignant. Several samples were obtained, most of which revealed extensive hypertrophic, isomorphic gliosis, with occasional nuclear abnormalities. Numerous abnormal vessels were also apparent, some of which were cuffed with small mononuclears, mineralized aggregates and fragments of tissue exhibiting coagulative necrosis. No evidence of tumour was found in any of the samples, and the tissue diagnosis was that of necrosis and gliosis. The ideal diagnosis of progressive post-radiation lobar necrotizing leukoencephalopathy, is derived from the logical composition of the clinical, therapeutic, imaging and pathological detail, and summarizes the disease process. Seven months after the biopsy, repeat scan showed persistence of temporal lobe signal alteration, with marked T2 signal inhomogeneity restricted to white matter, and delineated by a peripheral rim of subcortical enhancement, with a much finer, reticulated, internal component. The pathophysiologic basis of this picture has to be inferred from the documented evidence of the neuropathology of radionecrosis, being likely to represent a blend of necrosis, demyelinative phagocytic activity and gliosis, with the selective destruction of oligodendroglia and white matter vasculature forming the topographic determinants.

REFERENCES

1. Clasen RA, Torack RM. Computerised tomography and neuropathologists: two viewpoints. J Neuropath Exp Neurol. 1982;41:387–90.
2. Schild HS. MRI made easy (well almost). Berlin: Schering; 1990.
3. Young SW. Magnetic resonance imaging: basic principles. New York: Raven Press; 1988.
4. Zagzag D, Goldenberg G, Brem S. Angiogenesis and blood–brain barrier breakdown modulate CT enhancement: an experimental study in a rabbit brain-tumour model. AJNR. 1989;10:529–34.
5. Fullerton GD. Physiologic basis of magnetic relaxation. In: Stark DD, Bradley WD, eds. Magnetic resonance imaging. St Louis: Mosby; 1988:36–55.
6. Ehman RL. Interpretation of magnetic resonance images. In: Berquist TH, ed. MRI of the musculoskeletal system, 2nd edn. New York: Raven Press; 1990:27–51.
7. Ehman RL, Kjos BO, Hricak H et al. Relative intensity of abdominal organs in magnetic resonance images. J Comput Assist Tomogr. 1985;9:315–19.
8. Vogler JB, Murphy WA. Diffuse marrow diseases. In: Berquist TH, ed. MRI of the musculoskeletal system, 2nd edn. New York: Raven Press; 1990:491–516.
9. Modic MT, Steinberg PM, Ross JS et al. Degenerative disc disease: assessment of changes in vertebral body marrow with MR imaging. Radiology. 1988;166:193–9.
10. Fullerton GD, Cameron IL, Ord VA. Frequency dependence of magnetic resonance spin-lattice relaxation of protons in biological materials. Radiology. 1984;151:135–8.
11. Klatzo I. Cerebral edema and ischemia. Recent Adv Neuropathol. 1979;1:26–39.
12. Som PM, Dillon WP, Fullerton GD et al. Chronically obstructed sinonasal secretions: observations on T1 and T2 shortening. Radiology. 1989;172:515–20.
13. Egelhof JC, Ross JS, Modic MT et al. MR imaging of metastatic GI adenocarcinoma in brain. AJNR. 1992;13:1221–4.
14. Hirano A, Matsui T. Vascular structures in brain tumors. Hum Pathol. 1975;6(5):611–21.
15. Barkovich AJ, Atlas SW. Magnetic resonance imaging of intracranial haemorrhage. Radiol Clin N Am. 1988;26:801–20.
16. Chaney RK, Taber KH, Orrison WW et al. Magnetic resonance imaging of intracerebral hemorrhage at different field strengths. A review of reported intraparenchymal signal intensities. In: Hayman LA, Taber KH, eds. Neuroimaging clinics of North America. Nontraumatic intracranial hemorrhage. Philadelphia: WB Saunders; 1992:2:25–51.
17. Thulborn KR, Atlas SW. Intracranial haemorrhage. In: Atlas SW, ed. Magnetic resonance imaging of the brain and spine. New York: Raven Press; 1991:175–222.
18. Leestma JE, Martin E. An electron probe and histochemical study of the ferruginated neurone. Arch Pathol. 1968;122:597–605.
19. Duchen LW. General pathology of neurones and neuroglia. In: Hume Adams J, Duchen LW, eds. Greenfield's neuropathology. London: Edward Arnold; 1992:1–52.
20. Holland BA, Kucharcyzk W, Brant-Zawadzki M et al. MR imaging of calcified intracranial lesions. Radiology. 1985;157:353–6.
21. Chen JC, Hardy PA, Clauberg M et al. T2 values in the human brain: comparison of quantitative assays of iron and ferritin. Radiology. 1989;173:521–6.
22. Thulborn KR, Sorenson AG, Kowall NW et al. The role of ferritin and hemosiderin in the MR appearance of cerebral hemorrhage: a histopathologic biochemical study in rats. AJNR. 1990;11:291–7.
23. Boyko OB, Burger PC, Shelburne JD et al. Non-heme mechanisms for T1 shortening: pathologic, CT and MR elucidation. AJNR. 1992;13:1439–45.
24. Cote RA, Robboy S. Progress in medical information management. Systematised nomenclature of medicine (SNOMED). JAMA. 1980;243(8):756–62.
25. Yousem DM. Dashed hopes for MR imaging of the head and neck: the power of the needle. Radiology. 1992;184:25–6.
26. Adams JH, Graham DI, Doyle D. Brain biopsy: the smear technique for neurosurgical biopsies. London: Chapman and Hall; 1980.
27. Esiri MM, Oppenheimer DR. Diagnostic neuropathology: A practical manual. London: Blackwell Scientific Publications; 1989.

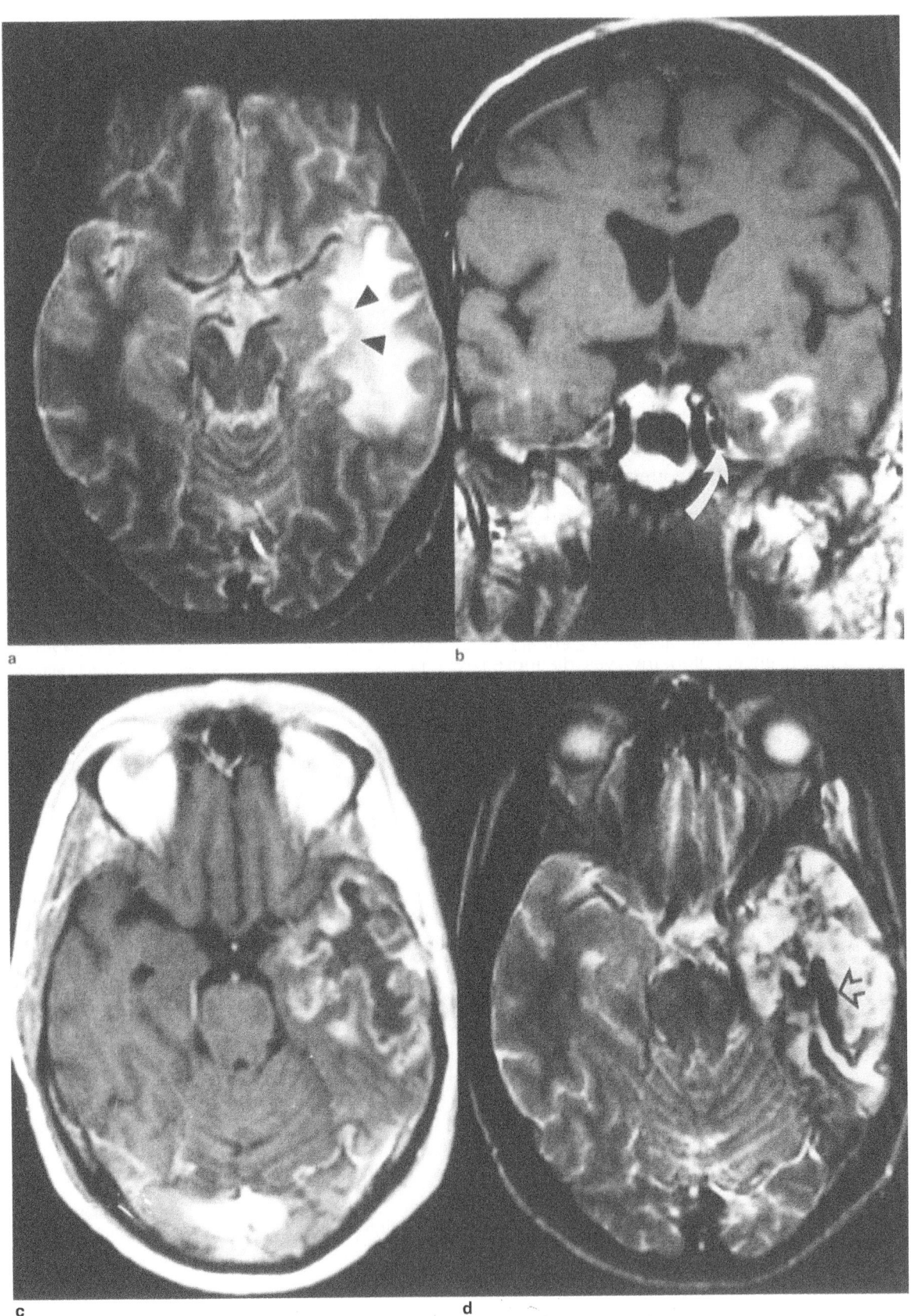

Figure 1.22 (*legend opposite*)

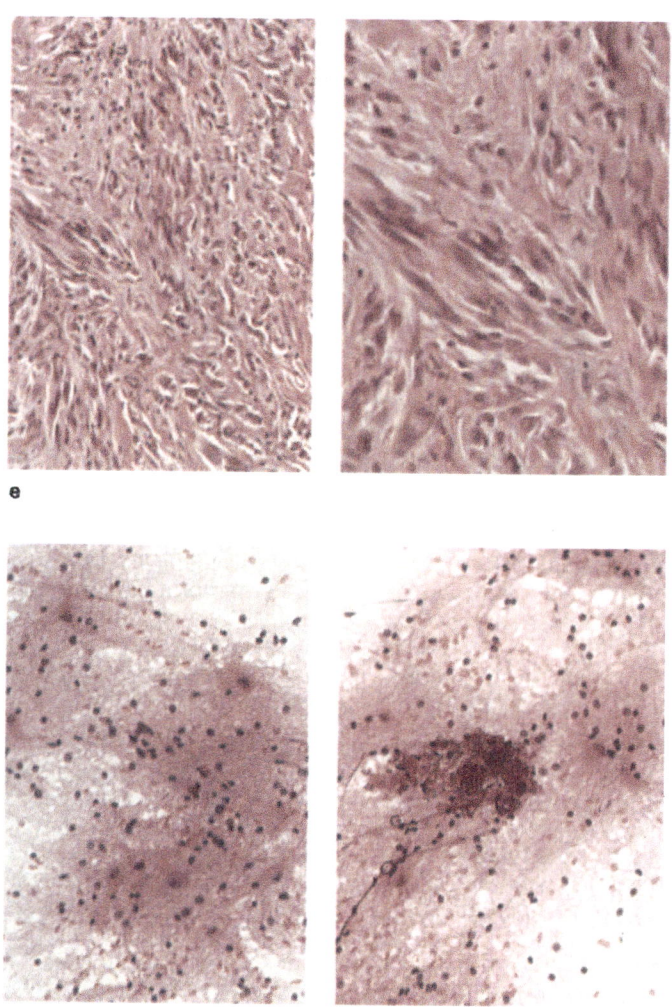

e

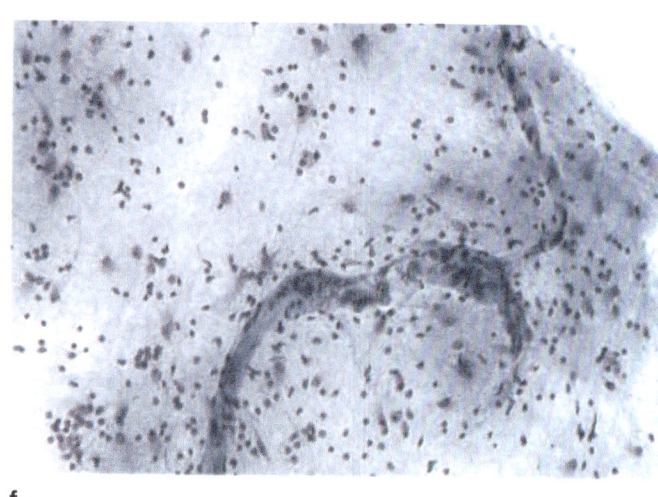

f

g

Figure 1.22 Progressive radiation encephalopathy (necrosis):
(a) T2WI, (b,c) T1WI + C, (d) T2WI, (e) HE ×200/×400, (f) Tol blue ×200, (g) HE ×200; initial 3-month post-radiation therapy images show white matter restricted T2 hyperintensity, and mild volumetric expansion with a central inhomogeneous component (a, arrows), corresponding to linear-ring enhancement in the centre of the temporal lobe (b); note slight enlargement of the adjacent 5th nerve (b, arrow). Original biopsy from left mandibular nerve showed a malignant schwannoma (e). Smear preparations from needle biopsy of temporal lobe show abnormal brain tissue with reactive astrocytosis, prominent reactive blood vessels (f) and mineralization (g); other samples showed coagulative necrosis, but no evidence of neoplasia. Third study, 9 months post-radiation treatment, shows persistent expansion of the temporal lobe, with white-matter hypointensity, which is sharply delineated by contrast (c). This alteration is now inhomogeneously hyperintense on the late echo (d). Nature of cortical hypointensity is unknown (d, open arrow), but could represent ferrugination (see also discussion under ideal diagnosis, Chapter 1). (Dr H Badenhorst, Panorama Hospital)

Lesions of the scalp and skull

2

The concentrated attention of a number of specialities, otorhinolaryngology in particular, has greatly enhanced the detail of clinical investigation in cranial lesions, but inevitably has had the effect of pathological compartmentalization, and access of the neuropathologist to many of these conditions tends to be restricted to cases involving the neurosurgeon. As is to be expected with epithelial and mesenchymal-proliferative lesions, signal characteristics are non-specific, approximating the common denomination of soft tissue in general, often with loss of differential contrast enhancement; thus meningioma invading muscle, for example, enhances less distinctively than usual (Figures 2.17 and 2.18). As a result the imaging approach, particularly with regard to the skull base, often has more to do with the anatomical location and extent of a lesion, rather than its signal intensities. This topographic approach, in which CT is essential, is currently well summarised[1-3] and, apart from considerations of bone pathology itself, anatomical sites providing a degree of diagnostic bias include the air sinuses (fungal infection, carcinoma), sphenoid wings (meningioma), posterior orbit–lateral sphenoid body complex (meningioma, schwannoma, granuloma), petrous apex (haemorrhagic retention (chocolate) cyst), acoustic–mastoid complex (schwannoma, dermal inclusion, rhabdomyosarcoma) and the clivus/basi-occiput (chordoma, meningioma). The combination of CT and MR has also made possible the precise identification of body foramina such as the internal meatus and jugular foramen, often providing the pathologist with a complete and accurate anatomical diagnosis (topography and morphology) in advance. It is also true, however, that in many instances the non-specific images of inflammation and neoplasia, particularly in relation to the air sinuses, leave the final say to histology, and the pathologist has to take particular care to ascertain the site of tissue sampling with a view to diagnostic correlation.

2.1. ENCEPHALOCELE (Cephalocele)

Excised cephaloceles are encountered fairly commonly in neuropathological practice, and in southern Africa seem to be mainly frontal[4]. Even in the presence of a midline body defect, CT gives no idea of the contents of these masses, which may be indistinguishable from dermal inclusion cyst (Figure 2.9). With MR the site and structure of the defect are apparent, but not the state of tissue disorganisation (Figure 2.1). Proliferation of meningeal vessels may lead to unexpected enhancement, which would also distinguish the tissue component of cephalocele from meningocele[5]. Acquired cephalocele, resulting from herniation through a traumatic dural defect, may present as an unexpected biopsy diagnosis (Figure 2.2).

2.2. MUCOCELE

Posteriorly placed mucoceles are of neurological interest when they compromise cranial nerve function[6] or present with intracranial extension, including effacement of the suprasellar cistern. Opacification is characteristically homogeneous on all sequences (Figure 2.3), T1 intermediate intensity, strong-T2 hyperintensity being a common appearance, together with peripheral, mucosal enhancement[7]. The very wide range of signal intensities, including soft tissue isointensity, has been shown to have an orderly dependence on protein concentration, with a remarkable signal loss on inspissation[8].

2.3. INFLAMMATION

Inflammation of the air sinuses and of the mastoid bones constitute regularly seen inflammatory conditions of the skull, the former sometimes displaying intracranial extension (see section 2.2). Infections situated primarily within the cranial bones are rare, and require biopsy principally in order to identify granulomatous disease and its aetiology. These lesions always have a pachymeningitic component which may contribute significantly to enhancement, particularly in the presence of necrosis.

2.3a. Sinusitis

The imaging approach aims to distinguish septic and aseptic obstruction and neoplasia, and although all are subject to a range of signal intensities, certain characteristics predominate in each. Inflammatory expansion is distinguished from tumour on grounds of CT inhomogeneous hyperdensity and T2 hyperintensity with limited, peripheral enhancement (Figure 2.4). When fungal elements are sufficiently aggregated, foci of signal shortening at both short and long TR may become apparent, possibly due to ferromagnetic substances[9]. By comparison, neoplastic tissue, mainly squamous carcinoma, conforms to the expected features of epithelial masses with homogeneous, low-intermediate signal intensities and diffuse enhancement[10] (section 2.6d.). The technical difficulties of specifying the location of biopsy material prevent any useful pathological correlation with regard to the problem of neoplastic versus granulation tissue.

2.3b. Tuberculosis

Lytic calvarial lesions present as a painless scalp swelling, with or without a sinus, and the bone margin is not sclerotic (Figures 2.5 and 2.6). Contents of these bone abscesses are T1 isointense, with an enhancing rim, and the aspirate appears purulent. Sphenoid involvement from adjacent focal pachymeningitis may cause hyperostosis, sometimes with associated carotid arteritis and ischaemia (Figure 3.11), but disease of the skull base elsewhere is not described[11,12].

2.3c. Madura skull

Painless, woody swelling of the cranial soft tissues characterizes the exceedingly indolent infection of *Streptomyces*. The skull is hyperostotic but also beset with sponge-like cavities, with both extra- and intracranial proliferative granulomatous inflammation which is hyperdense, T2 hypointense and strongly enhancing[13,14] (Figure 2.7).

2.3d. Parasites (see also section 3.3)

Hydatidosis occasionally involves the cranial bones, presenting as a poorly defined bony mass with characteristic coarse honeycombing on X-ray. Erosion of the inner table invariably leads to extradural cyst formation (Figure 2.8).

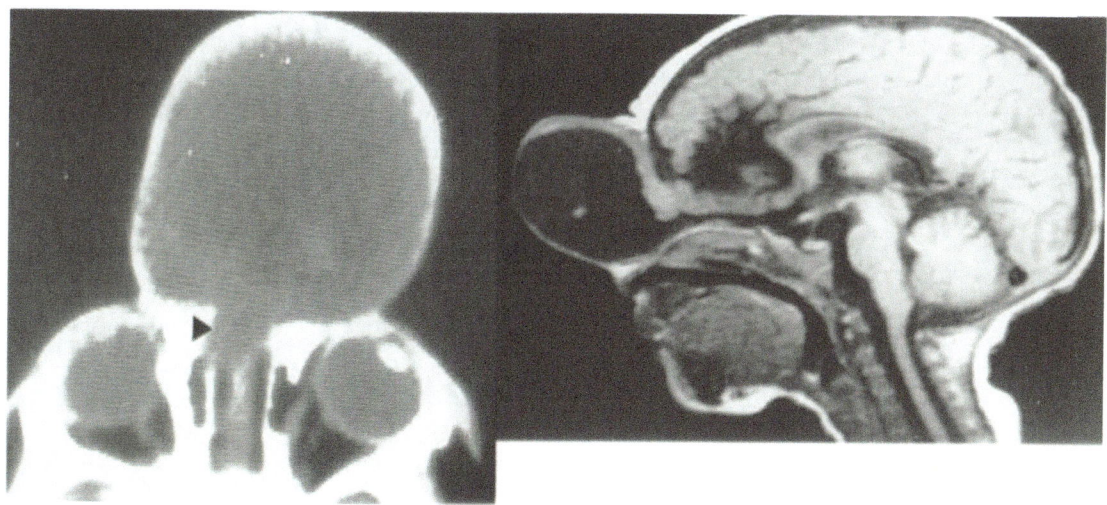

a

b

c

Figure 2.1 Encephalocele, frontal: (**a**) coronal CT, (**b**) T1WI, (**c**) HE ×200/VG ×100; prominent, homogeneously hypodense mass, overlying a supranasal defect (arrow). Sagittal T1WI shows the continuity with brain parenchyma, as well as cystic contents. Tissue component, although brain isointense, is disorganized and gliotic, containing excessive fibrovascular tissue (c)

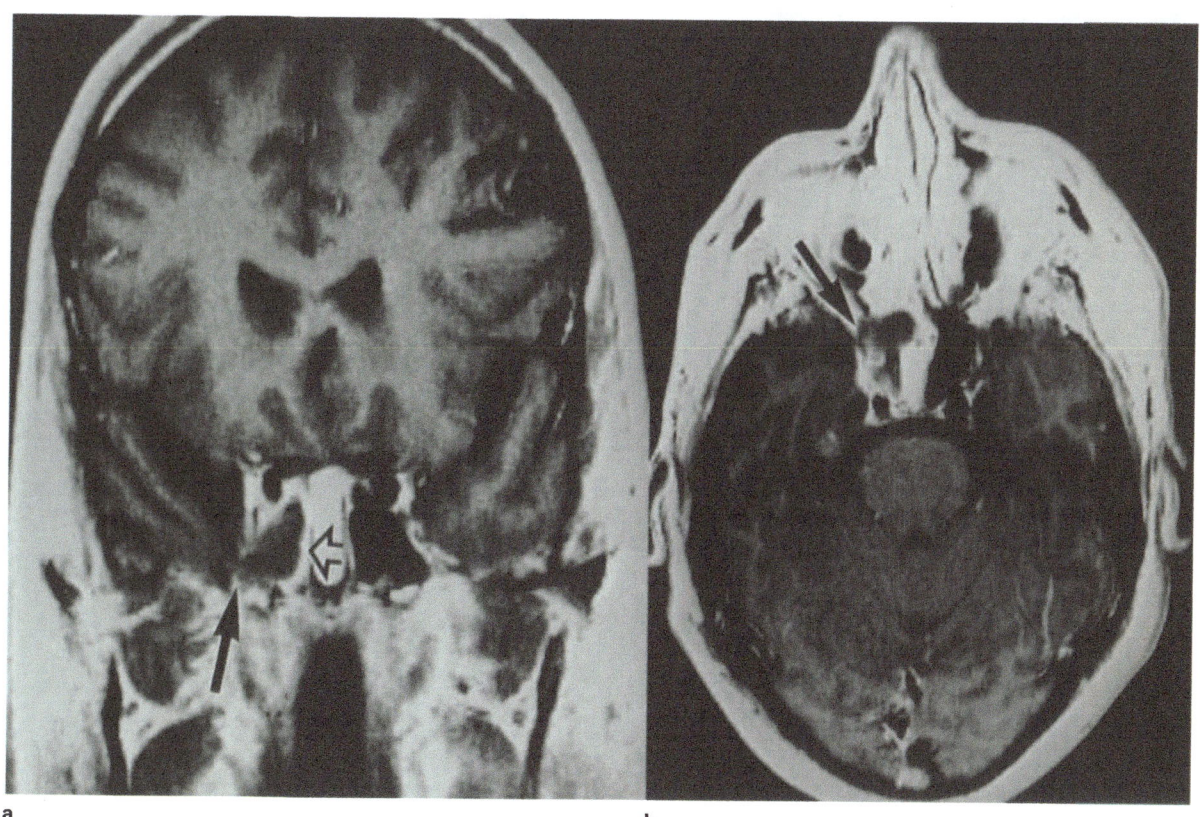

a

b

Figure 2.2 (*legend overleaf*)

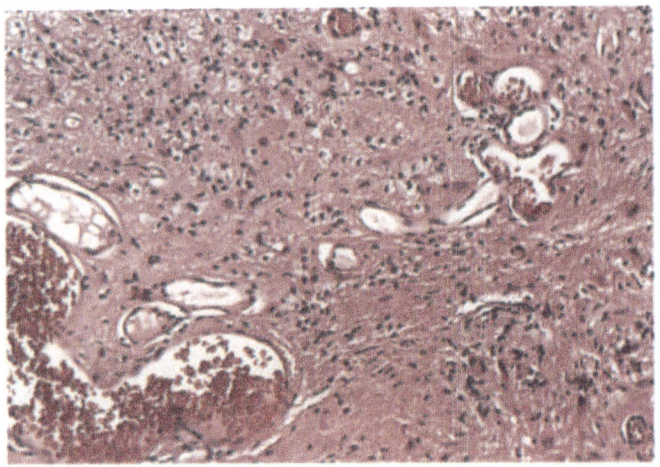

c

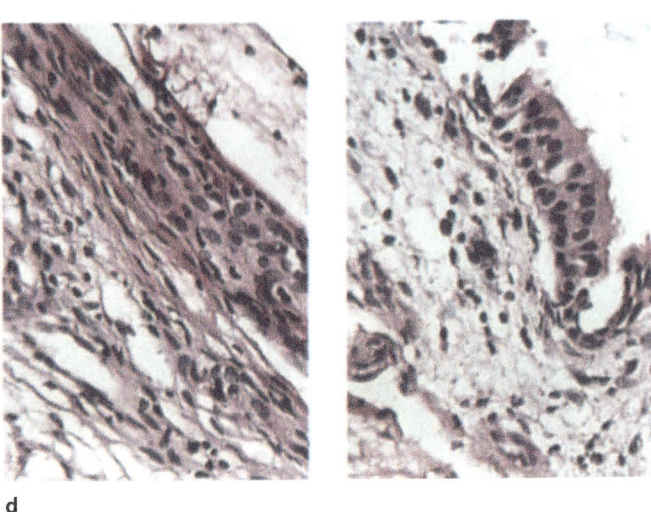

d

Figure 2.2   Brain–sphenoid hernia: (**a**) coronal T1WI + C, (**b**) axial T1WI + C, (**c**) HE ×400, (**d**) PAS ×200; male, 41 years, nasal CSF leak. Intra-operative histology revealed disorganized, gliotic brain tissue, to the surgeon's surprise. Postoperative MR shows soft tissue intensity obliteration of part of the sphenoid sinus, in continuity with temporal lobe (arrows). Intrasinus tissue is shown histologically to consist of disorganized neural tissue, with numerous thin-walled vessels (c), overlying meningothelial tissue (d, left) and respiratory epithelium (d, right). Strong peripheral enhancement (a, open arrow), is assumed to arise from mucosal and abnormal brain vessels. (Dr J Lotz, City Park Hospital)

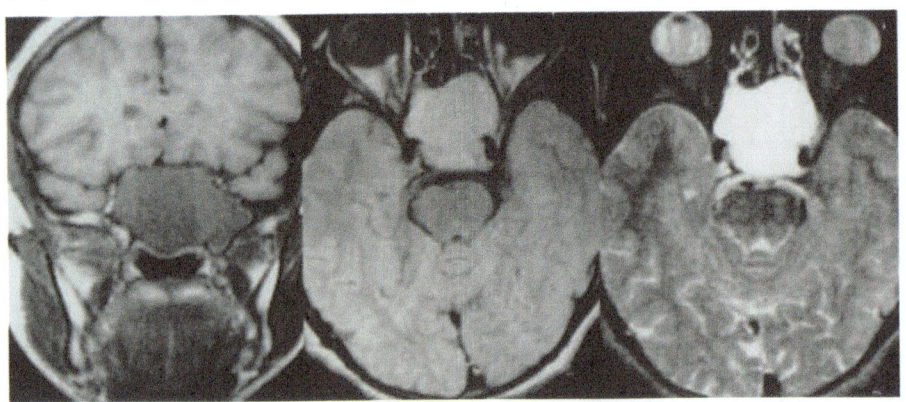

a   b   c

Figure 2.3   Sphenoid mucocele: (**a**) T1WI, (**b**) PDWI, (**c**) T2WI, (**d**) Giemsa ×400; very large cyst occupying and obliterating the sphenoid sinus and displacing the carotid vessels and hypophysis. Contents are T1 soft tissue isointense, T2 hyperintense. PDWI shows commencing T1 signal shortening due to macromolecular associated water, consistent with presence of mucin laden macrophages (d)

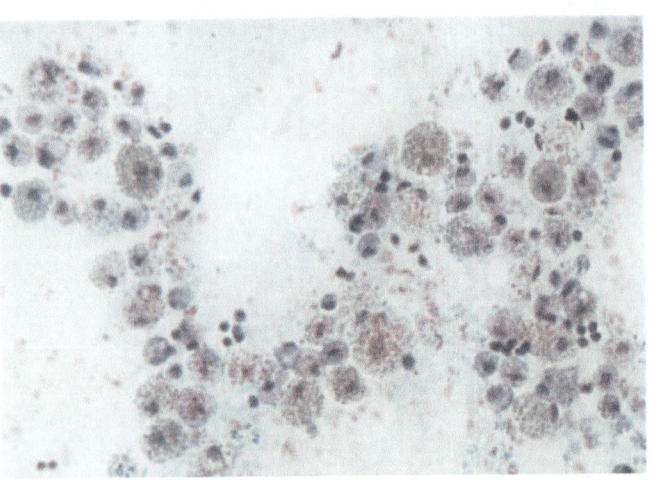

d

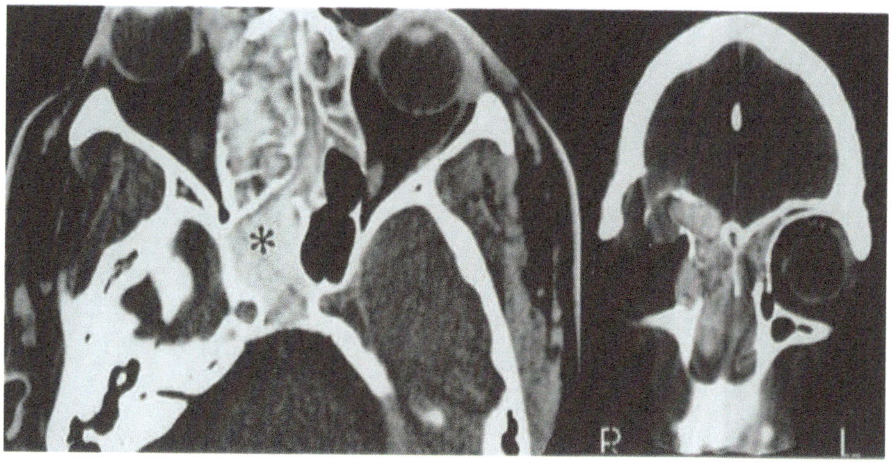

Figure 2.4   Sinusitis with intracranial extension (aspergillus): (**a**) axial CT, (**b**) coronal CT, (**c**) HE ×200, (**d**) methenamine silver ×400, (**e**) HE ×400; unenhanced CT shows expansion of the air sinuses, bone erosion and intracranial and intra-orbital extension. Inflammatory tissue (asterisk) is hyperdense without contrast. Histology shows necrotic acute exudate with fungal elements, degenerate red cells and focal mineralization (presumably the basis of the hyperdensity) and inflamed mucosa with granulation tissue, which does not contain fungi

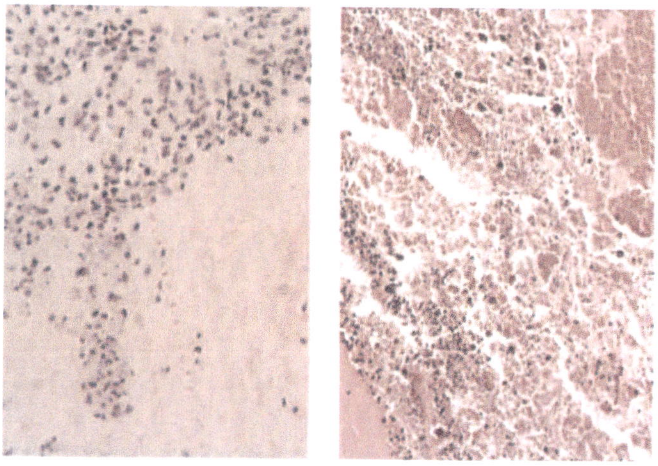

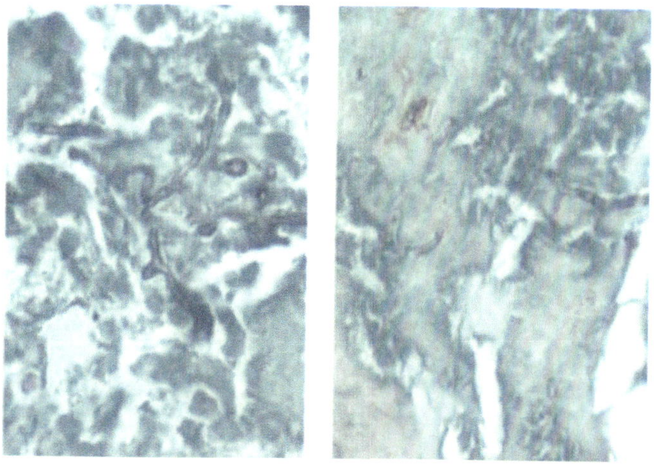

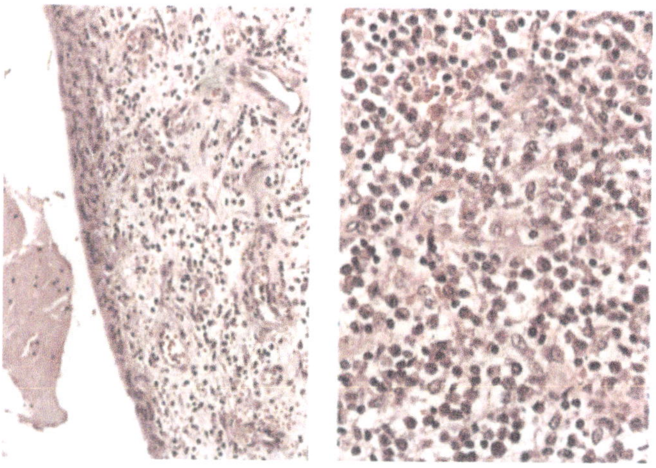

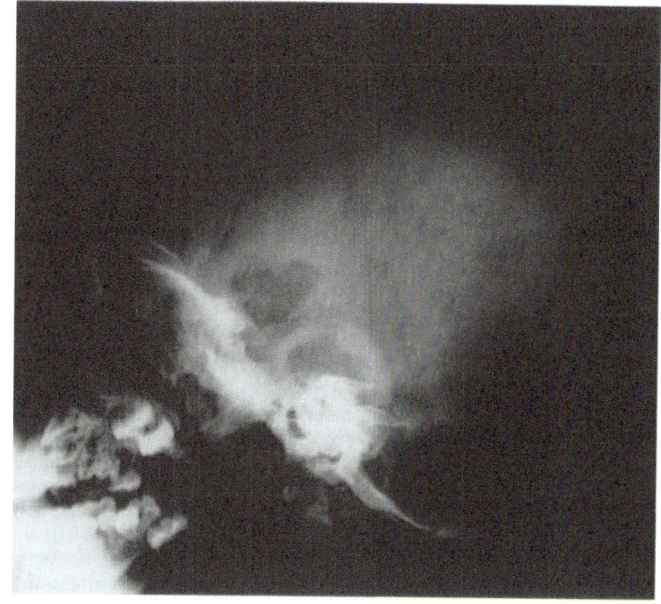

Figure 2.5   (*opposite*) **Tuberculosis, skull**: ill-defined lytic lesion of temporal bone, with untidy edge. (Professor ROC Kaschula, Red Cross Children's Hospital)

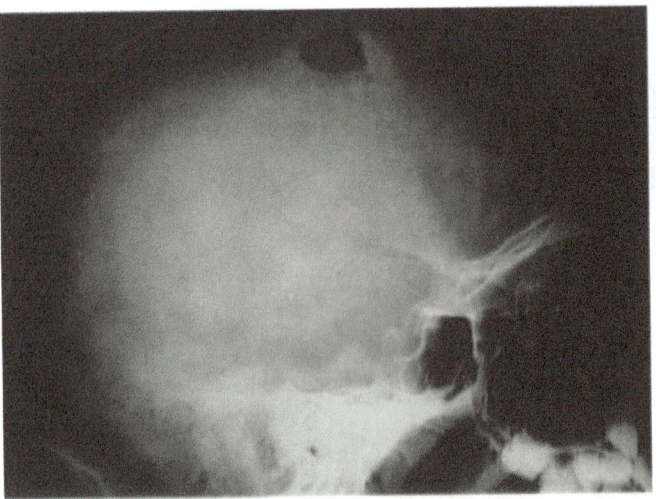

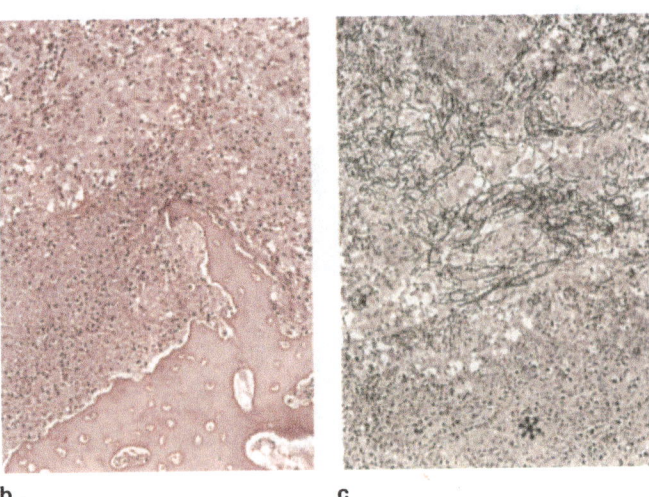

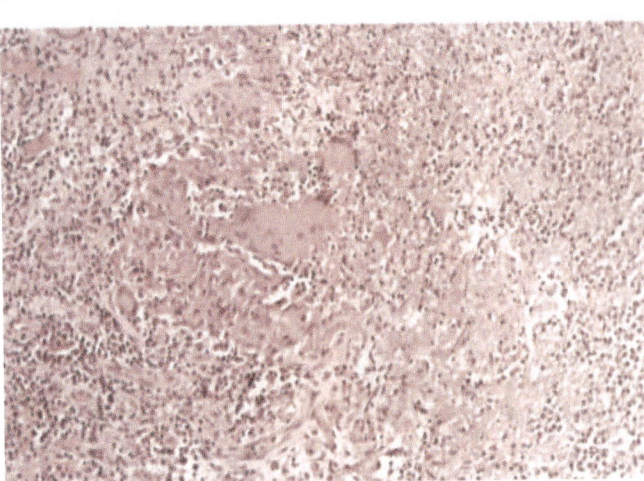

Figure 2.6   Tuberculosis, skull: (a) plain film, (b,d) HE × 200, (c) reticulin × 200; sharply circumscribed lytic lesions of the skull, with sclerotic edge. Histology shows granulomatous inflammation with adjacent caseous necrosis (asterisk), with necrosis of bone and marrow (d). Compare with **Figure 2.5.** (Professor ROC Kaschula, Red Cross Children's Hospital)

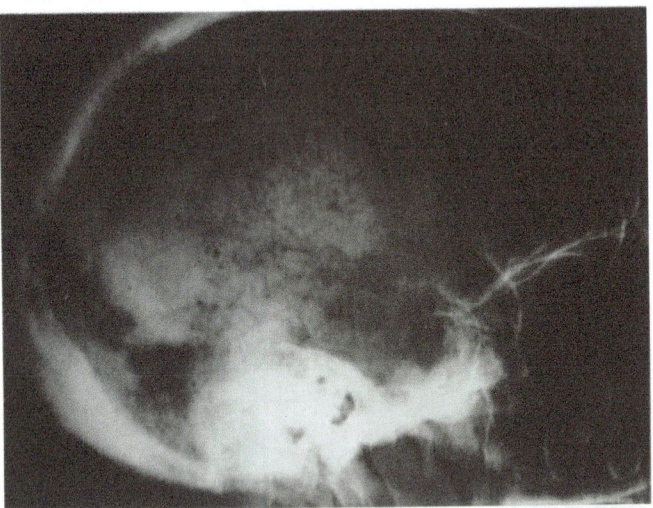

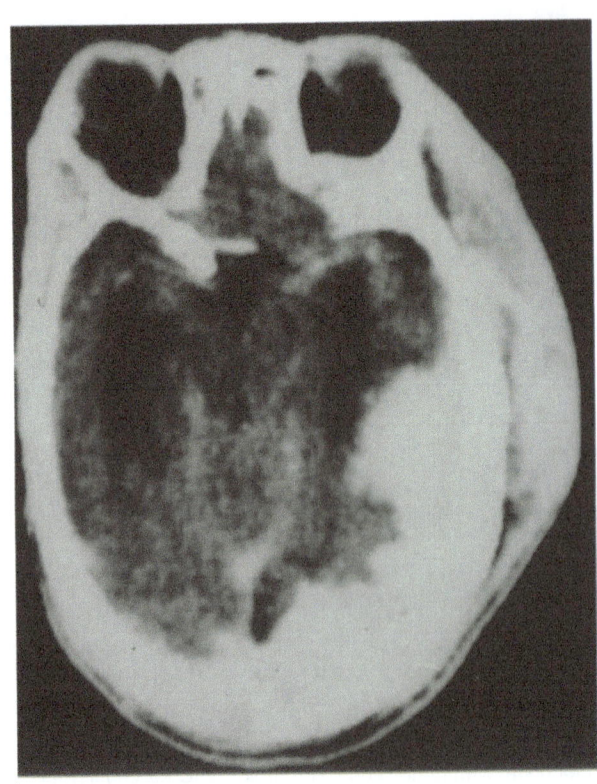

Figure 2.7   Granulomatous osteitis and meningitis (*Streptomyces somaliensis*): (a) plain film skull, (b) CT + C, (c) T2WI, (d) methenamine silver × 570; plain film shows hyperostotis with honeycombing. Intracranial component of mycetoma is hyperdense and strongly enhancing on CT; MR lesion is T2 inhomogeneous hypointense (T1 soft tissue isointense). This T2 signal shortening is assumed to be due to the mixture of collagen and fungal elements (d). Note elevation and penetration of dura (c, arrow) and marked indentation of brain, which shows T2 hyperintensity of vasogenic oedema. Parenchymal signal alteration reversed with treatment. (Reproduced with permission)

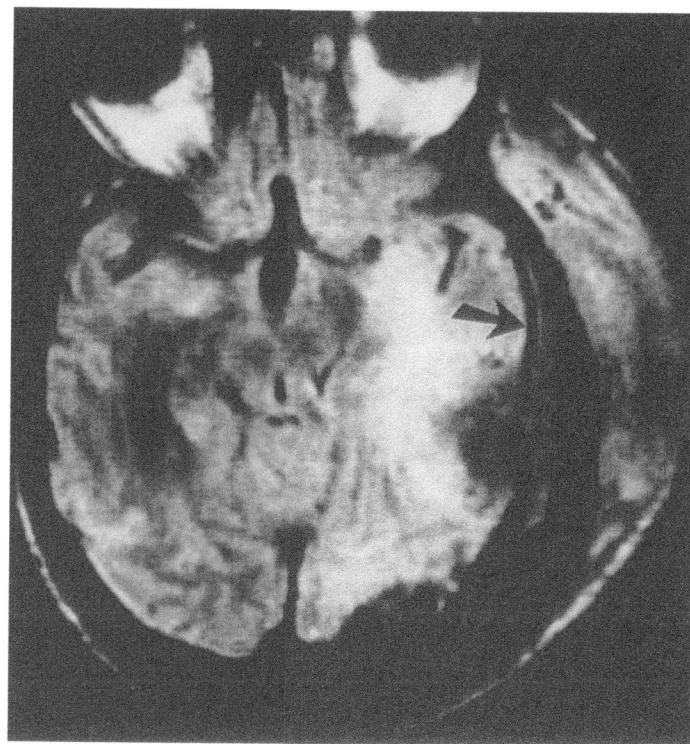

c

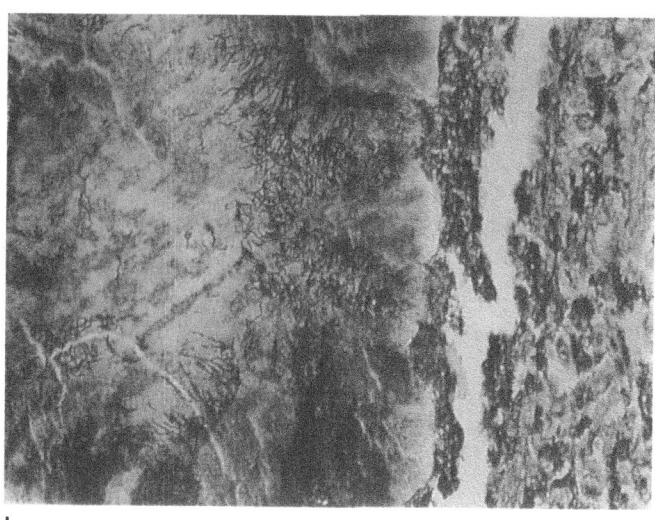

d

Figure 2.7 (*continued*)

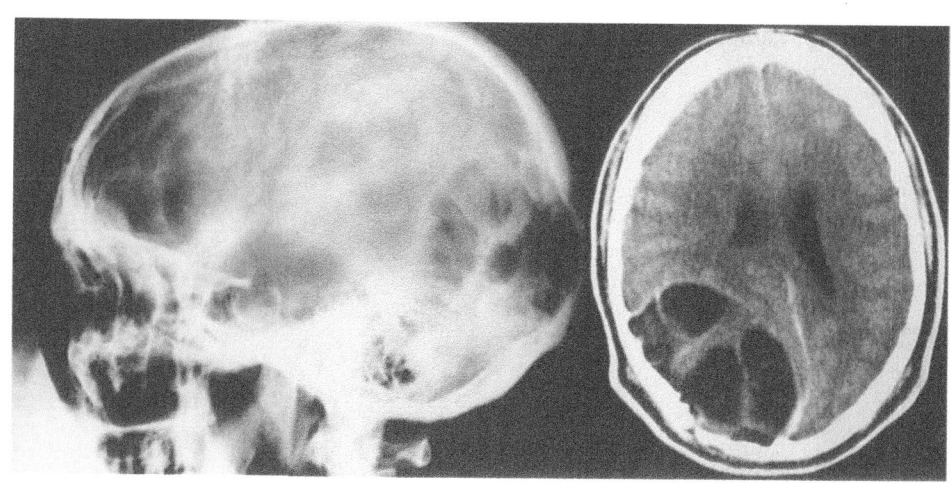

a
b

Figure 2.8   Hydatidosis, skull: (**a**) skull X-ray, (**b**) CT + C; skull X-ray shows cystic honeycombing with typical erosion of inner table on CT, and gross extraparenchymal cysts. At operation innumerable cysts were delivered, identical to those illustrated in Figure 7.23. (Drs J Gardiner and R. Melvill, Constantiaberg Hospital)

2.4.   DERMAL   INCLUSIONS
(epidermoidoma/cholesteatoma, dermoid teratoma) (See also sections 3.1a
(meningocerebral); 5.1a (suprasellar) and the discussion in section 6.1b for pathology.)

Both epidermoid and dermoid types of dermal inclusion tend to be located in and adjacent to the calvarial sutures[15], with dermoids being very much less common overall, as well as presenting in childhood (Figure 2.9). The bony profile of epidermoidoma (epidermoid cyst) on CT is characteristic, with marked atrophic expansion of the inner table, and irregularity of the outer table, which is sometimes breached[16]. Lesions may be very large, with peripheral dystrophic mineralisation[17] (Figure 2.10). The grey–white, flaky keratinous contents have a density of

about 25 HU, and are inhomogeneously T1 hypointense, T2 hyperintense (Figure 2.11). Marked T1 hyperintensity (increased lipid/protein content) and T2 inhomogeneity (Figure 2.9) usually serve to distinguish dermoid cyst from epidermoidoma.

Enhancement of the wall of a dermal inclusion denotes the complication of ulceration, granulation tissue formation and granulomatous inflammation in response to cholesterol–keratin debris. However, despite the close morphological association of cholesterol and keratin granulomas in some epidermoidomas (Figure 2.10), there is no scientific evidence for the belief[18] that cholesterol crystals are derived from the breakdown of keratin *per se*. Enhancement of an adult lesion raises the suspicion of malignant transformation[19].

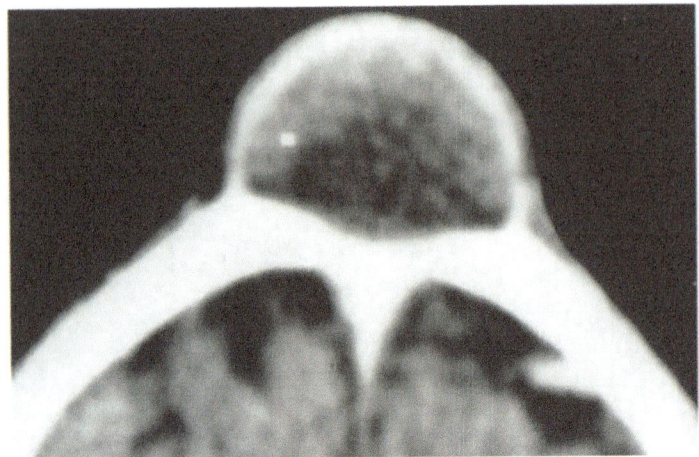

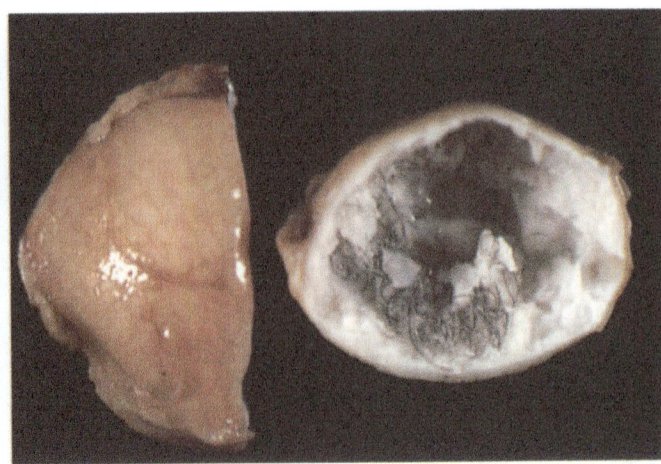

a

b

Figure 2.9 Dermoid cyst, frontal region: (**a**) CT + C, (**b**) fixed specimen, (**c**) HE × 100/ × 40; characteristic circumscribed mass indenting the frontal bone, with inhomogeneous hyperdense contents and rim enhancement. The excised cyst containing hair and degenerate keratin (b). Histology shows an ulcerated cyst lining with a granulomatous response and adnexal structures (c)

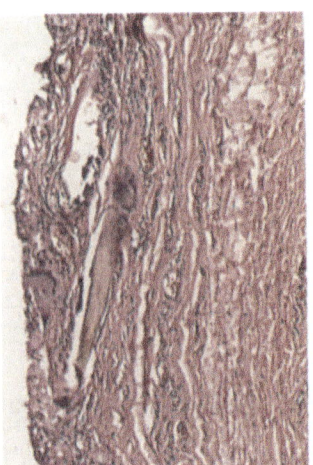
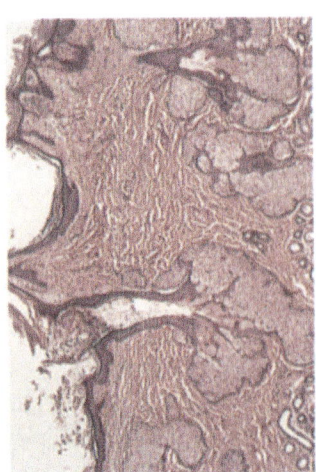

c

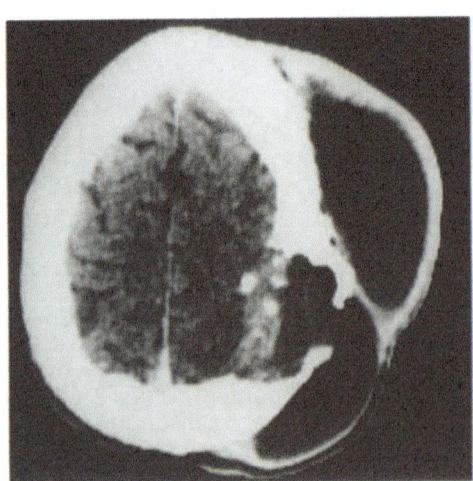
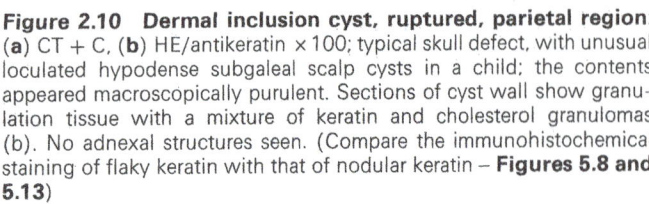

a

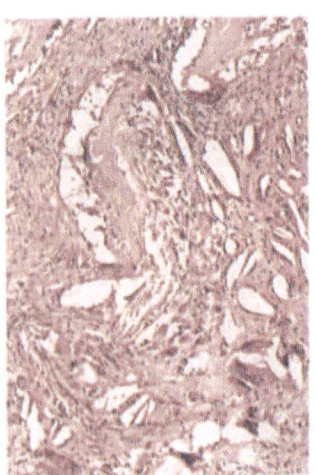
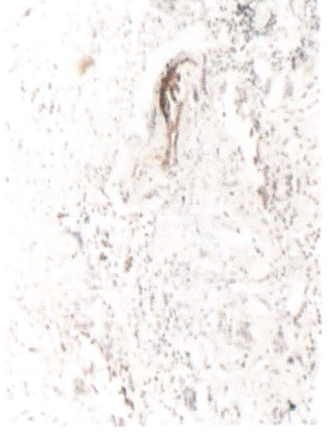

b

Figure 2.10 Dermal inclusion cyst, ruptured, parietal region: (**a**) CT + C, (**b**) HE/antikeratin × 100; typical skull defect, with unusual loculated hypodense subgaleal scalp cysts in a child; the contents appeared macroscopically purulent. Sections of cyst wall show granulation tissue with a mixture of keratin and cholesterol granulomas (b). No adnexal structures seen. (Compare the immunohistochemical staining of flaky keratin with that of nodular keratin – **Figures 5.8 and 5.13**)

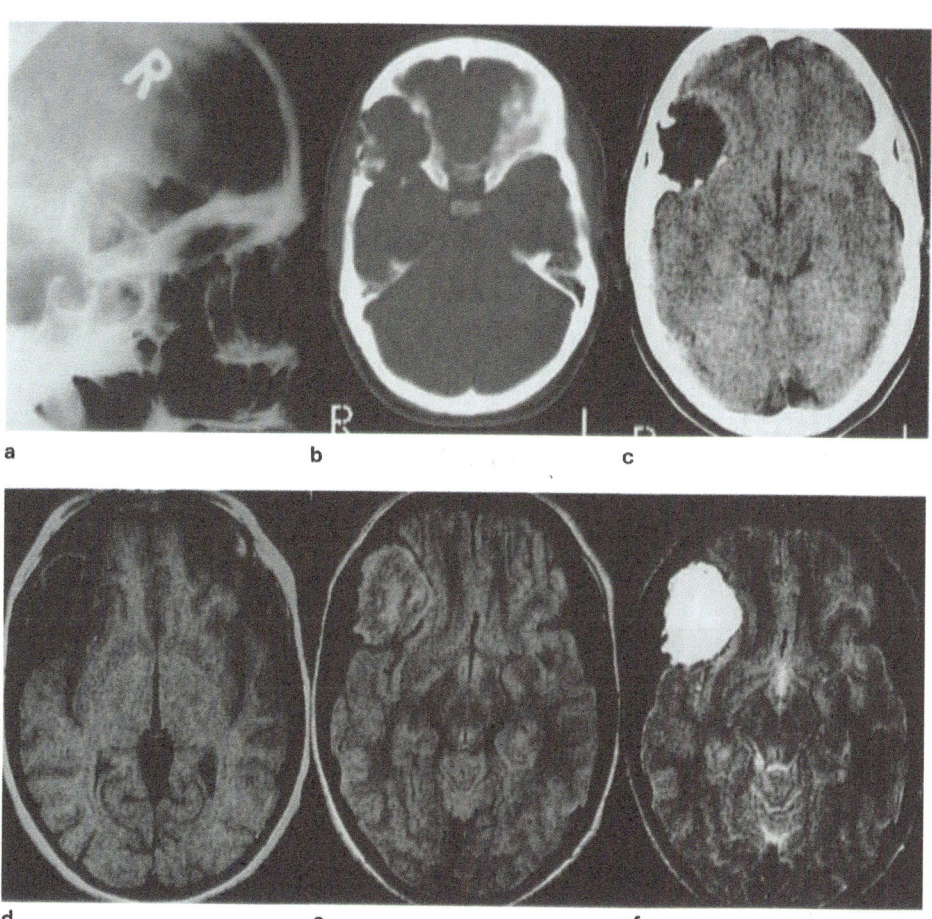

a   b   c

d   e   f

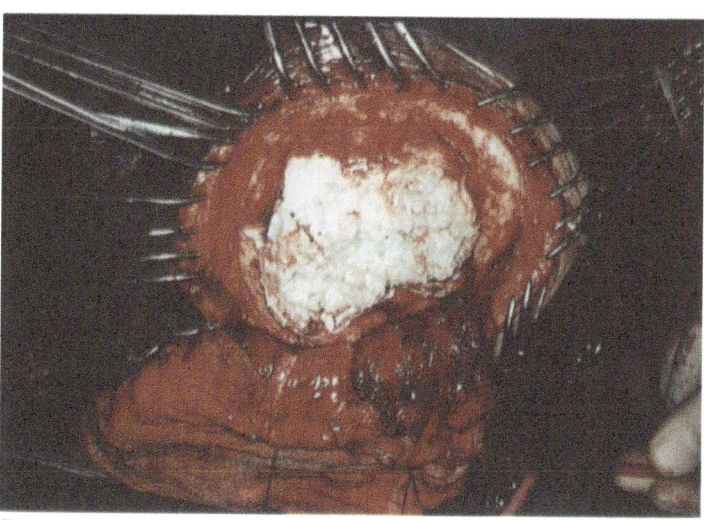

g

Figure 2.11 Epidermoidoma (pearly tumour), sphenoid wing: (**a**) plain film, (**b**) CT bone window, (**c**) CT, (**d**) T1WI, (**e**) PD, (**f**) T2WI, (**g**) operative specimen; CT-typical expansion of the sphenoid/frontal/orbit with inhomogeneous hypodense contents which are also T1 inhomogeneous hypointense; T2 sequences show isointensity on early echo (PD), marked hyperintensity on the late echo. The operative specimen shows the typical pearly white lobules of keratin. Histology showed contents to consist of laminated keratin only, with no epithelial lining

2.5. HAEMORRHAGIC RETENTION (CHOCOLATE) CYST OF THE PETROUS APEX

Also called mastoid cyst, epidermoid, mucocele and cholesterol cyst/granuloma[20,21], of which the last three designations are inappropriate or even incorrect. In particular, the use of the term 'cholesterol granuloma/cyst' as a diagnostic label is to be discouraged, as cholesterol crystal-associated granulomas have no specificity and may also be seen in Rathke's cleft cyst (Figure 5.4), haemorrhagic craniopharyngiomas (see section 5.2) and some epidermoidomas (Figure 2.10).

CT shows erosion of the petrous in various directions, including the sphenoid body, jugular foramen, internal auditory meatus and middle ear. The cyst may bulge into the posterior fossa and CP angle (usually covered with a thin rim of bone), and has a density similar to brain, sometimes with slight peripheral contrast enhancement. Contents are brown fluid with cholesterol iridescence and, as would be expected, the lesion is homogeneously T1/T2 hyperintense. Histology shows a fibrous wall, granulation tissue, amorphous debris, macrophages and giant cells (Figure 2.12); compare with the identical pathogenesis of haemorrhage in craniopharyngioma, section 5.2. The presence of respiratory type epithelium within one of these cysts (Figure 2.13), lends support to the contention that they are initiated by chronic obstruction to the ventilation and drainage of pneumatized spaces, complicated by ulceration and haemorrhage[22].

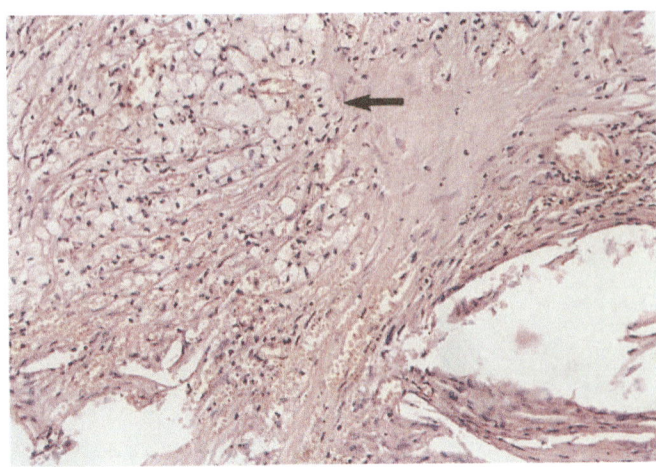

Figure 2.12   Cyst, haemorrhagic retention, petrous apex: biopsy of wall showing vascularised fibrous tissue, macrophages (arrow), pigment and cholesterol crystal clefts. HE ×200

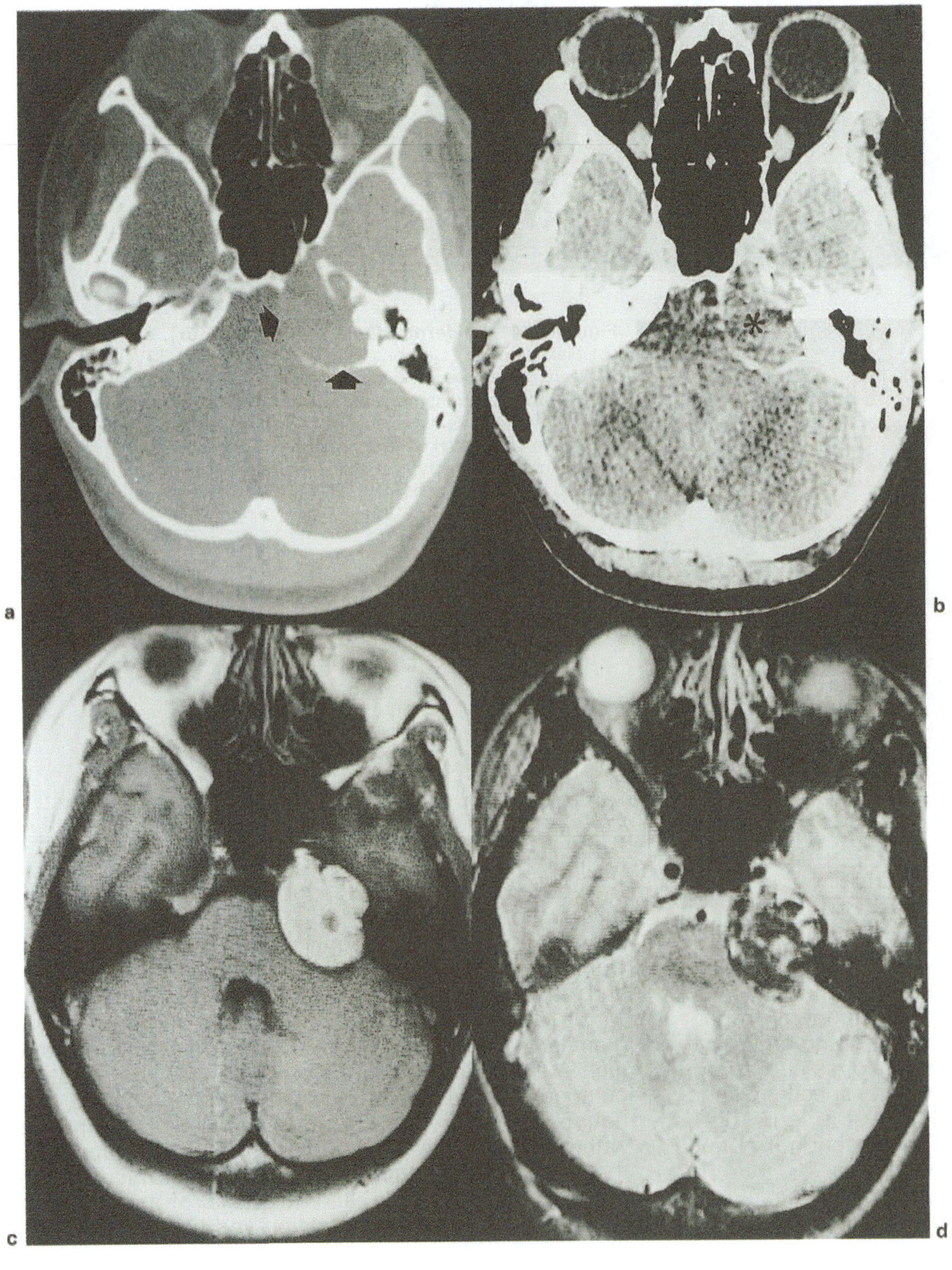

Figure 2.13   Cyst, haemorrhagic retention, petrous apex/CP angle: (**a**) CTBW, (**b**) CT, (**c**) T1WI, (**d**) T2WI, (**e**) HE ×200, (**f**) HE/Perls' ×200; there is typical ballooning of petrous apex occupying the CP angle, with preservation of a thin medial bony rim (a, arrow), and brain isodense contents (b, asterisk). MR shows cyst contents to be homogeneously T1 hyperintense (c), but markedly inhomogeneous at long TR/TE (d). At operation contents were yellow, almost inspissated material, with a mixture of fresh and degraded blood and cholesterol crystals (f); a tissue nodule found in the depths of the lesion is composed of effete respiratory epithelium and inflamed oedematous submucosa (e). (Cholesterol concentration of cyst contents 7.6 mmol/l) (compare with **Figure 5.13**)

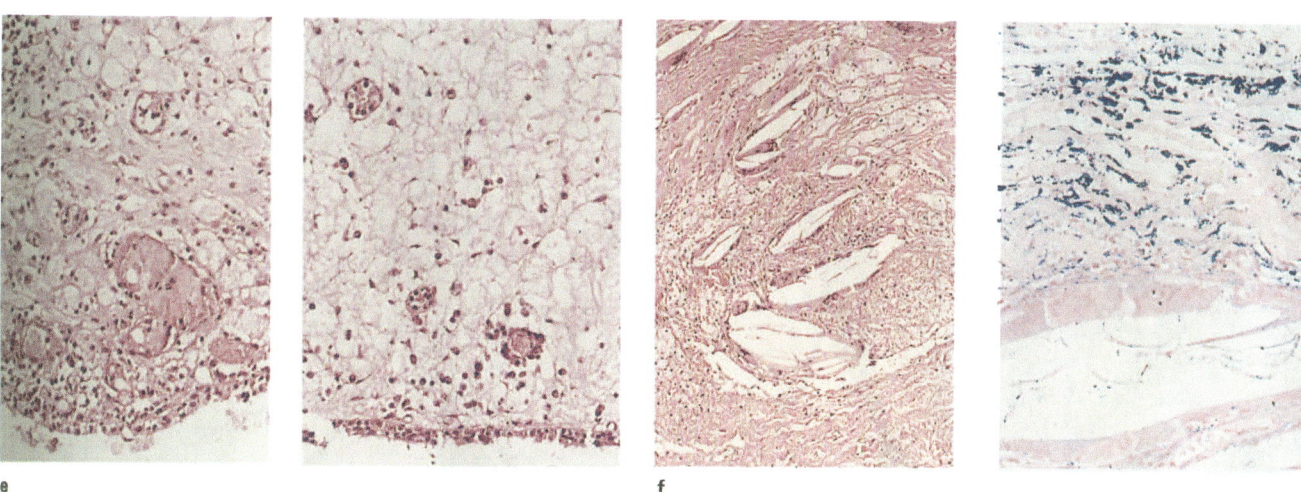

e

f

Figure 2.13 (*continued*)

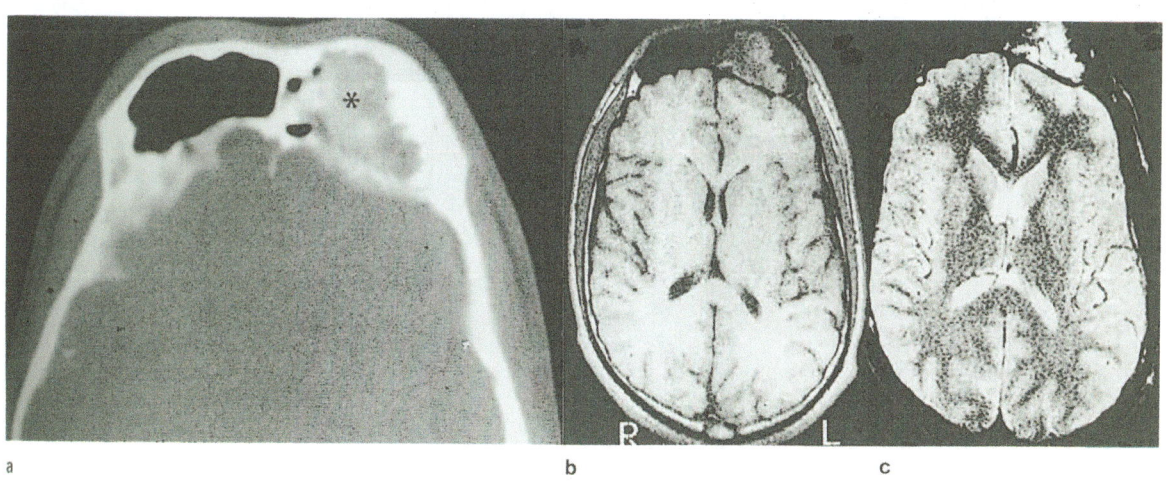

a

b

c

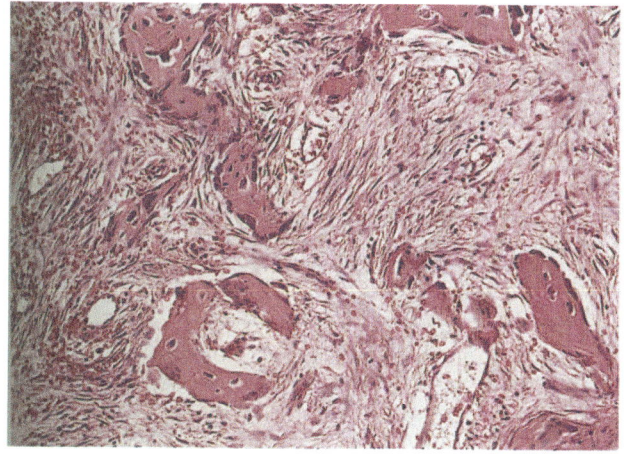

d

Figure 2.14 Ossifying fibroma (osteofibroma): (**a**) CT bone window, (**b**) T1WI, (**c**) T2WI, (**d**) HE ×200; left frontal sinus is irregularly hyperostotic and obliterated and filled by inhomogeneously hyperdense tissue (asterisk), which is T1 brain isointense and inhomogeneously T2 hyperintense. MR gives no indication of the considerable bone formation within the lesion; note abundant fibrous tissue and plentiful blood vessels (d), which explain the enhancement of this lesion

2.6. NEOPLASMS

2.6a. Benign fibro-osseous lesions (Ossifying fibroma/osteofibroma, fibrous osteoma, osteoma and fibrous dysplasia)

With the exception of ivory and mature osteomas, overlapping histological features and unsettled diagnostic criteria make differentiation of these lesions difficult[23,24]. There is also evidence which suggests that in the cranial bones, ossifying fibroma may undergo maturation towards an osteoma[25,26]. Radiographic examination in instances of air sinus involvement may show opacification, or the presence of a mass filling the sinus, the density of which will be proportional to the ratio of fibrous and mineralized osseous elements. Intertrabecular fibrous stroma predominates in the T1 brain isointense ossifying fibroma shown in Figure 2.14. Blood vessels are plentiful, accounting for strong enhancement, and an associated voluminous interstitial space could explain the T2 hyperintensity, since both osteoid and bone would be expected to have the reverse effect[27].

2.6b. Osteosarcoma

Cranial osteosarcomas, excluding the mandible, are rare neoplasms of the young, lacking site predilection and occasionally following upon radiotherapy, while in the elderly they may complicate Paget's disease. The usual finding of inhomogeneous signal hypointensity is a function of collagen production, matrix type and mineralization, the last being best appreciated with CT[28]; less

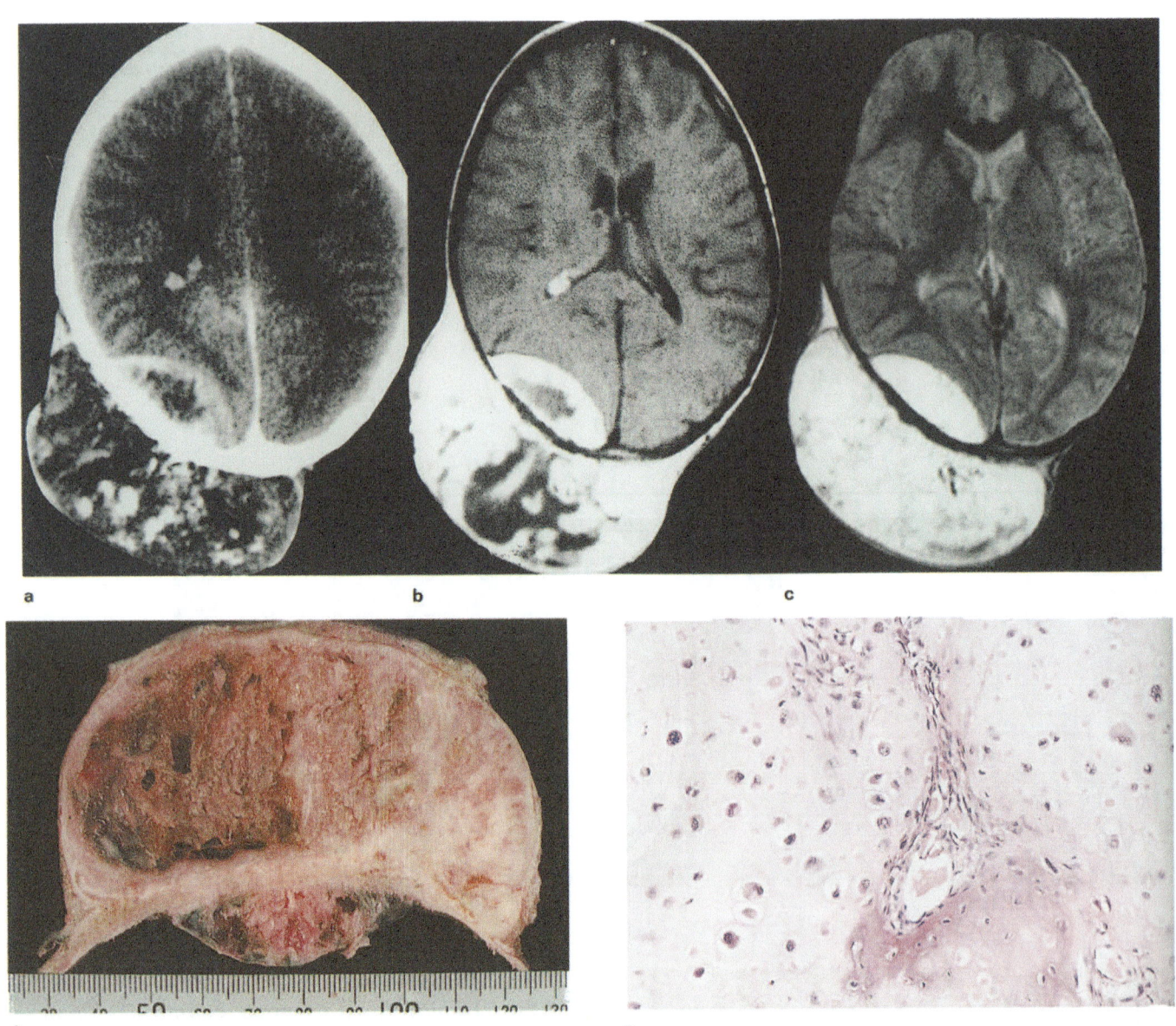

a   b   c

d   e

Figure 2.15 Osteosarcoma, occipital region, post-radiation therapy: female 2 years; surgical excision and craniospinal irradiation of thoracic ependymoma; 8 years of age, large occipital mass. (**a**) CT + C, (**b**) T1WI + C, (**c**) T2WI, (**d**) fixed specimen, (**e**) HE ×200; lesion is inhomogeneously T1 isointense (not shown), very strongly enhancing (b), and more or less diffusely T2 hyperintense (chondroid tissue (e). Long TR inhomogeneity is probable mineralization and necrosis, since distribution of mineral on CT does not correspond exactly.

Note weak inhomogeneous enhancement on CT (a), compared with MR (b). The macroscopic specimen (d) shows solid and vascular components, both of which appear to enhance equally (patient had chemotherapy between MRI and removal of tumour). Inner surface of intracranial component is a pseudocapsule – dura was not obviously infiltrated. Typical chondroblastic osteosarcoma, with large vascular channels (e). The sections also showed abundant necrosis and degeneration with foci of calcification

common T2 hyperintensity reflects either a poverty of osteoid (and mineral) or conversely the production of a chondroid ground substance (Figure 2.15). Strong enhancement is consistent with the prolific vasculature.

2.6c. Hyperostosing meningioma (see section 3.4 for general discussion on meningeal tumours)

A presumably intraosseous origin accounts for this unusual but nevertheless characteristic form of meningioma, for which a CT grading system has been described, including homogeneous, periosteal, three-layer and diploic types[29] (Figure 2.16). MR may show hyperostosis as merely hypointense, although deformity of adjacent cortex is apparent. The meningioma itself may be confined to the calvarial medulla, with no extension beyond the hyperostotic inner and outer tables[30], leading to radiological misdiagnosis of fibrous dysplasia, whilst focal diploic expansion can resemble a mucocele[31]. Involvement of the

sphenoid trigone is a typical manifestation, presenting with proptosis, and occasionally an ill-defined swelling of the temporalis muscle. CT is essential, since it demonstrates the distinctly nodular thickening of the orbital and maxillary parts of the sphenoid, with a soft tissue component projecting into the anteromedial middle fossa (Figure 2.17). MR reveals the expansion of lateral rectus and temporalis muscles – these, together with the intracranial tumour, all exhibiting distinct enhancement, whilst the normal T1 marrow signal is lost (Figure 2.17). Histology is non-specific in the sense that these tumours (in the experience of this hospital) are commonly meningothelial. Usually, the operation of sphenoid excision is planned at the outset of treatment, and histology of bone and muscle is routine, but sometimes intraoperative scrapings from the external dura and temporalis may be required to convince the surgeon that bony transgression has occurred (Figure 2.18).

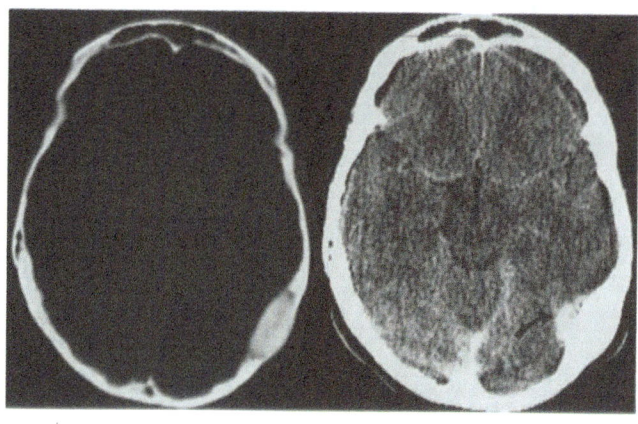

Figure 2.16 Hyperostosing meningioma, occipital region: (**a**) CTBW, (**b**) CT + C; characteristic diploic expansion of occipital skull, with a small enhancing dural component (arrow)

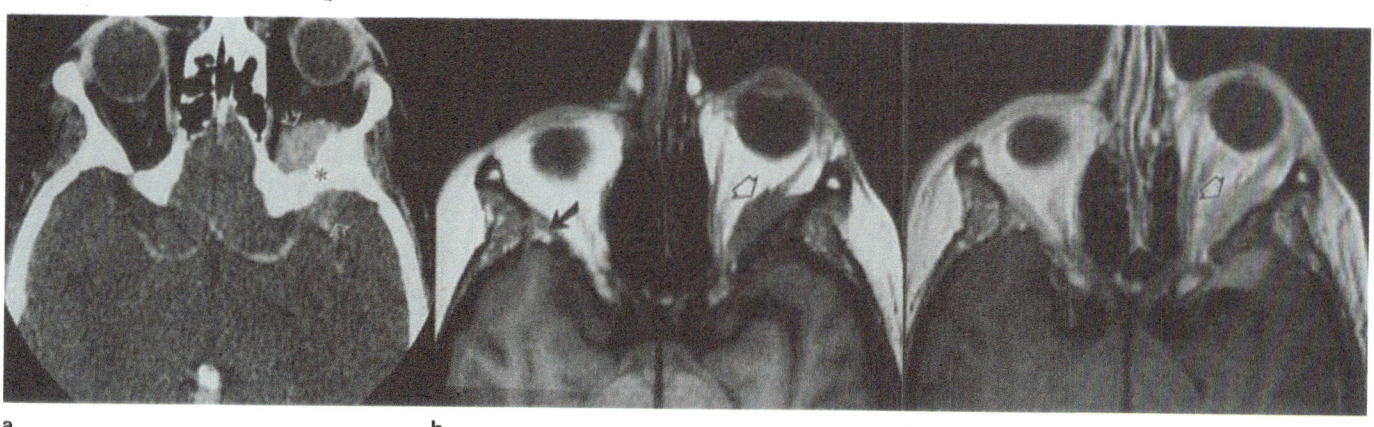

Figure 2.17 Hyperostosing meningioma, sphenoid wing: (**a**) CT + C, (**b**) T1WI, (**c**) T1WI + C; typical frontal/sphenoid hyperostosis (asterisk), with enhancing intracranial and intraorbital tumour growth (a, c, open arrows); T1 weighted image (b) shows extrinsic occular muscle involvement (open arrow), and note loss of normal marrow signal compared with opposite side (closed arrow)

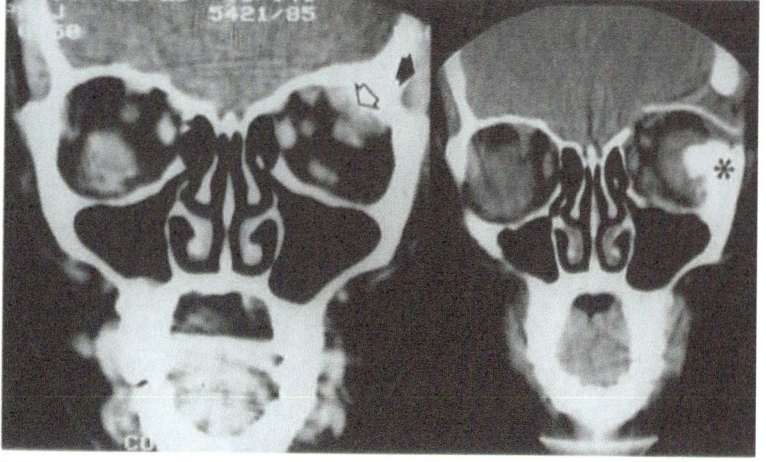

Figure 2.18 Hyperostosing meningioma, sphenoid wing and orbit: (**a**) coronal CT + C, (**b**) coronal CT, (**c**) Tol blue × 200/Bismark brown × 400, (**d**) HE × 200; original CT (a) shows sphenoid/orbit hyperostosis with intraorbital (open arrow) and temporalis (closed arrow) extension; follow-up scan 13 months later shows recurrence with gross intraorbital tumour and hyperostosis (asterisk), which also involves the maxilla. Smear preparation shows typical benign meningioma (c, left); note preponderance of mast cells in paraffin section (c, right) and invasion of temporal muscle and blood vessels (d)

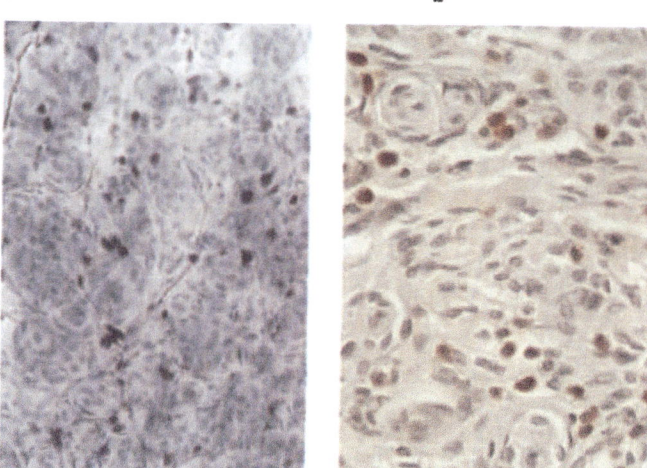
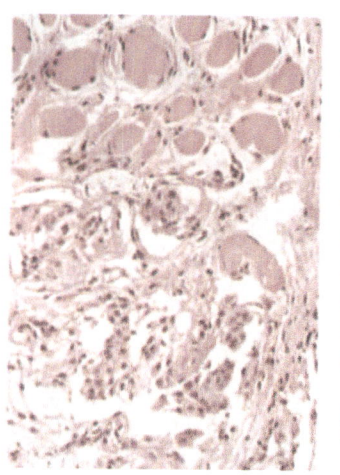
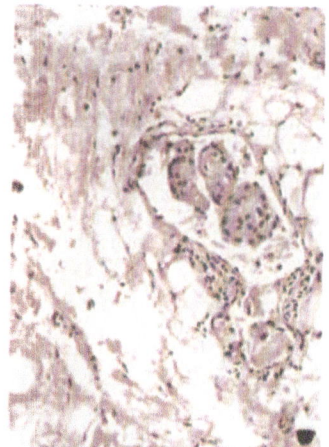

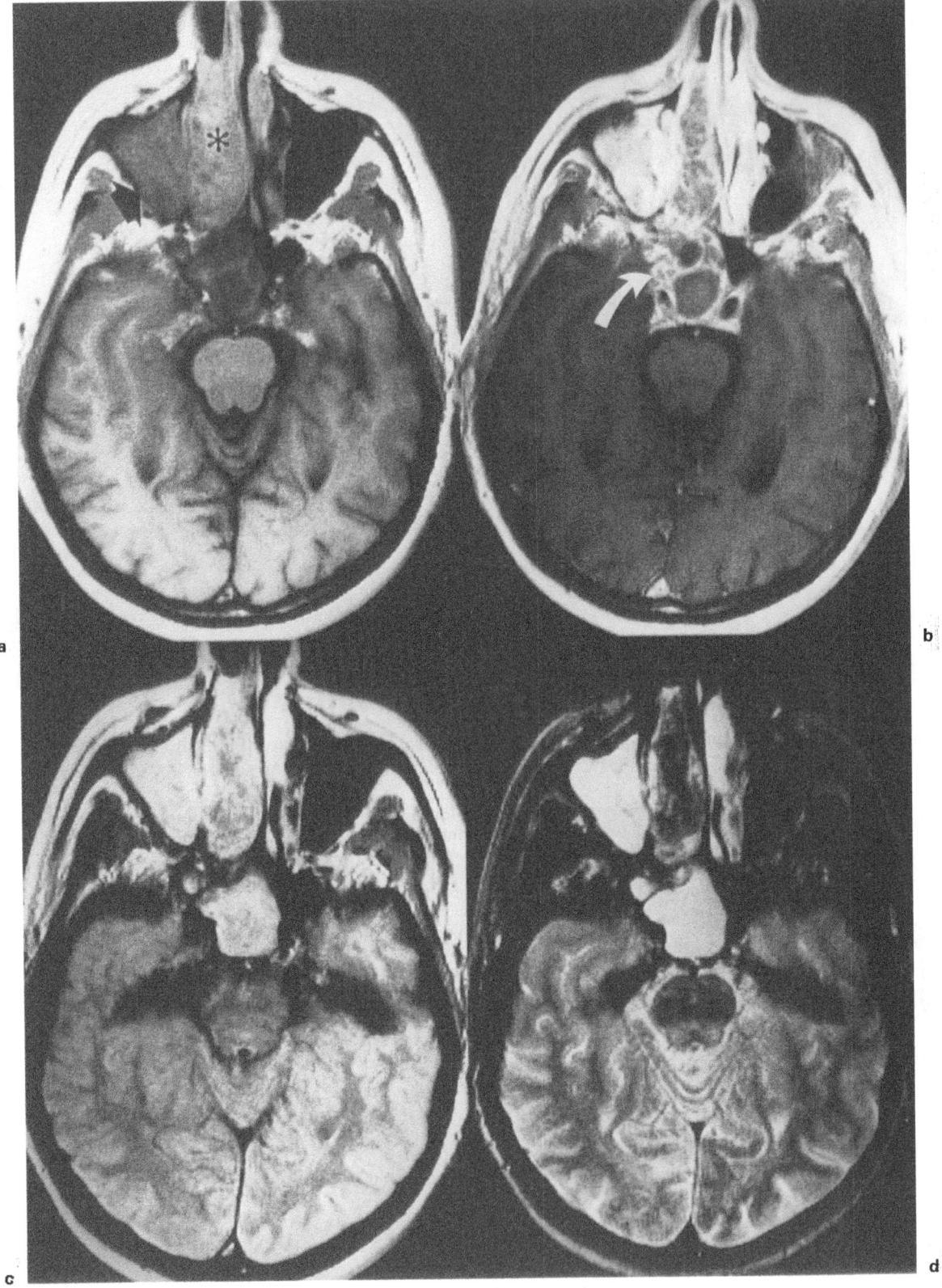

Figure 2.19 Squamous carcinoma, ethmoid and sphenoid sinuses: (**a**) T1WI, (**b**) T1WI + C, (**c**) PDWI, (**d**) T2WI; tumour tissue (asterisk) and reactive sinus mucosa (arrow) are of similar intermediate signal intensity at short TR (a, c), becoming differentiated after contrast and at long TR (b, d). Note sphenoid sinus invasion is apparent only in the contrasted image (b, white arrow)

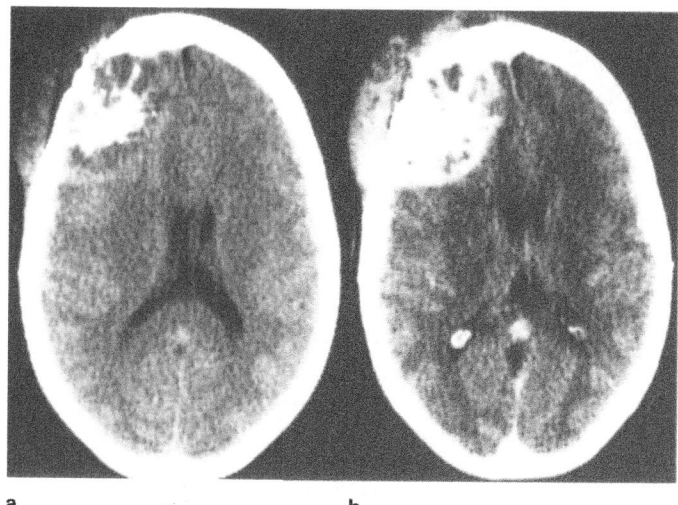

Figure 2.20 Metastatic carcinoma, skull: (**a**) CT, (**b**) CT + C; erosion of frontal skull with adjacent intracranial mineralization/ossification. Bony alteration forms the centre of an intra/extracranial nearly isodense mass, exhibiting strong but inhomogeneous enhancement. Brain is compressed but not oedematous. (Biopsy showed an undifferentiated carcinoma)

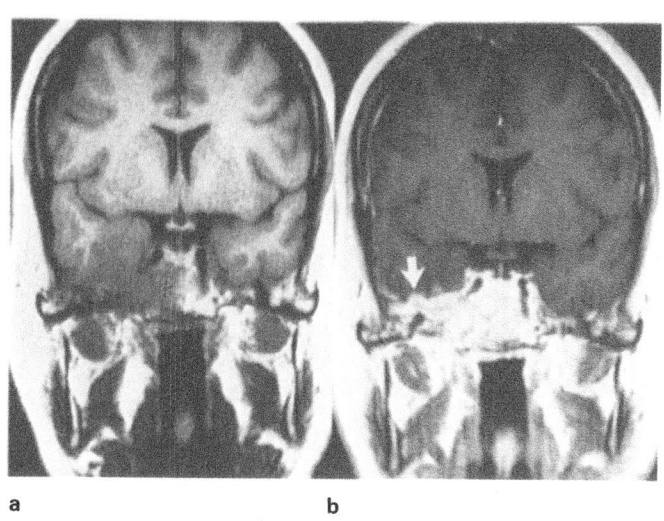

Figure 2.21 Metastatic carcinoma, skull: 57-year-old female with known primary carcinoma of the breast; (**a**) T1WI, (**b**) T1WI + C; the lesion is brain isointense, strongly enhancing, eroding the floor of the middle fossa sphenoid (asterisk) and invading the meninges (arrow)

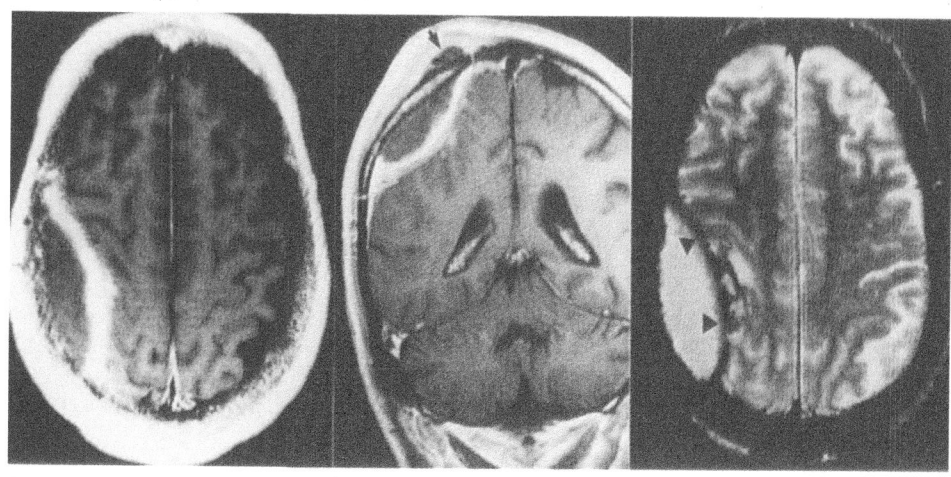

Figure 2.22 Malignant extradural effusion (pachymeningitis carcinomatosa): (**a**) axial T1WI + C, (**b**) coronal T1WI + C, (**c**) T2WI; typical lens-shaped lesion with marked extradural enhancement and adjacent soft tissue subgaleal nodule (b, arrow). Note that the protein-rich/blood-stained effusion and extracranial deposit have the same signal intensity, with normal intervening skull. T2 hypointensity (c, arrow heads) is due to a combination of dural collagen and haemosiderin deposition. (**Figure 3.35** illustrates the dense vascularity responsible for the intense enhancement)

2.6d. Carcinoma, including metastatic disease
(see also sections 3.5 and 4.12)

Primary carcinoma involving the skull, is usually associated with the nasopharynx, air sinuses or external auditory meatus (malignant otitis)[32], with neurosurgical interest in the event of intracranial or perineurial extension[33]. These are usually squamous carcinomas or adenocarcinomas, whose imaging features are characteristically soft-tissue isointense at both short and long TR, and diffusely enhancing (Figure 2.19). Adenoid cystic carcinoma, in comparison with other epithelial tumours, has been observed by us to be strongly T2 hyperintense, a finding compatible with its extensive and organized interstitial space. Lesions of the skull convexity are biopsied when solitary or unassociated with known metastatic disease (Figure 2.20), whilst occasionally the clinician wants to know whether a metastatic scalp malignancy involves the meninges. Figure 2.21 shows the typical T1 brain isointensity and strong, diffuse enhancement of a poorly differentiated adenocarcinoma, involving bone and meninges. These extraparenchymal, *en-plaque* tumours are not macroscopically necrotic (hence their intemediate T2 intensity), whilst their intracerebral counterparts almost always are. They may, however, present occasionally with extradural effusion (Figure 2.22). Rarely, metastatic disease presents in the skull base with selective involvement of a particular cranial nerve or bony fossa, adenoid

cystic carcinoma being the best known for this propensity[34]. Figure 2.23 shows metastatic carcinoma growing along the maxillary nerve, visible as marked enlargement of the neural canal.

2.6e. Lymphoreticular neoplasms[35] (see also sections 3.6 and 4.13)

Plasmacytoma[36] and non-Hodgkin's lymphoma[37,38] are rare but well-described primary, solitary, erosive tumours of the skull, exhibiting strong and diffuse enhancement, as a result of their prominent vascularity (Figure 2.24). Calvarial lesions typically have a scalp component, whilst the intracranial growth involves the meninges and sometimes the brain parenchyma (Figures 2.24 and 2.25). These lesions resemble meningioma except for the bone changes. Lymphoma, presumed to originate in the nasopharynx, may present as a large destructive, strongly enhancing, sphenoid body–sella mass (Figure 2.26); compare this lesion with the destructive pituitary adenoma illustrated in Figure 5.27.

2.6f. Chordoma

About one-third of chordomas are reported to be intracranial, occurring in and around the sphenoid and clivus[39], whence indiscriminate invasion of bone, air sinuses and dura occurs, with displacement and even invasion of

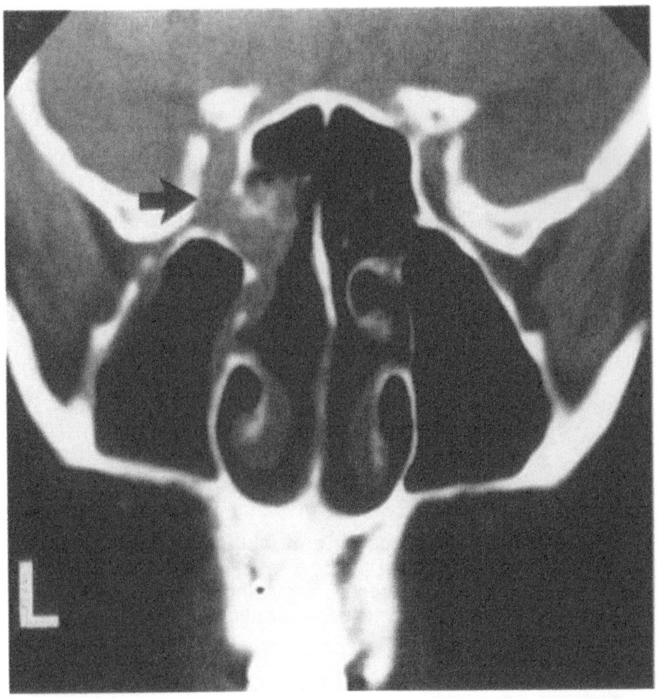

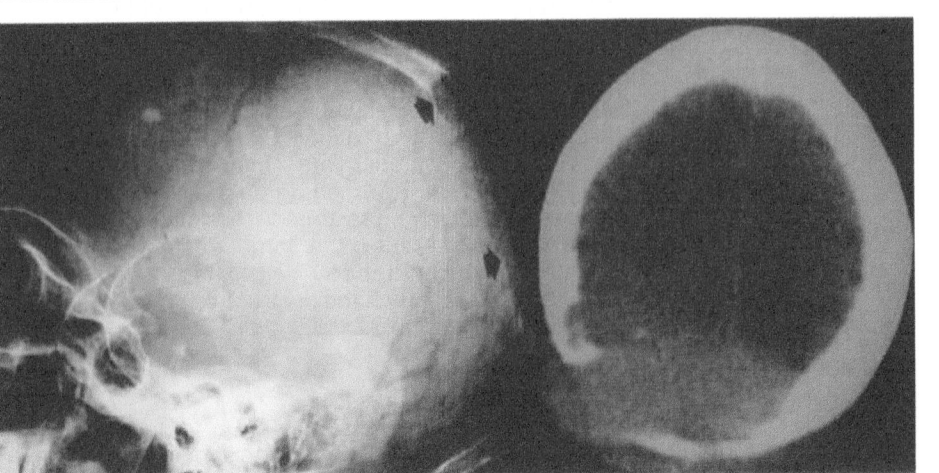

Figure 2.23 Carcinoma, pterygopalatine fossa, infraorbital nerve extension: (**a**) coronal CTBW, (**b**) T1WI + C, (**c**) T1WI, (**d**) HE × 100; CT shows expansion of inferior orbital fissure/pterygopalatine fossa (arrow) with ethmoid erosion. Extension into foramen rotundum (b, arrow) and infraorbital canal (c, arrow). Biopsy of infraorbital nerve (d) shows infiltrated nerve fasciculus

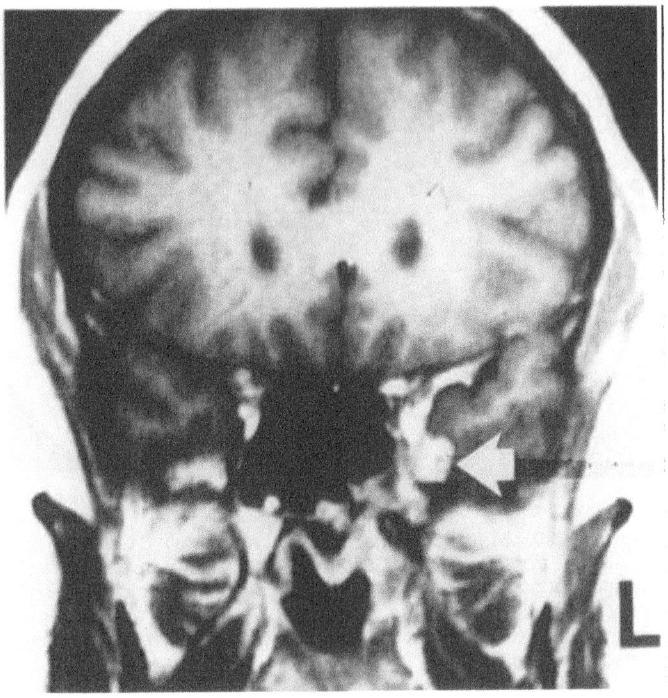

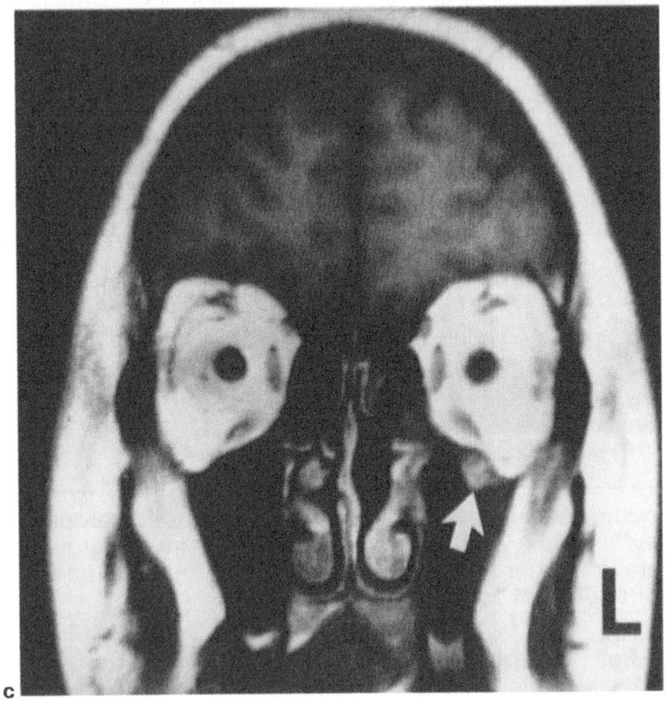

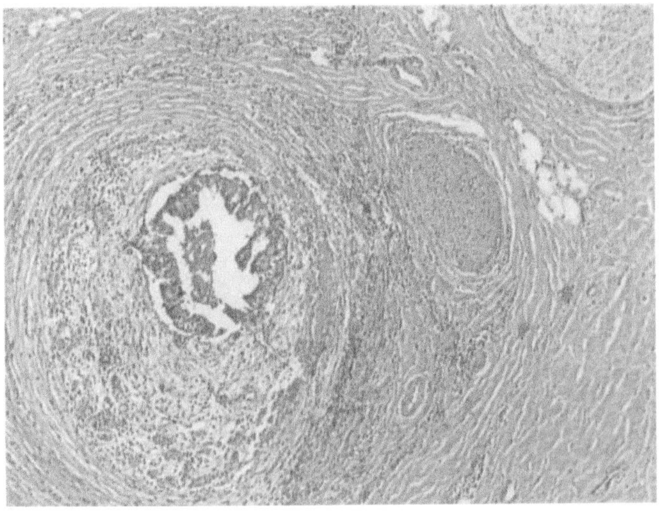

Figure 2.24 Plasmacytoma, occipital skull: (**a**) skull X-ray, (**b**) CT + C, (**c**) HE/MGP × 400, (**d**) reticulin × 200; solitary convexity lesion with extensive bone destruction (arrows) and moderate enhancement on CT scan (b). Histology shows sheets of neoplastic plasma cells (c), with a prominent vasculature, apparent only with reticulin staining (d)

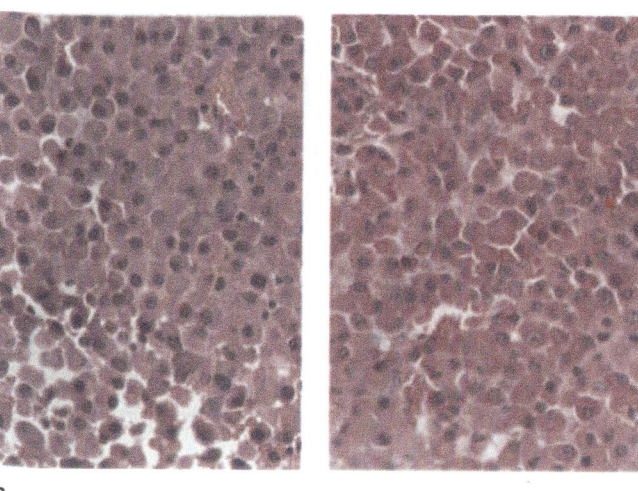

c

d

Figure 2.24 (*continued*)

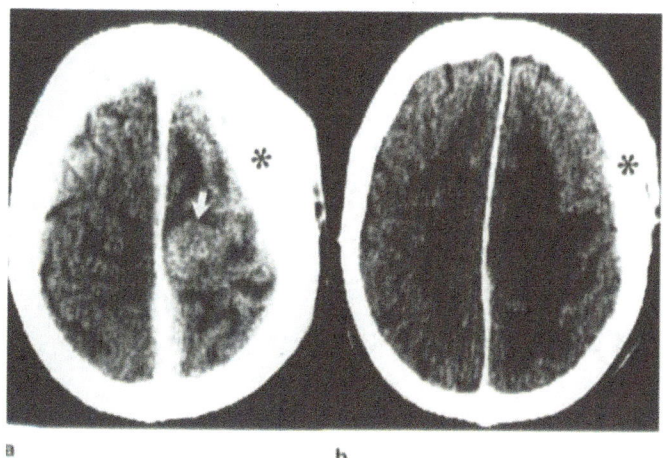

a   b

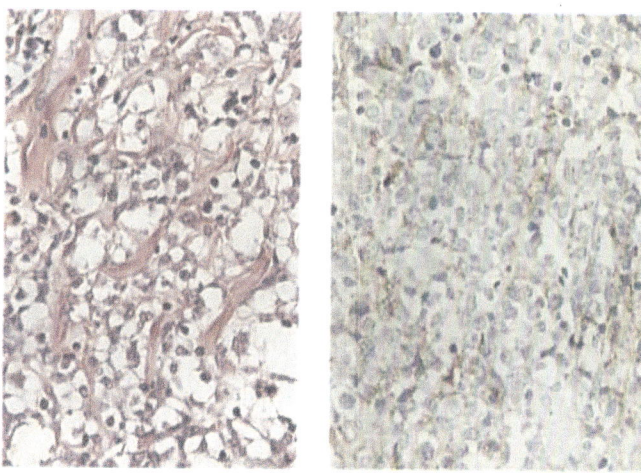

c

Figure 2.25 Lymphoma, primary, scalp, skull and brain: (**a,b**) CT + C. (**c**) HE/L26 × 400; CT shows expansion of skull (asterisk) with weakly enhancing, poorly defined meningocerebral mass (arrow), and adjacent white-matter hypodensity (b) (oedema). Histology is of a sclerosing large B-cell lymphoma. Poor enhancement of meningocerebral component is probably a combination of the high axial cut and the lesion sclerosis (c, left). (Compare with strong enhancement of parenchymal lymphomas, **Figure 4.97**)

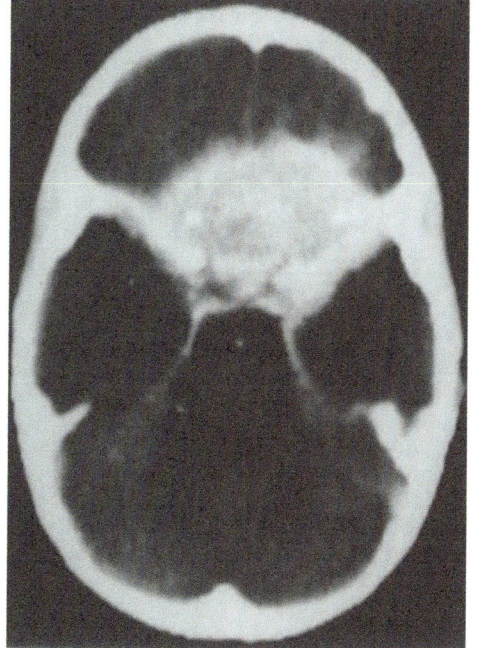

Figure 2.26 Lymphoma, central skull base: child presenting with proptosis and obtundation; contrasted CT shows strongly enhancing central, symmetrical mass, with indistinct edges, which has destroyed jugum and sphenoid wings. Origin from nasopharynx presumed. Cytology yielded sheets of obviously neoplastic mononuclear cells, paradoxically indicating a paucity of vessels and reticulin (see comment in **Figure 2.24**)

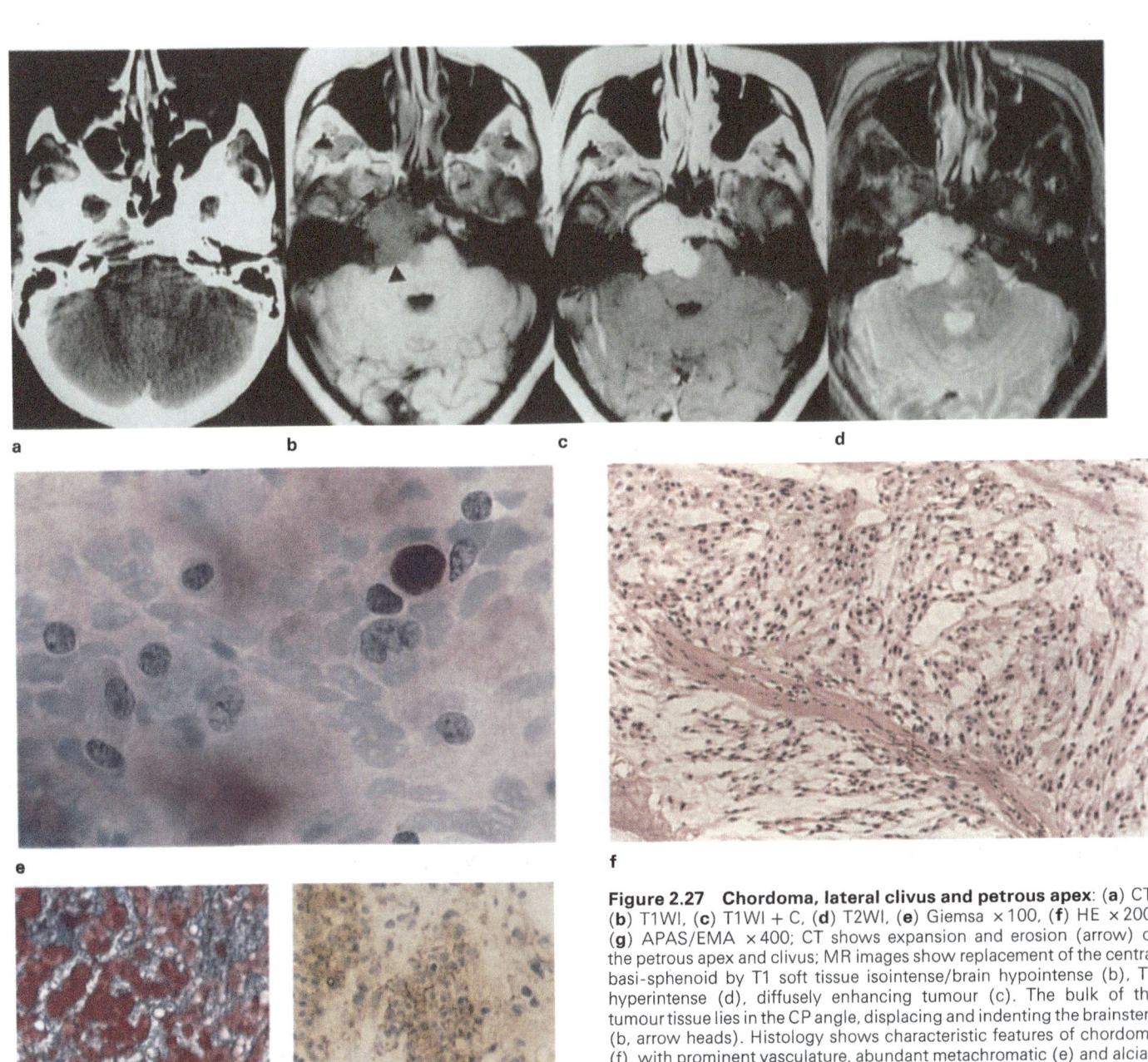

Figure 2.27   Chordoma, lateral clivus and petrous apex: (**a**) CT, (**b**) T1WI, (**c**) T1WI + C, (**d**) T2WI, (**e**) Giemsa × 100, (**f**) HE × 200, (**g**) APAS/EMA × 400; CT shows expansion and erosion (arrow) of the petrous apex and clivus; MR images show replacement of the central basi-sphenoid by T1 soft tissue isointense/brain hypointense (b), T2 hyperintense (d), diffusely enhancing tumour (c). The bulk of the tumour tissue lies in the CP angle, displacing and indenting the brainstem (b, arrow heads). Histology shows characteristic features of chordoma (f), with prominent vasculature, abundant metachromatic (e) and alcian blue/PAS positive material (g, left)

neural parenchyma (Figure 2.27). Tumours are generally hyperdense, T1 soft tissue isointense/brain hypointense and T2 hyperintense, strongly diffusely enhancing, MR features which are fairly specific for chordoma, chondrosarcoma and chondroid osteosarcoma (Figure 2.15), but which cannot differentiate between them[40]. The T2 hyperintensity, unusual for an 'epithelial' tumour[41], is possibly accounted for by the plentiful alcian blue-positive myxoid matrix and/or intracellular PAS-positive material (of whatever nature) (Figure 2.27). CT hyperdensity is paradoxical; nor is there any correlative study on the histomorphology of occasionally CT hypodense tumours. Typical absence of necrosis also favours homogeneity of enhancement (compare with images of chondroid osteosarcoma, Figure 2.15).

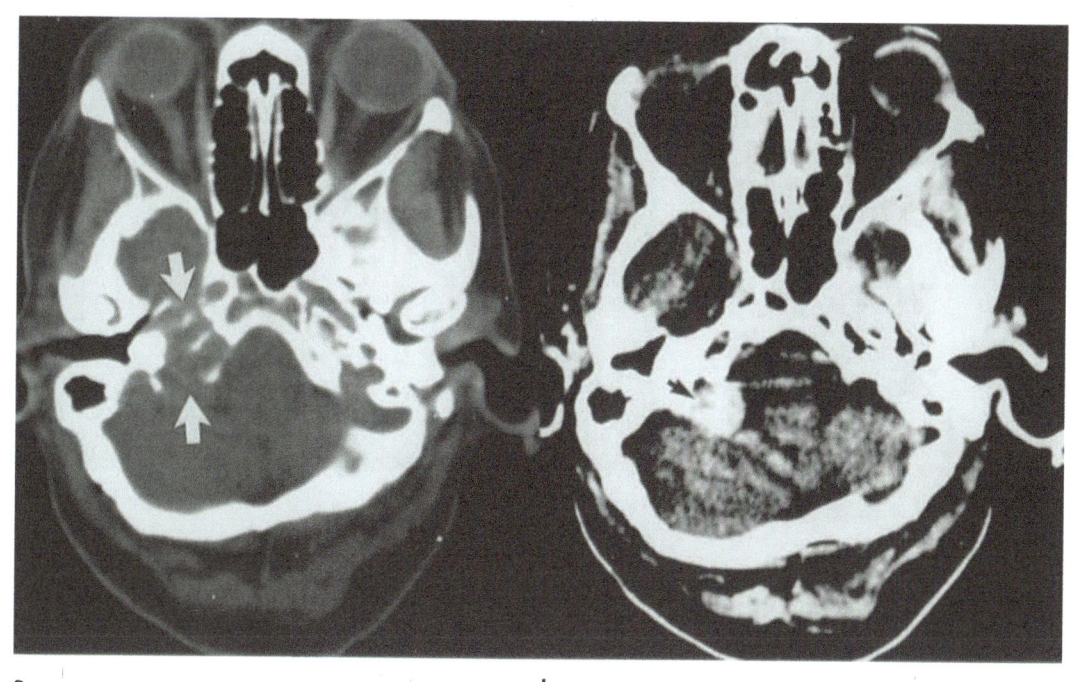

a   b

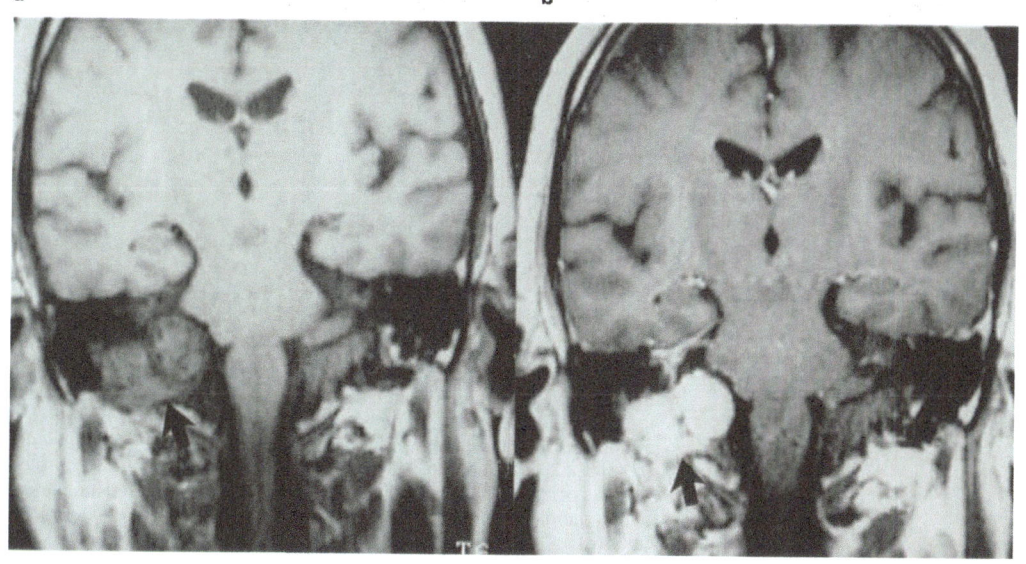

c   d

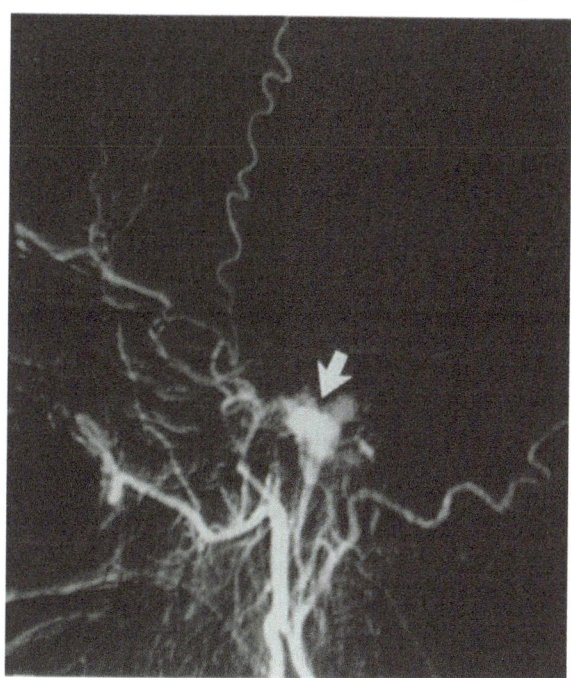

e

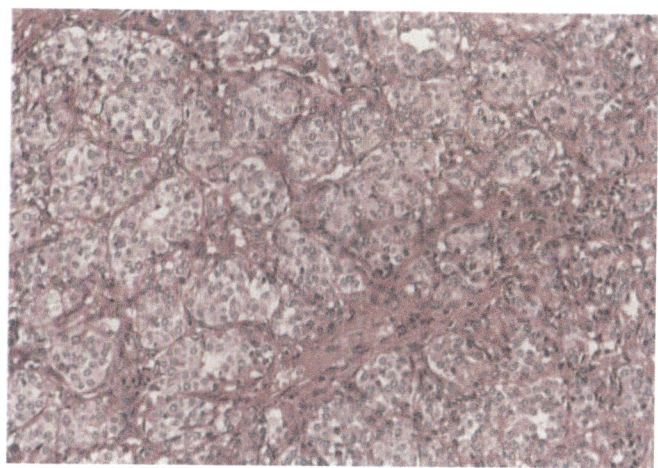

f

Figure 2.28 Paraganglioma, jugular foramen: (a) CTBW, (b) CT + C, (c) T1WI, (d) T1WI + C, (e) angiogram, (f) HE × 200; CT shows expansion and erosion of the jugular foramen and petrous bone, with enhancing mass in the cerebello-medullary cistern (arrows). MR shows bony and intracranial components to be cortex isointense and strongly enhancing (arrows c, d), with intense arterial blush on angiogram (indicative of vascularity and high blood flow). Deformation of the pons is similar to acoustic schwannoma. Histology shows characteristic nests of cells and prominent vasculature. (Drs M Wright & RM Bowen, Groote Schuur Hospital)

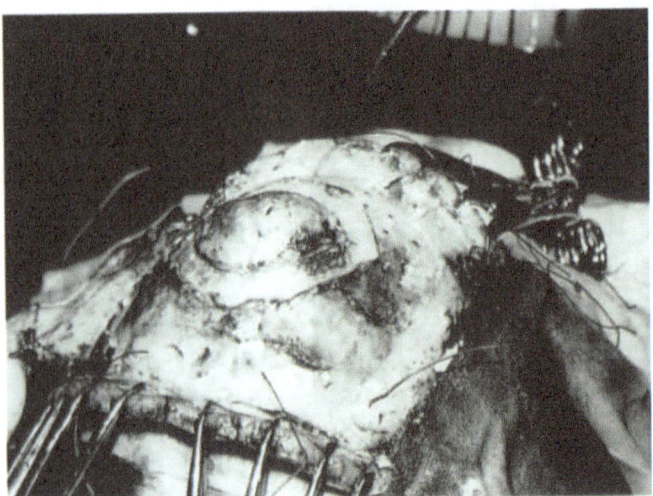

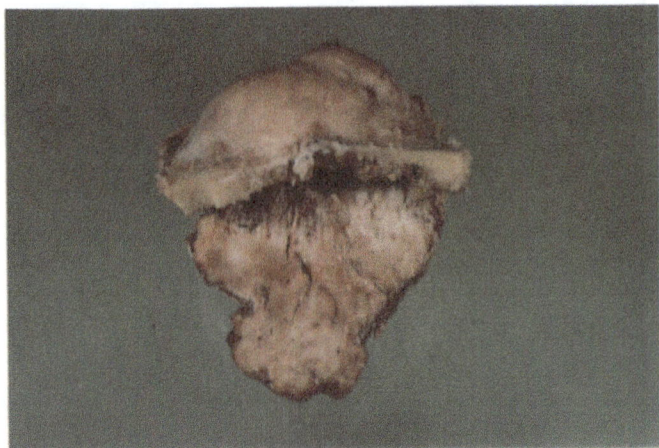

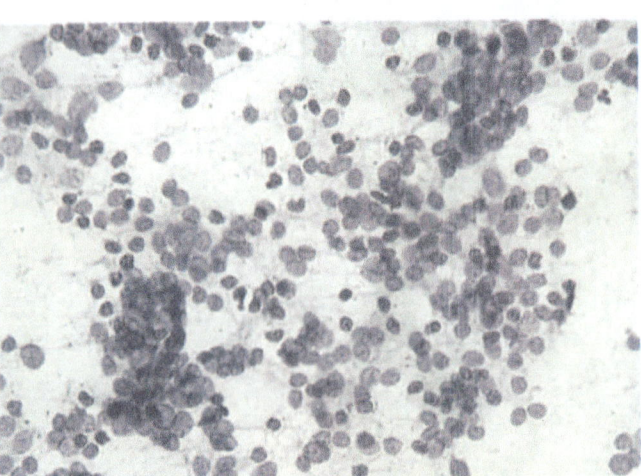

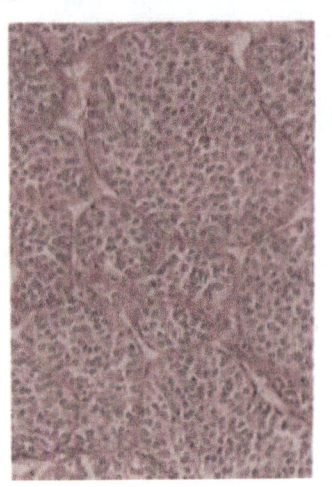
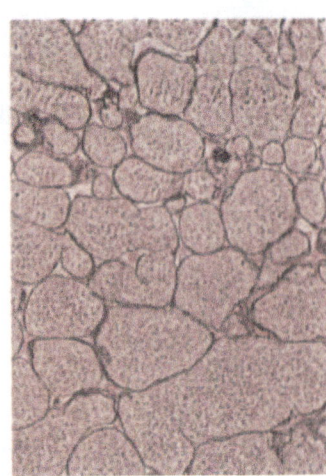

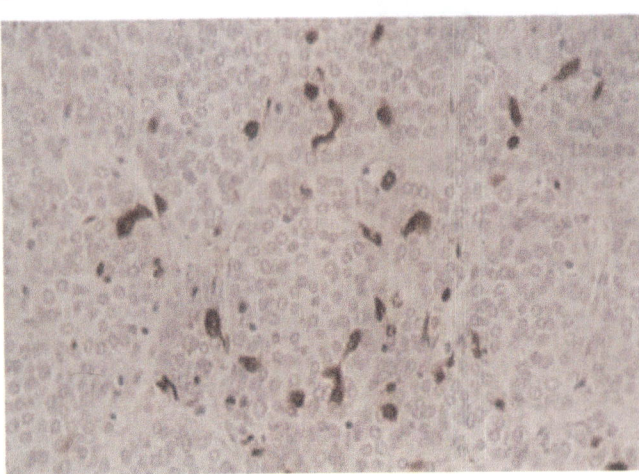

Figure 2.29 Paraganglioma, skull vault: images were indistinguishable from meningioma; (**a**) operative view of bony mass protruding from the convexity, (**b**) operative specimen showing hyperostosis and intracranial mass with prominent blood vessels, (**c**) Tol blue × 400, (**d**) HE × 200/reticulin × 100, (**e**) S100 × 400; intraoperative cytology (c) was perplexing but paraffin sections (d) show characteristic features of paraganglioma, including the presence of S100-positive sustentacular cells (e)

2.6g. Paraganglioma (glomus jugulare, chemodectoma)

The rather typical features of jugular foramen paraganglioma, including its clinical presentation and localization, may be complicated by a more rostral and intracranial extension. In the event, lateral expansion of the foramen is said to be a constant finding[2], combined with T1 brain isointensity, T2 hyperintensity and strong enhancement (Figure 2.28). The mass may contain flow voids, and is diffusely hyperintense on the gradient echo sequences. The imaging appearances of calvarial paraganglioma are indistinguishable from meningioma, including hyperostosis (Figure 2.29). Cords and islands of tumour cells[42] are separated by a striking vascular network.

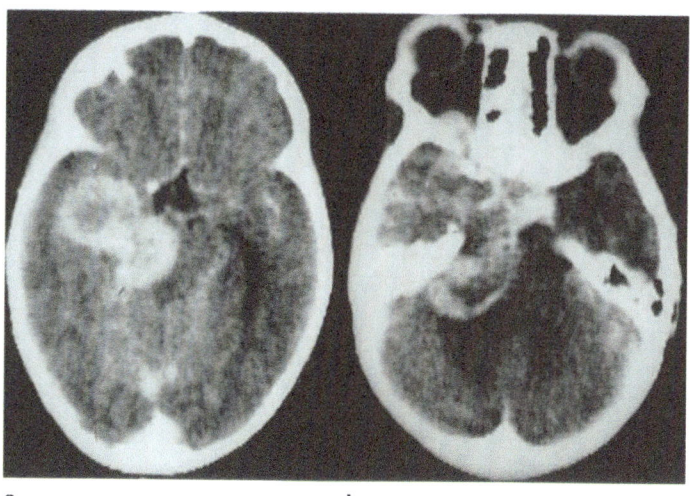

a   b

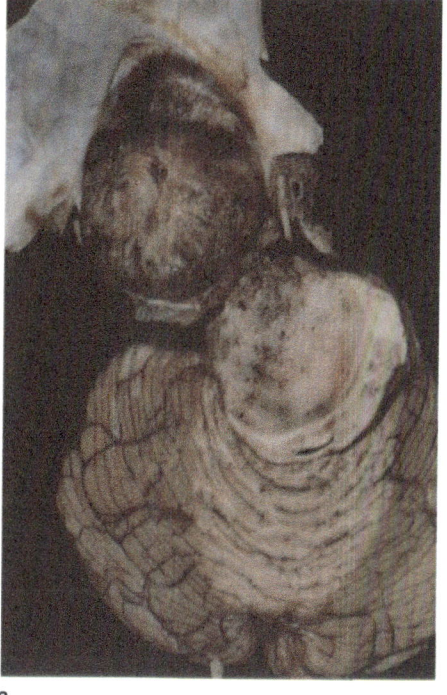

Figure 2.30   Rhabdomyosarcoma, petrous apex/CP angle: (a,b) CT + C, (**c**) post-mortem specimen, (**d**) HE ×200, (**e**) PTAH ×400/SMA ×100; enhanced CT shows strong peripherally enhancing mass eroding petroclivus and compressing brainstem and temporal lobe. Fixed specimen (c) exhibits a smooth lobulated non-invasive surface with prominent stromal vessels. Histology shows focal tumour necrosis (d), responsible for lack of central enhancement, and diagnostic histology (e)

c

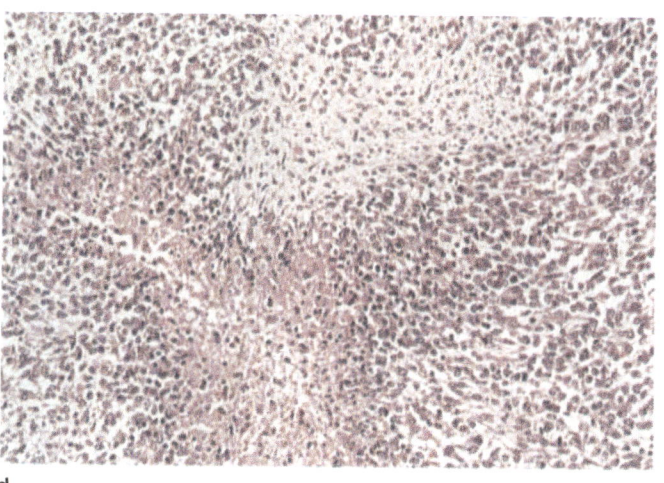

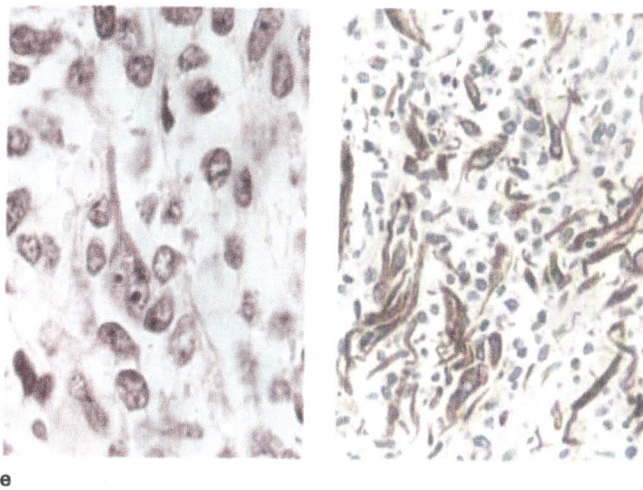

d   e

2.6h.   Rhabdomyosarcoma

Origin from the middle ear constitutes an important childhood tumour[43], usually presenting as a spurious complication of local infection, but occasionally as an intracranial growth with obvious erosion of the supero-medial petrous. Imaging features are of soft tissue-epi-thelial type (brain isodense and isointense at short and long TR), with strong, usually diffuse enhancement becoming inhomogeneous when extensive necrosis manifests[44] (Figure 2.30). Admixed, spotty T2 hyperintense foci in the petrous is due to associated air cell obstruction (Figure 2.31).

2.7.   LANGERHANS CELL HISTIOCYTOSIS
(histiocytosis X, eosinophilic granuloma)

This condition is usually encountered as a solitary calvarial lesion, with a painful scalp mass and sharply circumscribed bony lysis on plain films. Skull base involvement is rarer, as is meningocerebral LCH. Most cases occur in the first two decades, and the prognosis depends mainly on the extent of disease at diagnosis, and patient age[45]. As with lymphoma, from which it may be indistinguishable on imaging, the tissue mass is brain and soft-tissue T1 isointense/T2 hyperintense, and strongly enhancing[46,47] (Figure 2.32). Early lesions are cellular and locally destructive, composed of aggregates of Langerhans cells admixed with macrophages, eosinophils and lymphocytes (Figure 2.32); older lesions have fewer Langerhans cells and tend to fibrosis[48]. The differential diagnosis of early bone disease includes chronic osteomyelitis, where the presence of plasma cells, uncommon in LCH, may be a clue. Despite usual S-100 positivity and cytoplasmic halo formation with peanut agglutinin, only Birbeck granules are pathognomonic (Figure 2.32).

2.8.   LESIONS NOT DISCUSSED

Aneurysmal bone cyst[49]; esthesioneuroblastoma[50]; Ewing's sarcoma[51]; fibrous dysplasia; giant cell tumour[52]; haemangioma[53]; malignant fibrous histiocytoma[54]; melanotic neuroectodermal tumour of infancy (Figure 2.33); metastatic neuroblastoma.

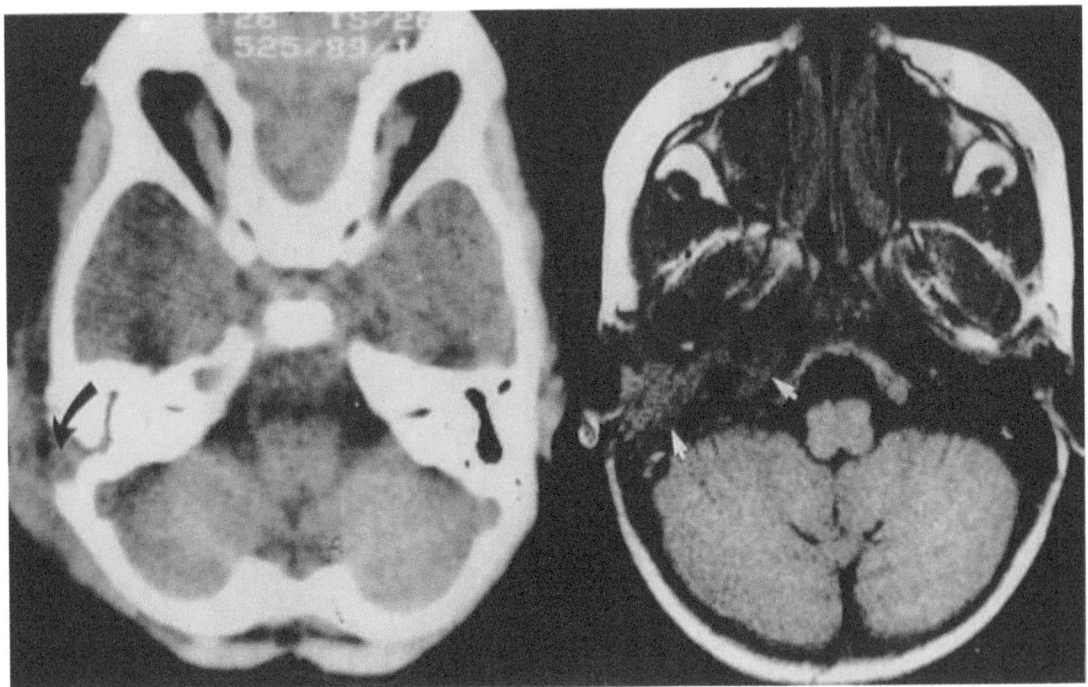

a   b

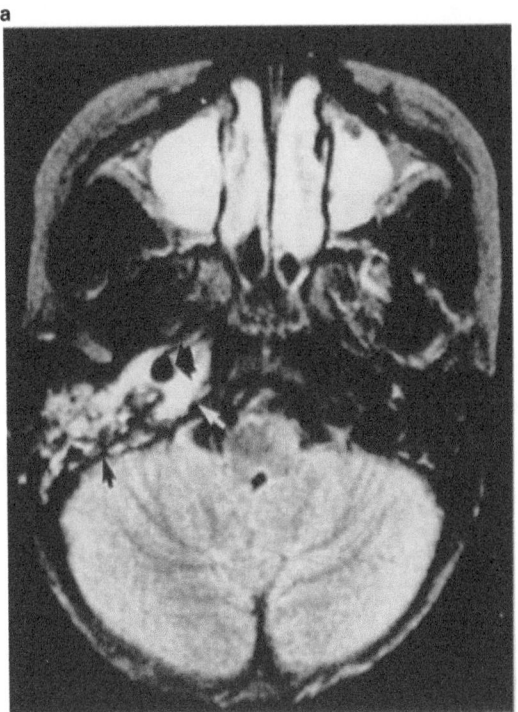

c

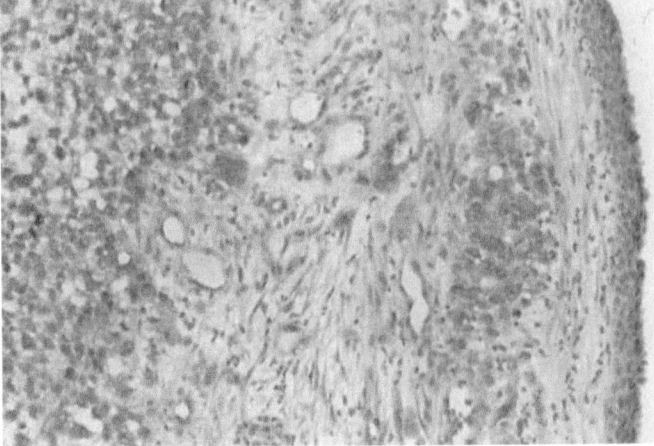

d

Figure 2.31   Rhabdomyosarcoma, external meatus and petrous: (**a**) CT, (**b**) T1WI, (**c**) T2WI, (**d**) HE × 200; CT shows soft tissue mass eroding and obliterating external meatus (arrow) with opacification of mastoid air spaces (compare with opposite side). Tumour is T1 soft tissue isointense, but is inhomogeneously T2 hyperintense. The T2 inhomogeneity is spurious and is probably mainly due to obstructed bony air spaces (arrows b, c). Note carotid artery (c, broad arrow). Biopsy from external meatus shows infiltrated meatal soft tissue and lining (d)

REFERENCES

1. Daniels DL, Houghton VM, Czervionke LF. Skull base. In: Stark DD, Bradley WG, eds. Magnetic resonance imaging. A comprehensive text. St Louis: CV Mosby; 1988:524–69.

2. Curtin HD, Hirsch WL. Base of the skull. In: Atlas SW, ed. Magnetic resonance imaging of the brain and spine. New York: Raven Press; 1991:669–707.

3. Laine FJ, Nadel L, Braun IF. CT and MR imaging of the central skull base. Part 2. Pathologic spectrum. Radiographics. 1990;10:797–821.

4. Barkovich AJ. Congenital malformations of the brain. In: Pediatric neuroimaging. Contemporary neuroimaging, vol. 1. New York: Raven Press; 1990:86.

5. Friede RL. Developmental neuropathology. Wien: Springer-Verlag; 1975:236–9.

6. Yve CP, Mann KS, Chan FL. Optic canal syndrome due to posterior ethmoid sinus mucocele. J Neurosurg. 1986;65:871–3.

7. Lanzieri CF, Shah M, Krauss D et al. Use of gadolinium-enhanced MR imaging for differentiating mucoceles from neoplasma in the paranasal sinuses. Radiology. 1991;178:425–8.

8. Som PM, Dillon WP, Fullerton GD et al. Chronically obstructed sinonasal secretions: observations on T1 and T2 shortening. Radiology. 1989;172:515–20.

9. Zinreich SJ, Kennedy DW, Malat J et al. Fungal sinusitis: diagnosis with CT and MR imaging. Radiology. 1988;169:439–44.

10. Som PM, Dillon WP, Sze G et al. Benign and malignant sinonasal lesions with intracranial extension: differentiation with MR imaging. Radiology. 1989;172:763–6.

11. Prinsloo JG, Kirsten GF. Tuberculosis of the skull vault. S Afr Med J. 1977;57:248–50.

12. Le Roux P, Griffin GE, Marsh HT et al. Tuberculosis of the skull: a rare condition: case report and review of the literature. Neurosurgery. 1990;26:851–6.

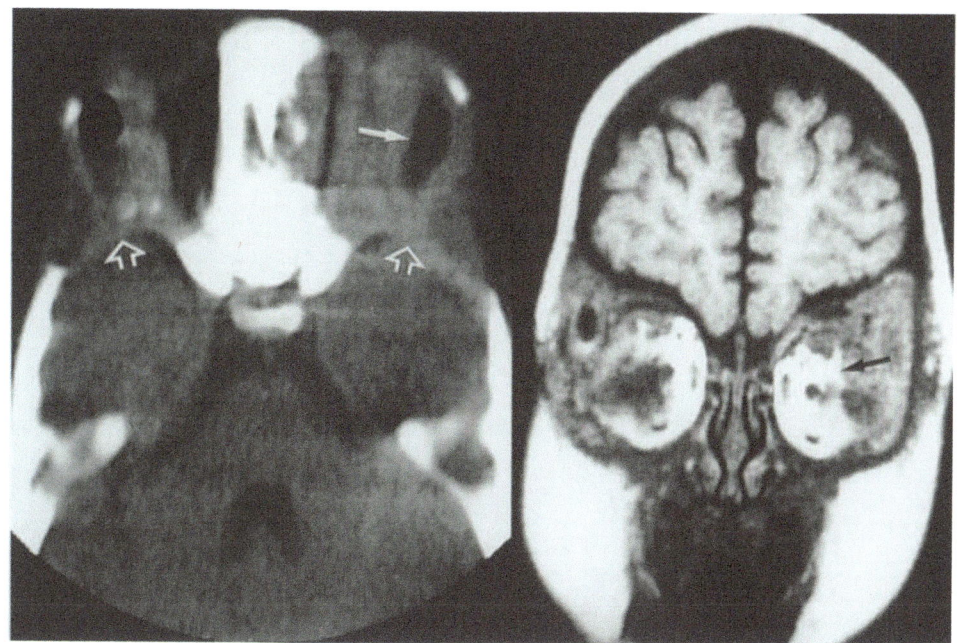

a   b

Figure 2.32 Langerhans cell histiocytosis: female, 3 years, proptosis and draining sinuses from both orbits; (a) CT, (b) coronal T1WI, (c) HE ×1000, (d) EM ×56000; CT shows hyperdense tissue eroding and replacing orbital roof and sphenoid greater wings (open arrows). (On CT tissue was also strongly enhancing.) MR shows slightly inhomogeneous soft tissue isointense mass compressing orbital contents bilaterally (b, arrow). The central hypodensities (a, arrow), which were abscess-like cavities containing necrotic tumour, are T1 isointense (T2 hyperintense). Histology shows a mononuclear infiltrate, including pigment-laden macrophages and cells with 'coffee-bean' nuclei (c, arrow). Ultrastructure illustrates diagnostic Birbeck granules (d, arrow)

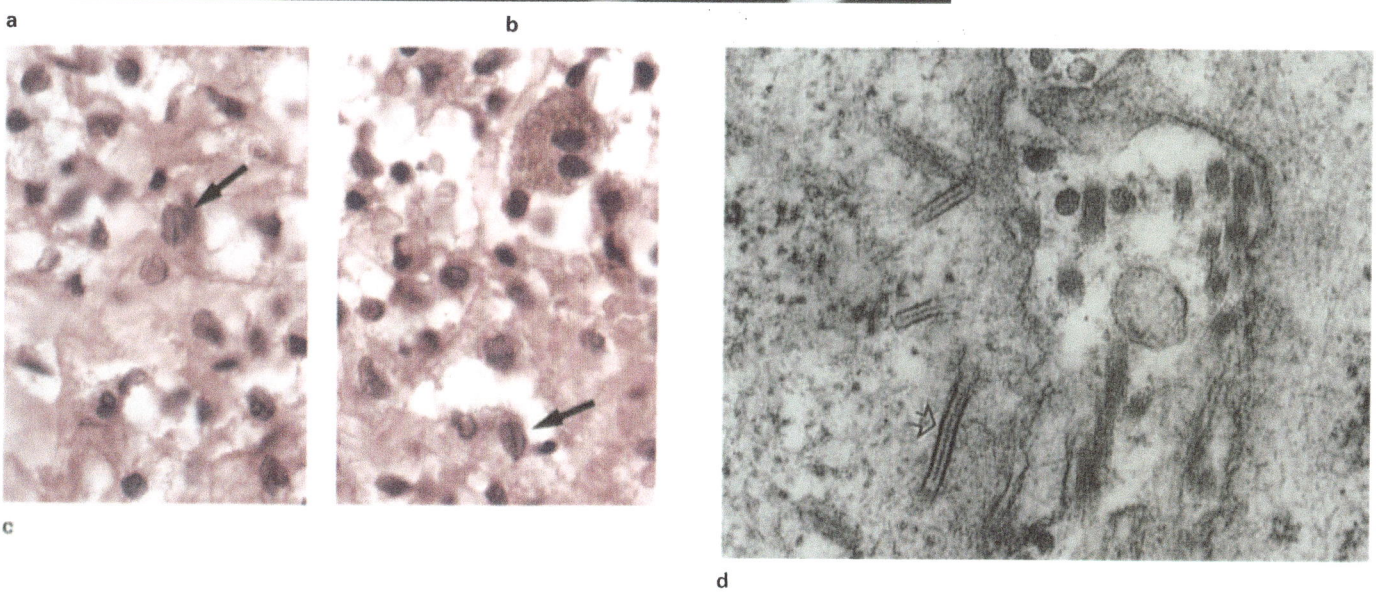

c   d

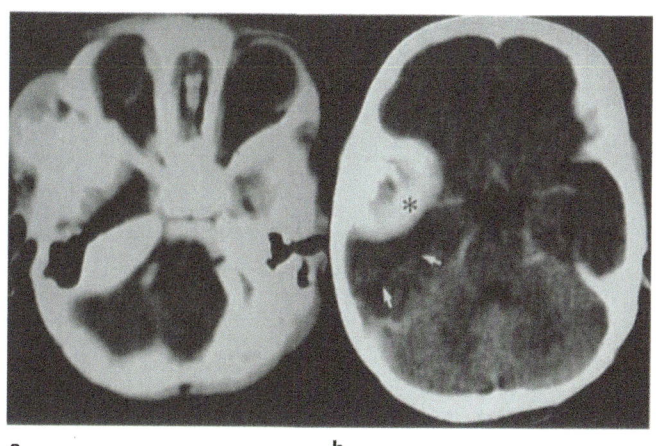

a   b

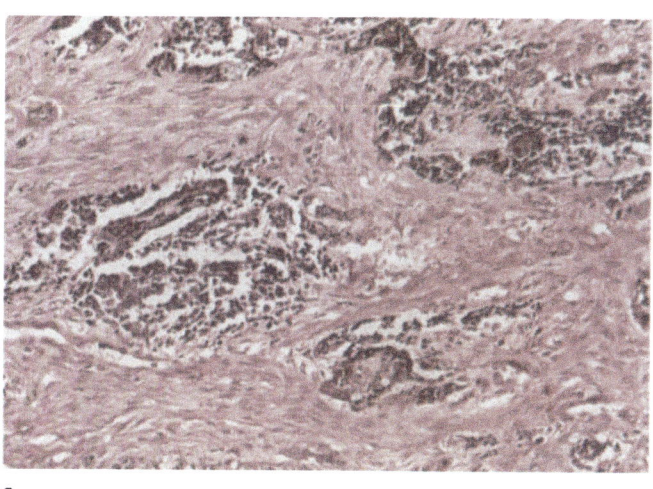

c

Figure 2.33 Melanotic neuroectodermal tumour of infancy (progonoma): female, 4 months; (a,b) CT + C, (c) HE ×200; images show gross sclerotic calvarial expansion, with prominent enhancing soft tissue component (b, asterisk), which is inducing cerebral oedema (b, arrows). Histology shows islands of small neuroectodermal cells, adjacent to melanin-pigment containing cells, with a conspicuous connective-tissue stroma; vasculature appears to be mainly stromal. Scan suggests origin from skull base

Supratentorial extraparenchymal and meningocerebral lesions

3.1. PRIMARY CYSTS (Developmental)

It appears from the literature on this subject[1-4], most of which is in neurosurgical journals, that the difficulties in classifying developmental intracranial cysts, particularly those having a simple epithelial lining, are mainly the result of investigative inconsistencies, such as the application of a particular antibody, the use or lack of electron microscopy, and so on. It is clear, however, that whilst a correlative approach is essential, no combination of topography, imaging features and morphology is specific for any particular cyst, even with a distinctive lesion such as colloid cyst of the third ventricle.

Ideally[5], and in most instances, cyst contents are iso-dense and isointense with cerebrospinal fluid (CSF) on all sequences; hyperintensity on the T1 and proton density images (T1 shortening) without significant alteration of long TR/TE signal usually characterizes the moderate increases in protein (albumin) concentration encountered in these cysts (Figure 5.4). Non-paramagnetic T2 hypointensity is currently assumed to be the effect of water perturbation by glycoproteins[6] (mucins) (Figure 5.4), whilst laminar keratin renders distinct inhomogeneity to an otherwise CSF-like T1 signal (Figure 4.3). Enhancement is almost always absent, but may occur when the wall becomes contiguous with meninges or choroid plexus. Parenchyma adjacent to or partly surrounding a benign cyst is usually normal in density and signal intensity; however, atrophic spongiosis may lead to minimal T2 hyperintensity. Topography, assessed by means of short TR in three planes, sometimes exerts the principal diagnostic bias, particularly with regard to cysts lying within the cisterns and ventricles, and some lesions are now assumed to have a particular morphology simply on account of their location[7]. Within the spinal canal, terminology is modified according to dural and nerve root relationships (see section 7.2).

In practical neuropathological terms, tissue diagnosis is complicated by the particular need for correct specimen orientation and fixation. Morphology has to include glial and epithelial cell markers, as well as ultrastructure, and even then may prove inconclusive[8,9]. Allowing for the prevailing nosological difficulties we have divided this group of cystic mass lesions into the following histomorphological categories, and individual examples of each category are discussed at appropriate sites:

(1) *Dermal inclusion (cyst)*: still referred to as cysts in many sources[10] despite their semi-solid and relatively waterless contents, comprise *epidermoid* (i.e. having a wall of keratinized squamous epithelium only), and *dermoid-teratomatous* (i.e. having epithelium, skin adnexae and, infrequently, mesenchymal tissues) types. Although epidermoidoma has been described as lacking geographic restraint[10], intracranial forms both tend to occur more commonly in the posterior fossa and suprasellar space, with intraparenchymal, hemispheric lesions being rarest (see section 3.1a, below).

(2) *Arachnoid (leptomeningeal) cyst*: characteristic sites favour a developmental origin in most cases, and the cyst wall is typically leptomeningeal, on both light and electron microscopy[11,12], sometimes with a fibrovascular component. Some cysts accumulate contrast or radioisotopes after a delay, evidence cited in favour of a secretory function, which could also explain enlargement (see section 3.1b below).

(3) *Simple epithelial cyst*:
  (a) neuroepithelial (ependymal, glioependymal, choroidal);
  (b) neurenteric (enterogenous, endodermal, foregut);
  (c) ectodermal;
  (d) colloid (paraphyseal);
  (e) Rathke's cleft;
  (f) indeterminate.
The present controversy surrounding this category of developmental cysts has to do with the identification of the lining epithelium, and in the consequent inferences with regard to (neur)ectodermal and endodermal origin. *Neuroepithelium* is accepted by us in its original context[13], to include cells of varying morphology lining the ventricles and choroid plexus; *neurenteric* cysts are lined by epithelium assumed to be derived from the foregut, of which ciliated columnar and goblet cells are the most distinctive elements. However, ultrastructural morphologies of both tissues are variable, overlapping, and sometimes uncertain[14], although broad distinction is becoming apparent using antibodies for GFAP, specific cytokeratins, epithelial membrane antigen and carcinoembryonic antigen[15,16]. The presence of strong mucin and PAS reactivity is generally regarded as favouring neurenteric epithelium, and currently, *colloid cyst* is being increasingly regarded as belonging to this category[17].

(4) *Benign brain cyst*: a term which is restricted to a rare intraparenchymal cavity cyst, devoid of any lining (see section 4.2).

3.1a. Dermal inclusion cyst (epidermoidoma and dermoid-teratoma)

The imaging characteristics and pathological correlates of *epidermoidoma* are discussed under extraparenchymal posterior fossa lesions, section 6.1b. Meningocerebral location appears to be the most uncommon intracranial site (Figure 4.3). The implications of T1 hyperintensity sometimes common to the suprasellar epidermoidoma, craniopharyngioma, Rathke's pouch and haemorrhagic retention cyst (cholesterol granuloma) of the petrous apex are discussed under suprasellar lesions, section 5.2.

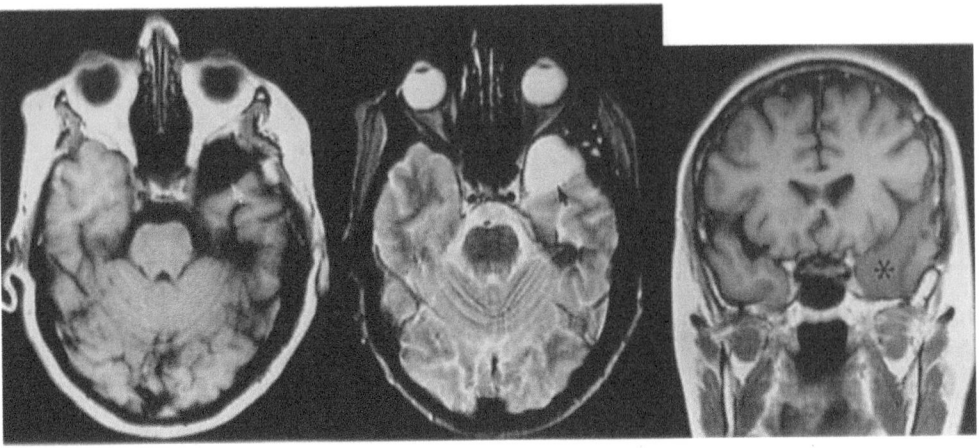

Figure 3.1   Arachnoid cyst, middle fossa: (**a**) T1WI, (**b**) T2WI, (**c**) coronal T1WI + C; cyst is CSF isointense on all sequences, and apparently separated from temporal lobe by a membrane (a,b, arrows); delayed study (4 h) shows distinct concentration of intravenous contrast within cyst (c, asterisk) (compare density of cyst contents with that of ventricular CSF)

a   b   c

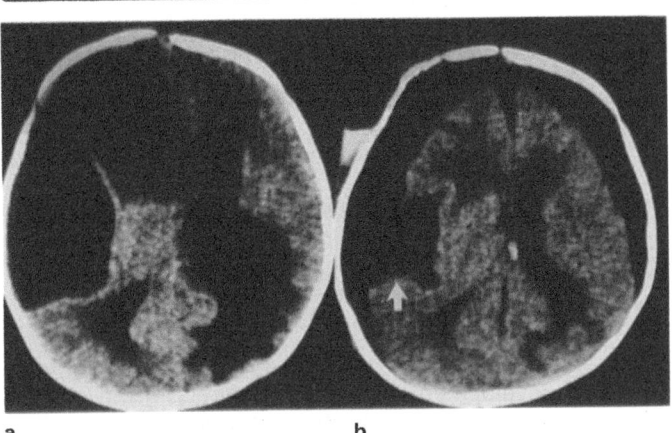

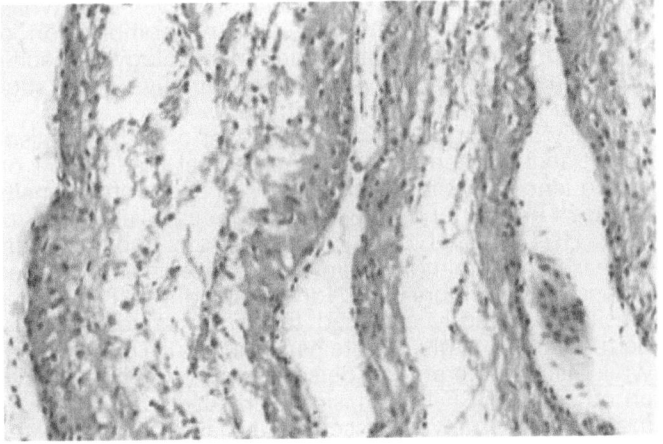

Figure 3.2   Arachnoid cyst: (**a**) preoperative CT, (**b**) postoperative CT, (**c**) HE × 200; CT shows two meningocerebral cysts, with skull moulding and marked hydrocephalus. Tissue from external wall of cyst shows only arachnoid (c). Note cyst base conforms to the insula in

c

follow-up scan (b), whilst temporal operculum appears deficient. Anterior cyst may have been a sequestrated anterior horn. (Dr D Le Roux, East London)

The rarity of intracranial *dermoid-teratoma* is attested by the imaging literature, as well as the experience in these hospitals where no case has been recorded in 15 years. An extracranial lesion is illustrated in Figure 2.9. The images are described as characterizing fat, but with dense internal inhomogeneity on T2 weighted sequences[18], resulting presumably from adnexal inclusions; neither these nor the nature of T2 hyperintensity within the cyst have been properly correlated so far.

3.1b.   Arachnoid cyst

Supratentorial cysts occur most commonly in the middle fossa, and are usually asymptomatic, despite displacement and sometimes hypogenesis of the temporal pole (Figure 3.1); the Sylvian fissure is also a distinctive location (Figure 3.2). Cyst fluid is, by definition, CSF-identical on all sequences, and the lining is devoid of focal thickening and non-enhancing, but contrast accumulates within the cavity after a delay[19]. Histology reveals arachnoid tissue, with typically flattened nuclei and ill-defined eosinophilic cytoplasm; some fibrosis may be present in relation to the meningeal part of the cyst wall, but does not constitute a genuine fibrous capsule.

3.1c.   Simple epithelial cyst

Rare at this site, the lesion illustrated was meningocerebral in location, lined by EMA and GFAP-negative, cuboidal epithelium, having a pseudoacinar organization in areas (Figure 3.3).

3.2.   GRANULOMATOUS MASS LESIONS

In the past, surgical intervention for a number of enhancing mass lesions resulted in excision of granulomas which were subsequently shown by serial imaging, in similar cases, to have a natural history of improvement on therapy or even spontaneous resolution; in addition, morbidity was often exacerbated by surgery. Based on this experience, granulomas are now seldom excised unless there is doubt as to the differential diagnosis, or when suspected fungal aetiology requires confirmation.

The differing aetiologies of granulomatous inflammation, including variable reactions to a specific agent such as *Mycobacterium tuberculosis*, present well-known difficulties in any account of intracranial granulomatous disease. In addition, the classical pathology[20,21], as well as correlation of imaging and morphological features of granulomatous inflammation[22,23], makes unlikely the notion[24] that even tuberculous granulomas will necessarily evolve stepwise from one form to another. Apart from its highly significant tendency to meningocerebral location, usually more vigorous proliferative component and the presence of epithelioid cells, the gliomesodermal response in granulomatous inflammation, which is the basis of both contrast enhancement and T2 signal shortening, does not differ significantly from that seen in chronic pyogenic infection (Chapter 4). Thus the wall of a granuloma tends to be thicker and more irregular (nodular, crenated) than in conventional abscess. A major divergence between this text and the accounts of others, however, concerns the definition[25,26] and imaging implica-

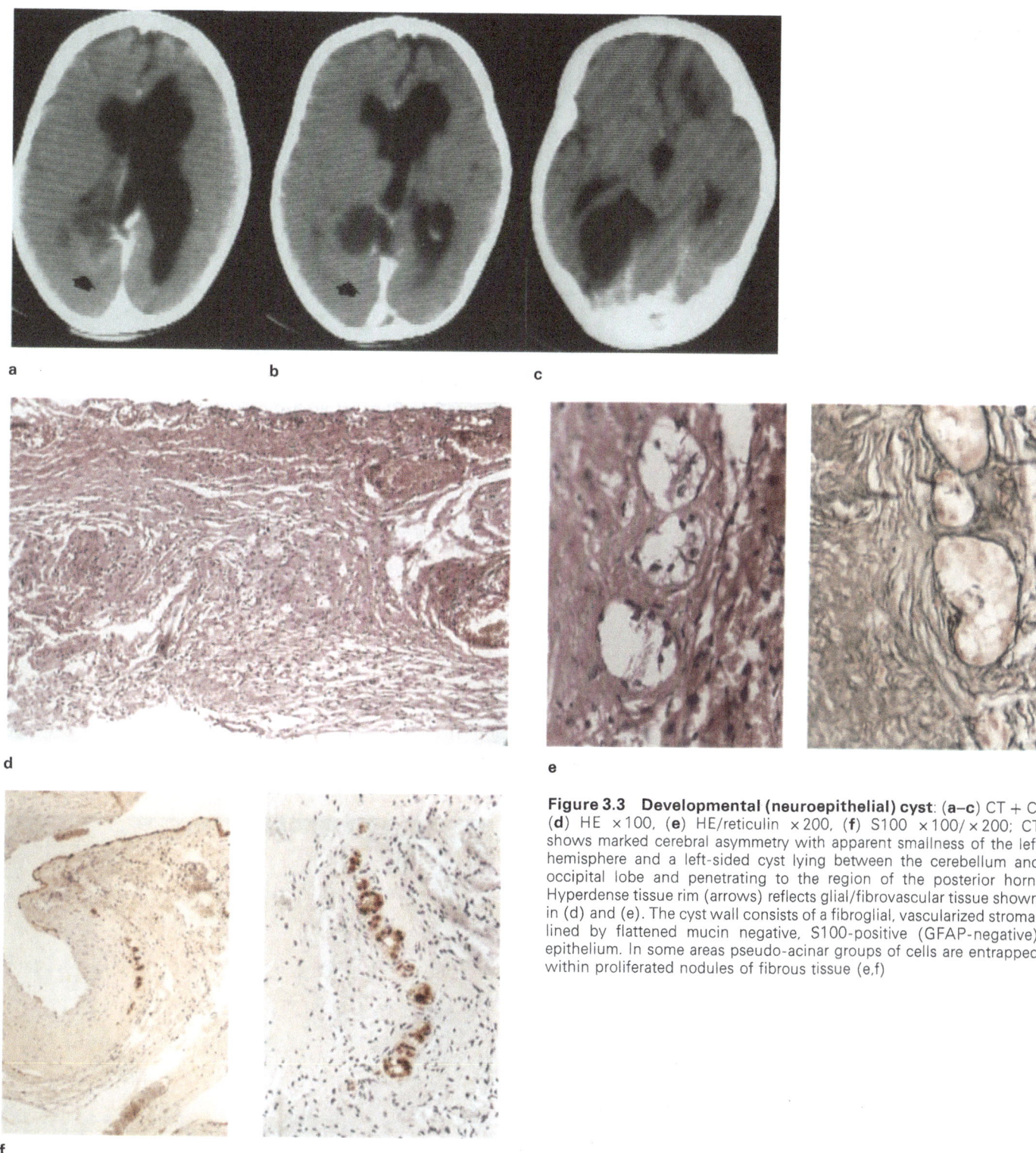

Figure 3.3   Developmental (neuroepithelial) cyst: (**a–c**) CT + C, (**d**) HE ×100, (**e**) HE/reticulin ×200, (**f**) S100 ×100/×200; CT shows marked cerebral asymmetry with apparent smallness of the left hemisphere and a left-sided cyst lying between the cerebellum and occipital lobe and penetrating to the region of the posterior horn. Hyperdense tissue rim (arrows) reflects glial/fibrovascular tissue shown in (d) and (e). The cyst wall consists of a fibroglial, vascularized stroma, lined by flattened mucin negative, S100-positive (GFAP-negative) epithelium. In some areas pseudo-acinar groups of cells are entrapped within proliferated nodules of fibrous tissue (e,f)

tions[27] of the necrotizing process. Based on work done at Stellenbosch University Medical School the writers believe that, in the CNS, the commonest type of necrosis is not caseous, but in fact gummatous, where inflammatory granulation tissue (together with all components of the infiltrate) undergoes ischaemic necrosis (Figure 3.4), usually in successive waves, as the lesion enlarges, identified macroscopically in the fixed specimen, on account of its firm texture and distinctly lamellated appearance (Figure 3.5). In caseation, by contrast, a purely cellular infiltrate consisting predominantly of macrophages and varying numbers of neutrophils, and lacking any fibrovascular stroma (Figure 3.6), undergoes necrosis which varies in consistency, being sometimes inspissated or caseous, and sometimes frankly liquefied or 'purulent' (Figure 3.7). As a rule the two processes (which may also be mixed) are indistinguishable macroscopically, as well as microscopically, using the HE method, and can only be reliably differentiated with the reticulin stain (Figure 3.4). Beside the obvious immunological and possible therapeutic implications, the significance of understanding these distinct necrotizing processes lies in their imaging attributes: gummatous necrosis is CT iso- or hyperdense, MR T1 isointense, T2 hypoin-

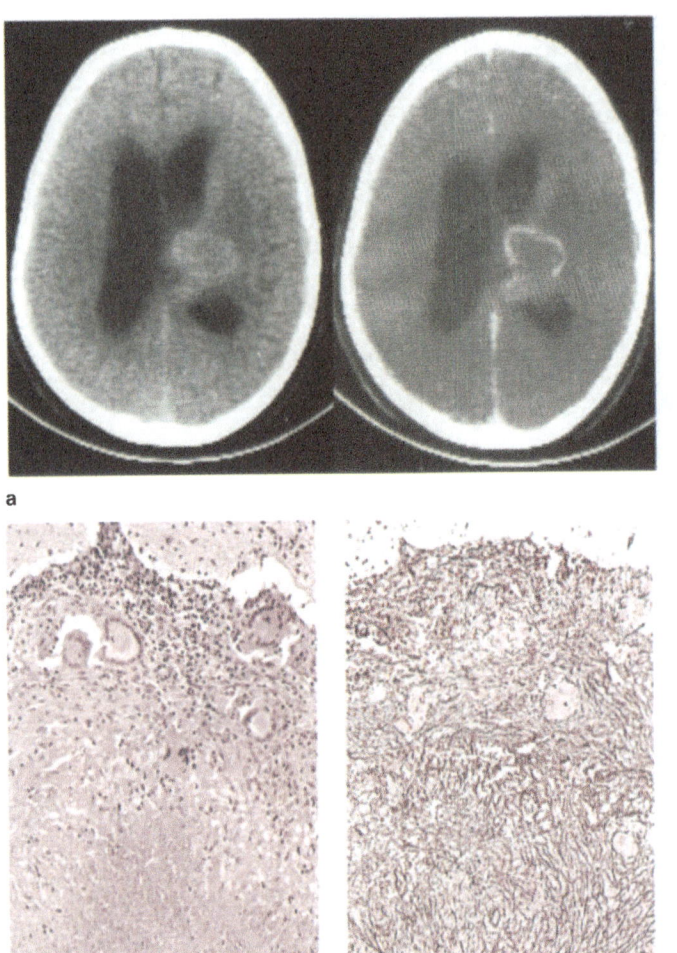

a

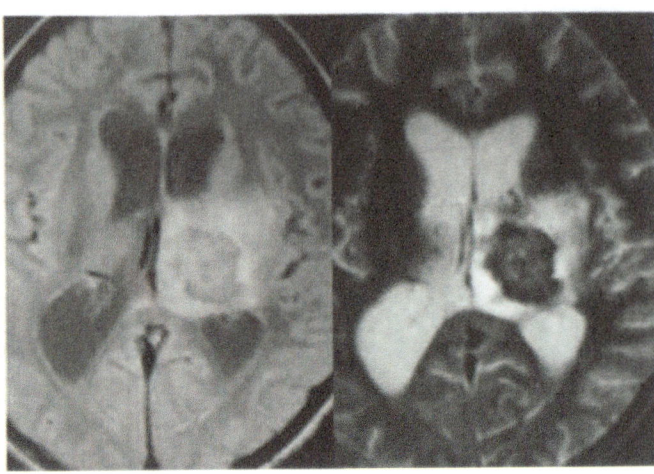

b

c   d

Figure 3.4 Gummatous necrosis/granuloma: (**a**) CT/CT + C, (**b**)
PDWI/T2WI, (**c**) HE ×200, (**d**) Retic ×200; lesion is brain isodense
(a, left), with peripheral (ring) enhancement (a, right); corresponding
T2 weighted MR images show the wall of the granuloma to be relatively
hypointense (white-matter isointense), with slightly brighter, lamellated
contents. Surrounding parenchymal hyperintensity is vasogenic oedema.
Comparative sections (c,d), illustrate gummatous necrosis; the vascular/
proliferative reticulin component is identifiable only following silver
staining (d)

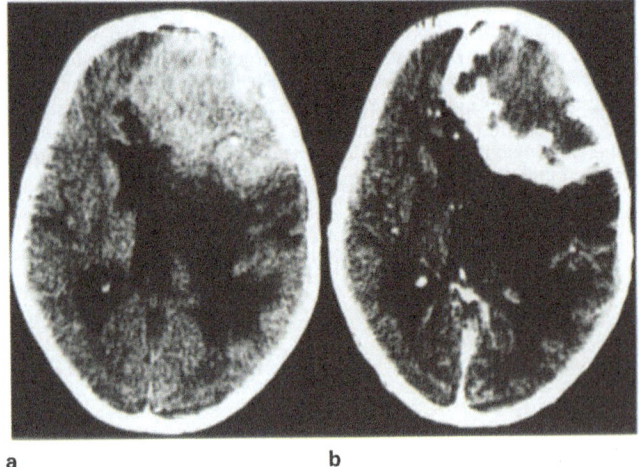

a   b

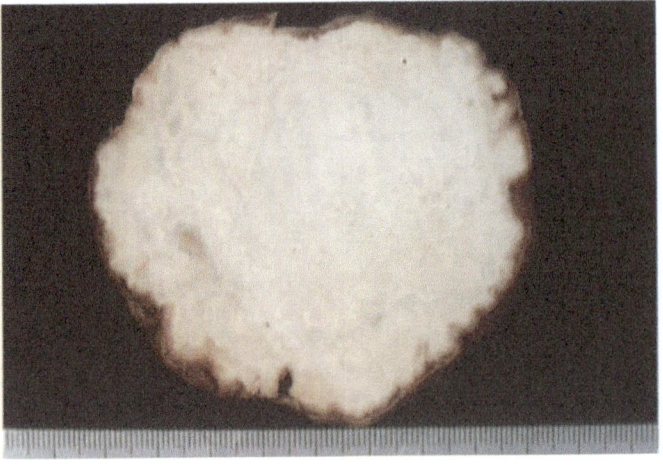

c

Figure 3.5 Gummatous granuloma: male 10 years; progressive
monoparesis and aphasia; (**a,b**) CT + C, (**c**) fixed specimen; images
show a large hyperdense meningocerebral mass, with a thick irregular/
lobulated enhancing wall and associated parenchymal hypodense
alteration; surgical specimen was exceptionally firm, with adherent meninges (arrow); cut surface shows characteristic blend of pale and
opalescent tissues having a whorled appearance. Histology showed
predominantly gummatous necrosis (see Figure 3.4), with focal caseation.
Mineralization was not apparent and all special stains were negative

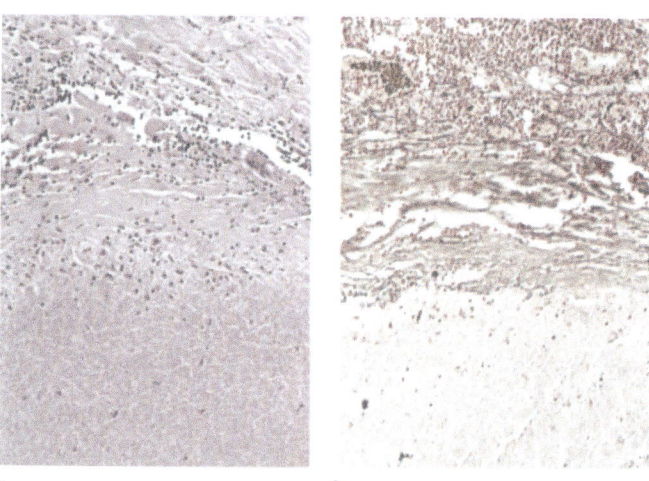

a   b

Figure 3.6 Caseous necrosis: (**a**) HE ×200, (**b**) reticulin ×200; comparative sections showing reticulin confined to capsule and absent from within the necrotic tissue

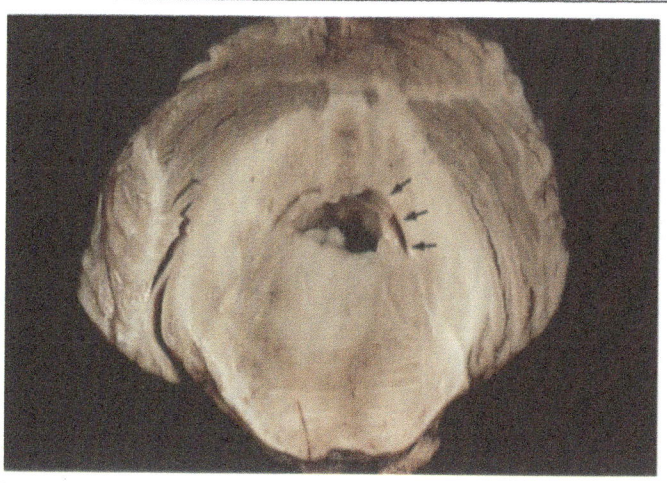

a

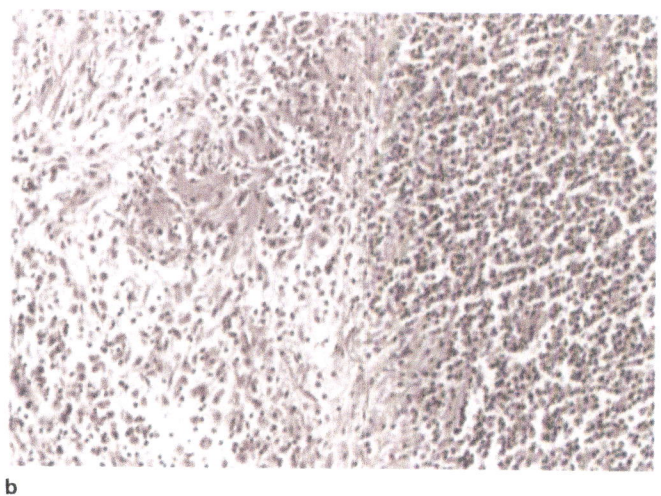

b

Figure 3.7 Tuberculous abscess, pontine/ventricular: male, 1 year, treated TBM; (**a**) autopsy specimen showing abscess with poorly defined capsule, with purulent contents, artefactually cavitated – the

4th ventricle (arrows) is effaced; (**b**) section showing granulomatous inflammation with 'pyogenic' component. HE ×400

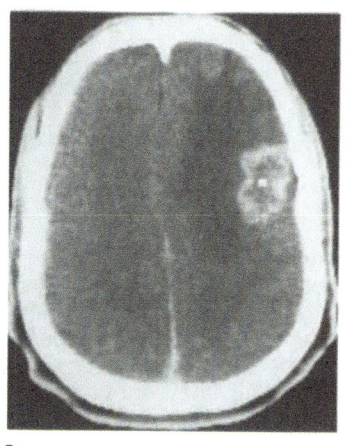

a

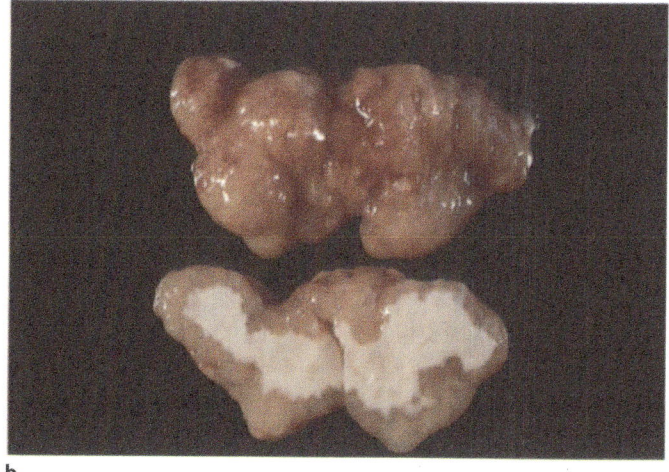

b

Figure 3.8 Gummatous granuloma: male 30 years; headache and seizures. (**a**) CT + C, (**b**) fixed specimen; image shows superficial convexity, irregularly shaped ring enhancing lesion with brain isodense contents and associated white-matter oedema. Lesion was invisible

before contrast. Excised specimen exhibits marked lobulation with a periphery of thick granulation tissue and creamy homogeneous contents, suggestive of classical caseation. Histology showed gummatous necrosis (see **Figure 3.4**). Special stains negative

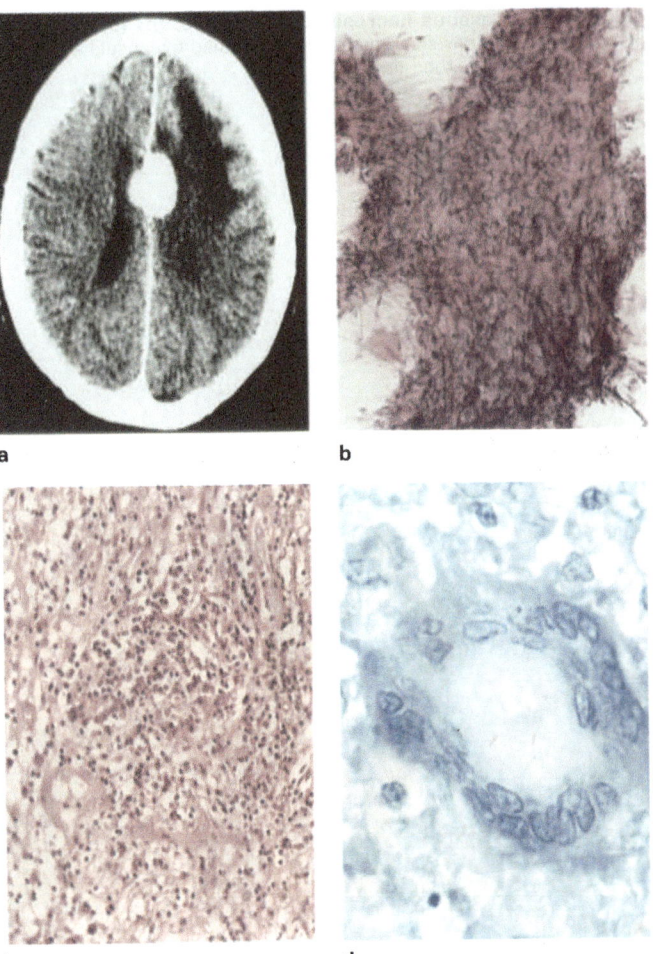

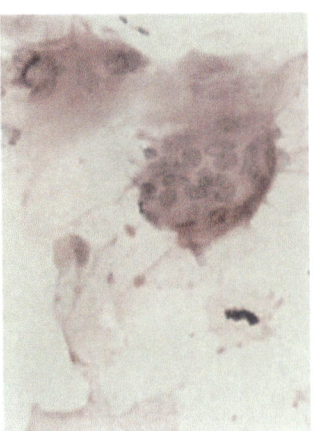

Figure 3.9   Proliferative meningocerebral granuloma (type IIIa): 52-year-old presenting with headache and seizures; (**a**) CT + C, (**b**) HE ×200/×400, (**c**) HE ×200, (**d**) Zn ×100; CT shows a circumscribed strongly diffusely enhancing parafalcine mass with adjacent vasogenic oedema. Radiological diagnosis was meningioma. Smear (b) shows typical untidy cellular fibrous tissue with isolated clearly defined multinucleate cells. Histology (c) shows non-necrotizing, proliferative granulomata with multinucleate giant and epithelioid cells; positive Zn (d) is unusual

tense, whilst caseous necrosis is CT hypo- or isodense, MR T1 iso- or hypointenase, T2 hyperintense – in other words identical to abscess. In an important variant referred to below as *proliferative granuloma*, necrosis of granulation tissue tends to remain microscopically focal, with a gross preponderance of viable, inflammatory vascular tissue, epithelioid cells and considerable interspersed collagen (Figure 3.9). When large numbers of organisms such as cryptococci or parasitic debris become sandwiched or layered between proliferative, non-necrotizing granulomatous tissue, another variety of granuloma forms, which we have called the *atypical/complex* type (Figures 3.16 and 4.15). Because the pathomorphology of these different forms of granuloma often correlates well with both CT and MR images of proven cases, a classification of CNS granulomatous disease is proposed, based on a combination of imaging and pathological features.

Type I: Gummatous granuloma
Presumed tuberculous (Figures 3.4, 3.5, 3.8 and 4.16) in most cases; 20–60 mm: meningocerebral and pachymeningeal lesions are largest, and irregular in outline; deeper lesions are rounded. CT hyperdense/isodense; ring enhancing, crenated or nodular wall; may show central calcification (target sign). MR T1 isointense–T2 hypo/isointense wall, contents mainly T2 white matter isointense, with hyperintense lamellae. (Pathological correlate: granuloma with central gummatous necrosis.)

Type II: Caseating/liquefying granuloma (pseudo-abscess)[28] and **granulomatous abscess** (tuberculous abscess[29,30], atypical abscess)
Parasitic or fungal (Figures 4.11, 4.12 and 4.13), rarely tuberculous (Figure 6.12); 10–50 mm: CT hypodense; ring enhancing; smooth wall. MR T1 isointense; T2 isointense wall, T2 hyperintense contents. (Pathological correlate: granuloma with caseous/liquefactive necrosis.)

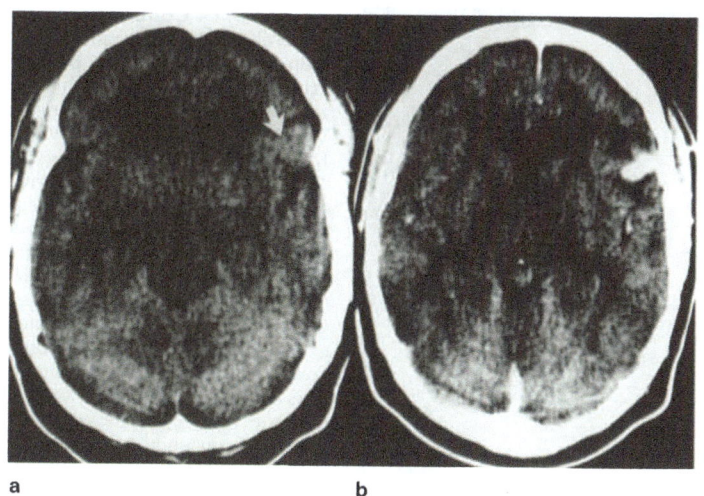
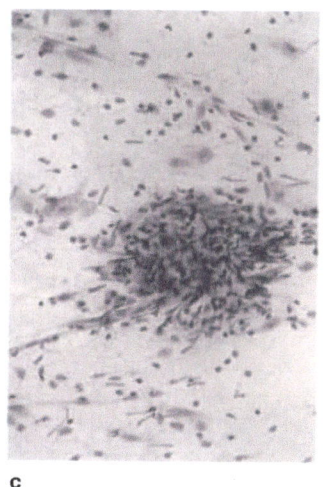
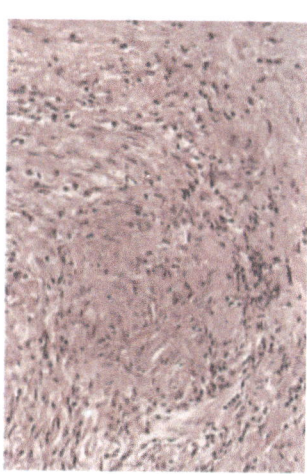

a   b   c

Figure 3.10 Proliferative meningocerebral granuloma, sarcoid: (**a**) CT, (**b**) CT + C, (**c**) Tol. blue/HE ×200; male 37 years; known pulmonary sarcoidosis, previously treated; images show cerebromeningeal, brain isodense, diffusely enhancing mass in the Sylvian fissure (a, arrow). Smear preparation (c, left) and paraffin section (c, right) shows non-necrotizing epithelioid granulomata. Lesion is not typical of neurosarcoidosis, but responded to treatment

Type IIIa: Proliferative meningocerebral granuloma

Usually tuberculous (Figure 3.9) or fungal[31], rarely luetic (Figure 7.19) or sarcoid (Figure 3.10); 10–20 mm: lesions are usually superficial (occasionally intraparenchymal), therefore lobulated or elongated. CT isodense; diffusely enhancing. MR T1 isointense–T2 grey matter isointense. (Pathological correlate: non-necrotizing epithelioid granulomatous inflammation; meningoparenchymal.)

Type IIIb: Proliferative pachymeningeal granulomatosis (also called hypertrophic pachymeningitis, sclerosing tuberculomatosis[20], tuberculoma en plaque)[32]. Various aetiologies (Figures 3.11, 3.12 and 3.13). CT iso/hyperdense; diffusely enhancing, MR T1 isointense/T2 hypointense. (Pathological correlate: non-necrotizing granulomatous inflammation; pachymeningeal.)

Type IV: Atypical/complex granuloma

Parasitic (Figure 3.16), fungal (Figure 4.15), or tuberculous; 10–50 mm: CT hyper/isodense; ring-like/linear, targetoid enhancement. MR T1 hypo/isointense-T2 inhomogeneous. (Pathological correlate: solid granulomatous inflammation admixed with necrosis, organism aggregates or debris (e.g. mycetoma, cryptococcoma, hydatidoma.)

Type V: Granulomatous cyst (also called complex cyst)

Parasitic; 40–70 mm (Figure 4.7): CT hypodense; thin rim enhancement. MR T1 hypointense–T2 hyperintense; separate T2 hypointense rim may be seen; may contain a smaller cyst(s) with different T2 hyperintensity. (Pathological correlate: parasitic cyst with peripheral granulomatous inflammation.)

In southern Africa at any rate, clinical evidence, therapeutic response and serial scanning show that the majority of gummata are tuberculous, and for this reason the same aetiology is inferred in surgical specimens where no organisms can usually be demonstrated; conversely, the majority of granulomatous abscesses have been shown to be fungal (Figures 4.11, 4.12 and 4.13) or parasitic, whilst cases of pachymeningeal proliferative granulomata show an even spread of specific and autoimmune aetiologies with a racial bias.

3.2a. Tuberculous gumma and abscess

We are aware, both from our clinical colleagues and from the current literature, that these terms or concepts are not generally accepted, and in a recent review of CNS tuberculosis[33] no mention is made of either gumma or abscess. Besides the implications of immunopathogenesis, experience in Cape Town is that both types of lesion may require surgical treatment under appropriate circumstances. The features which distinguish gummatous and caseous necrosis histopathologically and on the images, are summarized and illustrated above.

Gummatous tuberculoma qualifying for resection is meningocerebral, large and accessible (Figures 3.5, 3.8 and 4.16). The typically pale, hard and lamellated cut surface accurately reflects tissue which is dead, low in water content and incapable of enhancement. In other instances, probably to do with lesion age, the necrotic tissue, although T1 isointense/T2 hyperintense, has the colour and consistency of caseous necrosis, whilst the enhancing capsule may contain sizeable proliferative granulomata. Resolution of the gumma, as shown by serial scanning, is marked by the conversion of the contents to moderate, homogeneous T2 hyperintensity. This process, inferred from the examination of autopsy material, correlates histologically with loss of morphological detail (increasing eosinophilia), and presumably an increasing ratio of unbound water.

Tuberculous abscess: caseating tuberculoma may have contents varying in consistency from fluid to inspissated, depending on interrelated immunological factors in which polymorphonuclear cell infiltration appears to play a significant part. A tuberculoma containing liquid cell debris has all the macroscopic and imaging characteristics of an abscess[34], and when sufficiently large it is likely to benefit from initial drainage (Figure 6.12); satellite enhancing nodules are a clue to granulomatous aetiology. It has to be emphasized, however, that in most instances tuberculous abscesses are small (order of 8–20 mm), being diagnosed either on the images (where they are morphologically indistinguishable from solitary, small parasitic granulomatous abscesses (section 3.3 and Figure 3.17), or at postmortem. Doubtless these lesions will become commoner against the background of HIV infection.

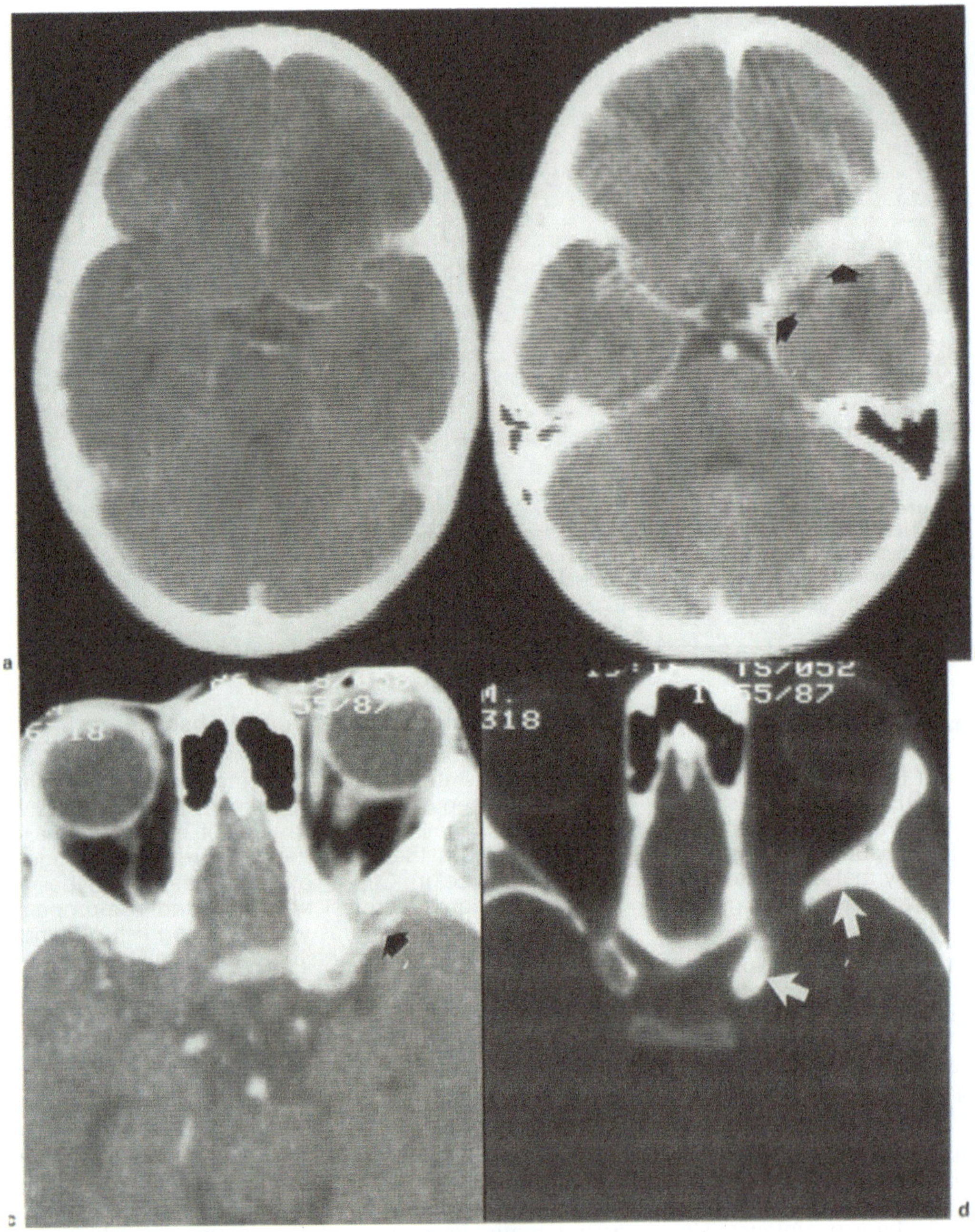

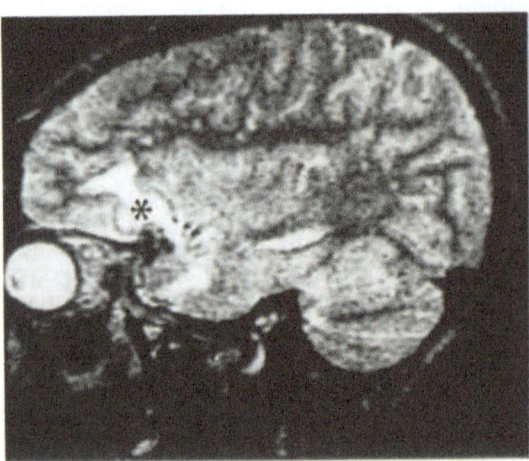
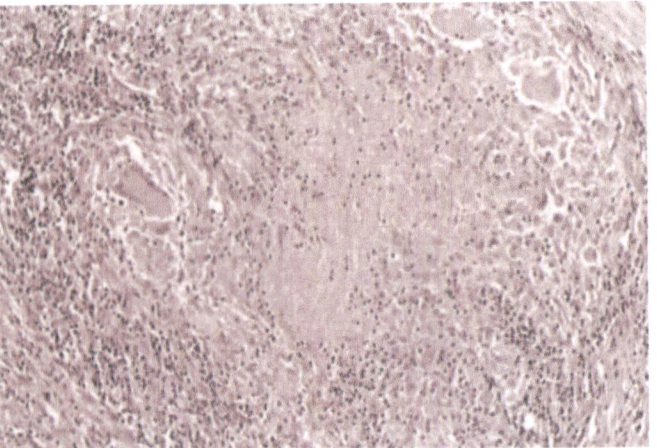

Figure 3.11 Combined meningocerebral (type IIIa) and pachymeningeal (type IIIb) proliferative granulomatosis: male, 6 years, presenting with proptosis; (**a**) CT, (**b,c**) CT + C, (**d**) CTBW, (**e**) T2WI, (**f**) HE × 200; CT shows patchy enhancement in the left Sylvian cistern (b, arrows), extending from the region of the terminal internal carotid to the lateral part of the great sphenoid wing, with adjacent parenchymal hypodensity (vasogenic oedema). The granuloma (c, arrow) extends through the superior orbital fissure, with surrounding hyperostosis (d, arrows; compare with the opposite side). MR shows a mass (asterisk) extending above the hyperostotic bone, with a brain isointense wall and T2 hyperintense contents. Biopsy of sphenoid dura shows multiple epithelioid granulomata, with occasional foci of caseous necrosis (presumably responsible for T2 hyperintensity), and scattered multinucleate cells. Cervical lymph node biopsy AFB positive. Intracranial lesion resolved completely on antituberculous therapy

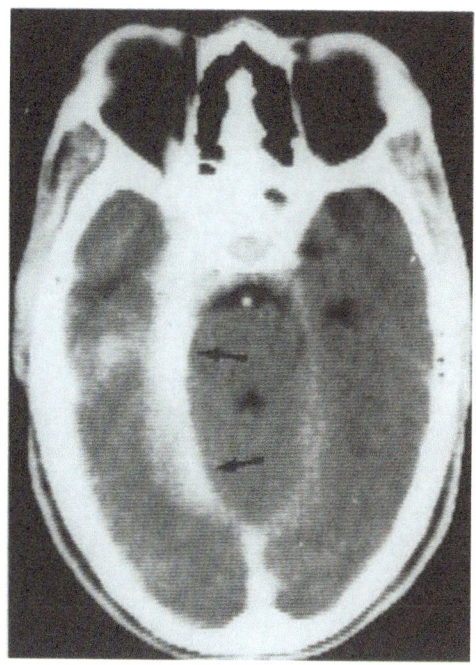

a

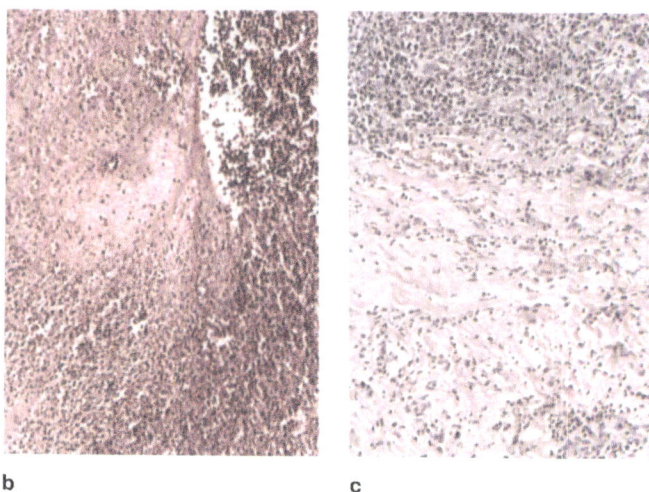

b c

Figure 3.12 Proliferative pachymeningeal granulomatosis: male, 30 years; 10-month history of delirium, blindness and proptosis of left eye. CSF culture negative, but there was a history of having been treated for syphilis 1 year previously; (**a**) CT + C, (**b**) HE ×200, (**c**) HE ×200; contrasted CT shows diffuse enhancement along the edge of the cerebellar tent, extending anteriorly to the dorsum sellae. The abnormality is bilateral but very much worse on the left. The histology shows non-specific subacute inflammation and vascularized fibrous tissue (c), with areas of acute inflammation showing degeneration and necrosis of exudate (b)

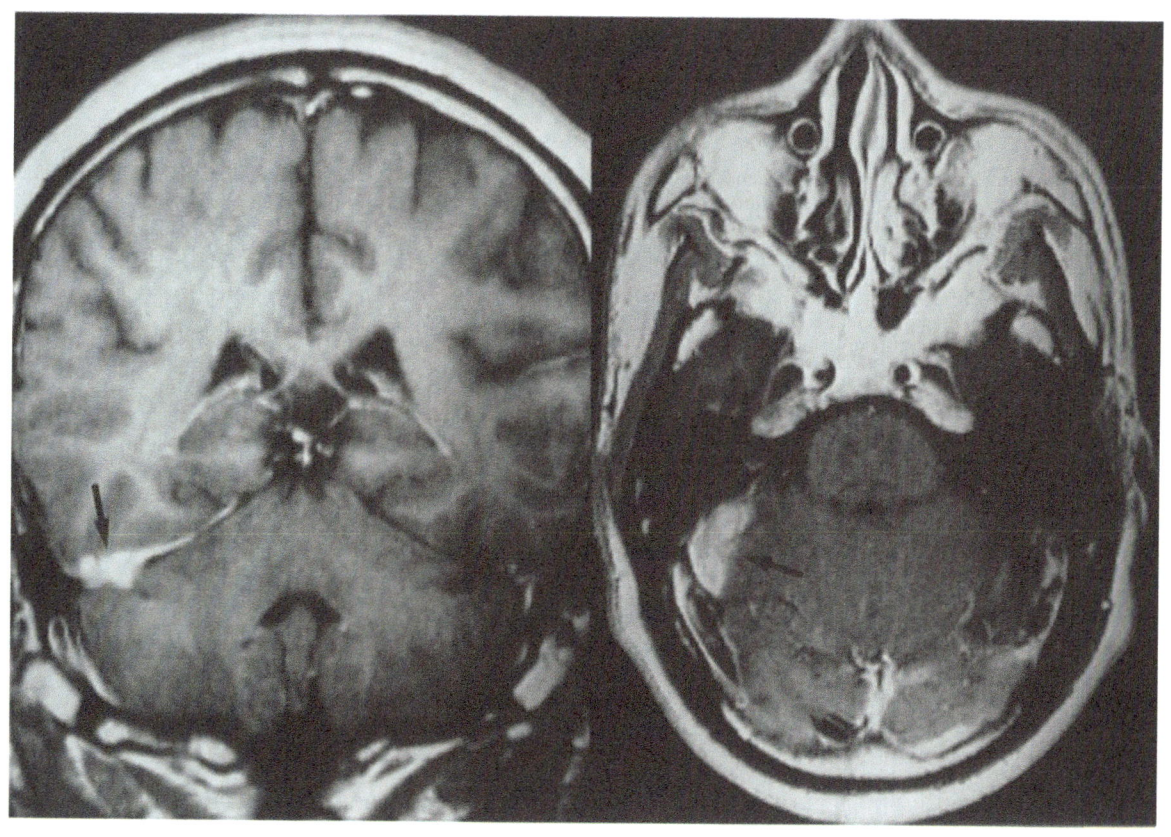

a b

Figure 3.13 Hypertrophic pachymeningitis, tentorium:male, 25 years; chronic headache with more recent painful third-nerve paresis. CSF and serology negative, but history of pulmonary tuberculosis; (**a**) coronal T1WI + C, (**b**) axial T1WI + C; images show slightly lobulated, diffusely enhancing mass involving the tentorium unilaterally (arrows). No abnormality of the cavernous sinus was shown. Resolution on steroids and antituberculous therapy

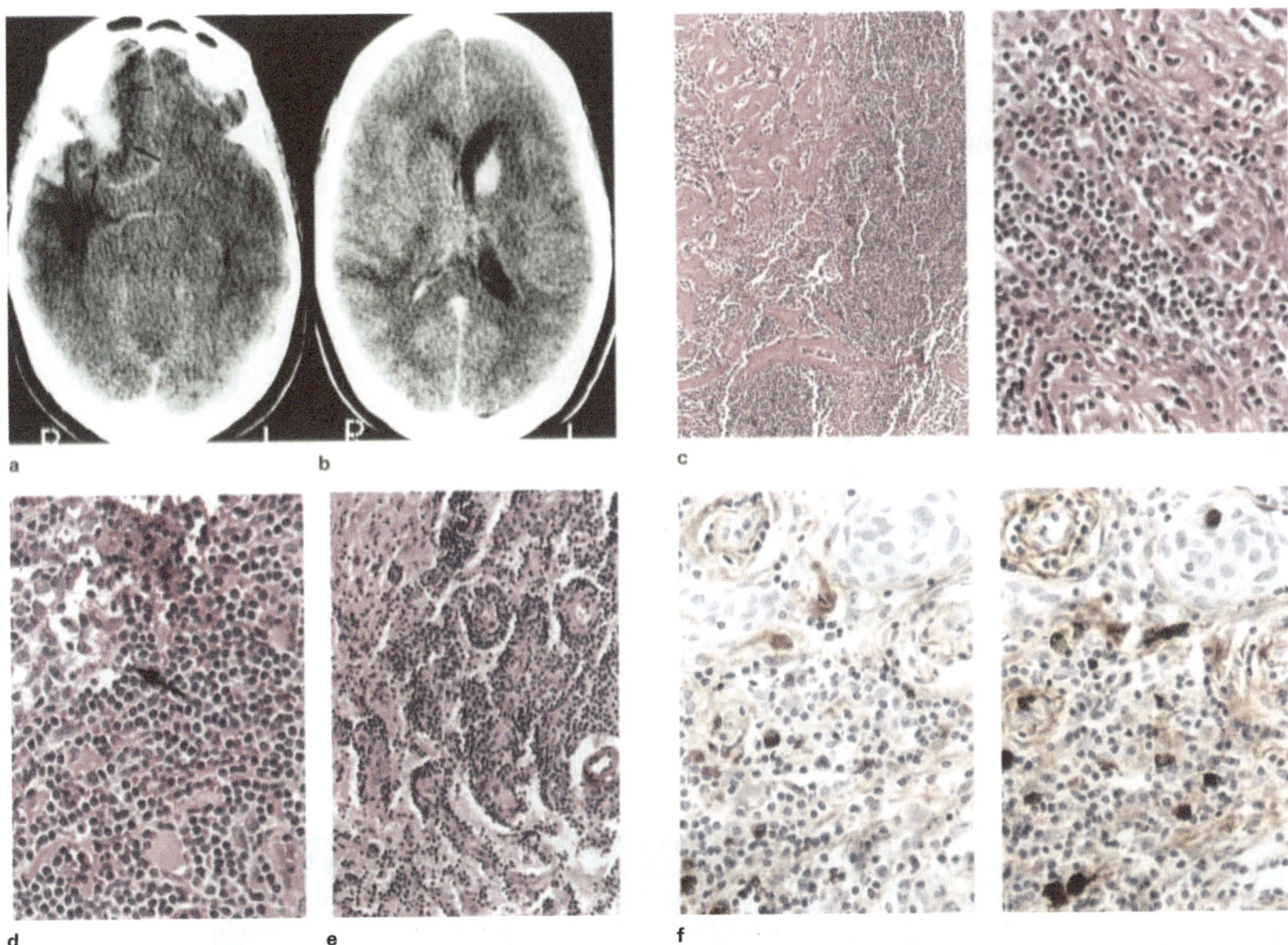

Figure 3.14 Plasma cell granuloma: female, 30 years; headache and progressive visual disturbance of approximately 11 months duration. (**a,b**) CT + C, (**c**) HE ×100/×200, (**d**) HE ×400, (**e**) HE ×200, (**f**) anti-kappa/lambda ×400; CT shows a frontotemporal poorly defined, enhancing meningocerebral lesion (a, arrows); cavernous sinus and orbit apex apparently uninvolved; separate diffusely enhancing mass in the L caudate head (b). Lesions remained unchanged over the 11-month period. At surgery abnormal, rubbery tissue found infiltrating bone, dura and brain (e). Histology shows florid sclerosing, vascular proliferative process (c), with a largely mononuclear, polyclonal (f) inflammatory infiltrate consisting predominantly of B lymphocytes and mature plasma cells, with poorly formed germinal centres (d, arrow), and a minority of T lymphocytes, macrophages and eosinophils. Note perivascular extension into adjacent brain parenchyma (e). Patient well 30 months later

3.2b. Hypertrophic pachymeningitis

Originally coined to describe a form of hyperplastic gummatous meningitis affecting the spine[35], this term has recently been adopted by neuroimagers and implies an expansile, diffusely enhancing, idiopathic inflammatory process affecting the cranial dura, and the tent in particular[36]. At surgery the abnormal tissue presents as a tough greyish-yellow membrane, grossly thickened. Microscopy reveals an admixture of dense collagenous fibrosis and granulation tissue, with a variable inflammatory cell infiltrate of lymphocytes, plasma cells, eosinophils and neutrophils, and sometimes epithelioid cells. Foci of necrosis may be present, either angiocentric, or gummatous (Figure 3.12). As may be expected, such sclerosing inflammation is T1 soft tissue isointense, T2 hypointense, and therefore only visualized with contrast (Figure 3.13). Although non-specific, both the pathological and imaging features are common to the idiopathic varieties of Tolosa–Hunt syndrome[37], and spinal pachymeningitis[38] (see section 7.3a) so that a pathoanatomical spectrum becomes readily apparent. The material collected by us in Cape Town also serves to emphasize the fact that, in the African context, hypertrophic cranial pachymeningitis continues to have diverse, sometimes specific aetiologies, of which tuberculosis remains the most important.

3.2c. Plasma cell granuloma

Intracranial[39] and spinal[40] plasma cell granuloma is rare, compared with occurrence in the lung and abdominal viscera. Lesions are usually meningocerebral, having intermediate density and signal intensity, with strong, diffuse enhancement and, when circumscribed, may be indistinguishable from meningioma and plasmacytoma. Microscopic differentiation from plasmacytoma is dependent on immunohistochemical demonstration of a polyclonal pattern (Figure 3.14). It may also resemble meningioma with conspicuous plasma cell–lymphocytic components[41].

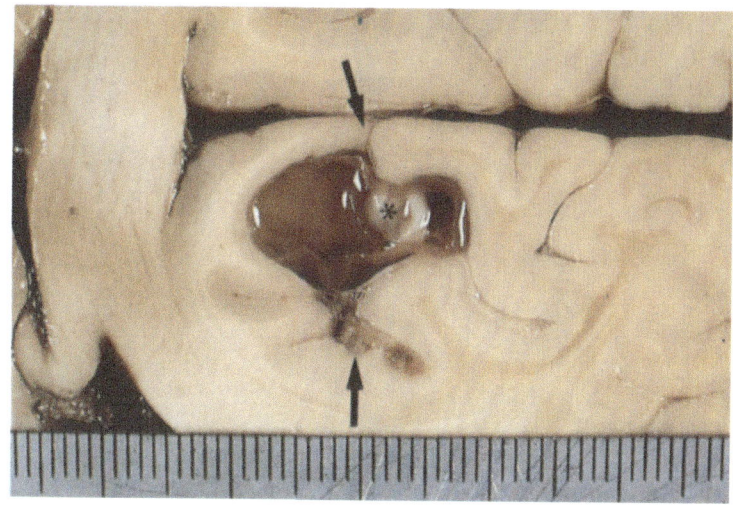

Figure 3.15 Cysticercosis, granulomatous cyst: bladder (germinal tissue) with dead, oedematous protoscolex (asterisk) lies within a sulcus which is sequestrated on account of early granulomatous inflammation (arrows)

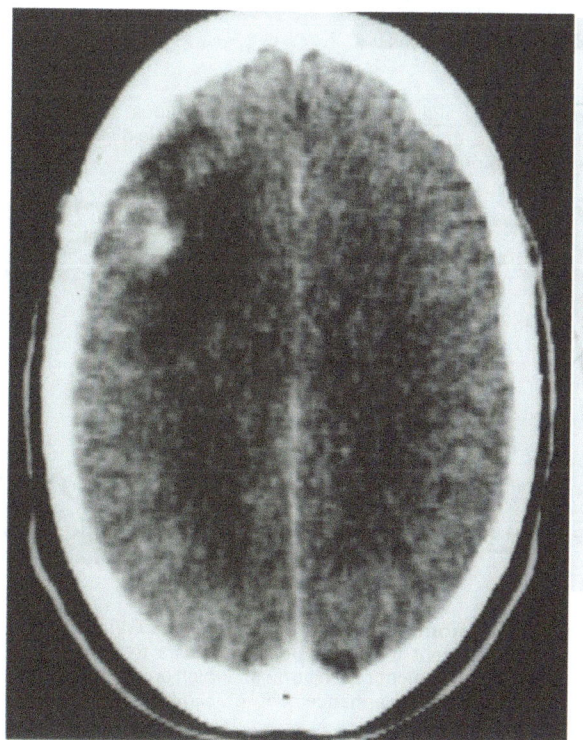

a

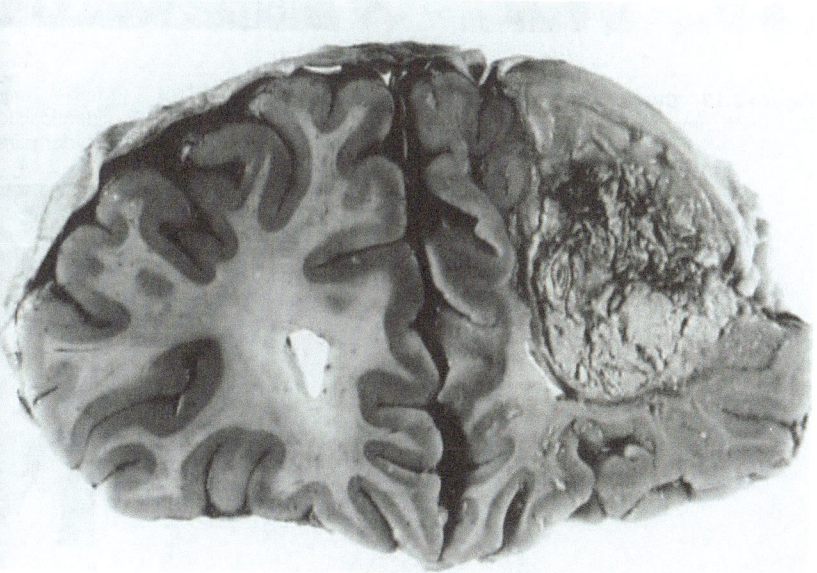

b

Figure 3.16 Hydatidosis, complex granuloma: (a) CT + C, (b) fixed brain slice; contrasted CT shows small ring lesion with brain isodense contents and solid diffusely enhancing component. Lesion in autopsy specimen (b), from another case illustrates the collapsed folded cyst wall with intervening amorphous and partly mineralized debris responsible for imaging characteristics

3.3. PARASITES

The imaging appearances of the major cystic metacestodes have been recently reviewed[42], and our correlative approach to the categorization of parasitic and other granulomata is presented and illustrated in section 3.2.

Apart from the occasional biopsy identification of granulomatous masses (of great neuropathological importance), neurosurgical intervention in craniospinal parasitic disease is aimed at the eradication of hydatid cysts in any location[43], and the removal of *Cysticercus* cysts giving rise to gross mass effect or acute intraventricular obstruction (section 4.3). Our experience with fixed brain material convinces us that the majority of parasitic lesions develop in the meninges (Figure 3.15) and superficial parenchyma, even though they may appear to be completely intraparenchymal on the images[23]. Cestode hexacanth larvae[44] have

a diameter of 30–50 µm, and must therefore arrest in the widest component of the arteriolar bed of grey matter, and the fact that many metacestodes are clearly extraparenchymal means that the meninges must also include a proportion of small vessels. As superficially placed bladders enlarge by means of parenchymal dissection, even in the case of very large hydatids a component of the cyst wall usually remains visible on the surface of the brain (Figure 4.7). With the onset of granulomatous inflammation the neural tissue interface is damaged (inflamed) and oedematous, emphasizing the apparent intraparenchymal imaging features. *Complex* hydatid granuloma owes its irregular appearance to isodense, folded contraction of the dead, lamellated cyst, with an intense giant cell response and early mineralization (Figure 3.16).

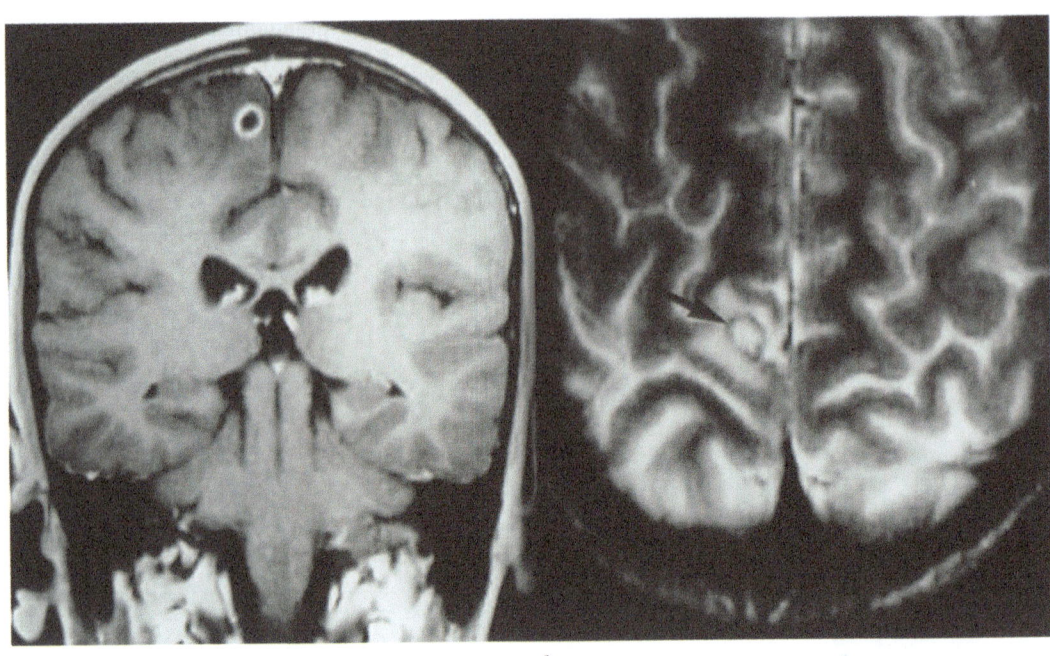

Figure 3.17 *Cysticercus* **granulomatous abscess**: (**a**) T1WI + C, (**b**) T2WI; images show a solitary ring-enhancing lesion with T1 hypointense/T2 hyperintense contents. The wall is relatively T2 hypoin- tense. Imaging features are non-specific and tuberculous abscess is identical; location, size, unifocality and absence of systemic disturbance favour parasitic aetiology

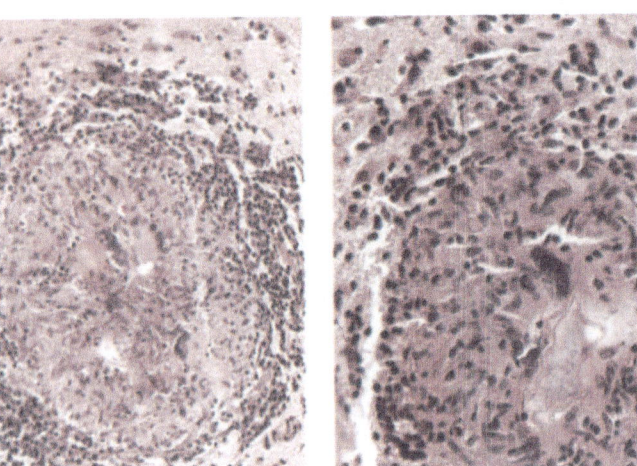

Figure 3.18 **Schistosomiasis**: numerous non-necrotizing micro-granulomata with parasitic remnants. HE × 100/ × 200

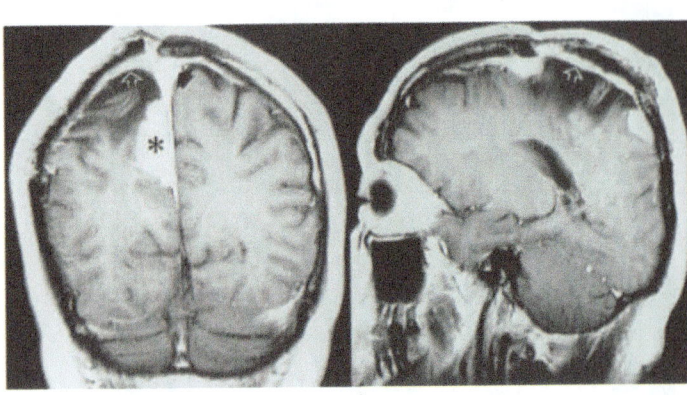

Figure 3.19 **Meningioma, recurrent**: (**a**) coronal T1WI + C, (**b**) sagittal T1WI + C; recurrent tumour (asterisk) appears to be distinct from thick epidural enhancement (open arrows), which could be entirely reactive. Note homogeneous enhancement of sagittal sinus (solid arrow), consistent with invasion

It must be emphasized that the preceding account excludes those small, non-specific ring-enhancing lesions of cysticercosis (Figure 3.17), which are infrequently biopsied, and are morphologically identical to other varieties of similarly sized granulomatous abscess, presenting a perennial differential diagnostic problem, particularly when solitary (section 3.2a). Their contents, being composed of macrophage and germinal tissue debris, are inevitably hypodense, T2 hyperintense and distinguishable on that account from gummatous necrosis.

AIDS-related *toxoplasmosis* is widely quoted as the cause of multiple, ring-enhancing cerebral lesions[45], whose hypodense, T2 hyperintense centres are assumed to be necrotic. Although indistinguishable from atypical or granulomatous abscess on the images, these lesions are ring-enhancing infarcts, initiated by a thromboangiopathy[46]. Such pathogenesis would explain the target-like enhancing cores illustrated in Figure 4.14. *Amoebiasis* and *schistosomiasis* may give rise to focal, non-necrotiz-ing, brain isodense and isointense, meningocerebral pro-liferative granulomata[47] (Figure 3.18), diffuse, homo-geneous enhancement also being consistent with this morphology. *Paragonimiasis*, whose images are so far reported only from eastern Asia, presents the appearance of multiloculated, cerebromeningeal abscess resembling fungal abscess[42,48].

3.4. PRIMARY MENINGOCEREBRAL NEOPLASMS

The fundamental imaging and surgical question 'is the mass intra- or extra-axial?', arising whenever a part of the lesion is superficial, has its natural consequence in the pathological distinction between cerebromeningeal and meningocerebral lesions, on the basis of histology and immunohistochemistry[49]. The imaging features denoting an extraparenchymal origin are characterized best in

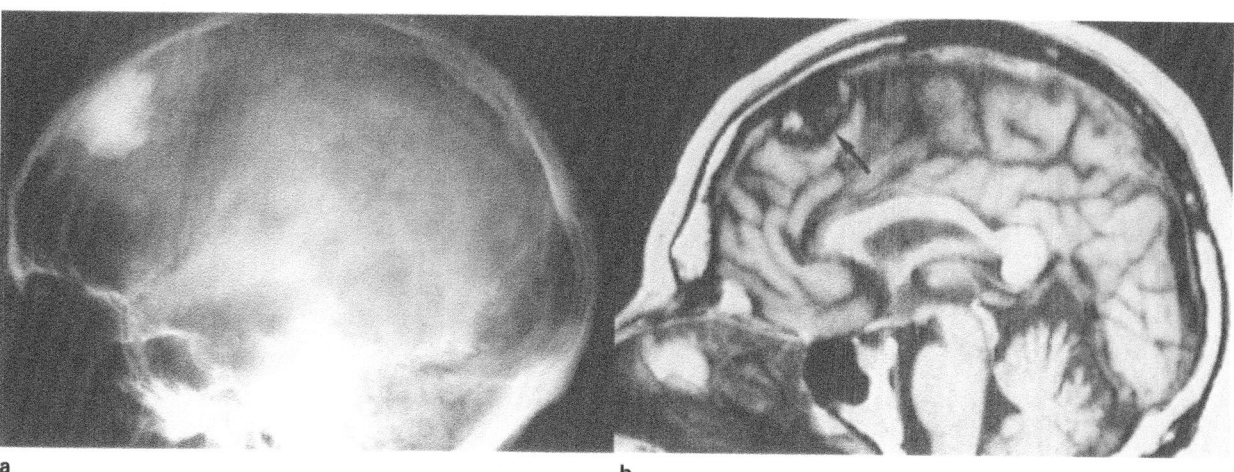

Figure 3.20 Meningioma, ossifying: (**a**) skull X-ray, (**b**) sagittal T1WI; heavily mineralized mass seen on plain film is inhomogeneous on T1W image (b, arrow), due to signal void of bone and intervening hyperintense marrow

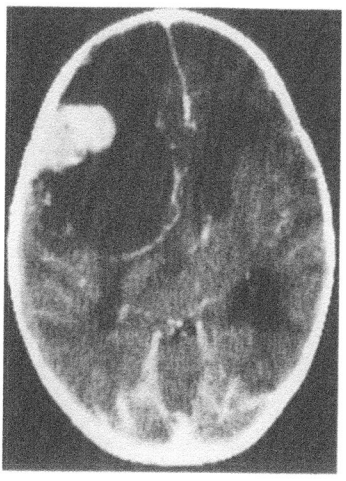

Figure 3.21 Meningioma, with brain cyst: contrasted CT shows a solid diffusely enhancing dural based mass separated from brain by a large cyst whose wall is partly enhancing. Nature of cyst wall enhancement is uncertain, but tumour has not recurred in spite of spinal metastases (see also **Figure 7.31**)

meningiomas, and include what the radiologists[50] have called a 'broad, dural-based margin' (Figures 3.19 and 6.16), a sharply defined tumour–brain interface (Figures 3.19 and 6.13) in which a fluid signal may be interposed, or the unmistakable presence of cerebral cortex encompassing the mass (Figure 3.20). Hyperostosis of the adjacent skull (Figure 5.29) is regarded as a diagnostic but uncommon sign of extracerebral neoplasia (see distinction from hyperostosing meningioma, section 2.6c). Not infrequently, these features (which are in any case strictly those of MR) may be absent or equivocal, or else they may occur in the context of a tumour cell type which is neither arachnoidal nor intrinsic to the brain parenchyma. Because of these and other inconsistencies, the term meningocerebral should be used in preference to extra-axial.

In a recently proposed modification of the WHO classification[51], primary meningeal neoplasms are divided into six categories, with the aim of more clearly defining their histological range, as well as improving clinico-radiologic correlation.

3.4a. Meningioma

Topographic localization constitutes one of the most characteristic features of meningioma, sites of most predilection including the sphenoid wing, falx and convexity, and clivus. A sharply circumscribed, extraparenchymal profile, and almost universal enhancement all combine to make an exceptionally firm imaging diagnosis. Even the peculiarities of en-plaque growth or associated brain cyst formation (Figure 3.21) are now considered characteristic in their own way (section 2.6c). It is therefore perplexing that little useful correlation exists between any clinical or imaging parameters, including biological behaviour, and the benign histological subtypes of meningioma; accounts of the microscopic diversity of these tumours remain entrenched in the literature, with meningotheliomatous, fibrous, transitional, psammomatous, angiomatous, microcystic[52], secretory[53], lipoblastic (vacuolated)[54], clear cell (glycogen rich), pseudoglandular[55], chordoid, lymphoplasmacytoid[56], and metaplastic types constituting the currently recognized variants. The main application of this descriptive subdivision lies in differentiating meningiomas from the numerous look-alikes.

Compared with the consistently iso- or mildly hyperdense, homogeneously enhancing lesions seen on CT (Figure 6.13), the MR appearances of meningiomas are much more varied, although generally conforming to the characteristics of tight-junction tissues (Figure 3.22) and therefore tending toward brain-isointensity at both short and long TR (Figure 3.23). The majority of tumours are T1 cortex isointense/white matter hypointense, T2 cortex iso- or hyperintense/white matter hyperintense. The principal factors responsible for heterogeneity are microcystic change (Figure 3.24), mineralization (Figure 3.20), fibrosis and the formation of wide-bore vessels. As with CT, strong enhancement is invariable in solid, non-mineralized tumours, reflecting dense angioarchitecture and vascular pooling (Figure 3.23). Multiple, prominent foci of signal void correlate with the large vascular spaces seen in some meningiomas (Figure 3.23), and are usually designated angioblastic on MR, though not always properly so histologically (see section 3.4d). Tumour morphology and signal intensity have been shown to exhibit some correlation in T2 weighted images, where cortical hypointensity is commonest with fibroblastic lesions, and hyperintensity with angioblastic and syncytial types[57]. A strongly and homogeneously T2 hyperintense tumour illustrated in Figure 6.14, is secretory in type, and similar signal characteristics may be expected of microcystic meningioma (Figure 3.24).

Whilst hyperostosis and sinus occlusion (Figure 3.19) are obvious indicators of dural invasion, microscopy remains the only reliable method of defining the extent of this form of growth in surgical specimens. Dural enhancement for a distance of 12–18 mm beyond the

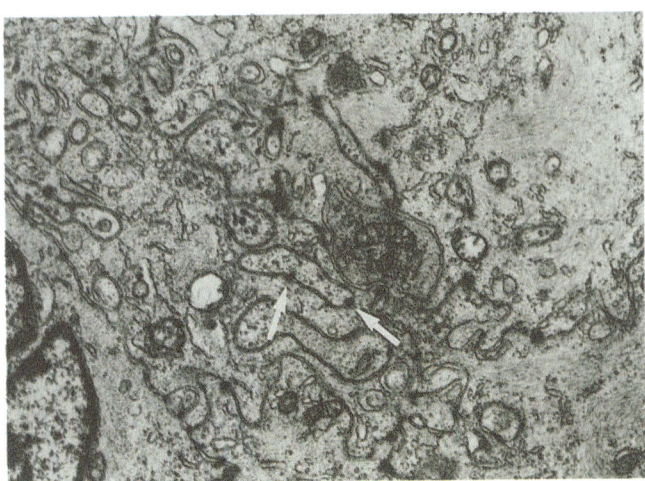

Figure 3.22 **Meningioma**: characteristic interdigitating processes and intercellular junctions (arrows), ultrastructural features assumed to be responsible for cortex and soft tissue isointensity on all sequences. EM ×10000

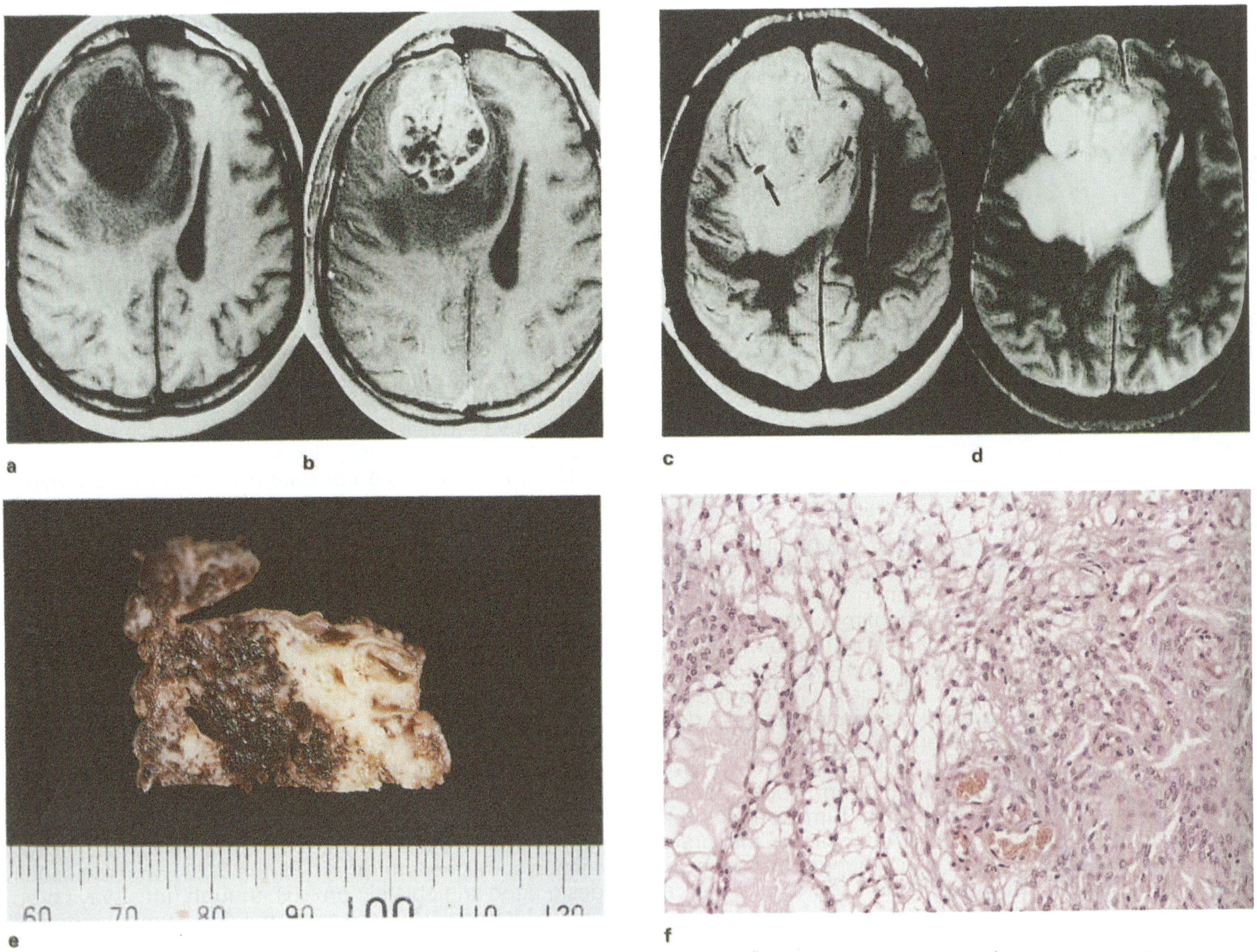

a   b   c   d

e   f

Figure 3.23 (*legend opposite*)

tumour margin – the 'dural tail' (Figures 3.25 and 6.16) has been suggested to be characteristic of meningioma[58], although not implying evidence of tumour invasion[59]; this feature, together with the extensive but non-specific enhancement of dura postoperatively, makes imaging assessment of local spread impossible (Figure 3.19). With the exception of inferred central necrosis (as opposed to cystic degeneration) there appear to be no imaging features which assist in predicting aggressive behaviour in a meningioma *ab initio*. The lack of a distinct brain–

tumour interface raises the possibility of parenchymal invasion, said to be an indication of potential 'malignant' behaviour in otherwise histologically benign tumours[60]. Usually, a tumour which exhibits microscopic features of malignancy including a papillary growth pattern (Figures 3.26 and 3.27), abundant mitotic activity, vascular invasion, etc., has no unusual features on the initial scan, and the prediction of biological malignancy can be made only on serial imaging. This is illustrated in Figure 3.26, where the neoplasm in the final stages of aggressive

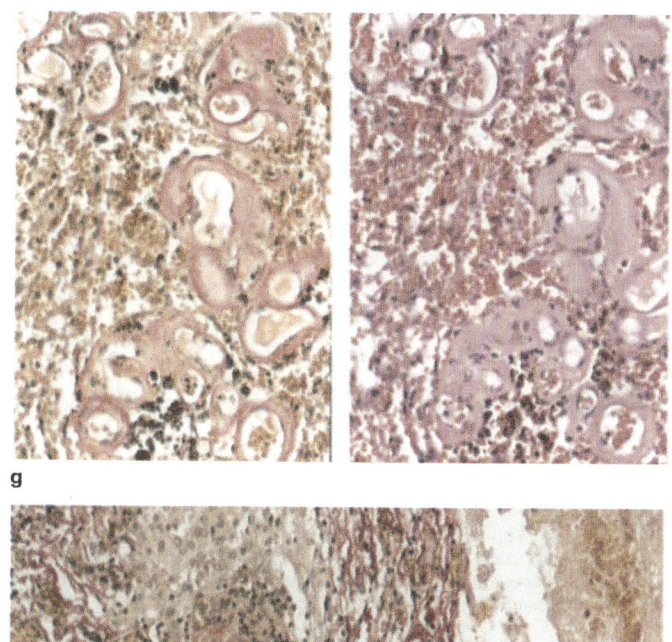

g

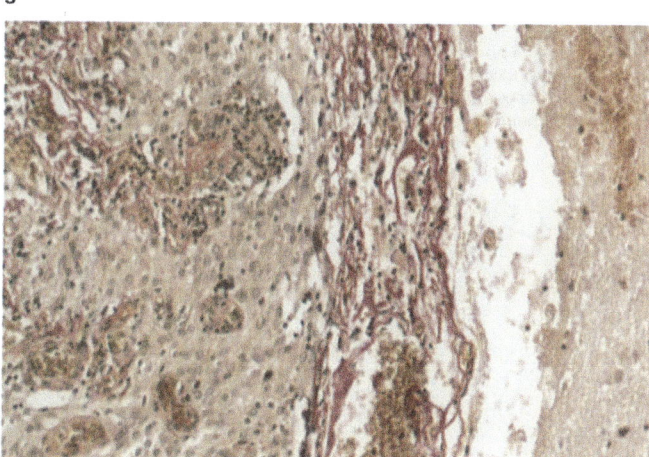

i

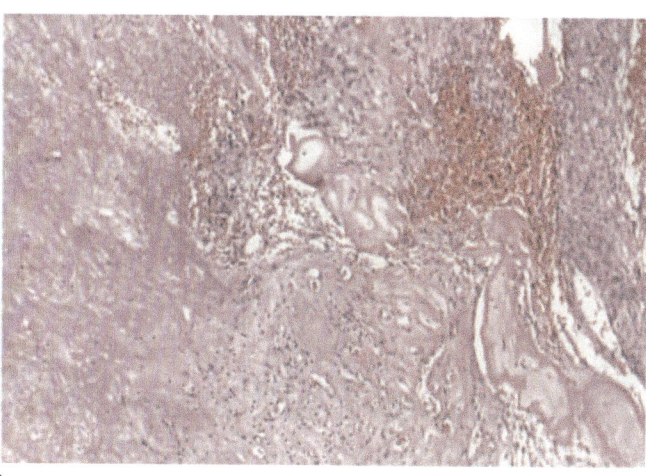

h

Figure 3.23 Meningioma, interhemispheric: (**a**) T1WI, (**b**) T1WI + C, (**c**) PDWI, (**d**) T2WI, (**e**) operative specimen, (**f**) HE × 200, (**g**) EVG/HE × 200, (**h**) HE × 100, (**i**) EVG × 200; lesion is unusually hypointense at short TR (a), mainly due to cystic degeneration which becomes apparent on enhanced T1 and T2W images (b,d). Cysts almost disappear on PDWI (c), presumably because of protein content. Note flow void evidence of large superficial and stromal vessels (c, arrows) and marked adjacent oedema. Cut surface of operative specimen confirms the presence of large vessels and cysts, the latter originating from confluent microcysts (f). Vascularity is consistent with enhancement but necrosis (h) was not predicted. Sharp tumour–brain interface shown microscopically in (i) is consistent with sharp post-contrast profile

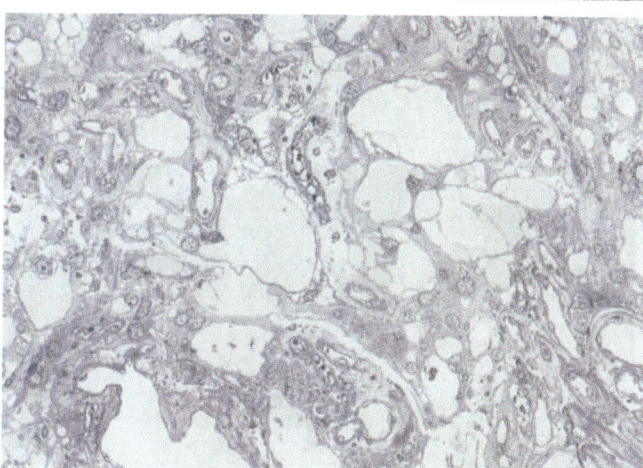

Figure 3.24 Meningioma, microcystic: epon section illustrating microcystic change, assumed to be responsible for T2 hyperintensity of some tumours. Tol blue × 200.

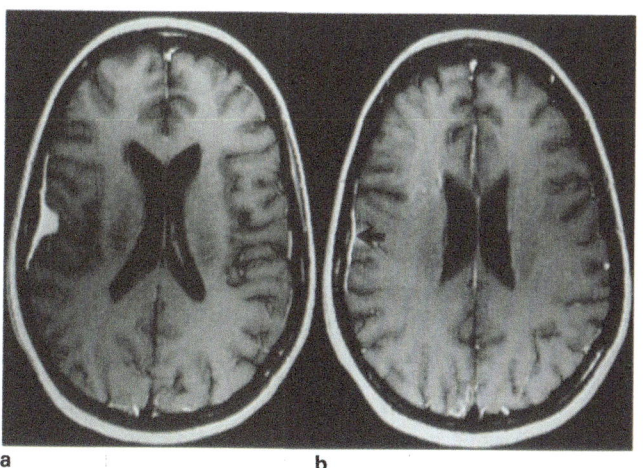

a　　　　　　　　　b

Figure 3.25 Meningioma, convexity, dural enhancement: (a,b) T1WI + C, (c) (*opposite*) HE × 100; images show a diffusely enhancing meningioma with extensive dural tail (arrow). Histology shows abrupt edge of tumour with prominent adjacent leptomeningeal proliferative alteration; vascular morphology suggests enhancement may be a reactive process akin to the subdural membrane.

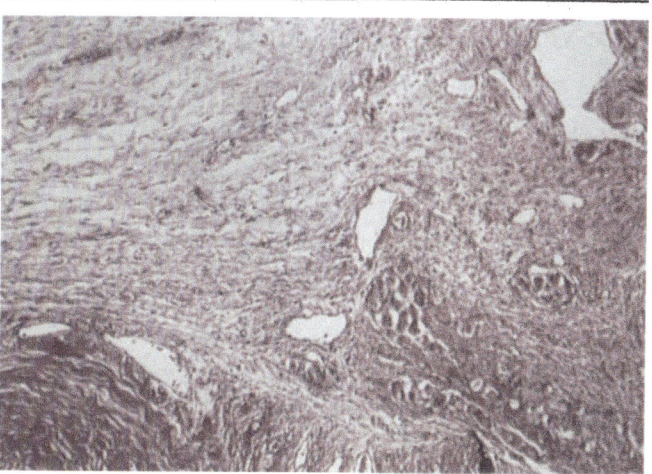

c

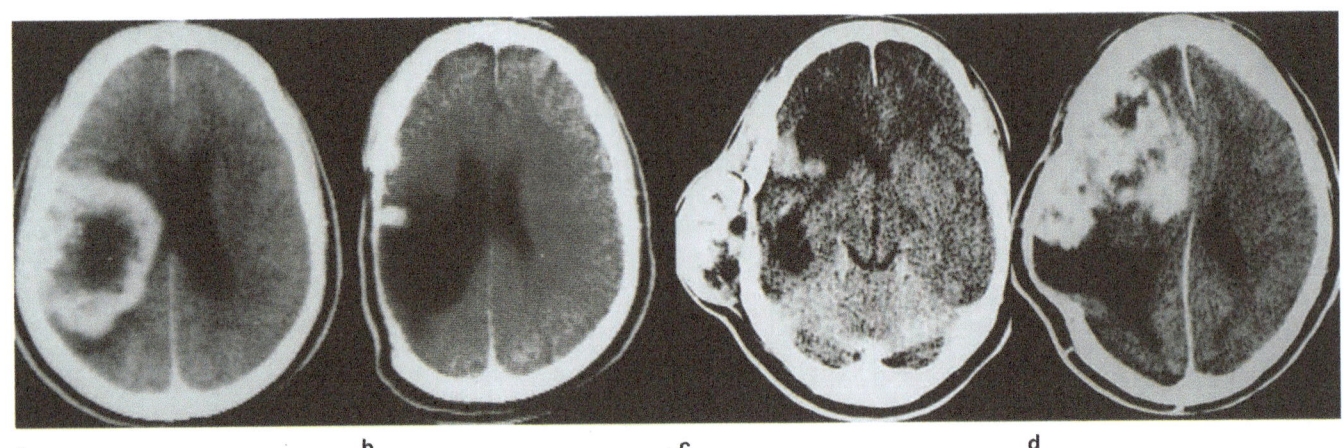

a   b   c   d

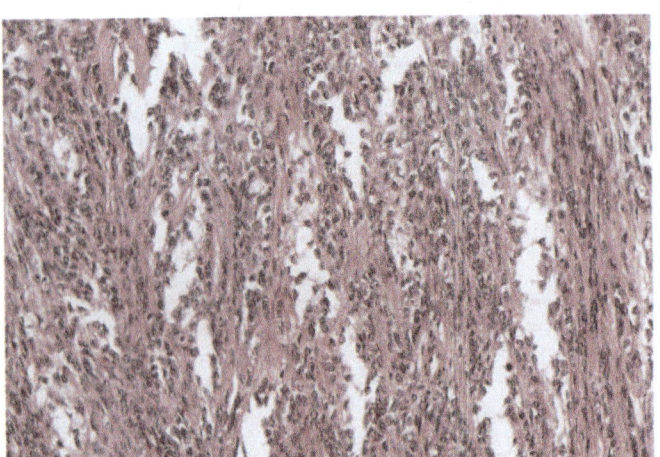

e

Figure 3.26 Meningioma, malignant: (**a–d**) CT + C, (**e**) HE ×200; initial image (a) shows enhancing tumour with central hypodensity. Follow-up study, 18 months later (b) shows two discrete enhancing nodules, progressing to massive intra–extracranial recurrence a further 6 months later (c,d). Morphology remained the same (e), including evidence of necrosis, in all biopsies

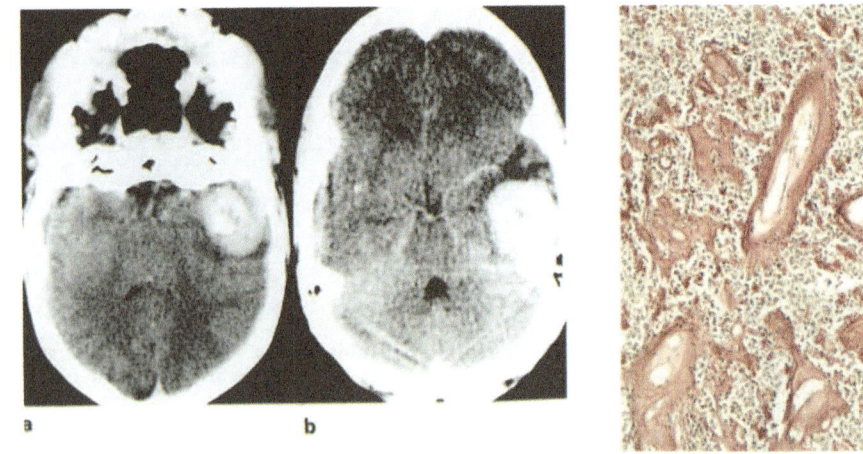

a   b

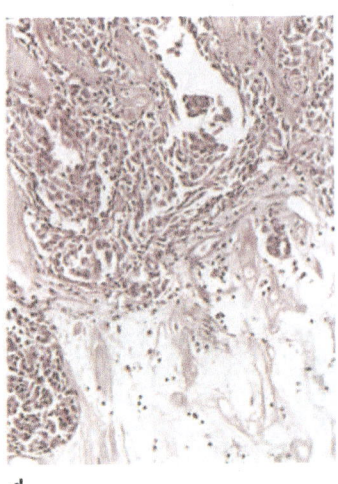

c   d

Figure 3.27 Meningioma, papillary, malignant: (**a**) CT, (**b**) CT + C, (**c**) VG ×100, (**d**) HE ×200; female, 26 years: images show the neoplasm to be hyperdense (a), as well as strongly enhancing (b), with central hypodensity and mineralization. Papillary morphology is associated with prominent sclerotic vasculature (c), presumably responsible for hyperdensity. Lucent part of tumour is due to degenerative change (d). Despite apparently total excision, tumour recurred after 10 months. (Histology reviewed by Prof. JJ Kepes, University Kansas)

recurrence still retains the usual signal characteristics, apart from central hypodensity.

3.4b. Hyperostosing meningioma

This entity, a lesion distinct from hyperostosis of the skull overlying a meningioma, is discussed and illustrated in section 2.6c.

3.4c. Meningeal sarcoma

The independent and unsatisfactory taxonomy of these rare tumours, as it recently existed in the neuropathological literature, has been revised by Jellinger so as to conform with the WHO classification of extracranial sarcomas[61,62]. Although fibrosarcoma (Figure 3.28) has previously been the most frequently diagnosed intracranial sarcoma, most such examples can now be more appropriately designated, particularly malignant fibrous

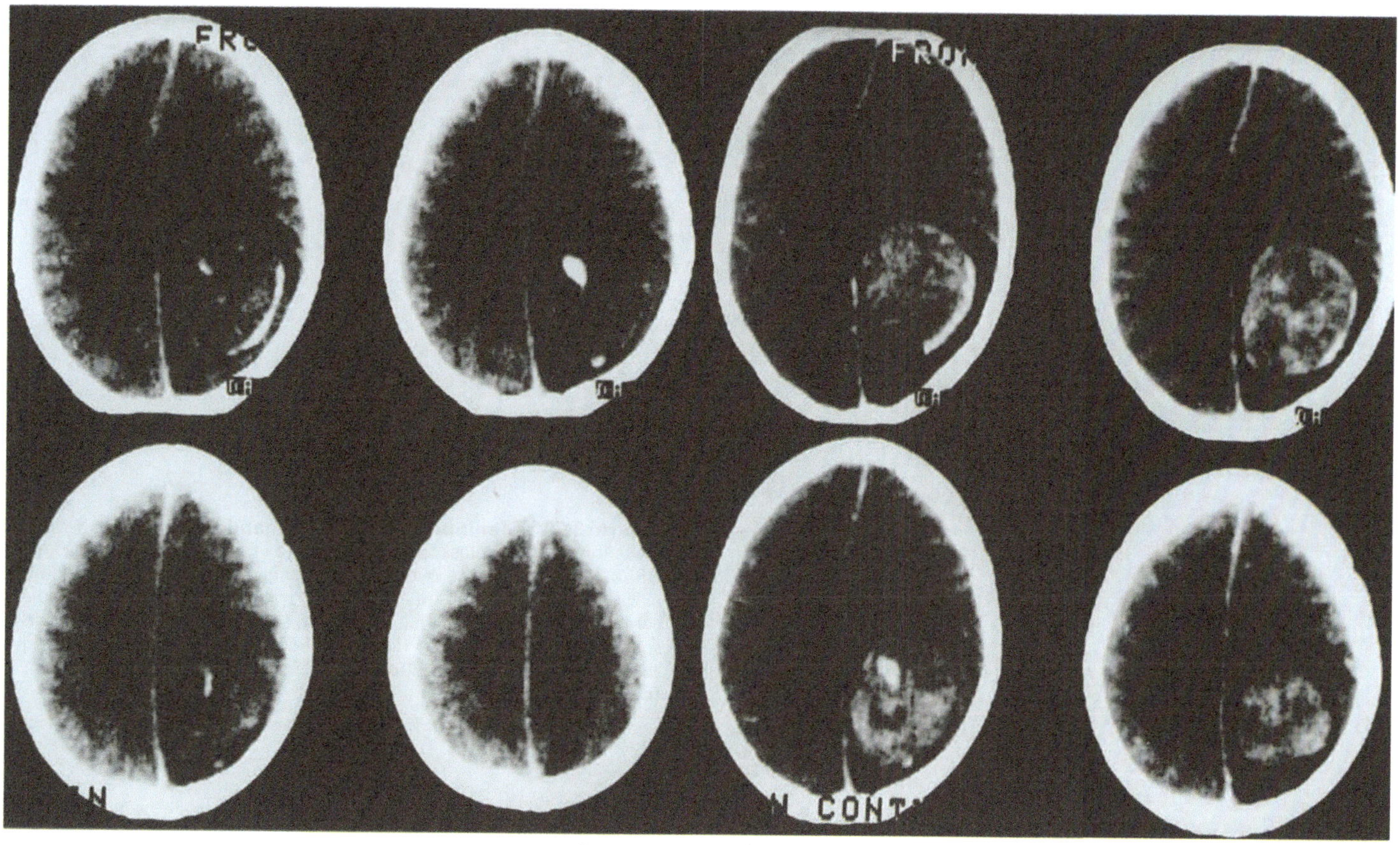

a

b

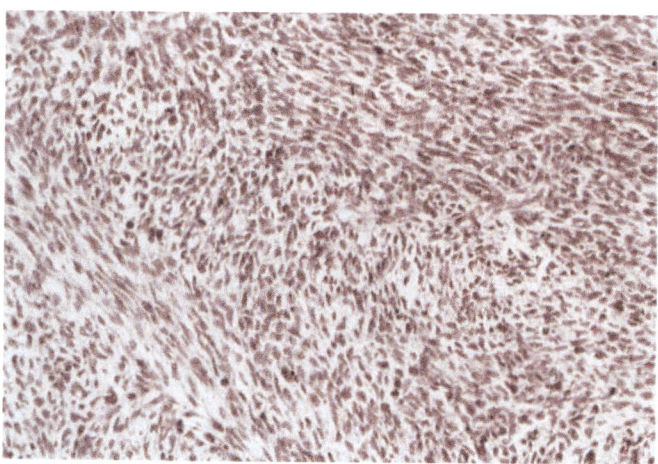

c

Figure 3.28   Meningeal fibrosarcoma: (**a**) CT, (**b**) CT + C, (**c**) HE × 200; CT shows large mainly intraparenchymal, brain isodense mass, with peripheral, focal and intraventricular haemorrhage. Enhancement is diffuse but inhomogeneous (b). Histology shows sheets of spindle-shaped cells sometimes having a herring-bone growth pattern, and a high mitotic index. Other areas showed intense vascularity, frequently associated with haemorrhage or extravasation of erythrocytes. (Histology reviewed by Prof JJ Kepes, University Kansas)

histiocytomas (MFH). Rare types are clearly derived from other mesenchymal tissues, including smooth or striped muscle, cartilage, vasoformative cells, and so on. A few entities reflect their uncertain origins, e.g. rhabdoid[63] (Figure 3.29) and ectomesenchymal tumours, whilst the term 'polymorphic cell sarcoma' is replaced by 'sarcoma NOS' (Figure 3.30), and is applied to those neoplasms whose morphology is quite non-specific. The neuroimaging literature does not appear to deal with meningocerebral sarcomas, and the CT/MR features of examples of various tumour types are to be found in neurosurgical journals. Occasionally this type of large, superficial, enhancing neoplasm is found to contain a significant population of GFAP-positive cells. Allowing for adequate tissue sampling this feature makes the diagnosis of glio-sarcoma (Figure 4.83) and/or sarcoglioma (Figure 7.56) a consideration.

We have not encountered examples of *meningeal sarco-matosis*, a term used to describe a diffusely infiltrating neoplastic process, without the formation of a tumour mass, occurring mainly in infants and children. *Haeman-giopericytoma* and *haemangioblastoma* are respectively discussed in sections 3.4d (below) and 6.6c.

3.4d.   Haemangiopericytoma

On grounds of light and electron microscopy[64], immuno-histochemistry[65,66] and biological behaviour[67], this tumour is now considered distinct from conventional meningo-thelial meningioma. Nevertheless, the historical confusion with angioblastic meningioma, combined with features of an enhancing extraparenchymal mass (Figure 3.31), accounts for the lack of a specific imaging identity.

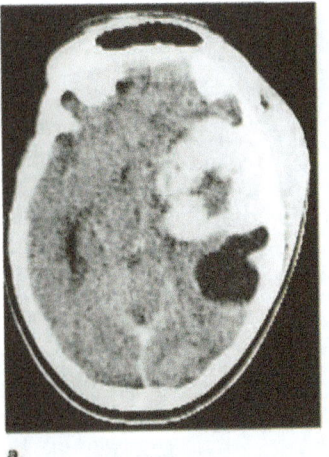

a

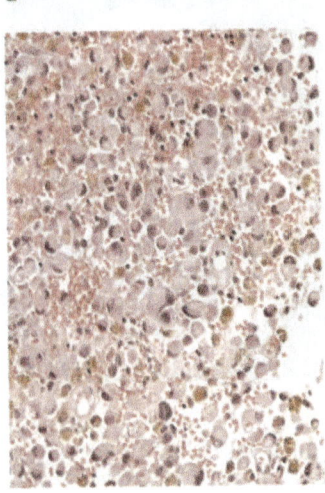

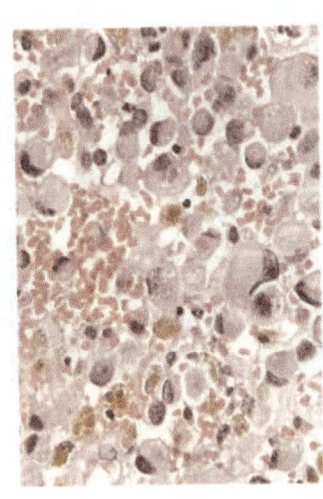

c

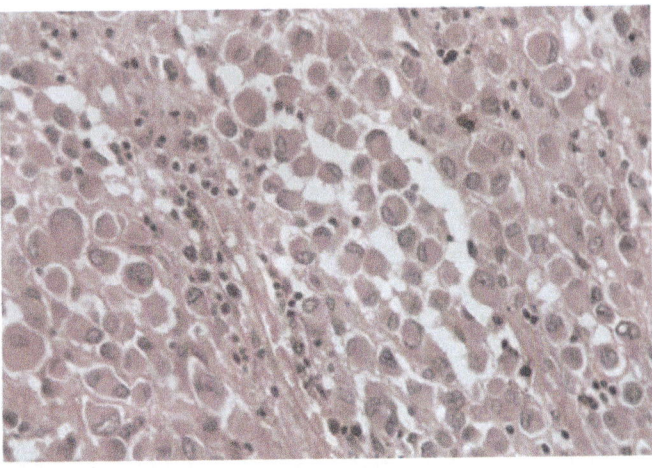

b

Figure 3.29 Meningeal, sarcoma, rhabdoid: female, 13 years, presenting with painless facial swelling; (**a**) CT + C, (**b**) HE × 400, (**c**) HE × 200/× 400; large hyperdense strongly enhancing temporal lobe mass, with central non-enhancing area (presumed necrosis) and adjacent brain cyst whose wall does not enhance. Tumour has eroded squamous temporal bone, with scalp soft tissue infiltration. Histology (b) shows characteristic rhabdoid sarcoma, with abundant haemosiderin (c)

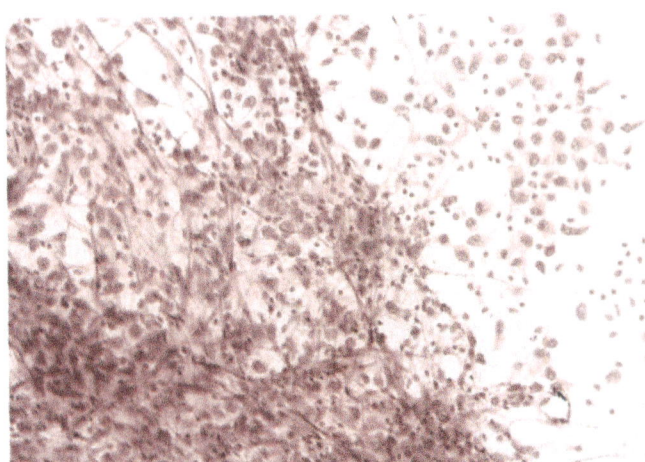

Figure 3.30 Meningeal sarcoma NOS: male, 16 years; presented with 8-year history of epilepsy. CT scan showed superficial occipital mass, identical to lesion shown in Figure 3.28. At operation tumour thought to be a meningioma, although there was evidence of central haemorrhage. Smear shows characteristic meningeal sarcoma. Patient died 5 months later; at autopsy there was diffuse cerebromeningeal spread. HE × 200

3.5. METASTATIC DISEASE

3.5a. Meningeal metastases (malignant meningitis)

Tissue diagnosis is occasionally sought in the syndrome of headache and progressive obtundation where imaging discloses evidence of a distal CSF block combined with diffuse meningovascular enhancement, usually most marked at the base. This picture, of course, is not specific, and is usually assumed initially to be due to some form of granulomatous inflammation (Figure 3.32). The diagnosis of malignancy is suspected and usually confirmed on CSF cytology, but this investigation may be equivocal (Figures 3.33 and 3.41), or even non-contributory, when meningeal biopsy is then undertaken. Lymphoma and melanoma exhibit this mode of spread more commonly than epithelial neoplasms, and of the latter, breast, bowel and lung are the usual primary sites. As is to be expected, MR has been described as considerably more sensitive than CT in the demonstration of abnormal meningeal enhancement[68], particularly over the convexity, and the mechanism has been shown to be blood–CSF barrier breakdown[69].

Metastatic spread of carcinoma to the pachymeninges, other than continuous extension of a superficial parenchymal lesion, is even rarer than involvement of the subarachnoid space. This form of growth is principally within the

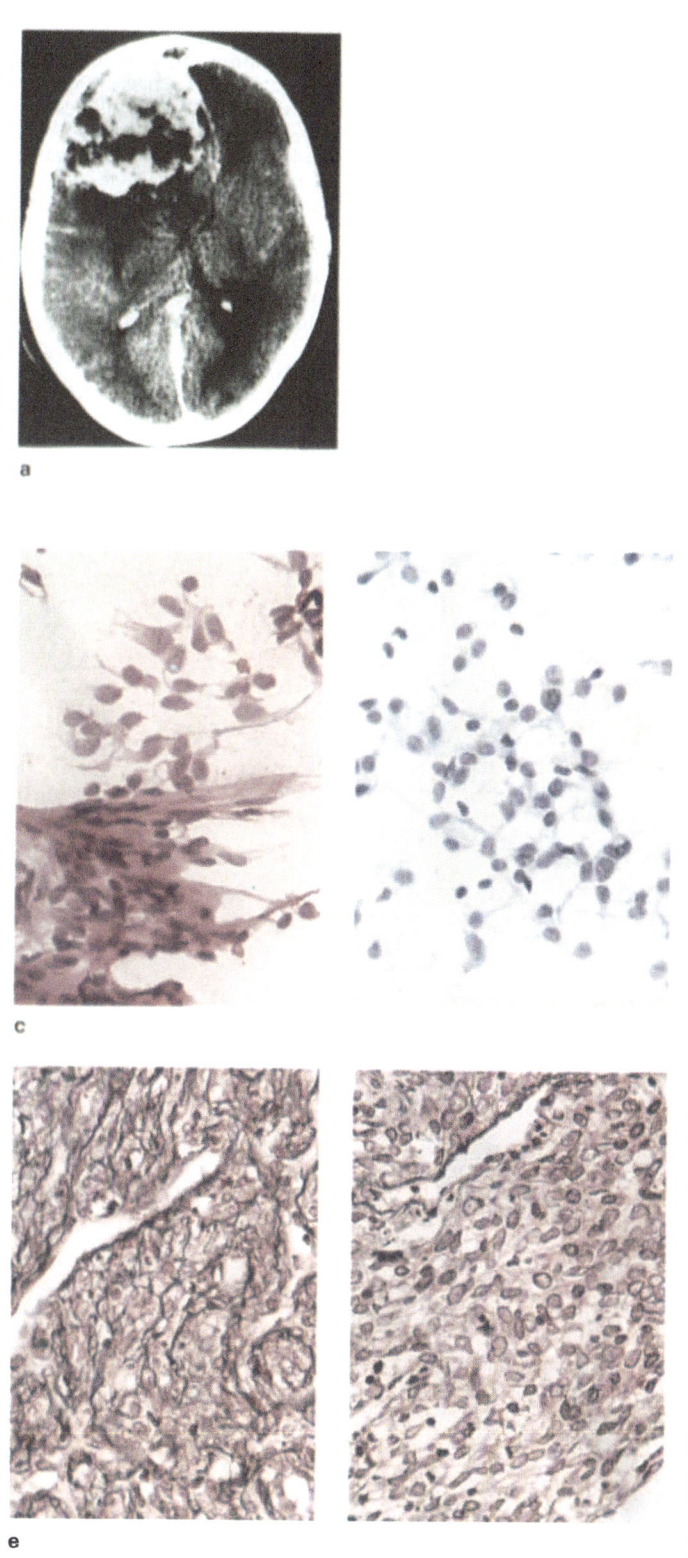

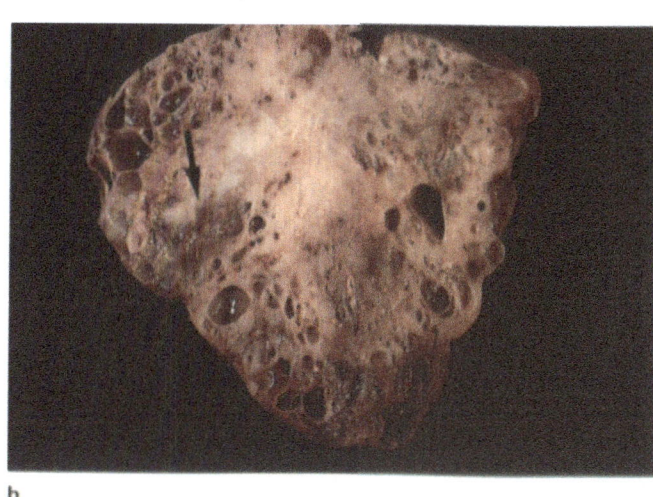

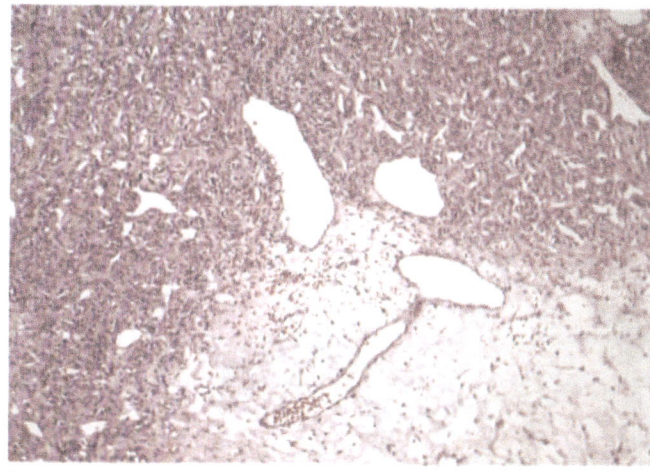

Figure 3.31 Haemangiopericytoma: (**a**) CT + C, (**b**) fixed specimen, (**c**) HE/Tol blue × 400, (**d**) HE × 100, (**e**) reticulin × 400; CT shows a large lobulated meningocerebral mass, with strong parenchymal enhancement interrupted by coarse cysts. The pale, more solid, component of the tumour as seen in (b) is represented by the cellular and vascular tissue shown histologically in (d). Myxomatous degeneration (d) presumably gives rise to cysts. Also seen in the fixed specimen are interspersed foci of organizing haemorrhagic necrosis (arrow). The imaging features are non-specific (compare with vascular meningioma, **Figure 3.23**). Characteristic pericellular reticulin (e) may not be uniform, explaining basis of alternate clumping and dispersal of cells on smear (c)

Figure 3.32 (*opposite*) **Malignant meningitis, medulloblastoma**: male, 3 years; (**a**) CT, (**b**) CT + C; images show coarse symmetrical meningocerebral spread of tumour which is hyperdense and strongly enhancing. Cerebellum was also diffusely involved by desmoplastic-type medulloblastoma, without a discrete mass, and picture was originally considered to be that of TBM

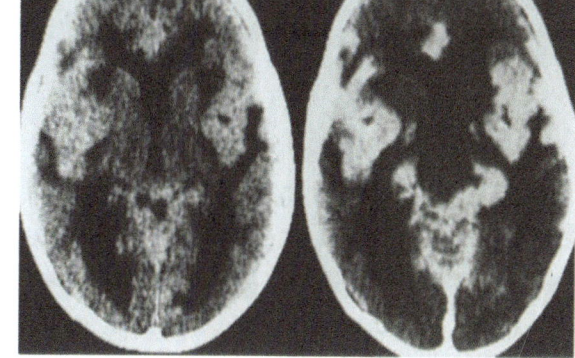

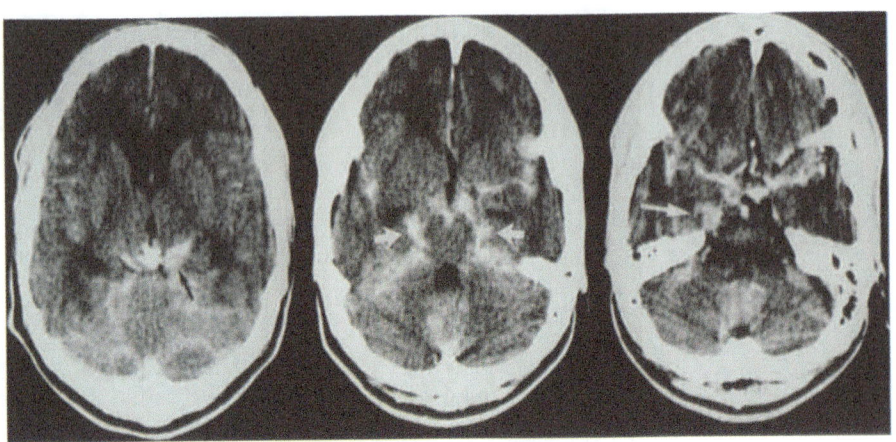

a b c

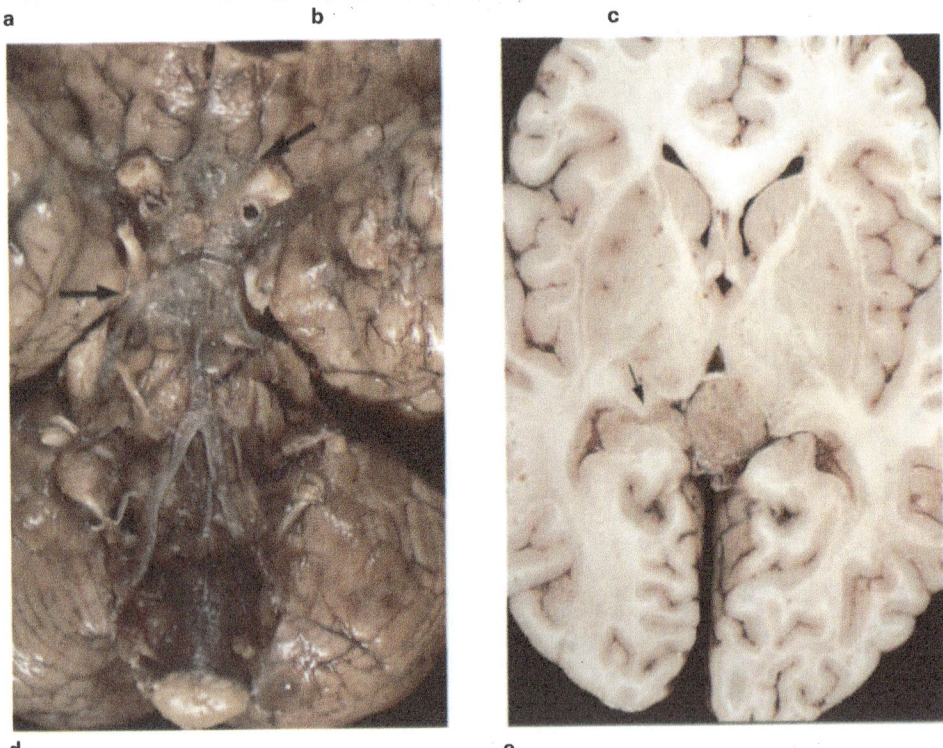

d e

Figure 3.33 Germinoma, diffuse subarachnoid spread: male, 17 years; presenting with headache and multiple cranial nerve palsies; (**a–c**) CT + C, (**d,e**) fixed brain; CT shows basal meningeal enhancement, particularly prominent in the ambient cistern (b,c, arrows). More localized lesions (a, arrow), in pineal region, were originally thought to be granulomata. Basal meninges of fixed specimen (d) exhibit innumerable plaque-like tumour deposits (arrows). Pineal lesion (e) is much more obvious than on the scan. Note extension of tumour into choroid fissure (arrow). Spinal meninges were involved at autopsy

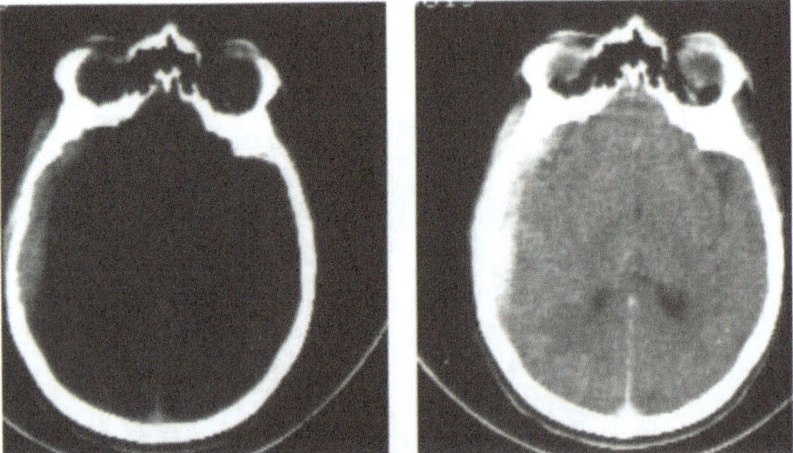

Figure 3.34 Metastatic disease, dural (primary breast carcinoma): CTBW/CT + C; shows diffusely enhancing en-plaque tissue with some mass effect and erosion of inner table of skull

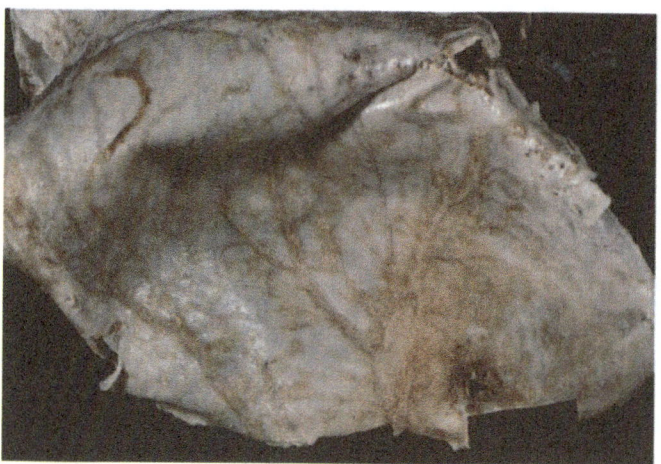

a

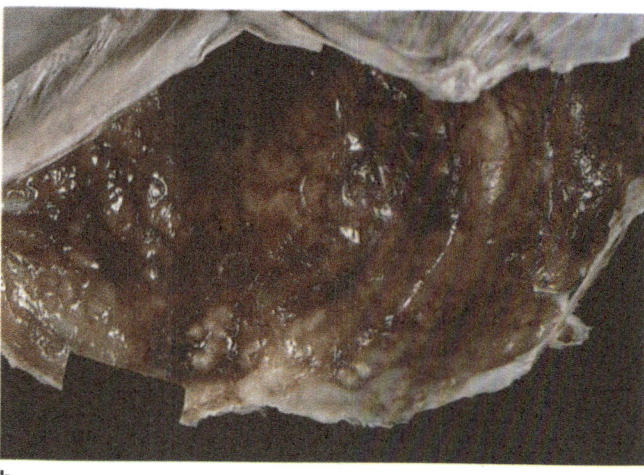

b

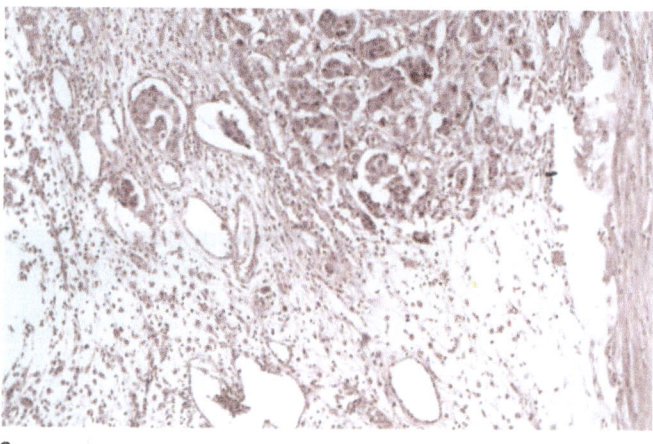

c

Figure 3.35   Metastatic disease, subdural: patient presented with a subacute subdural haematoma; (**a**) external dura with burr-hole and felt-like perivascular tumour growth, (**b**) subdural haematoma cavity with tumour nodules, (**c**) histology shows dura and adjacent tumour tissue, with surrounding vascular proliferative haematoma membrane, which would have enhanced independently. HE ×100

subdural space, presenting as plaque-like enhancement (Figure 3.34), sometimes with marked hypointensity due to desmoplasia, or occasionally as a haematoma (Figure 3.35). The enhancing lesion may be indistinguishable from a granuloma.

Both subarachnoid and subdural deposits (Figure 3.36) are typical of leukaemia, previously chloroma, now designated granulocytic sarcoma[70], when venous occlusion may occur (Figure 3.37). Although never a surgical histopathological problem, this may be of autopsy importance.

Carcinoma isolated to the lateral ventricular choroid plexus may be expected to present only when obstruction occurs (Figure 3.38); a tissue diagnosis precedes any attempt at removal, meningioma being the chief alternative.

3.6.   HAEMOPOIETIC AND LYMPHORETICULAR NEOPLASMS

Lymphoma may rarely draw clinical attention to itself as a solitary intracranial–extraparenchymal mass[71], but is then almost always found to be continuous with an adjacent extracranial primary source, most commonly the nasopharynx, orbit or scalp; usually, but not invariably, the skull exhibits expansion and lysis. The intracranial growth has en-plaque and focal mass components (Figure 2.25), both being strongly enhancing. As with most pachymeningeal infiltrates, desmoplasia may be considerable, with resulting hypointensity at short and long TR; however, when there is sufficient tumour bulk the stroma may become T2 hyperintense[72].

Solitary intracranial plasmacytoma is described[73,74], greatly resembling meningioma in morphology and enhancement, including hyperostosis of the adjacent skull. In some but not all instances there is progression to myeloma. This lesion must be differentiated from inflammatory pseudotumour of the meninges (plasma cell granuloma) (section 3.2c).

Other rare haemopoietic neoplasms involving meninges and/or the parenchyma include examples of neoplastic angioendotheliosis (section 4.13), metastatic mycosis fungoides[75], lymphomatoid granulomatosis (now recognized as an extranodal T-cell lymphoma)[76], which in rare instances may be confined to the CNS[77,78] (Figure 4.102), Langerhans cell histiocytosis (histiocytosis X) (section 2.7), familial lymphohistiocytosis and histiocytic medullary reticulosis (malignant histiocytosis). For practical purposes Hodgkin's disease of the CNS is secondary to widespread systemic disease. Primary leptomeningeal lymphoma, in which the neoplastic cells are confined to the leptomeninges and perivascular spaces[79] or nerve roots (neurolymphomatosis)[80] is exceedingly rare.

3.7.   UNCOMMON CONDITIONS

3.7a.   Trigeminal cave lesions

In recent years neuroimaging has contributed much to a long standing clinical interest in disease of the trigeminal nerve ganglion. Although a number of very rare conditions are documented[81,82] (Figure 3.40), those lesions of importance include schwannoma and meningioma, with T2 hyperintensity and cystic degeneration of the former constituting the main differentiating features (Figure 3.39). Coronal views are considered essential to the imaging diagnosis, and needle aspiration by the radiologist may mean exclusive cytomorphology[83].

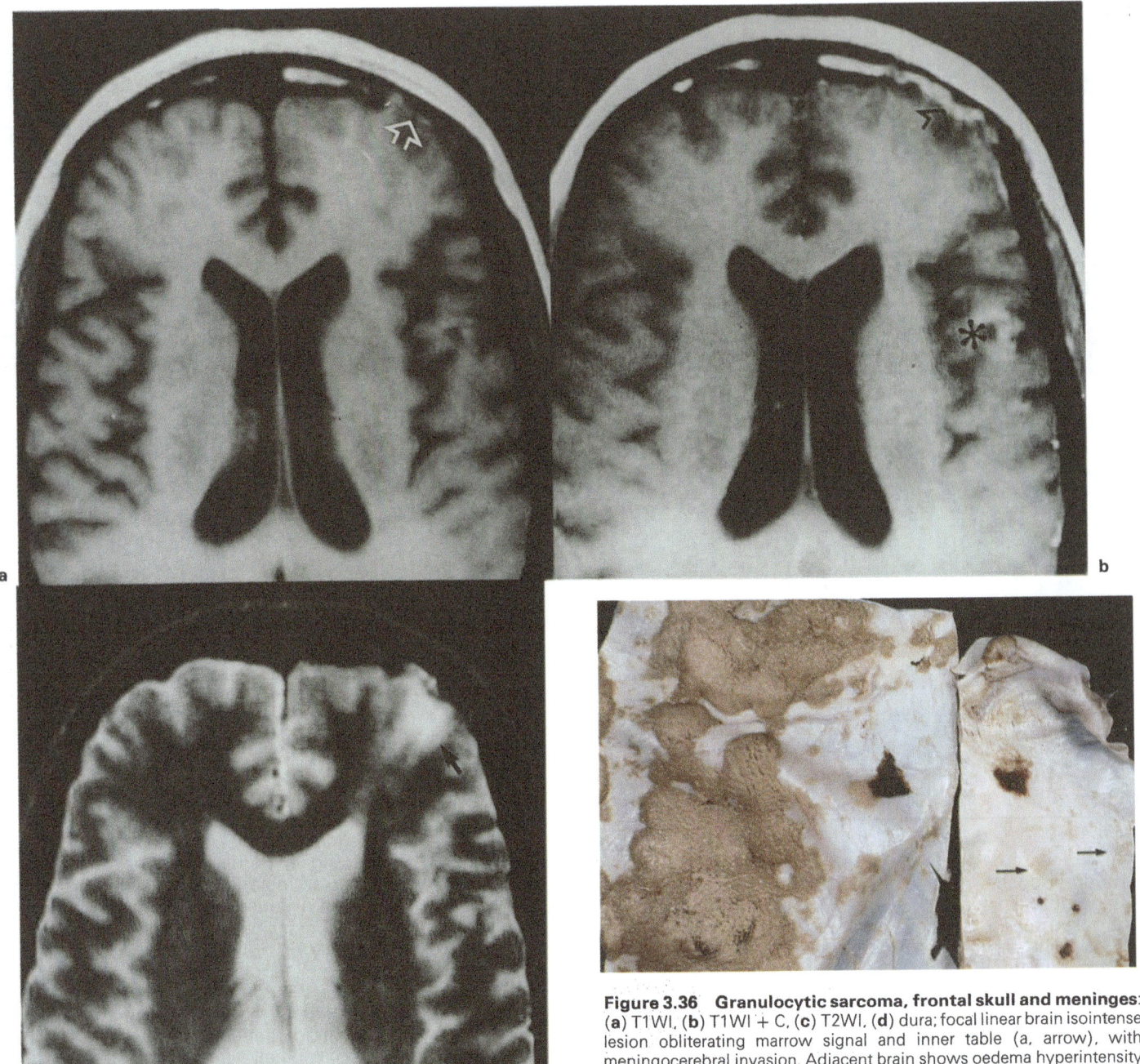

Figure 3.36 Granulocytic sarcoma, frontal skull and meninges: (a) T1WI, (b) T1WI + C, (c) T2WI, (d) dura; focal linear brain isointense lesion obliterating marrow signal and inner table (a, arrow), with meningocerebral invasion. Adjacent brain shows oedema hyperintensity (c). Tumour tissue enhances strongly (b, arrow). Second deeper meningeal lesion is visible in the temporal lobe (asterisk). Specimen (d) from an autopsy case shows extradural deposits, with much finer subdural penetration (arrows)

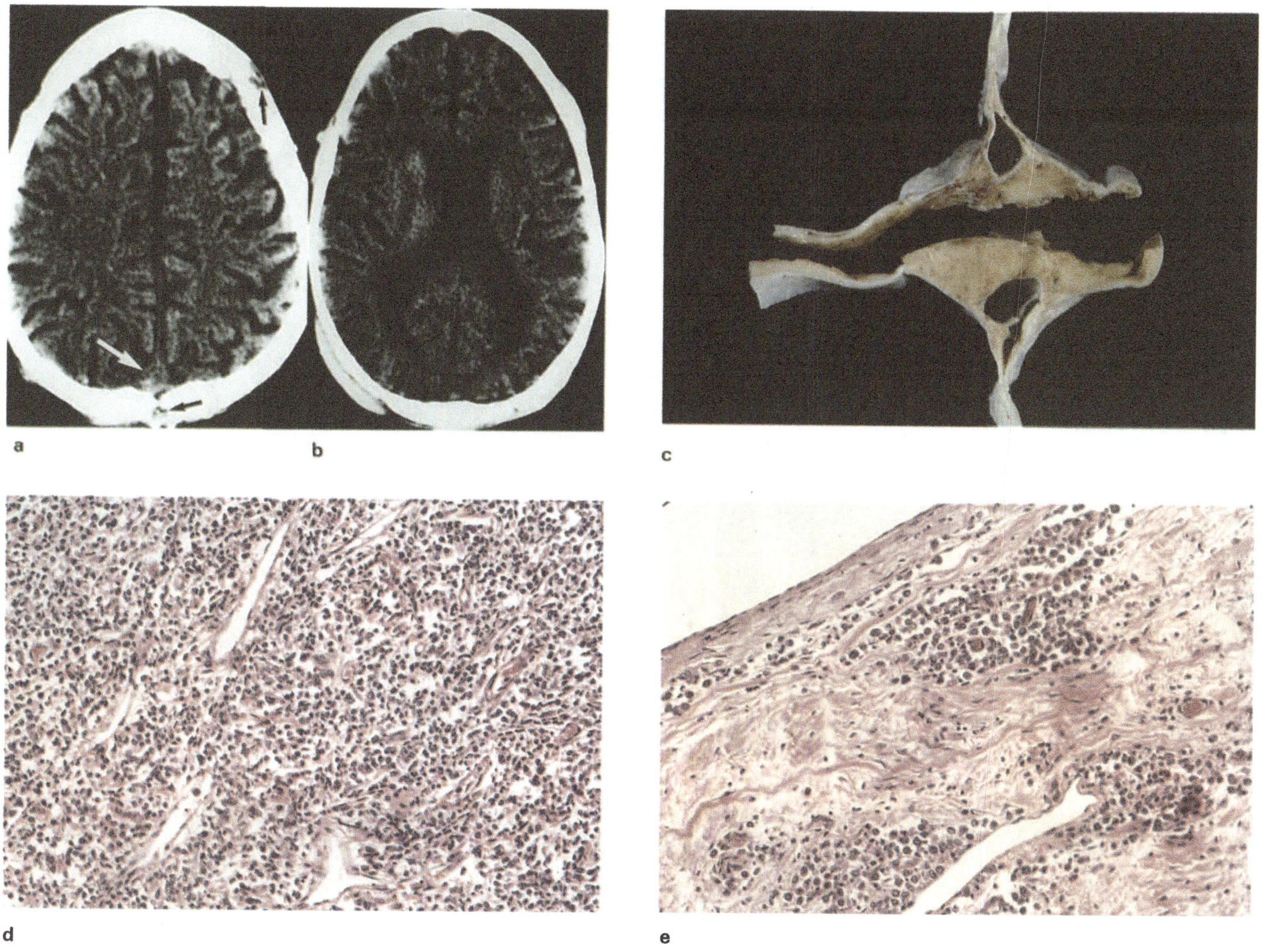

Figure 3.37 Granulocytic sarcoma, sagittal sinus involvement: (**a,b**) CT, (**c**) sagittal sinus, (**d,e**) HE ×200; CT shows focal lytic lesions of bone (a, black arrows), hyperdense sagittal sinus (a, white arrow) and sulcal ventricular dilatation (b), consistent with distal block, as shown in macroscopic section of dural sinus (c). Histology shows remarkably prolific capillary vasculature within the solid tumour (d), and possibly also within infiltrating dural cellular aggregates (e)

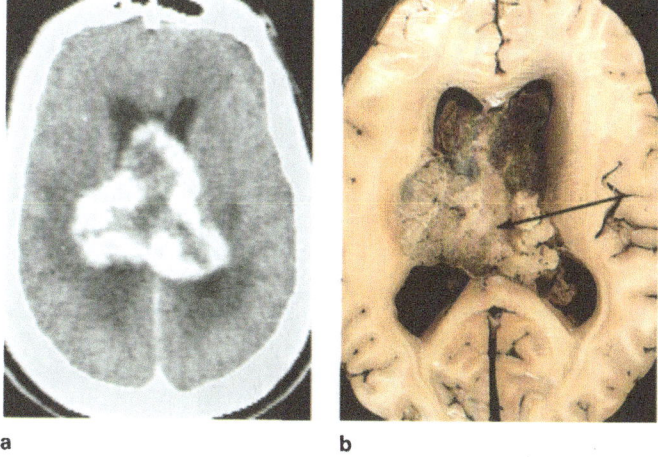

Figure 3.38 Metastatic disease, choroid/intraventricular adenocarcinoma: (**a**) CT + C, (**b**) fixed specimen; image shows large lobulated, peripherally enhancing intraventricular mass; central hypodensity corresponds to coagulative necrosis shown in fixed specimen (b, arrow). Discoloration of lobulated tumour is artefactual

3.7b. Primary malignant melanomatosis

Diffuse involvement of the leptomeninges and superficial cortex by melanin-producing cells is characteristic of neurocutaneous melanosis, and in a biopsy-proven case strong, diffuse enhancement is reported, with no significant alteration of T1 or T2 weighted images[84]. This appears to be indistinguishable from primary malignant melanomatosis of the leptomeninges[85] (Figure 3.41), or malignant meningitis in general (see section 3.5). Signal shortening (T1 hyperintensity/T2 hypointensity), when present, could probably be regarded as pathognomonic of melanin-related paramagnetism. On light microscopy the meningeal vessels are both dilated and increased in density (Figure 3.41); together with the morphological alterations implied by neoplastic cell encasement, these features are sufficient to account for diffuse contrast enhancement.

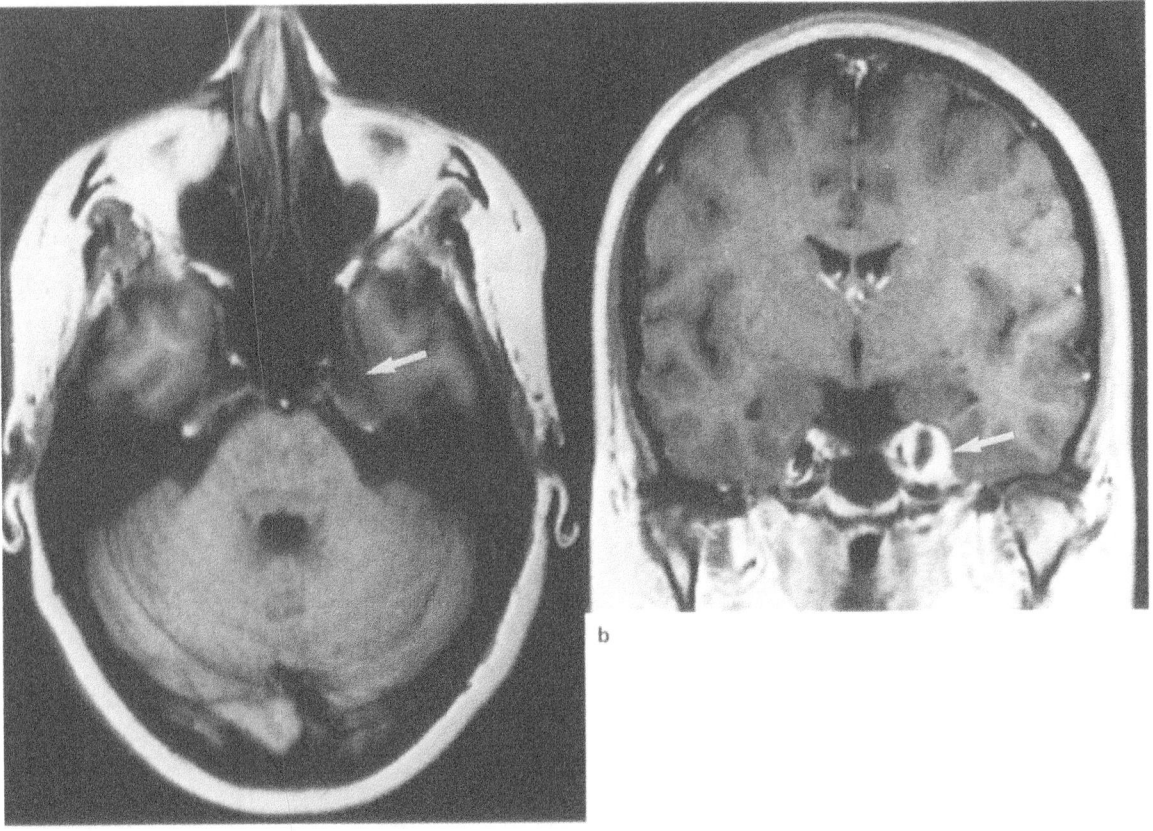

a

b

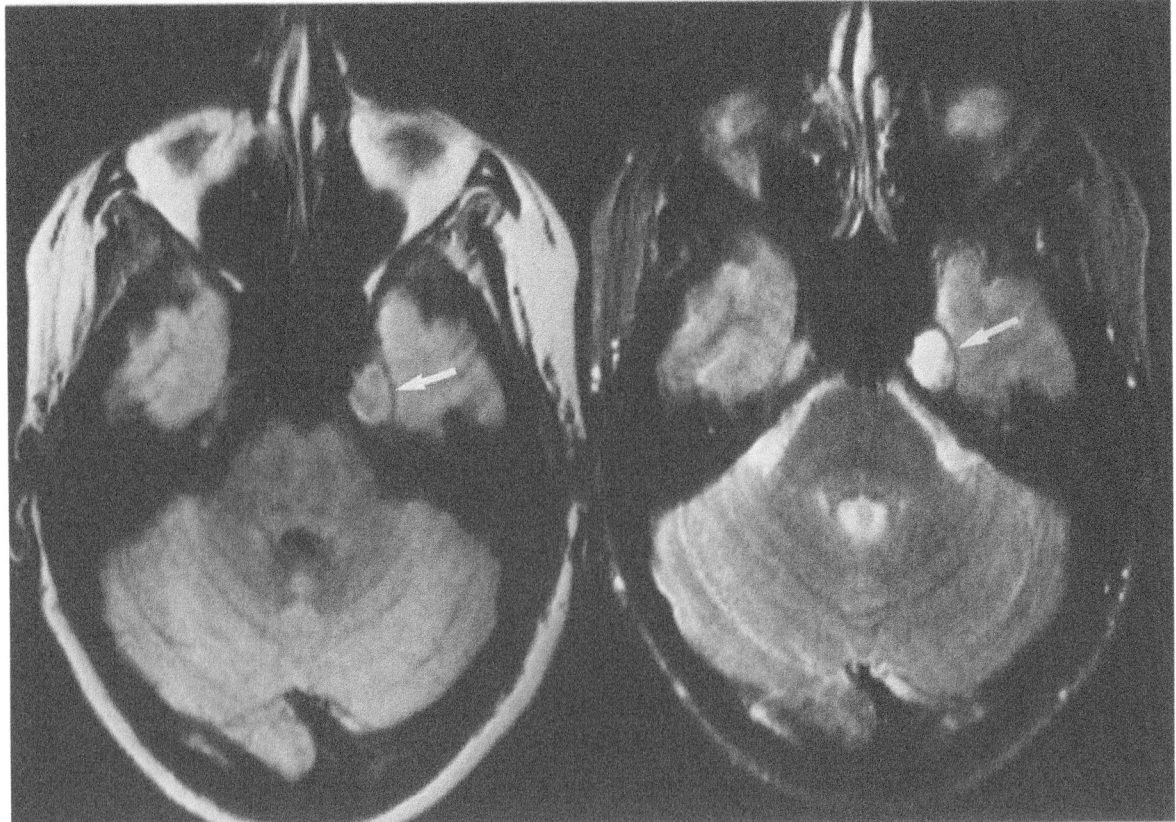

c   d

Figure 3.39 Schwannoma, trigeminal cave: female, 30 years; (**a**) T1WI, (**b**) T1WI + C, (**c**) PDWI, (**d**) T2WI; images show solid/cystic expansion of the left 5th nerve (a–d, arrows) with strong enhancement of solid component (b), which is also T2 hyperintense (d). Cyst contents are CSF-hyperintense on proton density weighted image (c). No histology, but site, images and progression are characteristic of schwannoma

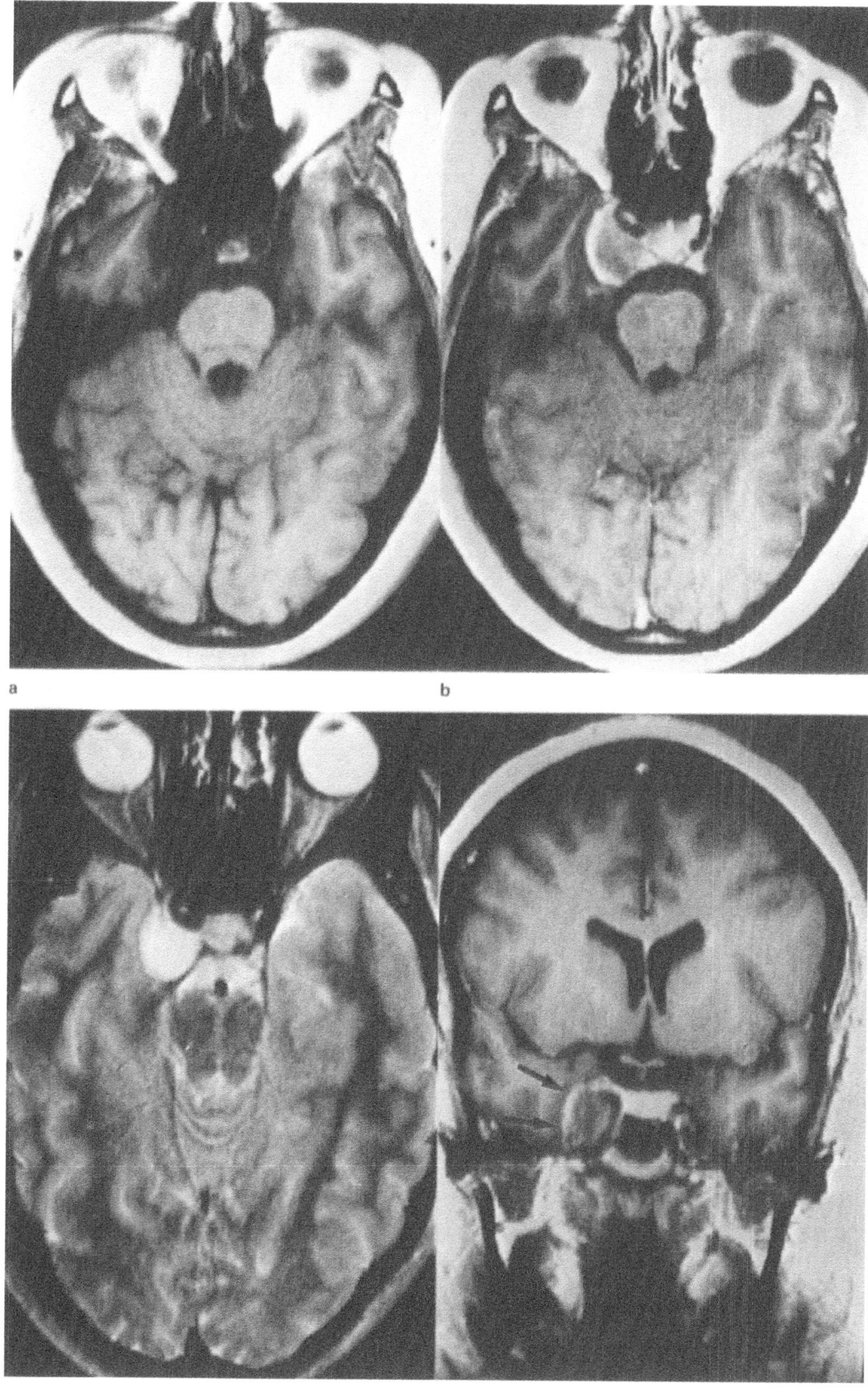

Figure 3.40 **Chordoma, trigeminal cave**: (a) T1WI, (b) T1WI + C, (c) T2WI, (d) coronal T1WI + C; sharply circumscribed mextraparenchymal mass centred on the trigeminal ganglion, which is infiltrated and expanded (d, arrow). Tumour impinges medially on the sella. Lesion is T1 hypointense/T2 hyperintense, exhibiting moderate homogeneous enhancement, strongest at the periphery. Signal characteristics are almost unique, other solid lesions (epithelial, meningothelial, schwannian) being T1 isointense

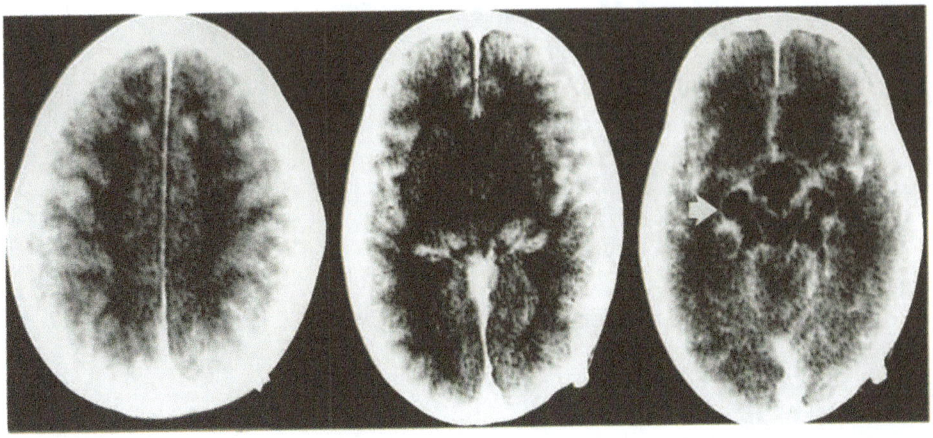

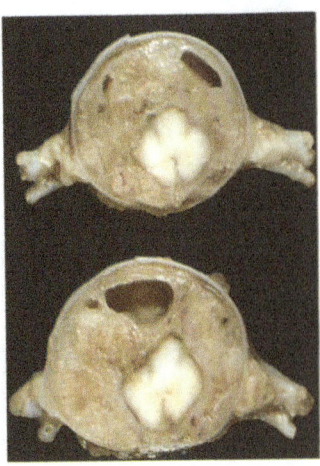

Figure 3.41 Primary malignant melanomatosis: (**a–c**) CT + C, (**d**) Giemsa × 900/Tol blue × 400, (**e**) fixed brain, (**f**) spinal cord, (**g**) HE × 400; CT shows generalized meningocerebral enhancement with meningeal CSF loculation in the basal cisterns (arrow). Differential diagnosis included TB and malignant meningitis. CSF cytospin (d) showed atypical cells with prominent vacuolation, considered suggestive of Burkitt's lymphoma, but pigmented cells were not appreciated. At operation meninges were distended and melanotic. Patient died shortly after. Brain shows generalized, diffuse pigmentation of cerebral cortex and diencephalic grey, with sparing of basal ganglia. Choroid fissures, basal cisterns and spinal subarachnoid space filled with non-pigmented tumour, containing CSF loculi. Histology of subarachnoid growth (g) shows diffuse capillary/sinusoidal neovasculature

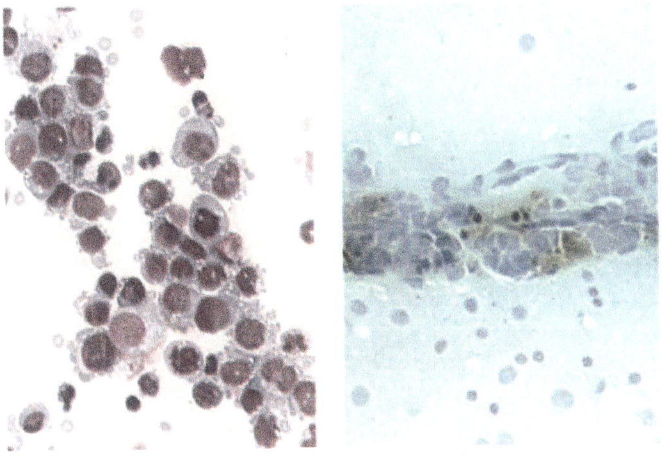

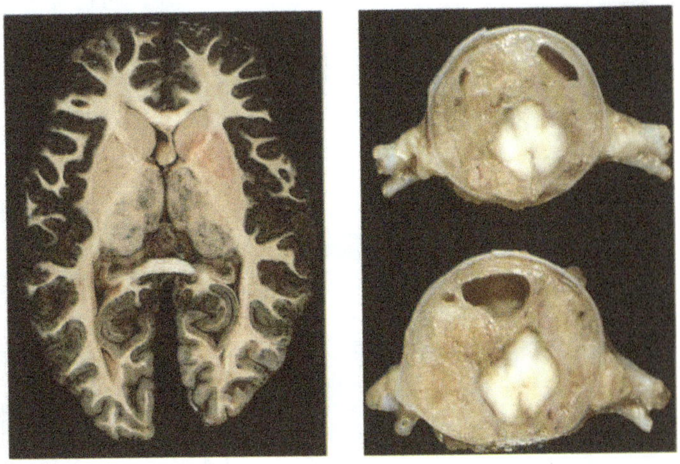

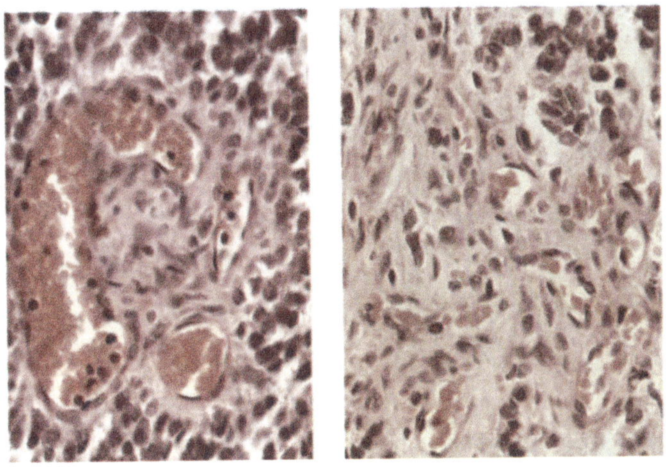

REFERENCES

1. Malcolm GP, Symon L, Kendall B *et al*. Intracranial neurenteric cysts. J Neurosurg. 1991;75:115–20.
2. Inoue T, Matshushima T, Fukui M *et al*. Immunohistochemical study of intracranial cysts. Neurosurgery. 1988;23:576–81.
3. Mackenzie IRA, Gilbert JJ. Cysts of the neuraxis of endodermal origin. J Neurol Neurosurg Psychiatr. 1991;54:572–5.
4. Uematsu Y, Rojas-Corona RR, Llena JF *et al*. Epithelial cysts in the central nervous system, characteristic expression of cytokeratins in an immunohistochemical study. Acta Neurochir. 1990;107:93–101.
5. Atlas SW. Intraaxial brain tumors. In: Magnetic resonance imaging of the brain and spine. New York: Raven Press; 1991:228.
6. Egelhoff JC, Ross JS, Modic M *et al*. MR imaging of metastatic GI carcinoma in brain. AJNR. 1992;13:1221–4.
7. Czervionke LF, Daniels DD, Meyer GA *et al*. Neuroepithelial cysts of the lateral ventricles: MR appearance. AJNR. 1987;8:609–13.
8. Fleming H, Murayama S, Dacey RG. Posterior fossa epithelial cyst of ectodermal origin. Neurosurgery. 1991;29:459–64.
9. Yoshida K, Nakamura S, Tsubokawa T *et al*. Epithelial cyst of the fourth ventricle. J Neurosurg. 1990;73:942–5.
10. Burger PC, Scheithauer BW, Vogel FS. Surgical pathology of the nervous system and its coverings, 3rd edn. New York: Churchill Livingstone; 1991:104–6.
11. Go KG, Houthoff HF, Blaauw EH *et al*. Morphology and origin of arachnoid cysts: scanning and transmission electron microscopy of three cases. Acta Neuropathol. 1978;44:57–62.
12. Rengachary SS, Watanabe I. Ultrastructure and pathogenesis of intracranial arachnoid cysts. J Neuropathol Exp Neurol. 1981;40:61–83.
13. Fulton JF, Bailey P. Tumors in the region of the third ventricle: their diagnosis and relation to pathologic sleep. J Nerv Ment Dis. 1929;69:1.

14. Burger PC, Scheithauer BW, Vogel FS. Surgical pathology of the nervous system and its coverings, 3rd edn. New York: Churchill Livingstone; 1991:306.

15. Kuchelmeister K, Bergman M. Colloid cysts of the third ventricle: an immunohistochemical study. Histopathology. 1992;21:35–42.

16. Kondziolka D, Bilbao JM. An immunohistochemical study of neuro-epithelial (colloid) cysts. J Neurosurg. 1989;71:91–7.

17. Maeder PP, Holtas SL, Basibuyuk LN et al. Colloid cysts of the third ventricle: correlation of MR and CT findings with histology and chemical analysis. AJNR. 1990;11:575–81.

18. Goldberg HI. Extraaxial brain tumors. In: Atlas SW, ed. Magnetic resonance imaging of the brain and spine. New York: Raven Press; 1991;327–78.

19. Robertson S, Wolpert S, Runge V. MR imaging of middle cranial fossa arachnoid cysts. AJNR. 1989;10:1007–10.

20. Dastur DK, Lalitha MD. The many facets of neurotuberculosis. In: Zimmerman HM, ed. Progress in neuropathology. New York: Grune & Stratton; 1973;11:351–408.

21. Sinh G, Pandya SK, Dastur MD. Pathogenesis of unusual intracranial tuberculomas and tuberculous space-occupying lesions. J Neurosurg. 1968;29:149–59.

22. Lotz J, Hewlett R, Alheit B et al. Neurocysticercosis: correlative pathomorphology and MR imaging. Neuroradiology. 1988;30:35–41.

23. Schoeman J, Hewlett R, Donald P. MR imaging in childhood tuberculous meningitis. Neuroradiology. 1988;30:473–7.

24. Loizou LA, Anderson M. Intracranial tuberculomas: correlation of computerised tomography with clinicopathological findings. Q J Med. 1982;51:104–14.

25. Huk WJ, Lotz JW, Hewlett RH. Inflammatory diseases of the central nervous system. In: Huk WJ, Gademann G, Friedman G, eds. MRI of central nervous system diseases. Berlin: Springer-Verlag; 1990:353.

26. Harriman DGF. Bacterial infections of the central nervous system. In: Adams JH, Corsellis JAN, Duchen LW, eds. Greenfield's neuropathology, 4th edn. London: Edward Arnold; 1984:248.

27. Draouat S, Abdenabi B, Ghanem M, Bourjat B. Computed tomography of cerebral tuberculoma. JCAT. 1987;11:594–7.

28. Harriman DGF. Bacterial infections of the central nervous system. In: Adams JH, Corsellis JAN, Duchen LW, eds. Greenfield's neuropathology, 4th edn. London: Edward Arnold; 1984:251.

29. Yang PJ, Reger KM, Seeger JF, Carmody RF. Brain abscess: an atypical CT appearance of CNS tuberculosis. AJNR. 1987;8:919–20.

30. Whitener DR. Tuberculous brain abscess: report of a case and review of the literature. Arch Neurol. 1978;35:148–55.

31. Jinkins JR, Siqueira E, Al-Kawi NZ. Cranial manifestations of aspergillosis. Neuroradiology. 1987;29:181–5.

32. Welchman JM. Computerised tomography of intracranial tuberculomata. Clin Radiol. 1979;30:567–73.

33. de Castro CC, Hesselinck JR. Tuberculosis. Neuroimaging Clin N Am. 1991;1:119–39.

34. Reichenthal E, Cohen ML, Schujman E et al. Tuberculous brain abscess and its appearance on computerised tomography. J Neurosurg. 1982;56:597–600.

35. Hughes JT. Pathology of the spinal cord, 2nd edn. London: Lloyd-Luke; 1978:117.

36. Martin N, Masson C, Henin D et al. Hypertrophic cranial pachymeningitis: assessment with CT and MR imaging. AJNR. 1989;10:477–84.

37. Curtin HD. Pseudotumor. Radiol Clin N Am. 1987;25:283–7.

38. Adler J, Sheridan W, Kosek J et al. Pachymeningitis associated with a pulmonary nodule. Neurosurgery. 1991;29:283–7.

39. West SG, Pittman DL, Coggin JT. Intracranial plasma cell granuloma. Cancer. 1989;46:330–5.

40. Eiomoto T, Yanaka M, Kurosawa M, Ikeya F. Plasma cell granuloma (inflammatory pseudotumour) of the spinal cord meninges. Report of a case. Cancer. 1978;42:1929–36.

41. Horten BC, Urich H, Stefoski D. Meningiomas with conspicuous plasma cell-lymphocytic components. Cancer. 1979;43:258–64.

42. Chang KH, Cho SY, Hesselink JR et al. Parasitic diseases of the central nervous system. Neuroimag Clin N Am. 1991;1:159–78.

43. Lunardi P, Missori P, Di Lorenzo N et al. Cerebral hydatidosis in childhood: a retrospective survey with emphasis on long term follow-up. Neurosurgery. 1991;29:515–18.

44. Morseth DJ. Ultrastructure of developing taeniid embryophores and associated structures. Exp Parasitol. 1965;16:207–16.

45. Bowen BC, Post MJD. Intracranial infections. In: Atlas S, ed. Magnetic resonance imaging of the brain and spine. New York: Raven Press; 1991:501–38.

46. Frenkel JK, Nelson BM, Arias-Stella J. Immunosuppression and toxoplasmic encephalitis. Clinical and experimental aspects. Hum Pathol. 1975;6(1):97–111.

47. Otofri-Kwakye SK, Sidebottom D, Herbert J et al. Granulomatous brain tumor caused by acanthameba. J Neurosurg. 1986;64:505–9.

48. Diaconita GH, Goldis G, Nagy P. Researches on histogenesis and anatomicopathological forms of distomiasis (paragonimiasis). Acta Med Scand. 1957;159:155–66.

49. Artlich A, Schmidt D. Immunohistochemical profile of meningiomas and their histological subtypes. Hum Pathol. 1990;21:843–9.

50. Goldberg HI. Extraxial brain tumors. In: Atlas S, ed. Magnetic resonance imaging of the brain and spine. New York: Raven Press; 1991;327–78.

51. Scheithauer BW. Tumors of the meninges: proposed modifications of the World Health Organisation classification. Acta Neuropathol. 1990;80:343–54.

52. Rutherfoord GS, Marus G. Microcystic meningiomas. Clin Neuropathol. 1987;6(4):143–8.

53. Alguacil-Garcia A, Pettigrew NM, Sima AAF. Secretory meningioma. A distinct subtype of meningioma. Am J Surg Pathol. 1986;10(2):102–11.

54. Lattes R, Bigotti G. Lipoblastic meningioma: 'vacuolated meningioma'. Hum Pathol. 1991;22:164–71.

55. Kepes JJ, Goldware MD, Leoni R. Meningioma with a pseudo-glandular pattern: a case report. J Neuropathol Exp Neurol. 1983;42(1):61–8.

56. Horten BC, Urich H, Stefoski D. Meningiomas with conspicuous plasma cell-lymphocytic components. Cancer. 1979;43:258–64.

57. Elster AD, Challa VR, Tucker TH et al. Meningiomas: MR and histopathological features. Radiology. 1989;170:857–62.

58. Schorner W, Schubeus P, Henkes H et al. 'Meningeal sign': a characteristic finding of meningiomas on contrast-enhanced MR images. Neuroradiology. 1990;32:90–3.

59. Tokumaru A, O'uchi T, Eguchi T et al. Prominent meningeal enhancement adjacent to meningioma on Gd-DtPA-enhanced MR images: histopathologic correlation. Radiology. 1990;175:431–3.

60. Russel DS, Rubinstein LJ. Pathology of tumours of the nervous system, 5th edn. London: Edward Arnold; 1989:479.

61. Paulus W, Slowik F, Jellinger K. Primary intracranial sarcomas: histopathological features of 19 cases. Histopathology. 1991;18:395–402.

62. Jellinger K, Paulus W. Mesenchymal, non-meningothelial tumours of the Central Nervous System. Brain Pathol. 1991;1:79–87.

63. Chou SM, Anderson JS. Primary CNS malignant rhabdoid tumor (MRT): report of two cases and review of literature. Clin Neuropathol. 1991;10(1):1–11.

64. Dardick I, Hammar SP, Scheithauer BW. Ultrastructural spectrum of haemangiopericytoma; a comparative study of fetal, adult and neoplastic pericytes. Ultrastruct Pathol. 1989;13:111–54.

65. D'Amore ESG, Manvel JC, Sung JH. Soft tissue and meningeal hemangiopericytomas: an immunohistochemical and ultrastructural study. Hum Pathol. 1990;21:414–23.

66. Winek RR, Scheithauer BW, Wick MR. Meningioma: meningeal haemangiopericytoma (angioblastic meningioma), peripheral haemangiopericytoma and acoustic schwannoma: a comparative immunohistochemical study. Am J Surg Pathol. 1989;13:251–61.

67. Russel DS, Rubinstein LJ. Pathology of tumours of the nervous system, 5th edn. London: Edward Arnold; 1989:474–9.

68. Sze G, Soletsky S, Bronen R, Krol G. MR imaging of the cranial meninges with emphasis on contrast enhancement and meningeal carcinomatosis. AJNR. 1989;10:965–75.

69. Frank JA, Girton M, Dwyer AJ et al. Meningeal carcinomatosis in the VX2 rabbit tumor model: detection with Gd-DTPA-enhanced MR imaging. Radiology. 1988;167:825–9.

70. Romaniuk CS. Case report: granulocytic sarcoma (chloroma) presenting as a cerebellopontine angle mass. Clin Radiol. 1992;45:284–5.

71. Jazy FK, Shehata WM, Tew JM et al. Primary intracranial lymphoma of the dura. Arch Neurol. 1980;37:528–9.

72. Crawford SC, Harnsberger HR, Lufkin RB et al. The role of Gd-DTPA in the evaluation of extracranial head and neck mass lesions. Radiol Clin N Am. 1989;27:219–42.

73. Kaneko D, Irikura T, Taguchi Y et al. Intracranial plasmacytoma arising from the dura. Surg Neurol. 1982;17:295–300.

74. Huk WJ, Heindl W. Intracranial tumors. In: Huk WJ, Gademan G, Friedman G, eds. MRI of central nervous system diseases. Berlin: Springer-Verlag; 1990:228–76.

75. Gold JH, Shelburne JD, Bossen EH. Meningeal mycosis fungoides: cytologic and ultrastructural aspects. Acta Cytol. 1976;20:349–55.

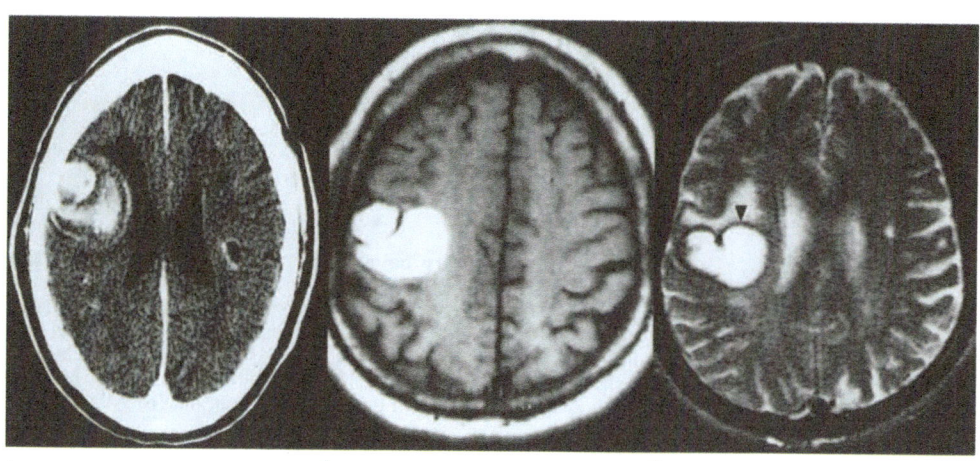

a   b   c

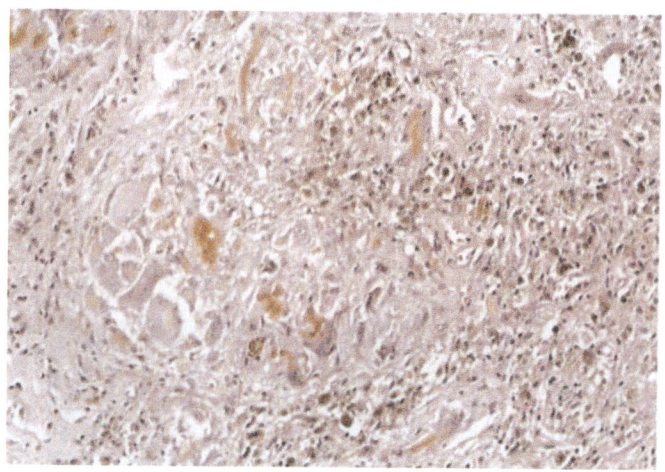

d

Figure 4.1 **Spontaneous haematoma, aetiology undetermined**: (**a**) CT + C, (**b**) T1WI, (**c**) T2WI, (**d**) HE × 200; CT shows ring-enhancing lesion containing two circumscribed hyperdense components suggesting two phases of haemorrhage. T1/T2 hyperintensity is consistent with subacute haemorrhage. Peripheral hypointense rim (arrow – c) is due to paramagnetic T2 signal shortening caused by haemosiderin pigment (d)

4.1. FOCAL VASCULAR LESIONS

4.1a. Spontaneous haematoma

Besides the crucial information of topography, imaging provides a dynamic view of haematoma morphology whose microscopic correlates are increasingly expected of the neuropathologist. The CT scanner has a particular and enduring use in the demonstration of clotted or sedimented blood (provided mineralization is not a consideration), but is being overtaken by MR, together with the extraordinary complexities which that modality has brought to the subject of intracranial haemorrhage.

Any spontaneous, non-ganglionic, parenchymal haematoma in a normotensive individual in whom (usually on account of topography or negative angiography) aneurysm is not suspected, raises the possibility of angioma, angiopathy or tumour. Such accessible, solitary haematomas are frequently evacuated for diagnostic or therapeutic reasons, the latter category including the so-called *'chronic, expanding haematoma'*[1] (Figure 4.1). The diagnosis of this lesion requires the demonstration of active granulation tissue with evidence of ongoing haemorrhage. The principal difference, when there is such,

between spontaneous haematoma of unknown but presumably angiopathic cause and the haemorrhage due to vascular malformation or tumour is in clot inhomogeneity – a feature very much more apparent on MR than CT. In addition, both these latter haemorrhages tend to exhibit contrast enhancement on CT (section 4.12). Although the presence of hypointense foci within an area of T1 hyperintensity, together with insignificant, or absence of, peripheral T2 shortening (haemosiderin) are quoted as useful pointers to haemorrhagic neoplasms[2], there is no doubt that haemorrhages of different aetiologies may have identical morphology, and in our own experience, age, blood pressure, chest X-ray and topography are crucial to the imaging diagnosis.

4.1b. Non-haemorrhagic (occult) angioma

For more than a decade, contrast-enhanced CT, almost invariably followed by angiography, has been the primary diagnostic means for identifying relatively large (20 mm across) arteriovenous malformations; pathological examination of the excised arteriovenous malfunction (AVM) is then a routine procedure, adding nothing to either diagnosis or management. However, the radiologic concept of angiographically occult cerebral vascular malformations (AOCVM)[3] has greatly increased both the morphological and therapeutic interest in a class of small, deep parenchymal angioma, usually of capillary-cavernous type. Some of these, as already mentioned, present as spontaneous haematomas, others with seizures or focal disturbance; whether haemorrhagic or not, the surgeon may use microscopic dissection in an attempt to locate an abnormal vascular structure, and will want a specific diagnosis. Non-haemorrhagic forms of AOCVM usually present as solitary hyperdense, sometimes mottled masses on CT, about 15 mm across, or larger, exhibiting mild

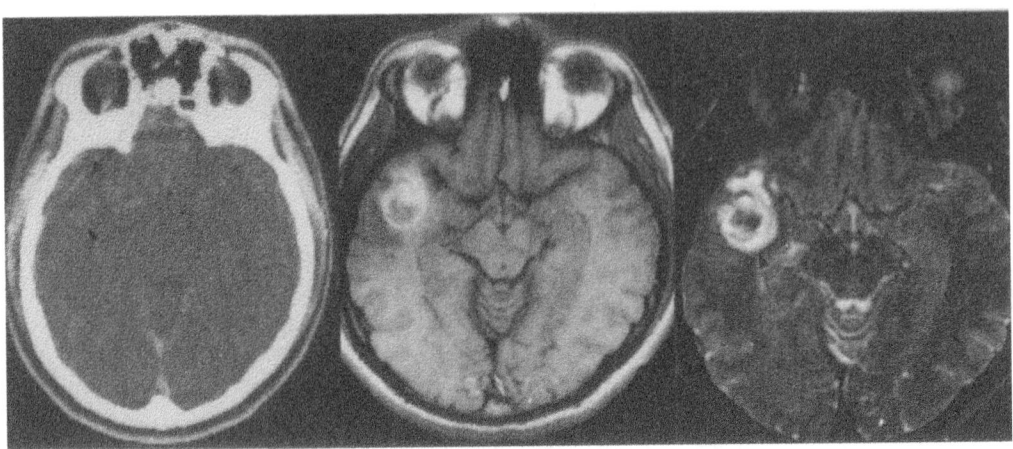

a   b   c

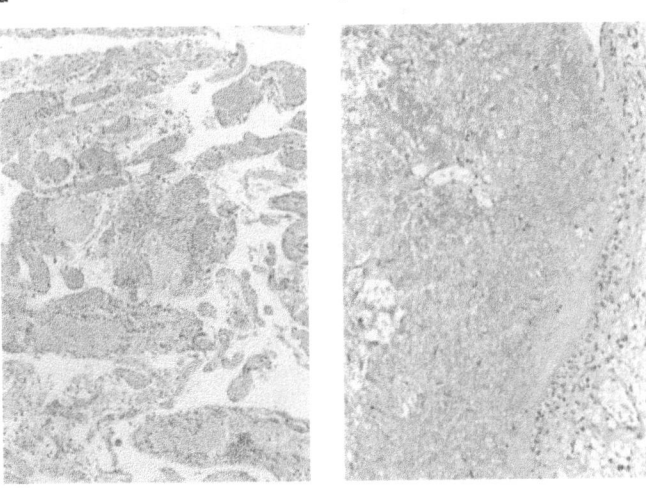

Figure 4.2 Capillary/cavernous angioma, angiographically negative: (a) CT + C, (b) PD, (c) T2WI, (d) EVG ×100, (e) HE ×200; CT shows poorly defined, feebly enhancing temporal lesions (arrows). MR features include T1/T2 hyperintensity (thrombus), with central signal void (flowing blood); surrounding parenchymal hyperintensity is oedema (c, arrows). Excision biopsy revealed a capillary/cavernous angioma (d) and organizing haematoma (e)

d   e

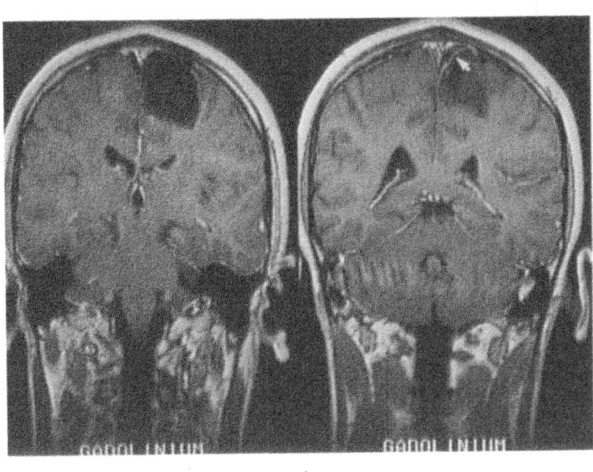

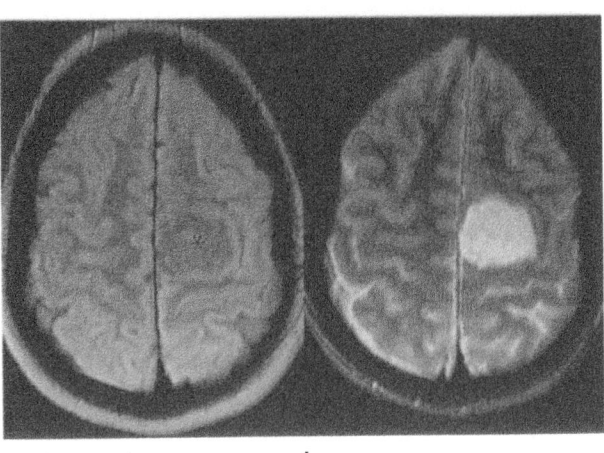

a   b   c   d

Figure 4.3 Epidermoidoma, hemisphere: (a,b) T1WI + C, (c) PDWI, (d) T2WI; convexity cyst, possibly continuous with the dura at the vertex; signal intensity of contents resembles CSF on T1 and T2 weighted images becoming characteristically inhomogeneously hyperin- tense (relative to CSF) on PD weighted image (c, asterisk). Superficial part of cyst shows slight enhancement (b, arrow). At operation surface of lesion was typically pearly, with flaky keratin contents (see Figure **2.11**)

diffuse or ring enhancement in about 75% of cases[4]. On MR there is a fairly characteristic mixture of signal intensities arising from combinations of blood stasis, thrombosis, collagen, iron and calcium deposition, and pathological alteration of surrounding brain parenchyma (Figure 4.2). Two of the most consistent features include central, sometimes lobular, hyperintense foci on both T1 and T2 images, presumed to be thrombosis (or methaemoglobin, at least), and a hypointense rim on the late T2 sequence, due to haemosiderin deposition[5]; if multiple, MR of these lesions is considered pathognomonic.

The classical separation of cavernous angioma and capillary telangiectasis[6] continues to be questioned because of the existence of mixed or transitional forms, i.e. the presence of dilated capillaries separated by brain parenchyma, in association with the aggregated, contiguous channels of cavernous type; or else cavernous channels which themselves are not contiguous. In a recent review of this problem the term 'cerebral capillary malformation' has been suggested[7]. The histology of a typical capillary–cavernous angioma is illustrated in Figures 4.2 and 5.32.

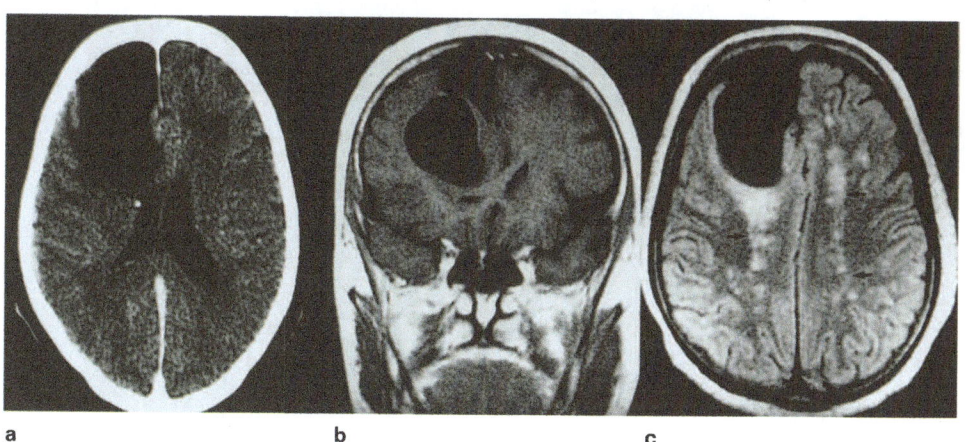

a   b   c

Figure 4.4 Benign brain cyst, frontal lobe: female, 60 years, presenting with chronic seizures. (**a**) CT + C, (**b**) coronal T1WI, (**c**) axial PDWI; MR shows lesions to be loculated, with superficial and deep components, deeper cyst appearing to be under pressure and exerting mass effect. T2WI shows bilateral signal abnormality in the boundary zones (arrows), hence cyst thought to have ischaemic pathogenesis. Surgeon found nothing to biopsy

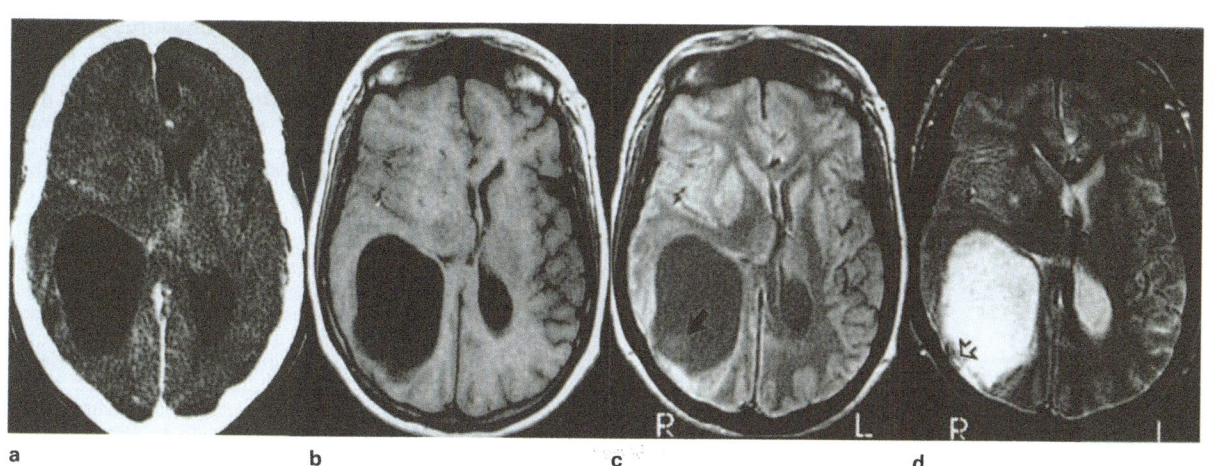

a   b   c   d

Figure 4.5 Cysticercosis, granulomatous cyst: (**a**) CT + C, (**b**) T1WI, (**c**) PDWI, (**d**) T2WI, (**e**) HE ×100; non-enhancing occipital lobe complex cyst, with small internal peripheral mass visible only on PDWI (c). This was part of a larger, invisible germinal tissue cyst which completely filled the cavity (e). A superficial nodule, excised from the meninges (d, arrow), showed granulomatous inflammation

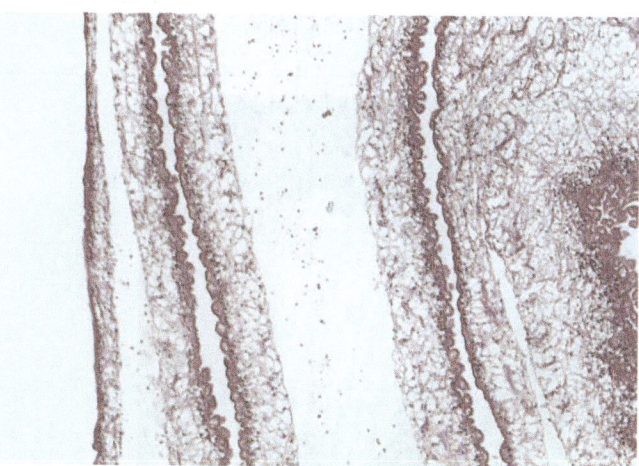

e

4.2. PRIMARY CYSTS (Developmental)

Our approach to the characterization of developmental cysts is discussed in section 3.1. Properly intraparenchymal lesions are occasionally reported, including dermal inclusion (Figure 4.3) and simple epithelial types[8,9], but without MR, the exact anatomical relationships of these cysts remain in doubt, and the majority of examples are found within the lateral and third ventricles, comprising particularly colloid and choroidal neuroepithelial types (see section 4.10h).

Benign brain cyst has been defined as intraparenchymal, having no lining except normal brain, and no communication with the subarachnoid space or ventricle[10,11]. The lesion may be solitary or loculated, CSF isodense/isointense, non-enhancing on CT, and typically exhibits mass effect (Figure 4.4).

4.3. PARASITIC CYSTS (see also section 3.3)

Cysticercosis, coenurosis and hydatidosis may all give rise to large, CSF isointense cysts, but the former are usually somewhat irregular, whilst solitary hydatid cyst has a uniquely tidy, almost circular profile (Figures 4.5, 4.6 and 4.7). Although all may contain smaller cysts, these have profoundly different surgical implications, since hydatid germinal tissue and protoscolices are transplantable, whilst the cysticercus bladder is invariably sterile, even if a mural nodule is demonstrable[12]. Coenurus is likewise frequently sterile. These large parasitic cysts may or may not exhibit enhancement which, when present, denotes granulomatous inflammation and, in the case of hydatid, forms an inflammatory pseudocapsule generally adherent to the lamellated ectocyst (Figure 4.7). The fluid accumulation between the brain and parasitic cyst is partly exudative, having a higher protein content than CSF, with signal shortening at short TR; similar changes in cyst content presage necrosis of germinal tissue. The morphology of intraventricular cyst growth and decay is similar to that of the extra–intraparenchymal environment.

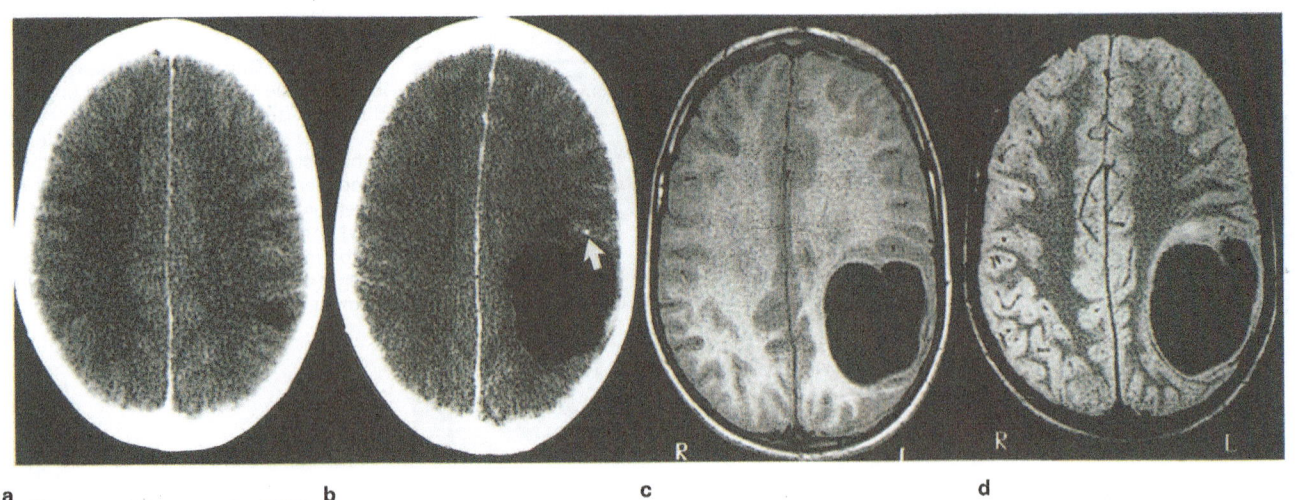

a   b   c   d

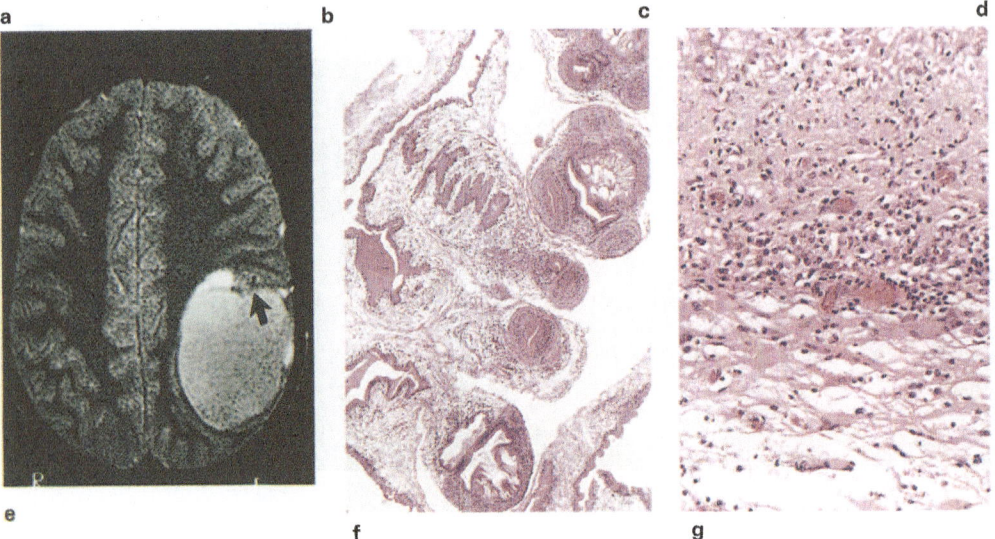

e   f   g

Figure 4.6 **Coenurus granulomatous cyst**: male, 11 years, presenting with seizures; (**a,b**) CT + C, (**c**) T1WI, (**d**) PDWI, (**e**) T2WI, (**f,g**) HE ×100; initial CT scan (a) shows a focal superficial non-enhancing hypodensity. Follow-up scans (b–e) 3 months later show a septated cyst with CSF isointense contents. Nodule (b, arrow) is partly mineralized on CT (signal void on all MR sequences (e, arrow) and is presumed to be a meningeal component of the granuloma. Contrast enhancement was negligible. At operation a single cyst with gliotic granulomatous inflammatory pseudocapsule was removed (g). The nodule (b, arrow) was not identified. Multiple protoscolices of indeterminate viability were present within the cyst (f)

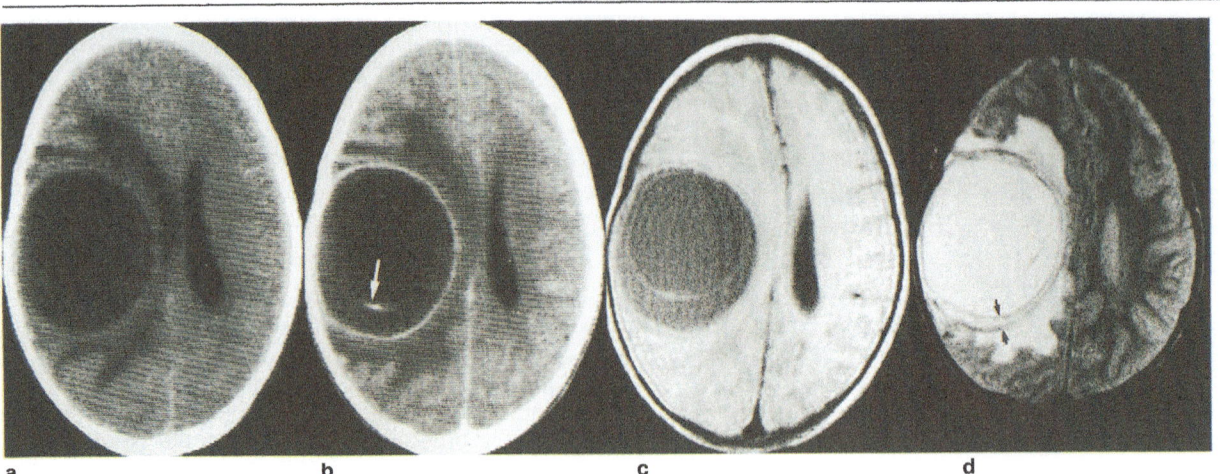

a   b   c   d

Figure 4.7 (*legend opposite*)

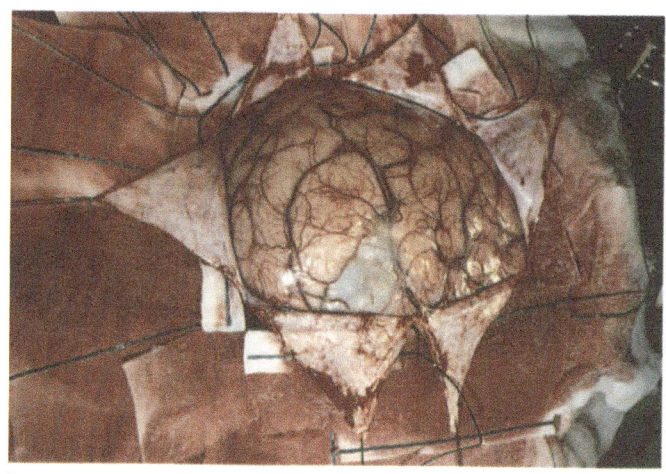

e

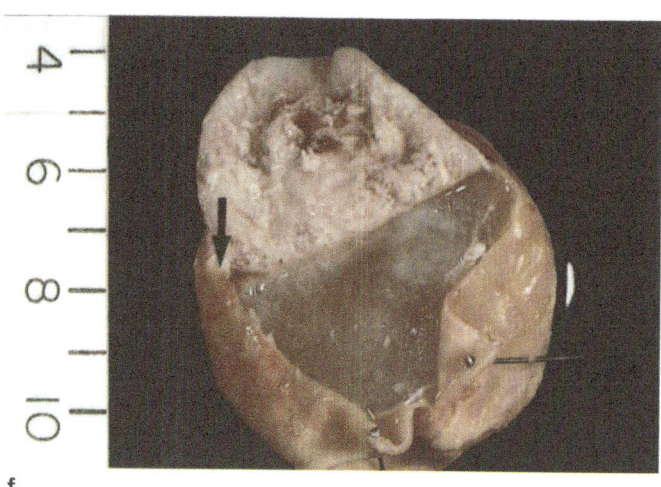

f

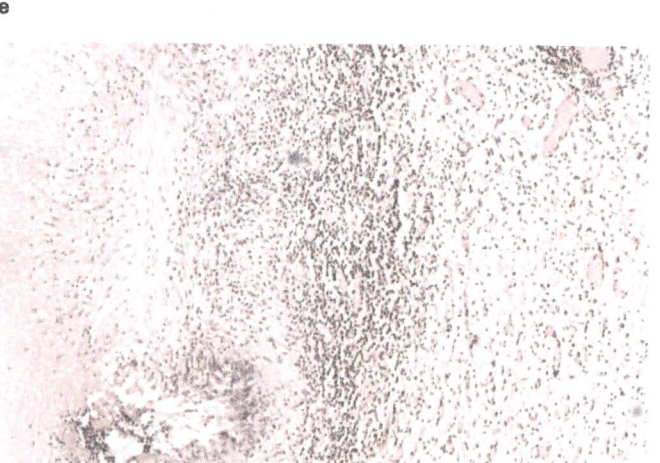

g

Figure 4.7 Hydatidosis, granulomatous cyst: (**a**) CT, (**b**) CT + C, (**c**) T1WI, (**d**) T2WI, (**e**) operative view, (**f**) fixed specimen, (**g**) HE ×100; CT shows large cyst reaching the surface of the brain with thin rim of enhancement and faintly visible internal cyst (b, arrow). T1WI shows differential signal intensity of internal and external cyst fluid. Ectocyst wall resolves as hypointense tram-lining on T2WI (d, arrow), with surrounding oedema hyperintensity. Operative view shows meningeal surface of cyst, with displaced cortex, possibly originally a sulcus. Sample from ectocyst wall (f, arrow) shows gliotic brain with a thick granulomatous inflammatory lining (g). Endocyst is viable hydatid, containing numerous protoscolices. (See section **4.4a** for discussion on tram-lining)

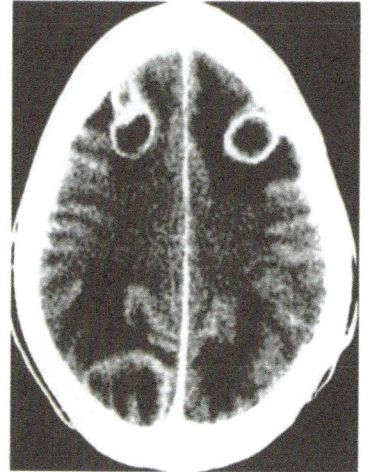

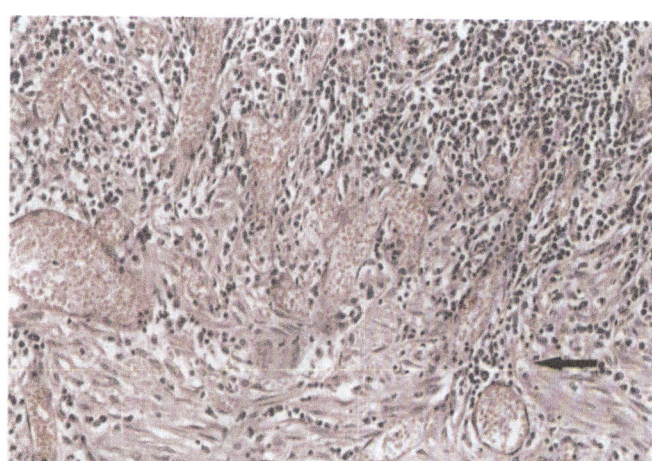

Figure 4.8 Pyogenic abscesses, haematogenous, boundary zone: patient with pulmonary TB and septic arthritis of the hip; enhanced CT shows variably shaped ring lesions with central hypodensity and vasogenic oedema. Boundary zone distribution is characteristic of haematogenous spread

Figure 4.9 Pyogenic abscess: biopsy of abscess wall showing prolific thin-walled vessels emanating from vasoformative tissue (arrow) and largely mononuclear inflammatory infiltrate. HE ×200

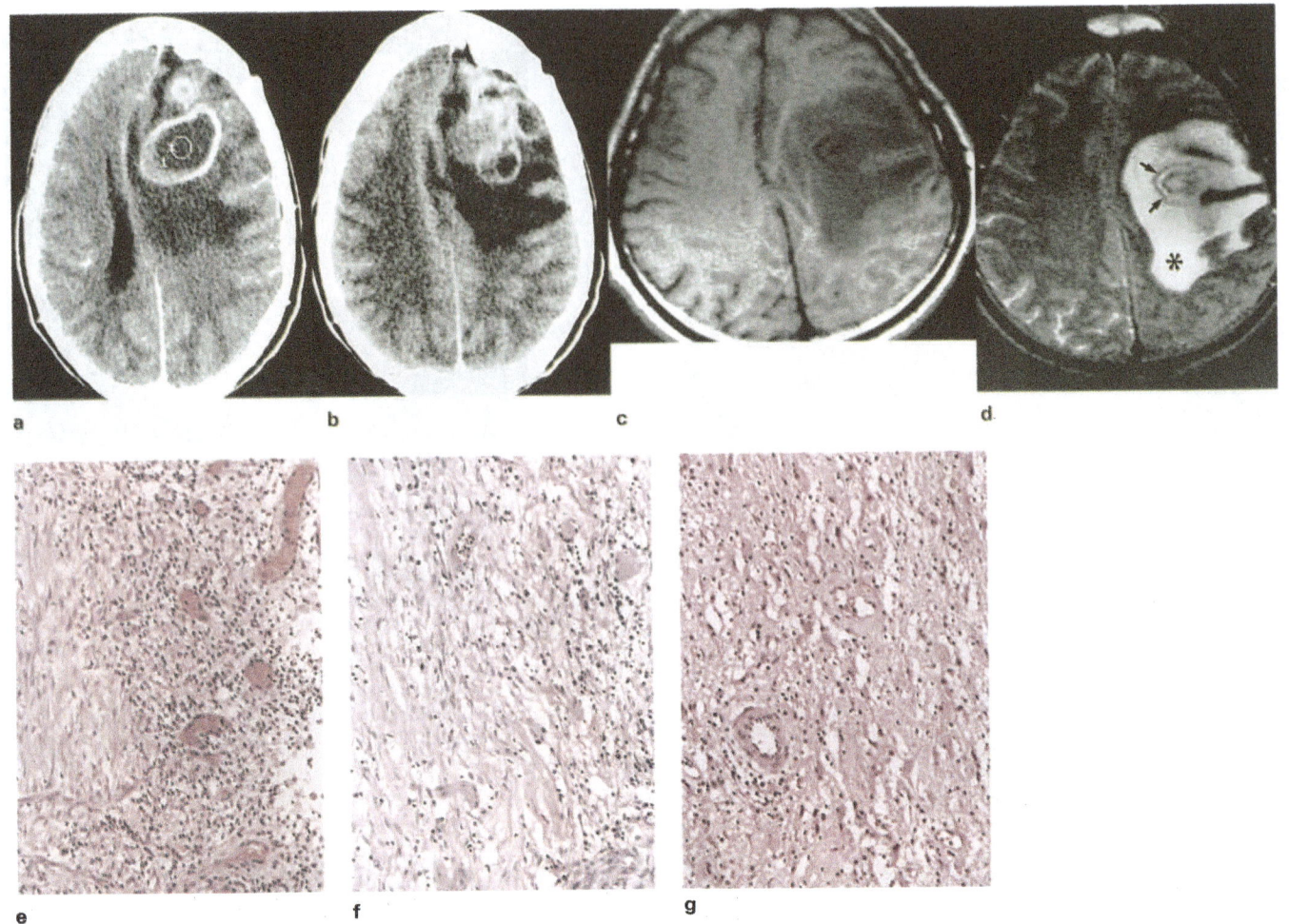

Figure 4.10 Abscess, post-traumatic, convexity: (**a,b**) CT + C, (**c**) T1WI, (**d**) T2WI, (**e–g**) all HE × 200; lesion site (superficial/convexity) and morphology (multilocular) are features which designate it as atypical; the penetrating component of the injury was not visible. MR shows concentric T2 hypointense bands with intervening hyperintense zone (arrows, d). T1 image is the reverse of this, i.e. tram-lines are isointense with intervening hypointense zone. Extensive surrounding T2 hyperintensity (asterisk) is vasogenic oedema. Excised abscess wall is 3–4 mm wide, and comprises a thin inner layer, approximately 200 μm width, composed of dilated capillaries with polymorph–macrophage infiltrate (e); external to this is a fibrovascular layer, 2 mm wide, mainly oedematous, but somewhat more compact internally (f); outermost zone consists of vascularized, oedematous brain, infiltrated by mononuclear inflammatory cells (g). T2 hyperintense band is presumably the oedematous, fibrous capsule. (See section **4.4a** for discussion on tram-lining)

4.4. INFLAMMATORY MASSES

4.4a. Abscess[13]

Pyogenic lesions of the frontal and temporal lobes, and cerebellum, which are derived from sepsis in the adjacent frontal and mastoid bones, are usually solitary, white-matter masses; when infection is haematogenous, lesions are characteristically multiple, distributed along the boundary zones (Figure 4.8), or rarely involve the diencephalon and brainstem. The capsules of these abscesses are routinely submitted to histology and show stereotyped features of collagenous granulation tissue infiltrated by polymorphonuclear and mononuclear cells (including variable numbers of plasma cells) (Figure 4.9). Vascularized collagen is always present, but varies according to chronicity, treatment and other factors, whilst the adjacent brain parenchyma is oedematous and contains reactive astrocytes. Although enhanced CT demonstrates a range of size and capsule thickness in pyogenic brain abscess, parasitic or tuberculous aetiology should always be considered in smaller, round–oval lesions, less than 20 mm in diameter, and situated toward the cortex (section 4.4c).

The pathology of inflammatory liquefactive necrosis (suppurative encephalitis), as seen in autopsy material in association with acute infective endocarditis and septic embolism, is the same process demonstrated experimentally to be the initial stage of brain abscess, and correlates well with clinical CT[14]. Once the inflammatory gliomesodermal response or abscess wall is established, the lesion is characterized on CT by its tidy, enhancing rim, hypodense contents and surrounding hypodense, volumetric expansion of brain (vasogenic oedema)[15] (Figure 4.10). MR reveals the abscess capsule as slightly T1-hyperintense, but strikingly hypointense on the late T2 sequences, owing to the signal hyperintensity externally of vasogenic oedema, and internally of liquefactive necrosis. Enhancement on MR is practically identical to CT. Although the physical basis of capsular T2 signal shortening is unsettled, examination of the wall of the lesion shown in Figure 4.10, in which hypointense tramlines are apparent, indicates that the fibrovascular component is in fact T2 hyperintense, supporting the suggested paramagnetic effect of some component of the inflammatory infiltrate[16].

4.4b. Atypical abscess (see also section 4.4c)

The designation of brain abscesses (or focal, necrotizing infection) as typical or atypical, arising from characteristics of morphology and topography on imaging, serves as a useful pointer to unusual infections[17]. In the cerebellum,

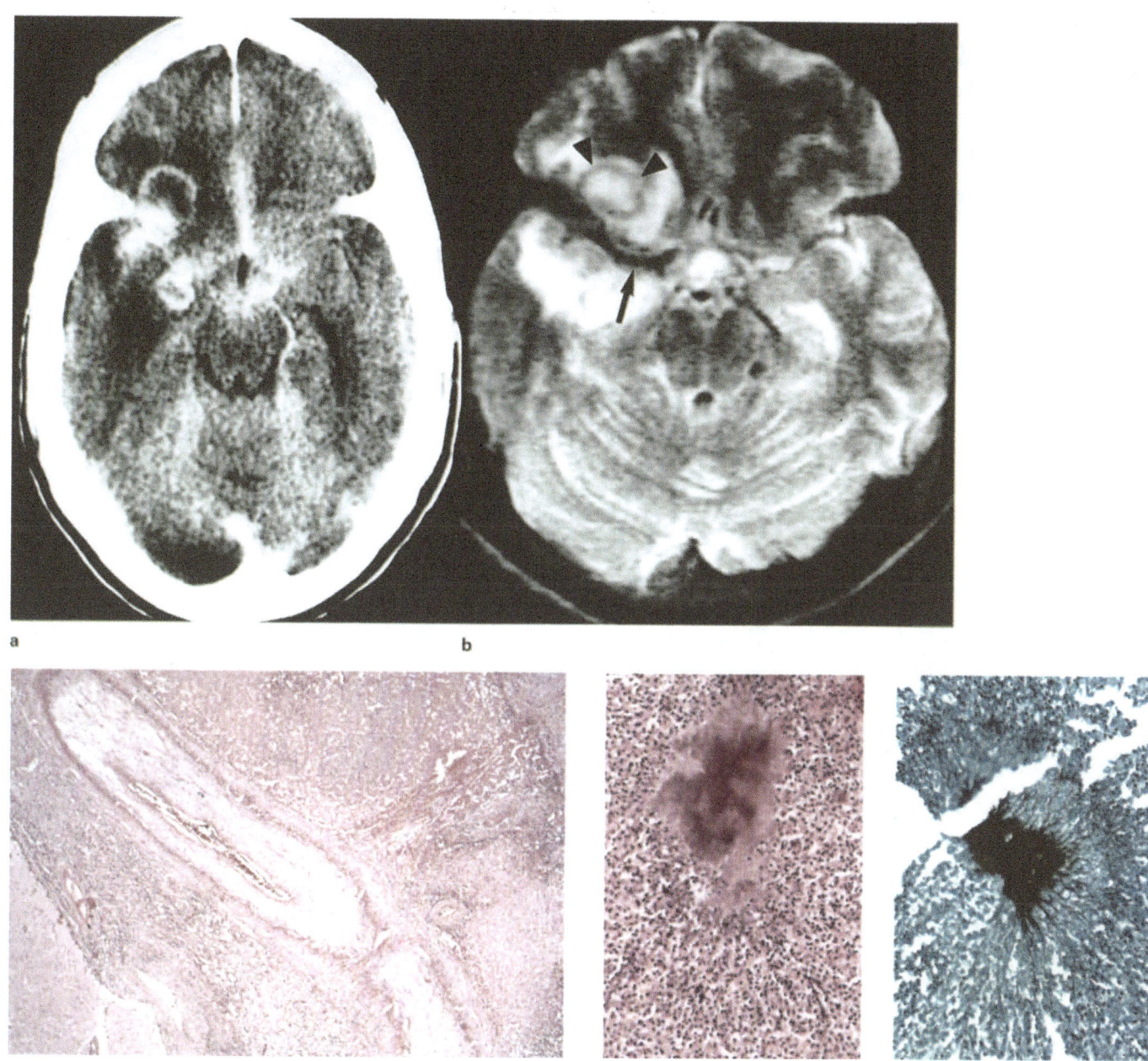

Figure 4.11 Granulomatous abscess, actinomycosis: male, 55 years; subacute meningitic illness and axillary lymphadenopathy; (**a**) CT + C, (**b**) T2WI, (**c**) HE ×40, (**d**) HE/MS ×200; contrasted CT shows basal enhancement, with solid/ring-enhancing lesions in Sylvian fissure and adjacent frontotemporal parenchyma, and vasogenic oedema. T2 image shows inflammatory granulation tissue-hypointensity of the fissure (arrow) and abscess walls (arrow-heads), delineated by diffuse hyperintensity of oedematous parenchyma. Low-power view of Sylvian fissure (c) shows obliteration of the subarachnoid space by inflammatory granulation tissue, endarteritic vessel and focally necrotic exudate; colonies present within exudate (d), but not granulomatous tissue, do not appear to have shortened the T2 signal of abscess contents

multilocularity of primary pyogenic abscess is usual (Figure 6.11), but with the exception of trauma this is much less obtrusive in the hemispheres. Thus, features denoting atypicality include inappropriate topography, such as basal meningocerebral and deep grey-matter sites, multiloculation and targetoid enhancement (Figures 4.11, 4.12, 4.13, 4.14, 4.15 and 6.12). The importance of this imaging concept to surgical neuropathology is that it implies the need to identify granulomatous inflammation and its aetiology. Under these circumstances management is likely to be based on histopathological findings sooner than microbiology (Figure 4.14).

4.4c. Granuloma

Examination of granulomas of different aetiologies in fixed brain specimens leaves us in no doubt that, contrary to imaging opinion, the majority are meningeal or cerebro-meningeal in location (Figures 3.9 and 3.10). Properly intraparenchymal lesions, by comparison, are rare (Figures 4.16 and 4.17).

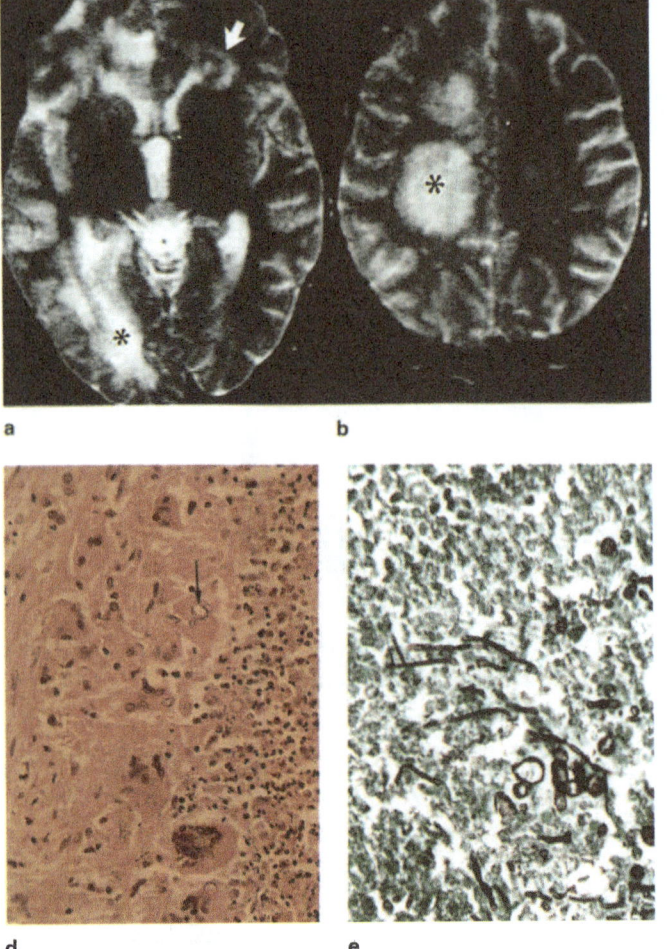

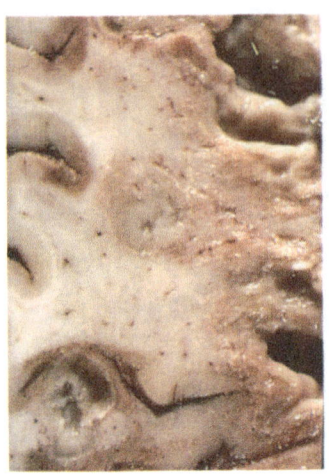
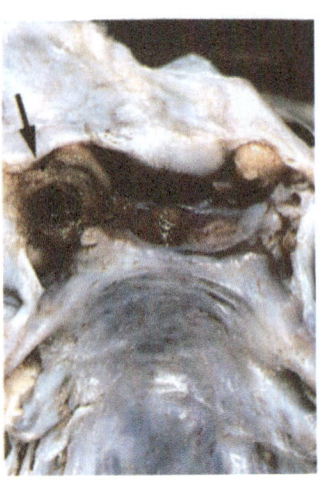

Figure 4.12 Granulomatous abscess/necrotizing encephalitis, aspergillus: (a,b) T2WI, (c) fixed brain slice/internal carotid artery, (d) HE ×400, (e) MS ×400; images show multiple areas of signal abnormality, including vasogenic oedema (a, asterisk), abscess (a, arrow) and circumscribed white matter lesions (b, asterisk), subsequently shown at autopsy to consist of diffusely proliferating fungus (e). Fixed autopsy specimens show focal and confluent white-matter abscesses (c, left) and internal carotid artery thrombosis (c, arrow). Histology shows organisms to be both within abscess walls (d) and exudate (e)

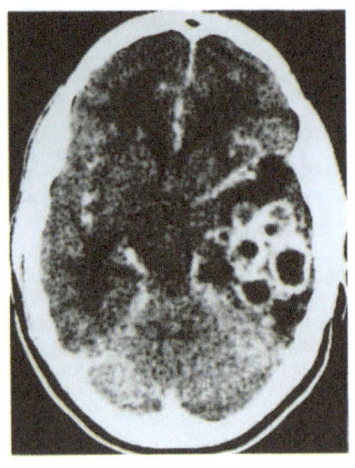

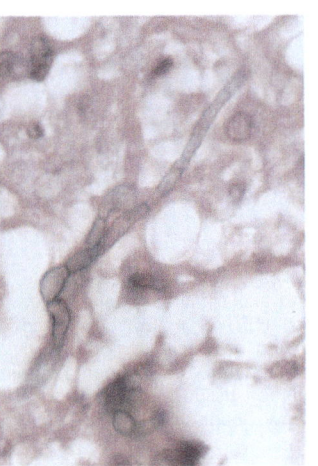
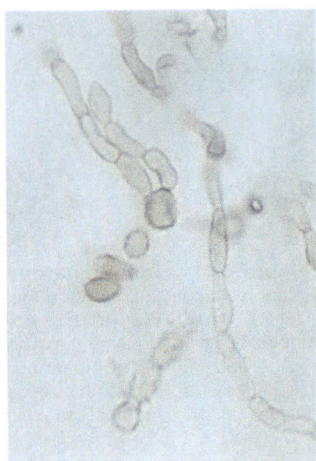

Figure 4.13 Granulomatous abscess, cladosporiosis: male, 20 years; headache, seizures, inflammatory CSF; (a) CT + C, (b) HE/ unstained ×1000; abscesses occupy the basal temporal lobe (meningo- cerebral), forming a honeycomb-like cluster, with contiguous cavities of different size. Definitive diagnosis was made only on histology, where pigmented fungal elements were seen (b)

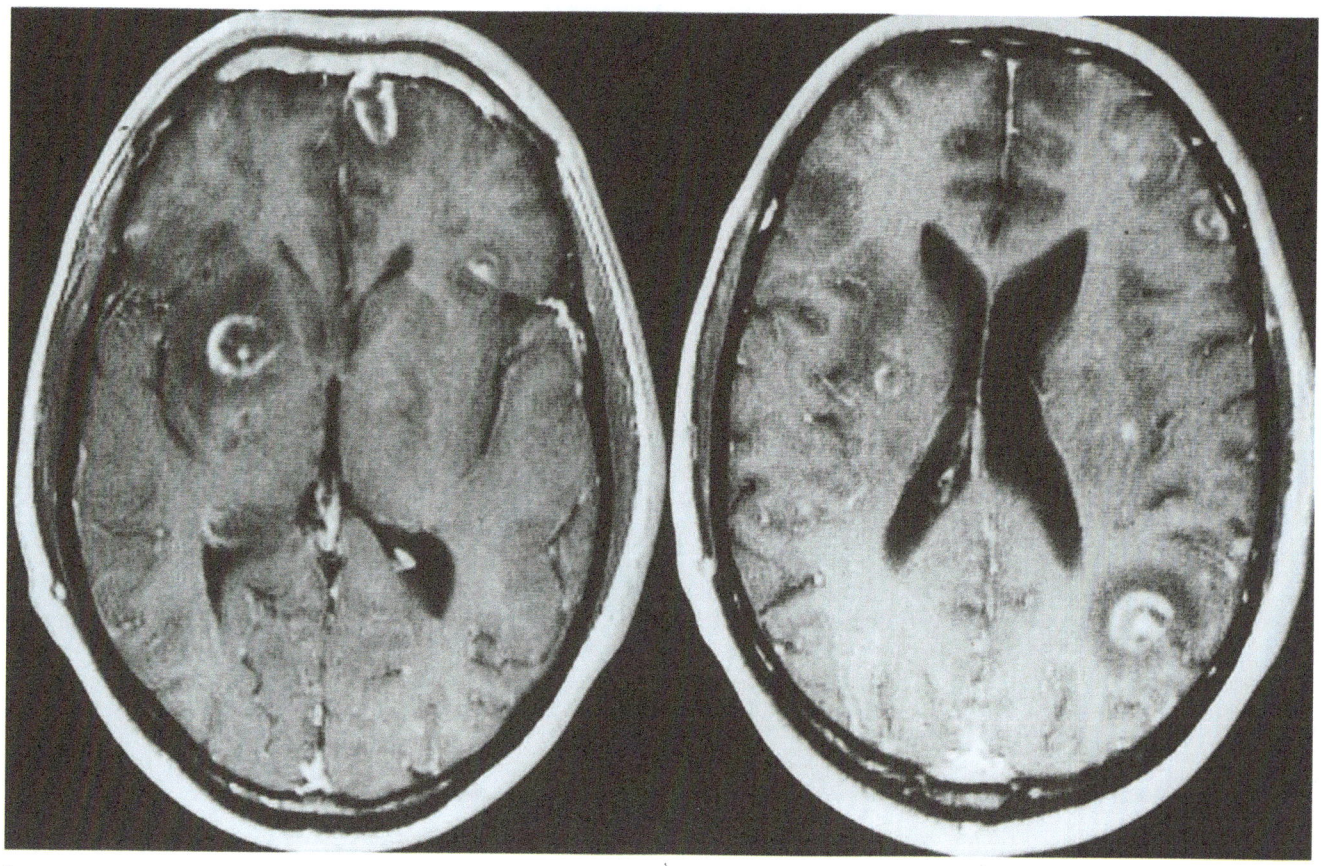

a

b

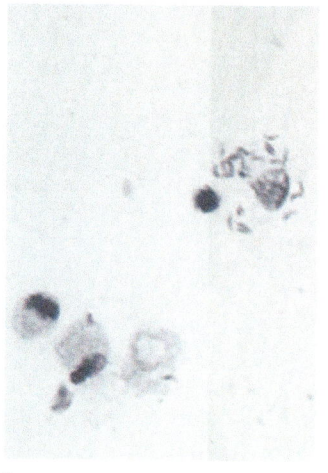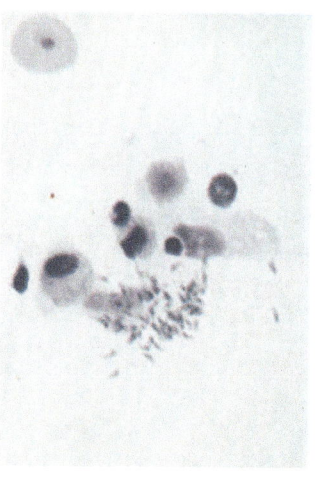

c

Figure 4.14 Enhancing target lesions, AIDS-related toxo-plasmosis: (a,b) T1WI + C, **(c)** Tol blue × 100; multiple ring lesions, some with internal target-like enhancement. The presumptive diagnosis of toxoplasmosis was made on positive serology and response to therapy; in the event such lesions are likely to be ring-enhancing infarcts, centred on thrombosed and inflamed blood vessels. (Smear preparation from a similar case shows tachyzoites being shed from unidentified cells – c)

4.5. DEMYELINATION[18]

Solitary demyelinative lesions constitute a significant imaging diagnostic problem, and may occasionally be indistinguishable from neoplasm or granuloma, including strong diffuse or peripheral enhancement and mass effect[19] (Figure 4.18). Active lesions, identified by sequential and correlative studies[20,21], demonstrate enhancement over a period of 6–12 weeks, corresponding to an evanescent vasculopathy (probably venular) with parenchymal macrophage infiltration. T1 hypointensity/T2 hyperintensity is consistent with oedema in the initial phase of demyelination, and spongiosis in late active or healed lesions. Neutral lipid is proposed to account for central T2 hypointensity reported in some large ring-enhancing plaques, and may explain the weak signal abnormality in the spinal cord lesion illustrated in Figure 7.21.

4.6. GLIAL NEOPLASMS OF THE HEMISPHERE, HYPOTHALAMUS AND DIENCEPHALON
(excluding pineal region, section 4.8)

According to Russell and Rubinstein[22] about 40% of adult primary (CNS) neoplasms are gliomas, usually situated in the hemispheres; in childhood the same overall incidence applies, but distribution is almost equally divided between the supra- and infratentorial compartments. Paediatric tumours possess, in addition, a number of distinctive morphological and biological features associated with their origin from the phylogenetically older and more central secondary germinal areas of the CNS, where considerable postnatal cellular proliferation occurs[23,24]. These histogenetic factors account for the differences seen in childhood neuroepithelial tumours, compared to conventional adult gliomas, as exemplified by the topographic prevalence of midline[25,26], brainstem[27–29] and cerebellar lesions[30]; the frequency of pilocytic astrocytomas and medulloblastomas; and the occurrence of mixed gliomas, primitive neuroectodermal and cerebromeningeal tumours.

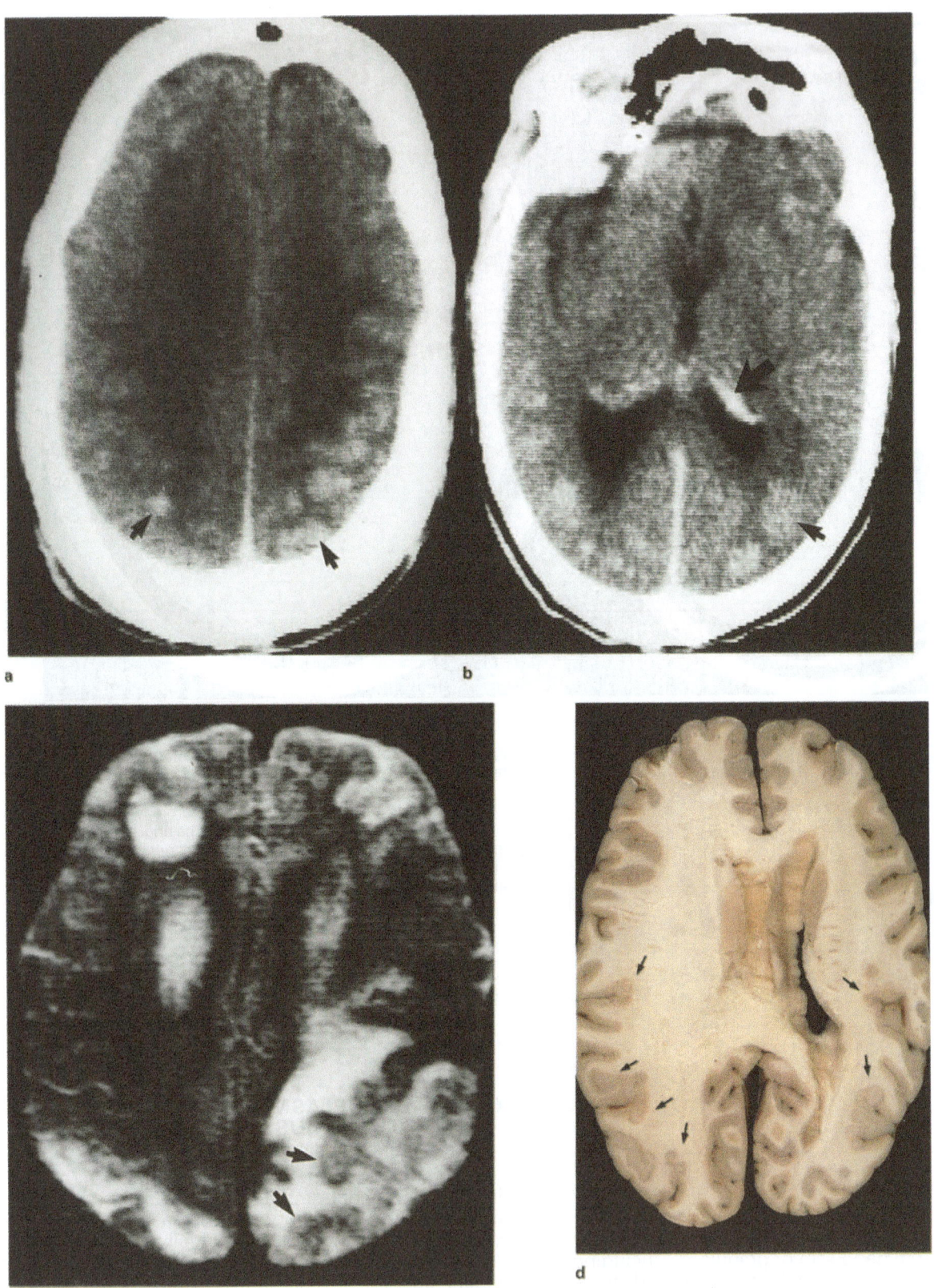

Figure 4.15 Atypical/complex granuloma, cryptococcoma and choroid plexitis: (**a,b**) CT + C, (**c**) T2WI, (**d**) fixed brain slice (sides reversed), (**e**) HE × 40; images show multiple poorly defined, enhancing, superficial nodules (a,b, arrows), with marked enhancement of choroid plexus (b, large arrow); T2 sequence (c) shows multiple inhomogeneous, targetoid lesions in the cerebral cortex, corresponding to discrete centrally punctate, cortical granulomata shown in fixed specimen (d); histology shows non-necrotizing perivascular cryptococcal aggregates and peripheral inflammation (e)

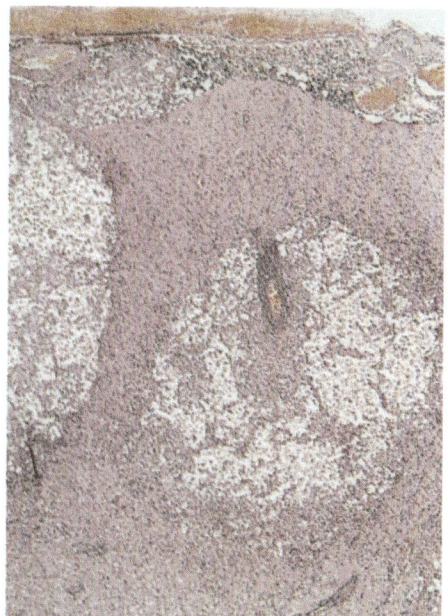

Figure 4.15(e)

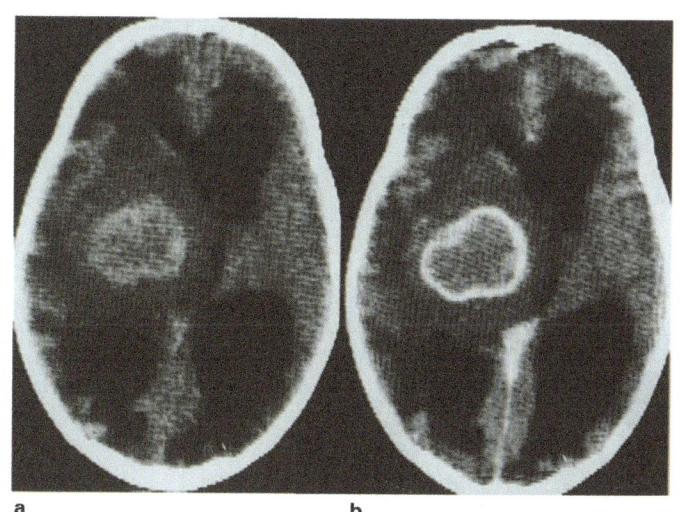

a   b

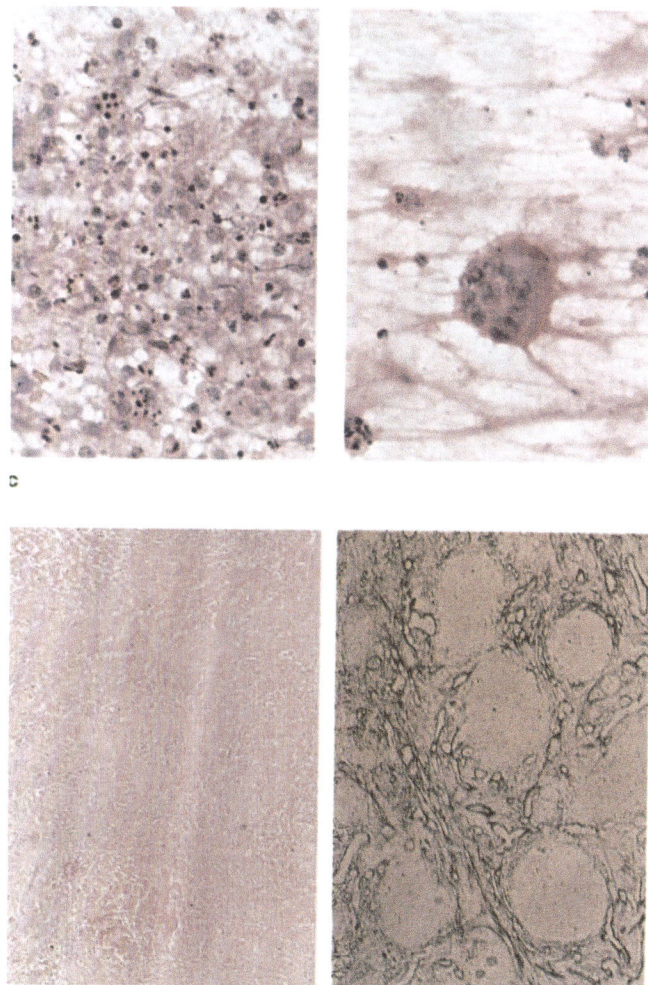

d   e

Figure 4.16 Gummatous granuloma, deep grey matter: (**a**) CT, (**b**) CT + C, (**c**) HE ×400, (**d**) HE ×200, (**e**) Retic ×100; images show cortex isodense mass (a), with strong peripheral enhancement. Smears show macrophages, nuclear debris and giant cells (c); necrosis is both gummatous and caseous (d,e)

However, although patient age provides an undeniably useful modifier in categorizing primary CNS neoplasms, it tends to hold true for glial tumours only at extremes, and the common microscopic morphologies of astrocytoma–malignant glioma–glioblastoma may be encountered from the first to the fifth decades. However, if topography, patient age and, where relevant, tumour size are taken together with imaging characteristics, microscopic morphology and immunohistochemistry, a set of parameters is obtained which may be said to constitute the ideal diagnosis (see the diagnostic approach). Furthermore, as is the experience of every neuropathologist, histological identification and grading of the gliomas is both restricted and complicated by the problem of sampling, particularly in the case of needle biopsy. Although the procedure of basing the poorest prognosis on features of anaplasia and necrosis remains sound[31], the assessment of well-differentiated glial cells, degrees of fibrillation, degenerative pleomorphism, and vascularity, in small (even tiny) tissue fragments, remains as problematic as ever. By comparison, the imaging diagnosis of glial neoplasia, including rough grading, is made with considerable confidence by contemporary radiologists and neurosurgeons, whose approach is increasingly eclectic, involving pathological and even ultrastructural considerations[32,33].

The correlative features of *glial neoplasms* are conveniently considered in terms of spin echo (T2) signal intensity and enhanced T1-weighted (short TR) images, even though these are manifestly interrelated.

Signal intensity
The basic tendency is to induce signal prolongation, most obviously in the long TR (T2) sequences (Figures 4.20 and 4.21). At short TR, hypointensity is often only a little more than grey matter. The mechanism is initially one of an expanded interstitial space resulting from the loss of the faculty of 'interstice occupation' (Figure 4.19), envisaged by us as it has been demonstrated in the experimental model[34]. Further, with alteration of structural specificity of tumour vessels (see below), particularly the capillary proliferation accompanying malignant transformation, the interstitial space is probably also widened by abnormal fluid accumulation (Figure 4.19). T2 hyperintensity is most marked in well-differentiated astrocytomas regardless of type, and is maximal in brightness and homogeneity with increasing parenchymal attenuation, or when the neoplasm undergoes microcystic degener

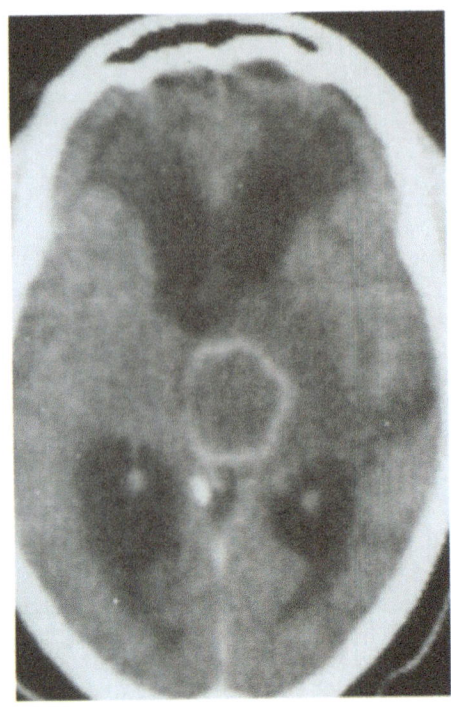

a

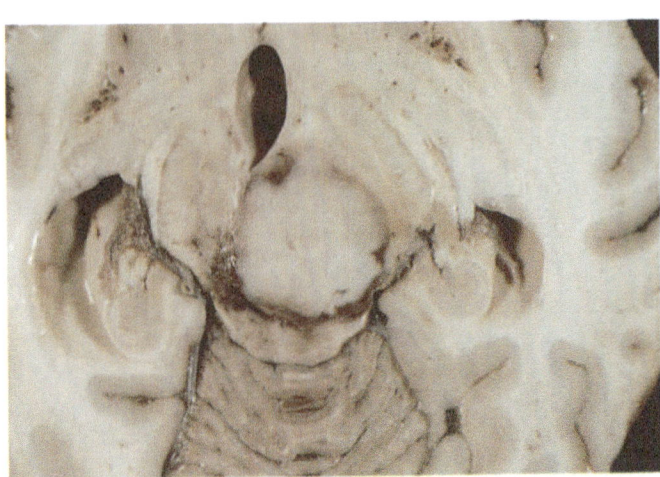

b

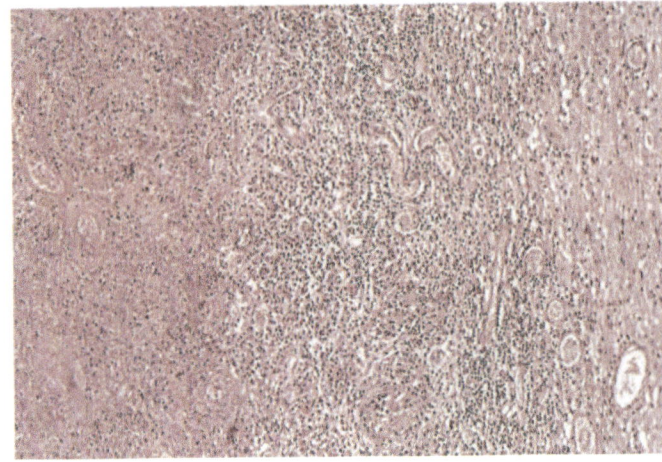

c

Figure 4.17 Gummatous granuloma, brainstem: (**a**) CT + C, (**b**) fixed autopsy specimen, (**c**) HE × 100; image shows characteristic ring-enhancing lesion with crenated outline and brain near isodense contents, matching the pale gummatous consistency of fixed specimen; histology shows vascularized, parenchymal granulomatous inflammation and gummatous necrosis

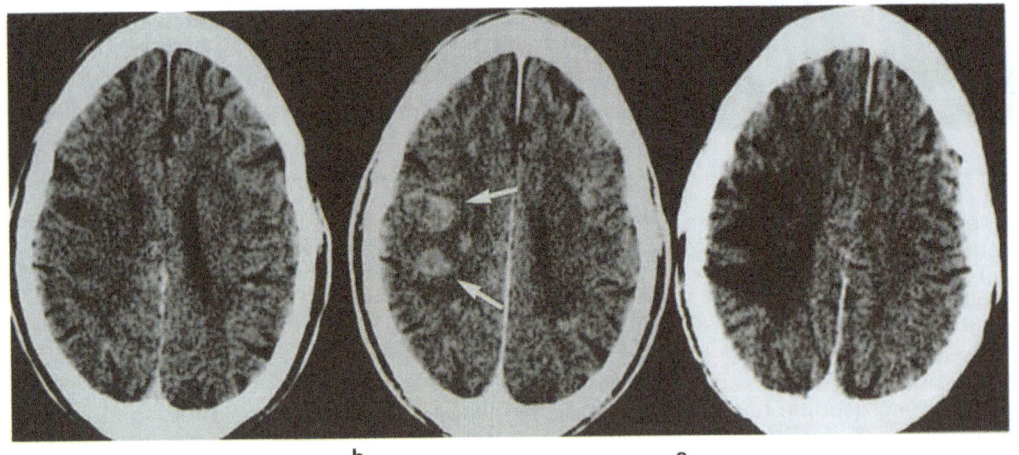

a   b   c

Figure 4.18 Demyelination: male, 48 years, acute paresis, headache and visual disturbance; CSF normal; (**a**) CT, (**b,c**) CT + C, (**d**) Tol blue × 400, (**e**) HELB × 200, (**f**) Palmgren × 200; multiple ill-defined hypodense foci, exhibiting feeble partial ring enhancement, with minimal mass effect (diagnosis of neoplasia was considered). Smear preparation (d) shows sheets of macrophages, with interlaced processes (axonal); characteristic demyelinative lesion is shown with combination stain (e): residual blue-staining myelinated fibres are seen at edge of plaque, separated by reactive macrophages and astrocytes; vein is surrounded by inflammatory cells and macrophages. Silver stain (f) reveals a network of surviving axons with intervening astrocytes. Follow-up scan at 8 weeks (c), showed resolution of lesions and residual spongiotic hypodensity

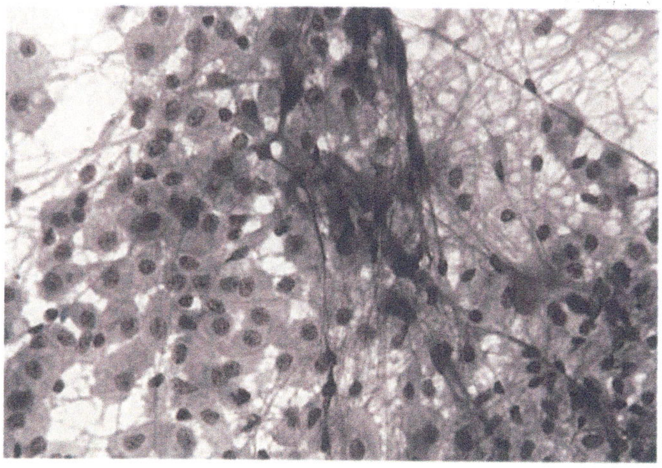

d

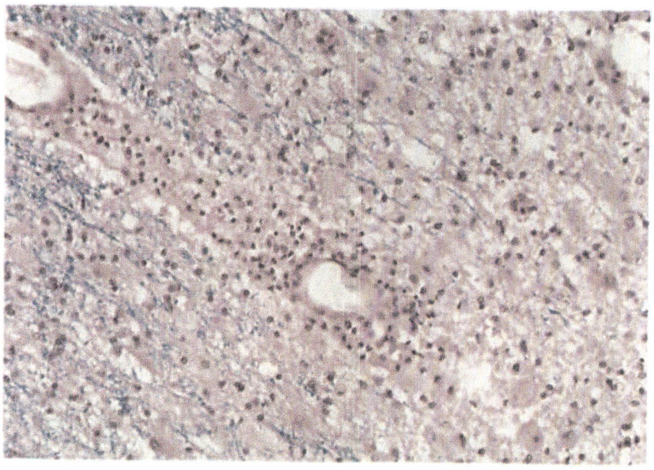

e

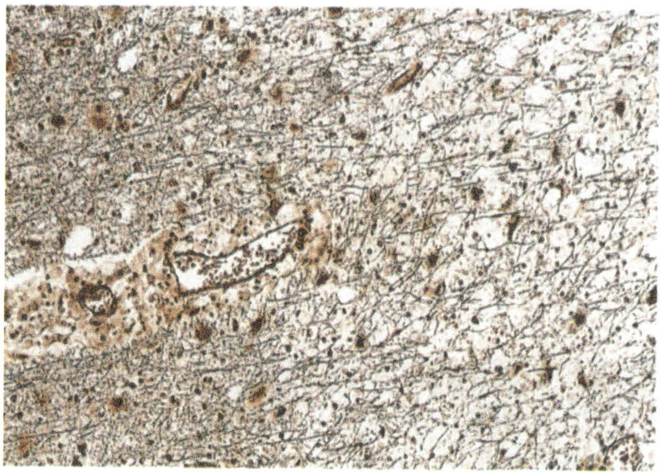

f

Figure 4.18 (*continued*)

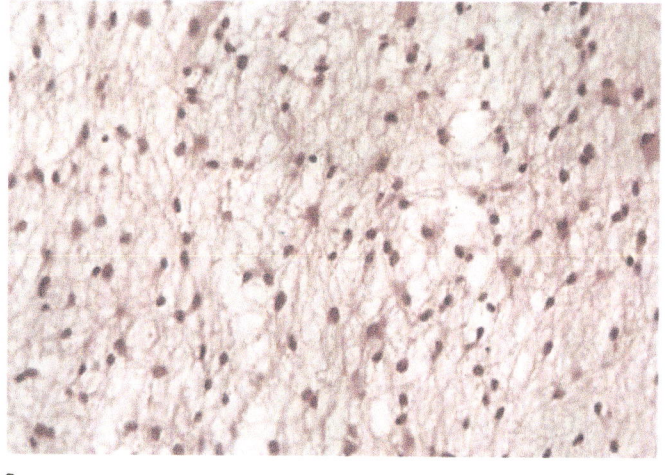

a

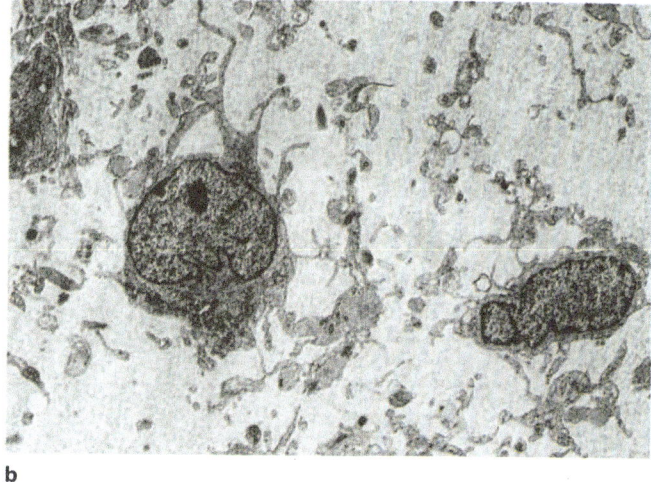

b

Figure 4.19 Astrocytoma: (a) HE ×400, (b) EM ×3250; paraffin section illustrates typical fibrillary astrocytes, whilst electron microscopy shows protoplasmic astrocytes with prominent intercellular space con-taining granular material having high spin density and protein hydration, responsible for hyperintensity on proton density and T2 weighted image

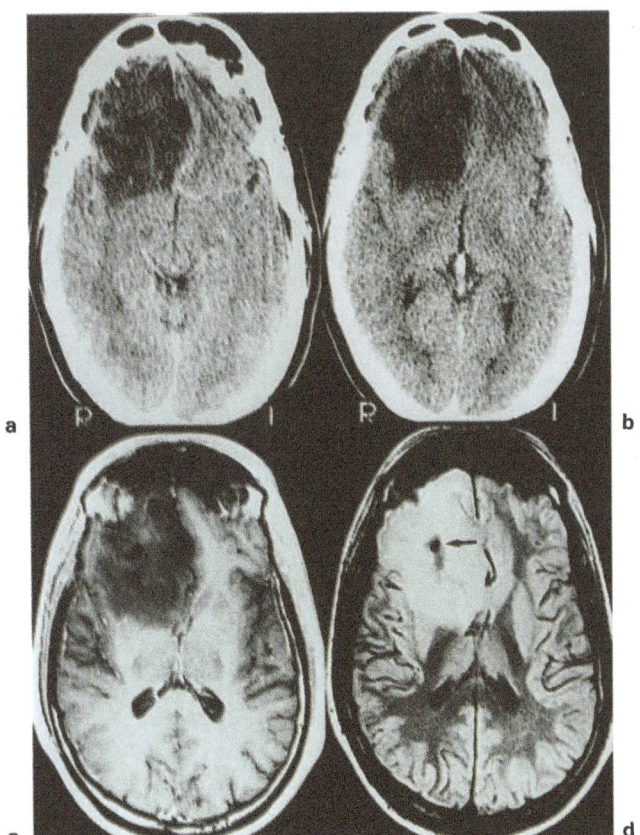

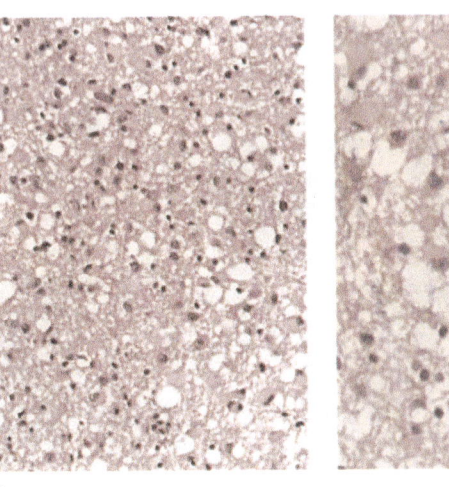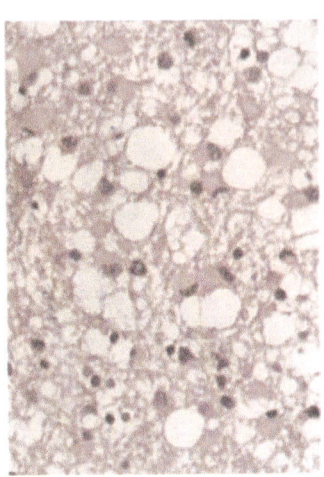

Figure 4.20 Astrocytoma, fibrillary, non-enhancing: (a) CT, (b) CT + C, (c) T1WI + C, (d) PDWI, (e) HE ×200/×400; large frontal, hypodense, T1 hypointense/T2 hyperintense, non-enhancing mass, with central cyst (d, arrow) (invisible at long TR/TE), involving grey and white matter. Histology shows fibrillary astrocytoma, with gemistocytic elements, microcystic change and striking absence of abnormal vessels. Combined imaging and morphological features are characteristic of astrocytoma of non-enhancing type

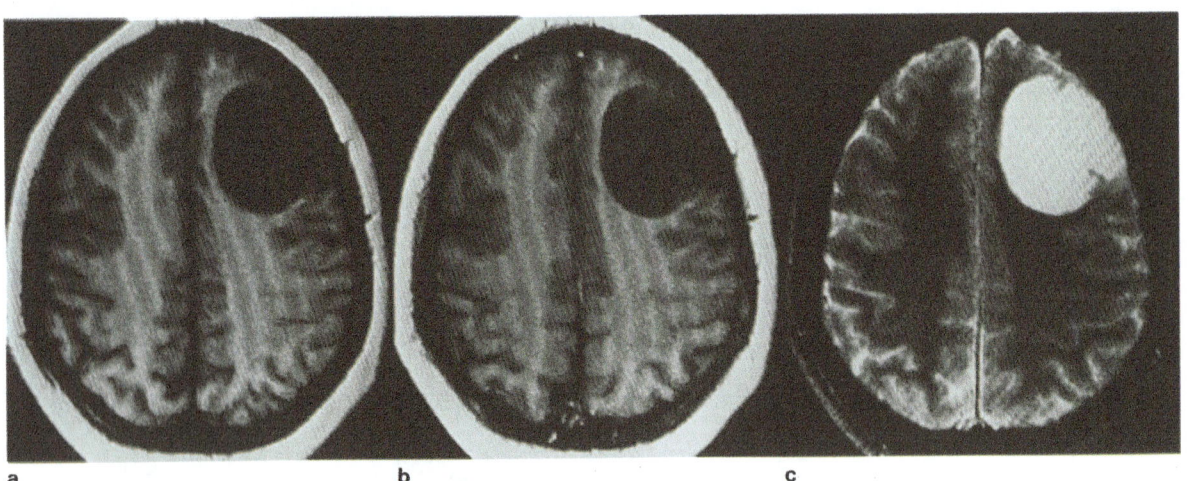

Figure 4.21 Astrocytoma, protoplasmic, non-enhancing: (a) T1WI, (b) T1WI + C, (c) T2WI; characteristic sharply circumscribed T1 hypointense/T2 hyperintense, non-enhancing tumour. Faintly structured inhomogeneity appearing on enhanced scan (b) is technical. Note absence of associated white matter oedema/hyperintensity in T2 weighted image (c). Histology typical of protoplasmic astrocytoma. (Dr RM Bowen, Groote Schuur Hospital)

ation. As is to be expected, the factors which diminish T2 signal intensity in an inhomogeneous manner include reticulin–collagen production and the effects of necrosis, haemorrhage and mineralization (Figure 4.29).

Enhancement
The gliomas exhibit three generally distinct responses to contrast administration: (1) no enhancement; (2) homogeneous enhancement, either diffuse or incomplete; (3) inhomogeneous enhancement (linear, serpiginous and ring forms). The basis of enhancement, comprising the triad of a vascular bed, capillary leakage and an

abnormal perivascular space[35,36], is discussed in Chapter 1. Our use of the term 'vascular structural specificity' refers mainly to the physical attributes of the blood–brain barrier, including tight junctions (zonulae occludentes), basal laminae and paucity of pinocytotic vesicles of parenchymal capillary endothelial cells. In tumours which are completely refractory to enhancement, including diffusely infiltrating or circumscribed astrocytoma (Figures 4.20 and 4.21), diffusely infiltrating oligodendroglioma (Figure 4.36), anaplastic astrocytoma (Figure 4.24) and gliomatosis, loss of structural specificity is precluded, in spite of a widened extracellular space. However, 'glioma vessel'

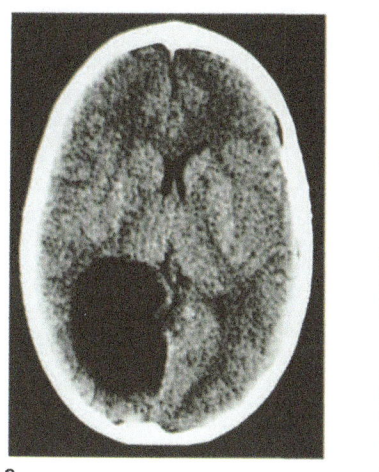
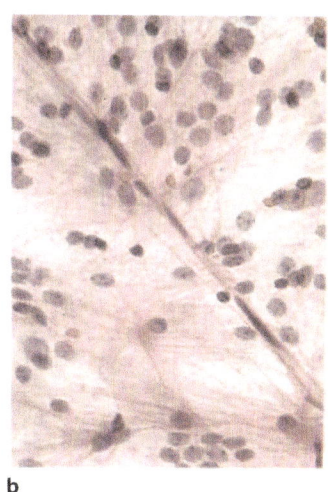
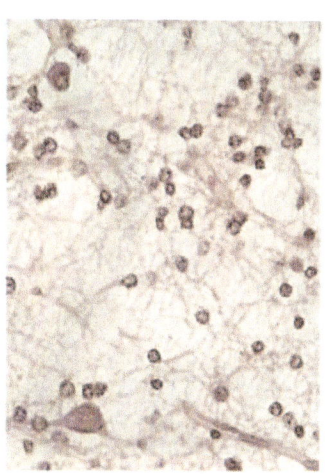

Figure 4.22   Astrocytoma, protoplasmic, non-enhancing: (a) CT, (**b**) HE × 400; sharply circumscribed, hypodense (non-enhancing), occipital lesion thought to represent a parasitic cyst. At operation biopsy yielded gelatinous tumour tissue, which smeared easily to show obvious astrocytes and a capillary vasculature (b, left). While cytological distinc-

tion between protoplasmic and fibrillary astrocytes is rarely possible, the histology is that of protoplasmic astrocytoma (b, right), and further diagnostic bias is provided by the imaging features. (For MR features see Figure **4.21**) See also addendum

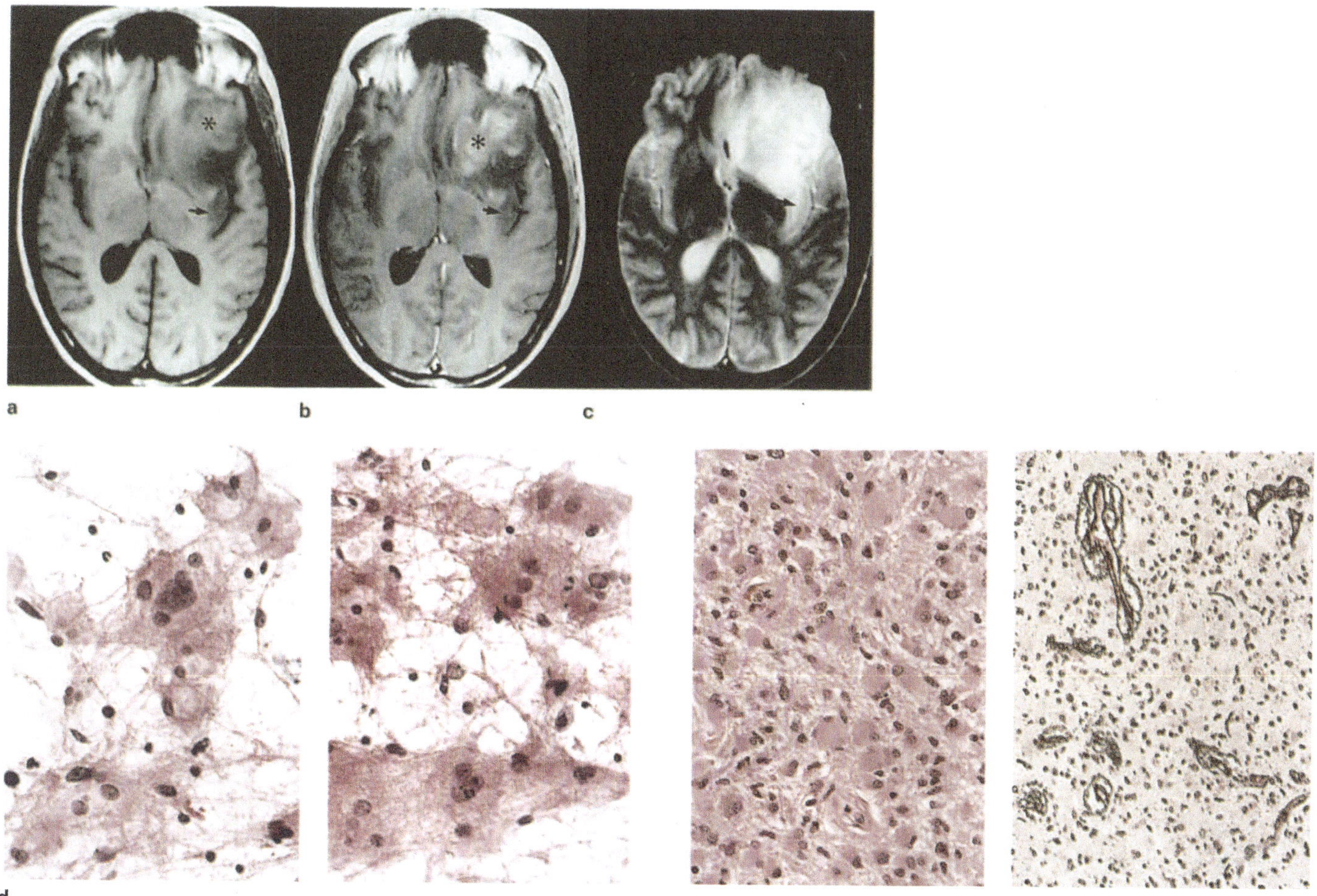

Figure 4.23   Gemistocytic astrocytoma, frontal lobe: male, 26 years; (**a**) T1WI, (**b**) T1WI + C, (**c**) T2WI, (**d,e**) HE × 400, (**f**) Retic × 200; white-matter component of lesion is T1 cortex isointense (a, asterisk) and enhances feebly (b, asterisk), whilst cortical component, which does not enhance (arrows), is relatively T1 hypointense (a), but remains T2 cortex isointense (c). Marked hyperintensity on T2 weighted

image probably includes oedema. Images are atypical for conventional astrocytoma (compare with Figure 4.21) so that gemistocytic cytology (d) and absence of malignant criteria may confer a degree of specificity to the signal characteristics. Paraffin sections from abundant sampling showed the tumour to be homogeneous (e), with relatively prominent but benign vasculature (f)

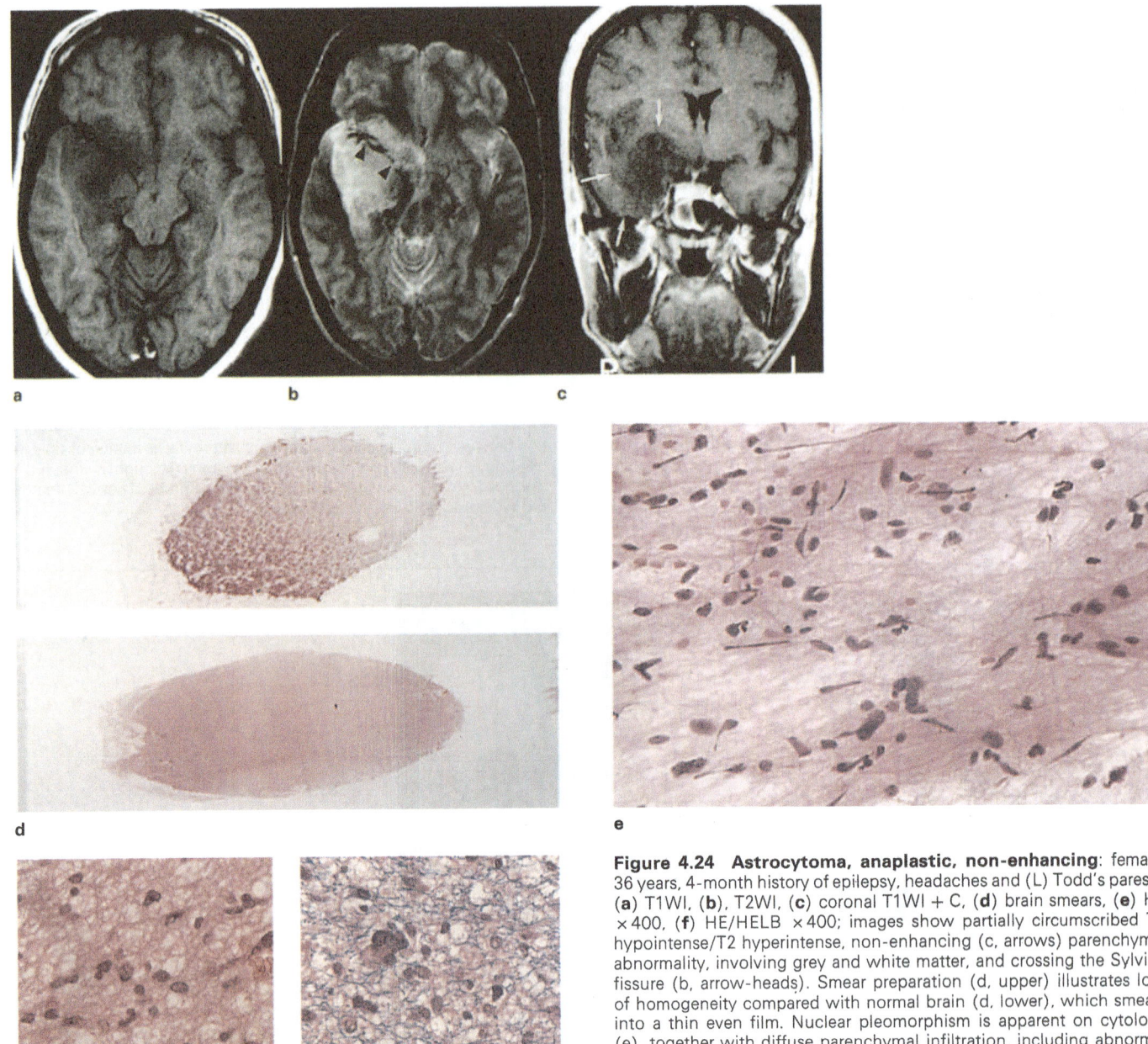

Figure 4.24 Astrocytoma, anaplastic, non-enhancing: female, 36 years, 4-month history of epilepsy, headaches and (L) Todd's paresis; (a) T1WI, (b), T2WI, (c) coronal T1WI + C, (d) brain smears, (e) HE ×400, (f) HE/HELB ×400; images show partially circumscribed T1 hypointense/T2 hyperintense, non-enhancing (c, arrows) parenchymal abnormality, involving grey and white matter, and crossing the Sylvian fissure (b, arrow-heads). Smear preparation (d, upper) illustrates loss of homogeneity compared with normal brain (d, lower), which smears into a thin even film. Nuclear pleomorphism is apparent on cytology (e), together with diffuse parenchymal infiltration, including abnormal mitoses (f, left) (note blue-staining myelin sheaths on right). Extensively sampled lobectomy specimen showed no additional features of malignancy

formation, is invariably associated with enhancement, mainly on the basis of generalized loss of tight junctions[37]; as is well known, this type of angioarchitecture tends to be patchy and necrosis-associated, giving the effect of linear-inhomogeneous forms of enhancement which are thus a sure indication of malignancy (Figures 4.29 and 4.32).

Diffuse or homogeneous enhancement is characteristic of juvenile pilocytic astrocytoma[38], and is consistent with an evenly dispersed tumour vasculature. In this category of tumour, increased vascular permeability is possibly due to the presence of fenestrated vessels, in association with a widened perivascular space[39], rather than a loss of tight junctions. (Fenestrated capillaries have also been reported in tumours of the pituitary and choroid plexus, schwannoma, meningioma, craniopharyngioma, and vascular tumours such as haemangioblastoma and haemangiopericytoma[40].)

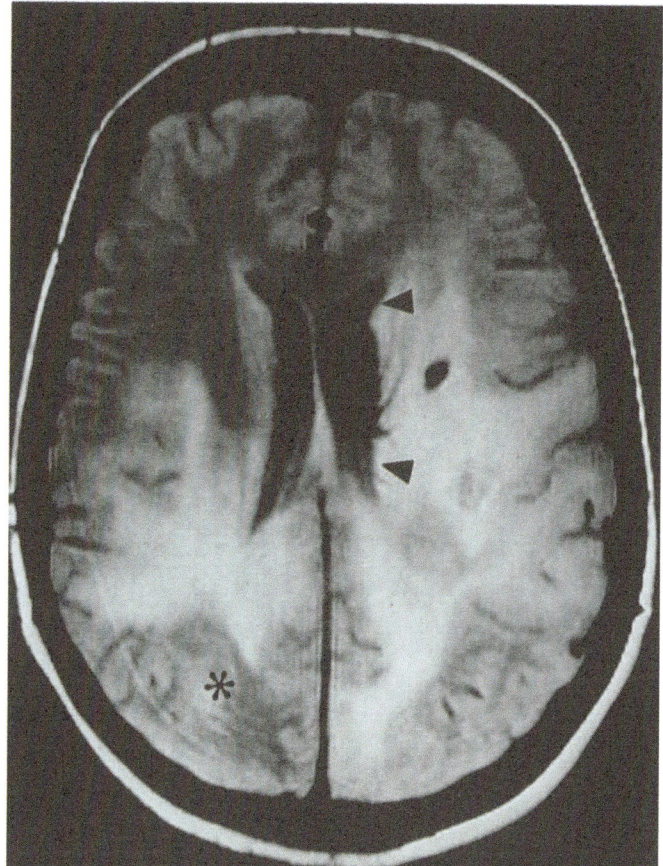

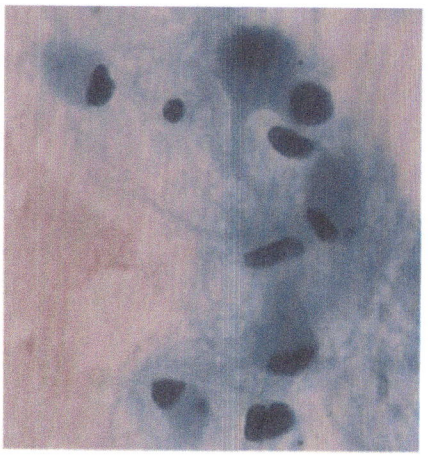

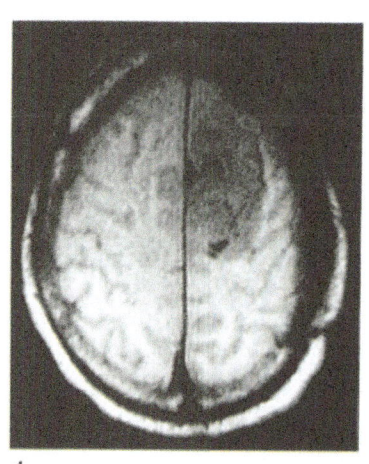

Figure 4.25 Gliomatosis cerebri: female, 40 years, slowly progressive hemiparesis and intellectual decline over 3 years; proton density weighted image shows diffuse, bilateral hyperintense signal abnormality, with cyst formation. Note irregular profile of ventricular wall (arrowheads), suggestive of subependymal growth. Patchy inhomogeneity (asterisk) is unexplained. Histological examination of a needle biopsy showed characteristic diffuse infiltration by anaplastic glia

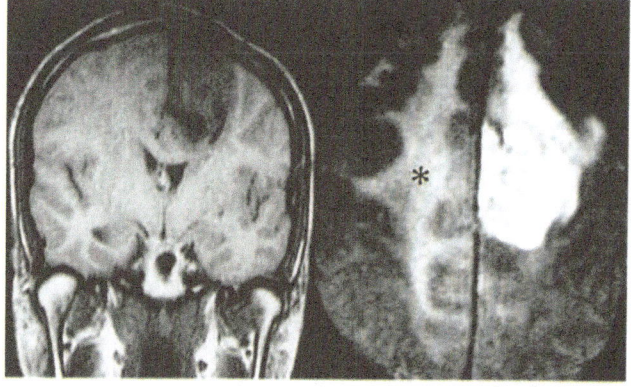

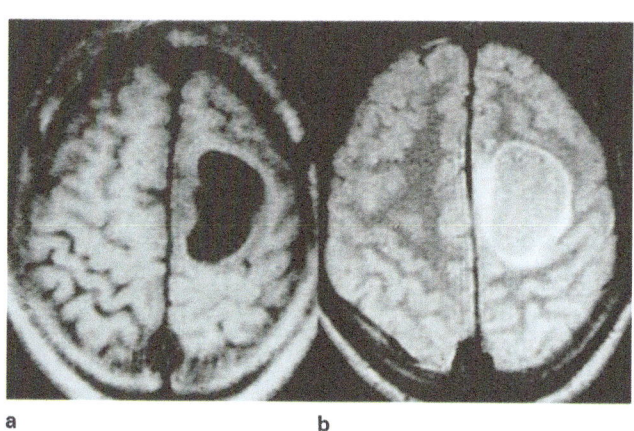

Figure 4.26 Gliomatosis cerebri: male, 34 years, presenting with seizures; (**a**) T1WI, (**b**) PDWI, (**c**) Giemsa ×1000, (**d**) T1WI, (**e**) coronal T1WI, (**f**) T2WI, (**g**) HE ×400/×200; initial images (a,b) show a large hemisphere cyst with T2 hyperintense rim and contents slightly denser than CSF (b). No enhancement seen on CT. Cytospin of aspirate showed glial-like cells (c). Follow-up scan 3 years later showed conversion of cyst site to T1 hypointense/T2 hyperintense mainly solid tumour (d–f), with T2 alteration of adjacent white matter and opposite centrum (f, asterisk). At autopsy, approximately 42 months after initial presentation, site of original tumour showed anaplastic astrocytoma/glioma, and elsewhere gliomatosis cerebri (g), including brainstem. (Drs M Wright and RM Bowen, Groote Schuur Hospital)

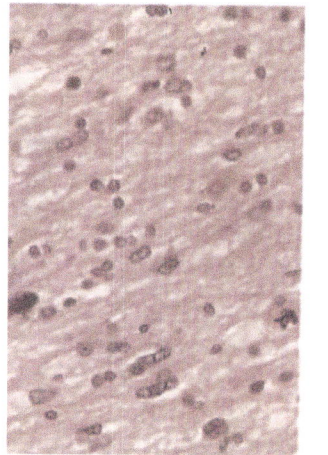

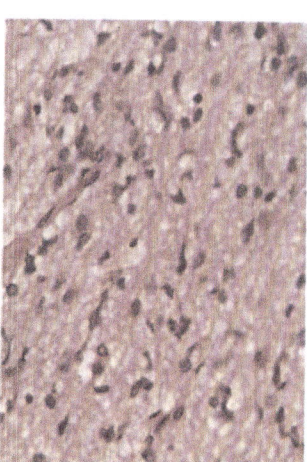

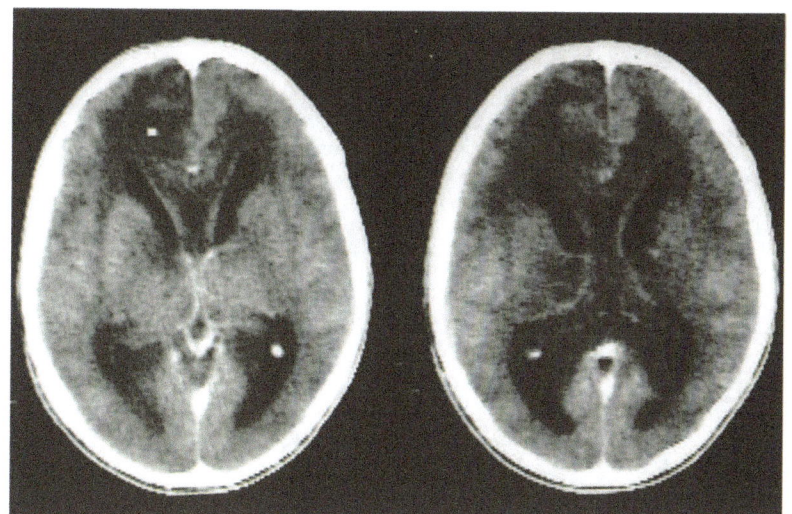

Figure 4.27 Gliomatosis cerebri: male, 19 years, juvenile diabetic presenting with seizures and subsequent coma; (**a**) CT + C, (**b**) fixed brain, (**c**) HE × 200, (**d**) HE × 400; CT shows non-enhancing, bilateral symmetrical hypodense alteration and expansion of septum/fornix, corpus callosum and frontal lobe white matter surrounding anterior horns. Fixed specimen (b) confirms topographic distribution of tumour, including frontal subependymal growth (arrow). Histology revealed predominant protoplasmic astrocytoma with prominent microcystic change (c), with areas of anaplastic change (d). Tumour also extended into the brainstem

a

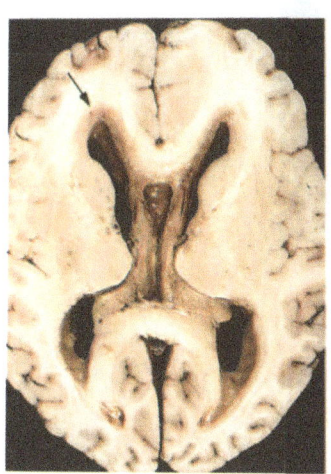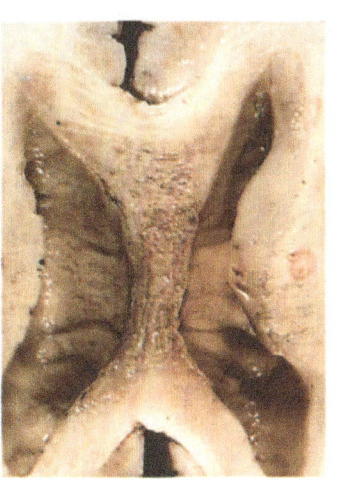

b

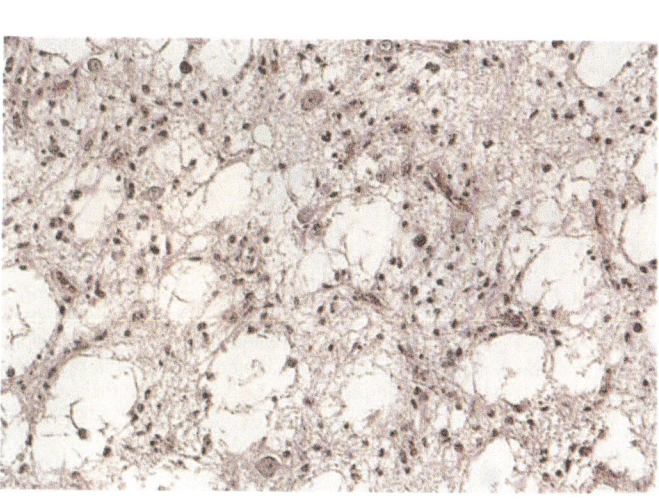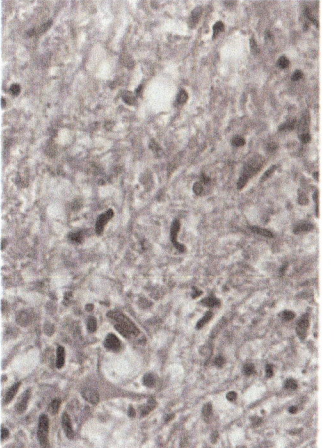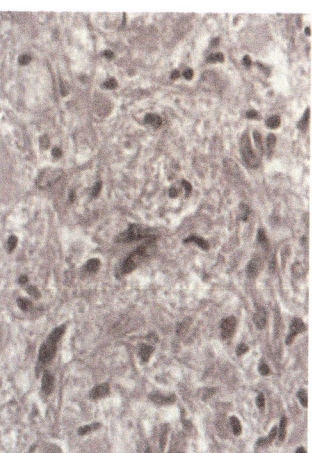

c

d

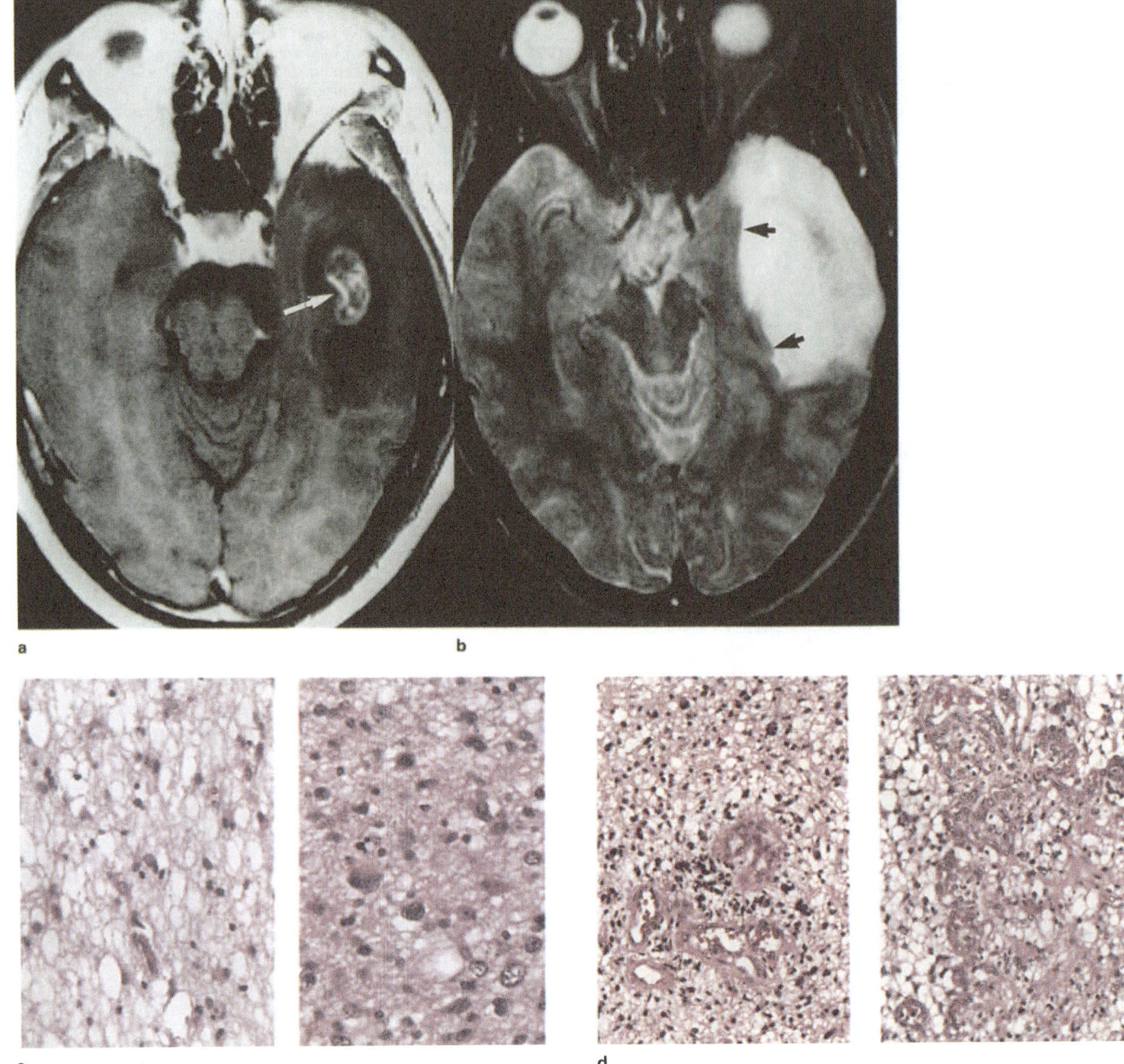

Figure 4.28 Astrocytoma, malignant change: (a) T1WI + C, (b) T2WI, (c) HE ×400, (d) HE ×200; images show T1 hypointense/T2 hyperintense expansion of the anterolateral temporal lobe, with central circumscribed enhancing component (a); note sharp delineation of tumour–brain interface (b, arrows). Histological examination of sample from peripheral non-enhancing area shows a gradation from benign astrocytoma (c, left), to cytologically anaplastic astrocytoma (c, right); the central circumscribed inhomogeneously enhancing nidus shows florid neoplastic vascular proliferative change and cytologically anaplastic astrocytoma. Inhomogeneity of enhancing tumour was considered to be consistent with histologically observed foci of necrosis

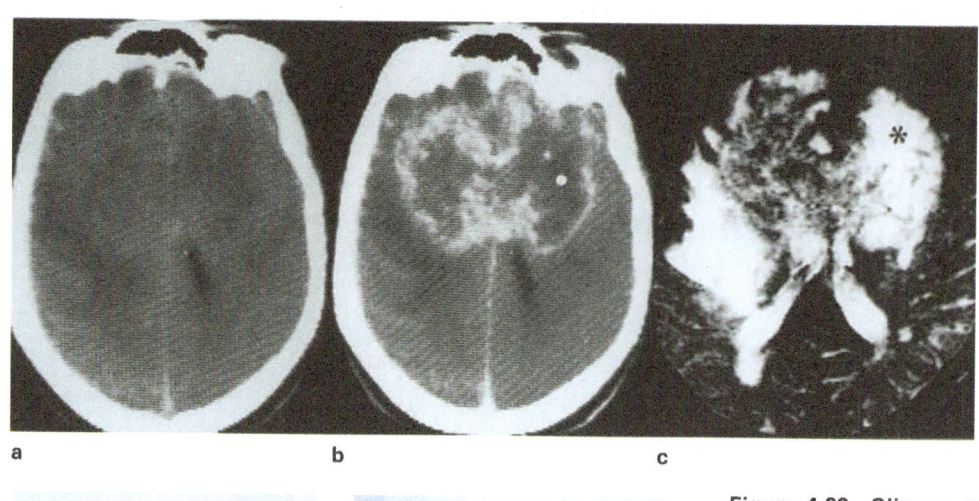

a   b   c

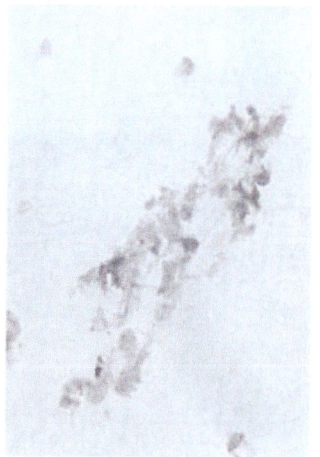
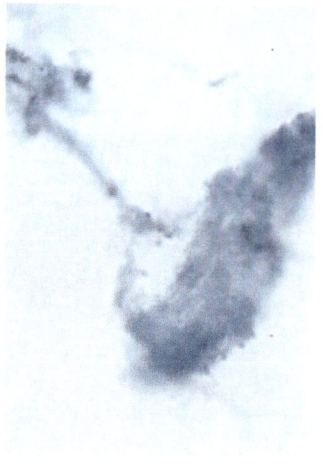

d

Figure 4.29   Glioma, malignant, corpus callosum: (**a**) CT, (**b**) CT + C, (**c**) T2WI, (**d**) HE/Tol blue × 400; images show an inhomogeneous, peripherally enhancing mass having a characteristic 'butterfly' configuration (a,b); T2 weighted image also shows diffuse signal inhomogeneity, assumed to be the effect of coagulative necrosis and haemorrhage, admixed with cystic degeneration. Note that more uniformly hyperintense component of tumour (c, asterisk) is also diffusely hypodense (b, dot) (presumably oèdema and/or less necrosis). Necrotic tissue obained by needle aspirate of right frontal lobe (d), is still 'diagnostic' in the context of the images. (**Figure 4.30**, from a similar case, shows the macroscopic appearance of such a tumour)

4.6c.   Malignant astrocytoma (malignant glioma) and glioblastoma; focal or topographic (callosal); inhomogeneously enhancing

As has been pointed out in the general discussion of gliomas, untidy inhomogeneity, in terms of both signal quality and enhancement, is characteristic of malignancy[45]. Our own material proves that malignant transformation, in the form of an enhancing nidus, may occur within a more extensive as well as cytologically benign tumour. Such foci are commonly untidy linear/ring lesions in which (mainly T2) signal shortening also occurs (Figure 4.28), and conform histologically to vascular proliferation, encompassing multiplication of endothelial lining cells, mitotic activity, increased numbers of vessels, as well as haemorrhage, thrombosis and necrosis. In other tumours, particularly the callosal 'butterfly' gliomas, the neoplasm is diffusely T2-inhomogeneous, *pari-passu* with enhancement, and accurately reflects the admixture of proliferative and necrotizing processes (Figures 4.29 and 4.30). On CT this morphological blend is often isodense and may even induce slight hyperdensity. As may also be expected, the same factors determine the presence or absence of enhancement of an associated cyst wall.

Except for a tendency to form relatively large, circumscribed ring lesions, *glioblastoma* has no other specific imaging features and remains a histological diagnosis (Figure 4.32). On the other hand, we contend that such a diagnosis cannot be made in the absence of enhancement (Figures 4.33 and 4.34). An unusual variant in terms of relatively diffuse enhancement has been encountered in the granular cell glioblastoma, illustrated in Figure 4.35.

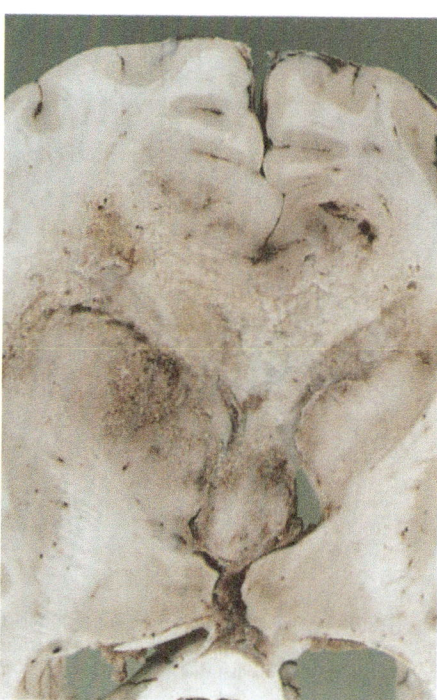

Figure 4.30   Glioma, malignant, corpus callosum: section of fixed brain illustrating the typical variegated appearance of a callosal glioma

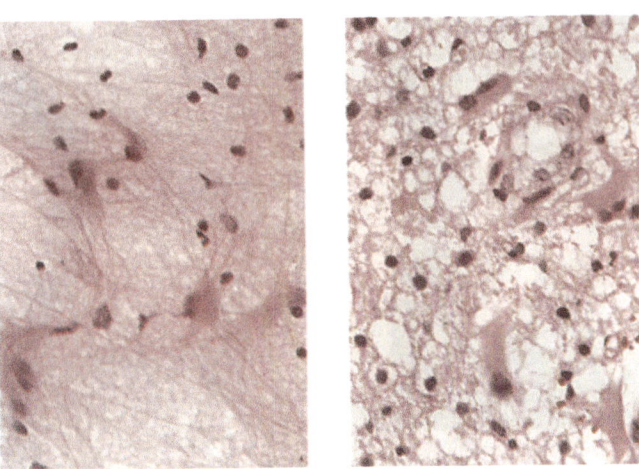

Figure 4.31 Astrocytes, reactive: smear left, paraffin section right. HE ×400

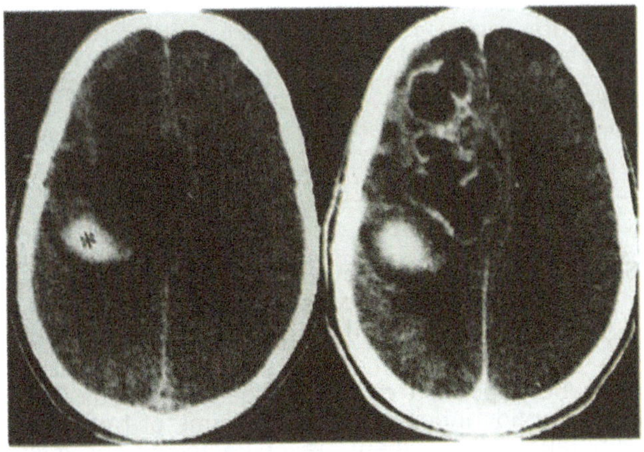

Figure 4.32 Glioblastoma multiforme, cystic: male, 60 years; (**a**) CT, (**b**) CT + C, (**c–e**) HE ×200; images show a frontoparietal, multiloculated cystic lesion with strong peripheral enhancement (hyperdense mass posteriorly is biopsy haematoma (a, asterisk). Images are non-specific and include atypical abscess (compare with **Figures 4.10** and **4.13**). Histology shows the spectrum of morphology required for the diagnosis of glioblastoma multiforme, including nuclear anaplasia and giant-cell formation (c), glomeruloid vascular proliferation (d) and necrosis with palisading (e)

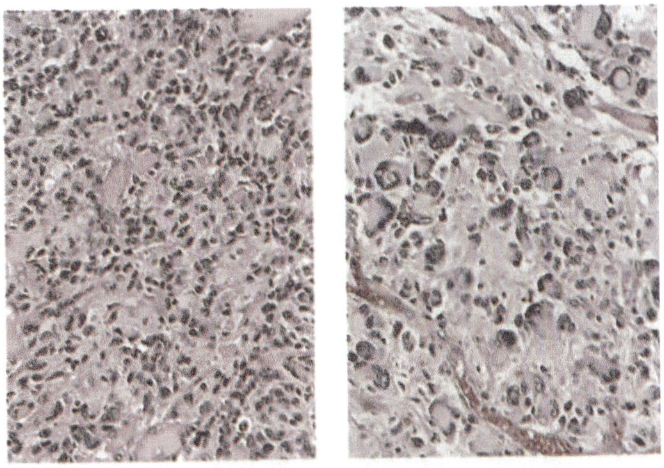

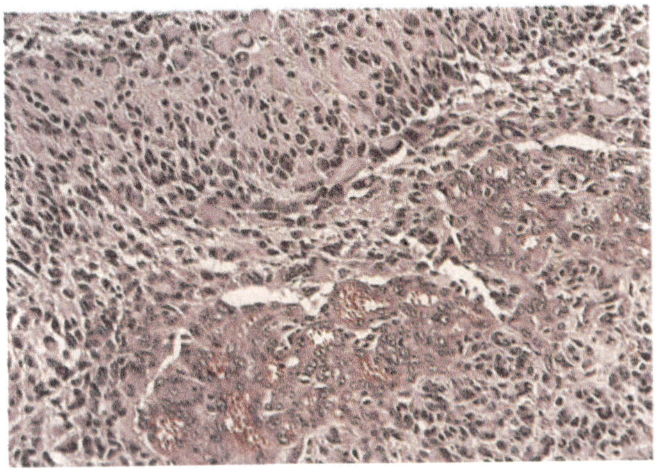

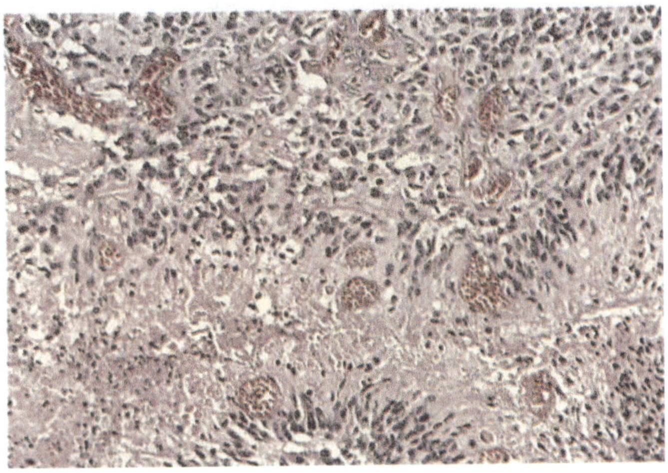

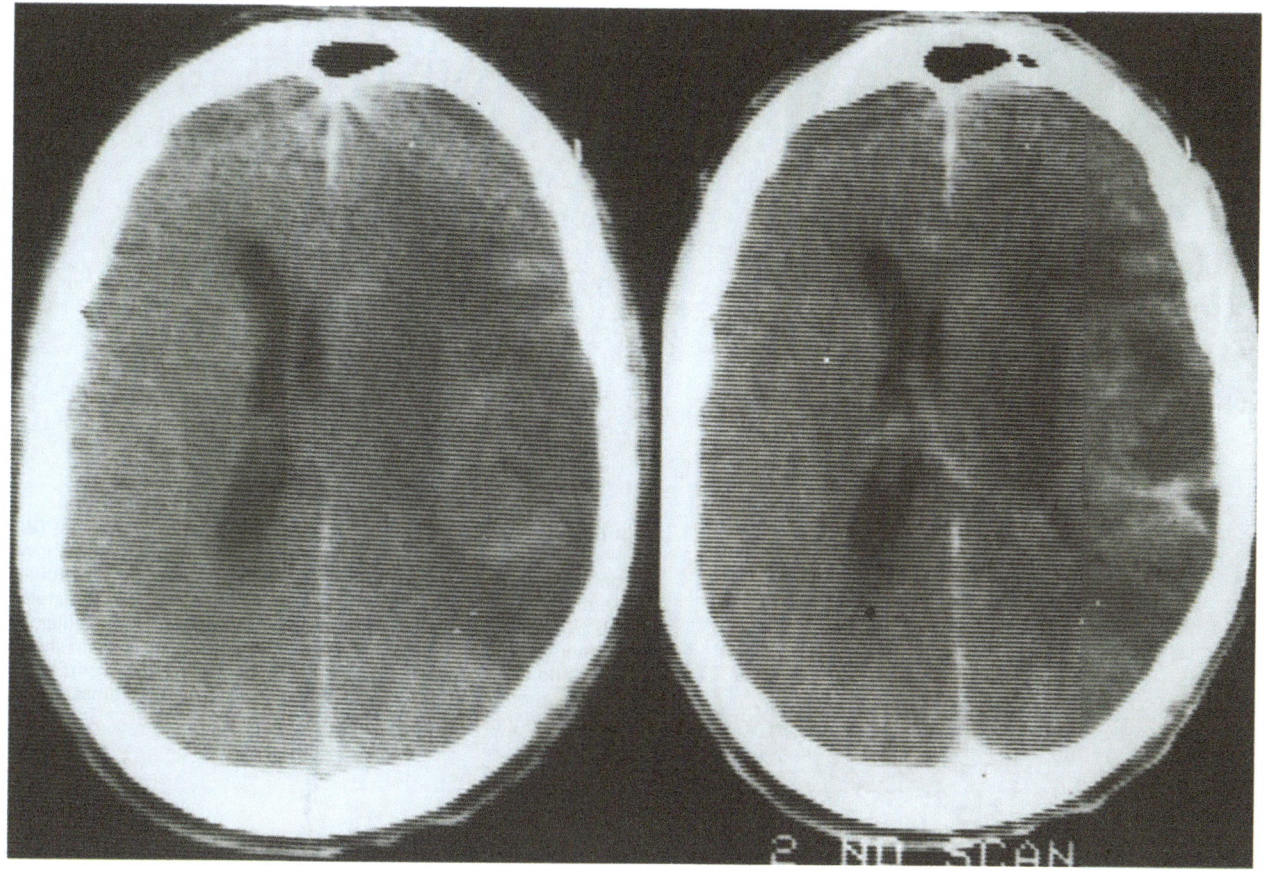

a   b

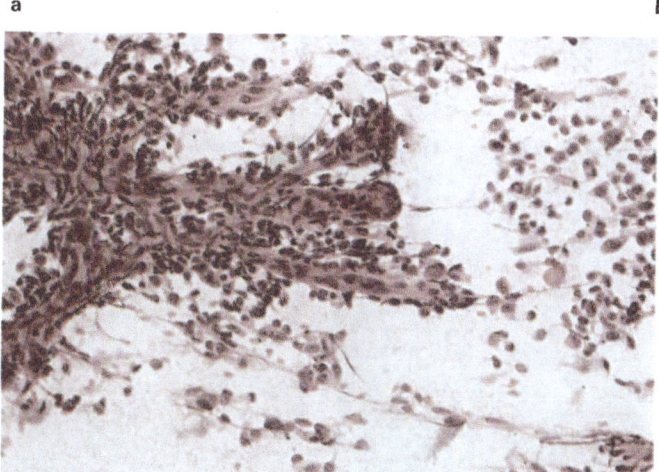

c

Figure 4.33   Glioblastoma multiforme: male, 62 years; (**a**) CT, (**b**) CT + C, (**c**) HE ×200; images show an inhomogeneously enhancing lesion, with spurious middle cerebral artery territory topography, somewhat resembling an infarct, although with excessive volumetric expansion. Needle biopsy smear preparation shows vascular leashes with poorly fibrillated neoplastic cells (c)

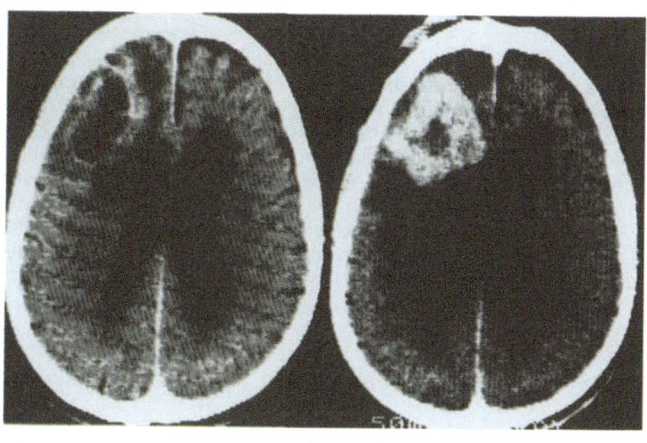

a   b

Figure 4.34   Glioblastoma multiforme, hemisphere: male, 60 years; (**a,b**) CT + C; initial scan (a) shows cyst with enhancing rim. Initial diagnosis was that of a cystic malignant astrocytoma. Follow-up study 25 days later shows remarkable enhancing tumour proliferation, with prominent circumspection. Histology showed a typical glioblastoma multiforme

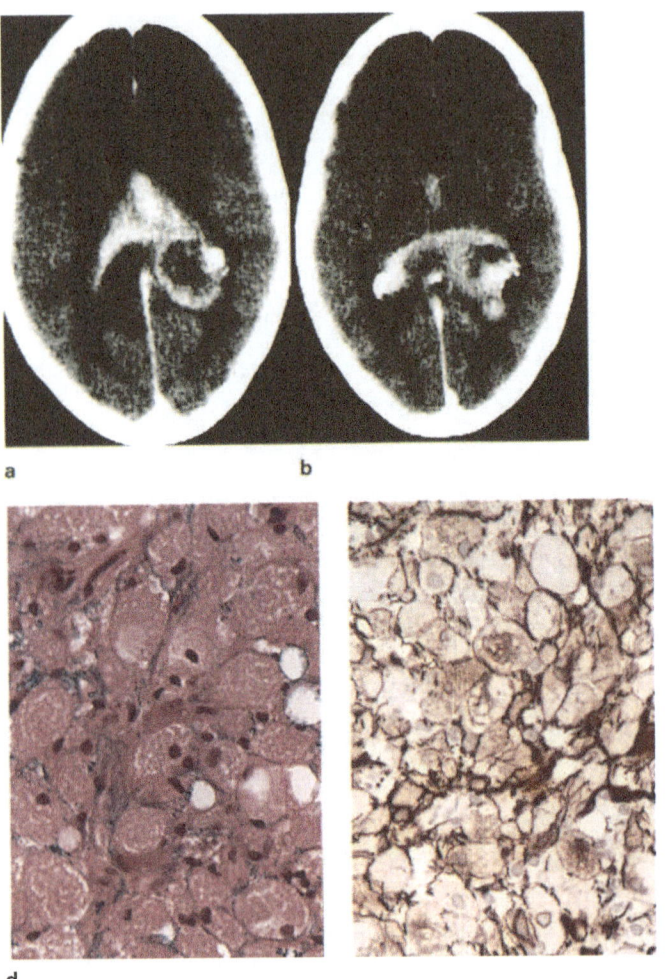

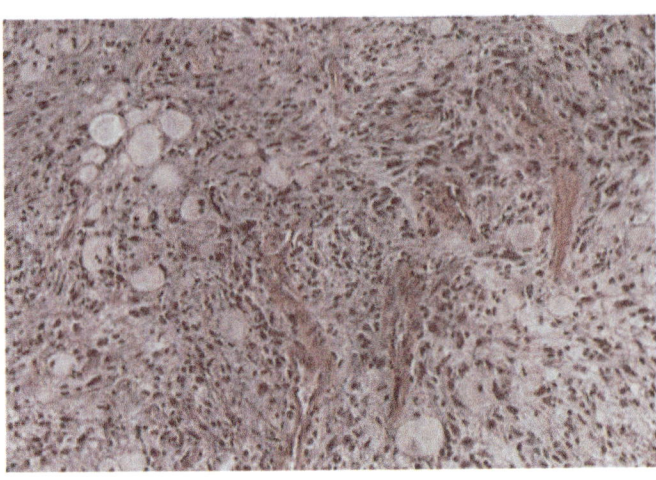

Figure 4.35 Glioblastoma, granular cell: female, 61 years; (**a,b**) CT + C, (**c**) PTAH ×200, (**d**) HELB/GFAP ×400; images show a lesion which has solid and ring-enhancing components, probably conforming to the posterior corpus callosum and fornix. Histology shows a cellular glial tumour (c), with a prominent granular cell component (d); infiltrative nature is illustrated by residual myelin sheaths (d, left), and GFAP positivity with demonstrable cell processes d, right); there is a prominent diffuse vasculature (c). In other areas tumour features were those of a conventional glioblastoma

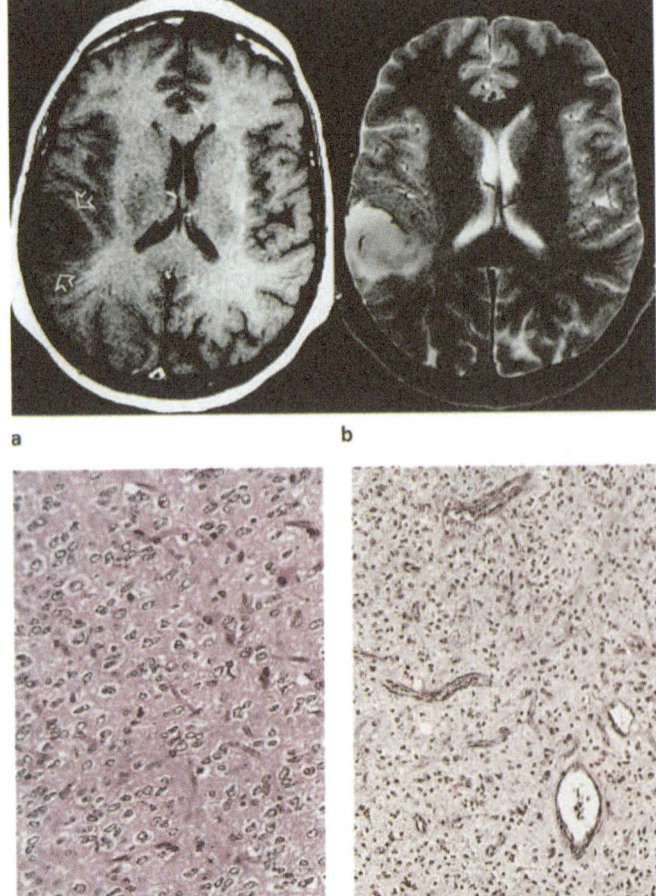

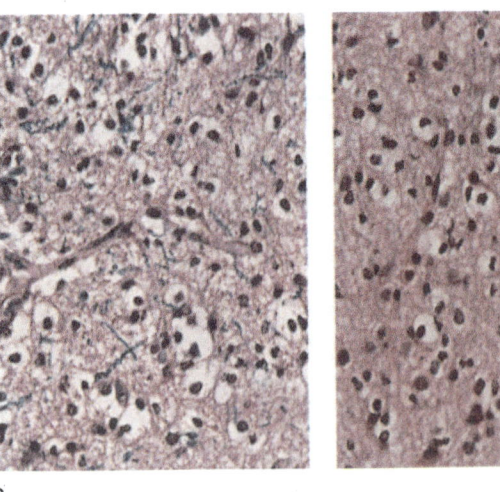

Figure 4.36 Oligodendroglioma, temporoparietal, circumscribed, non-enhancing: (**a**) T1WI + C, (**b**) T2WI, (**c**) HE/HELB ×400, (**d**) HE ×400, (**e**) Retic ×400; images show a T1 hypointense/T2 hyperintense, non-enhancing mass, mainly involving cerebral cortex (a, arrows); vasogenic oedema is minimal. Histology shows a typical oligodendroglioma, with perinuclear halos; widely separated myelin sheaths (blue) are typical of parenchymal infiltration. Vessels (d,e) are characteristically thin-walled and probably do not exceed normal cortical density

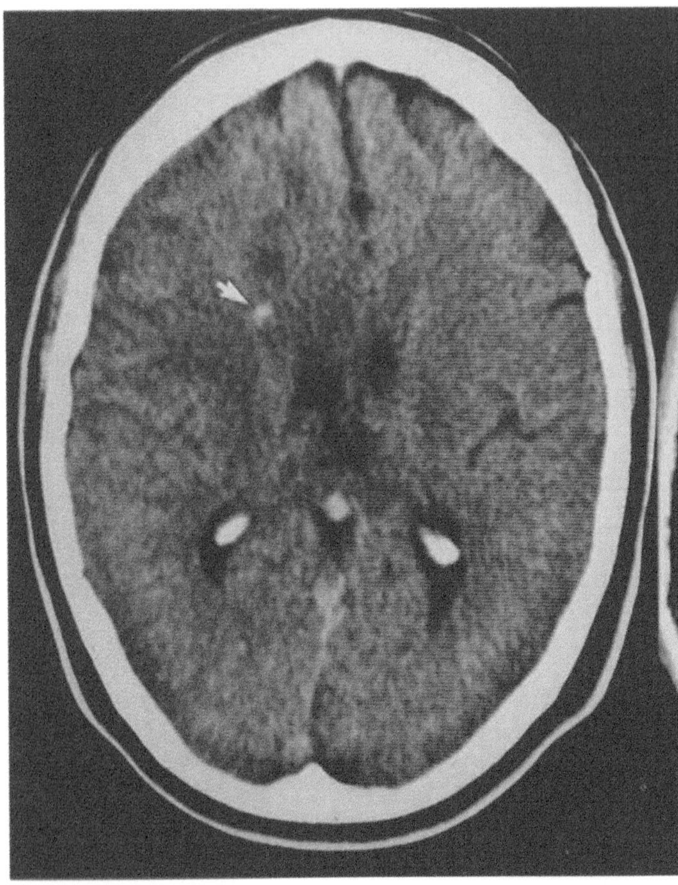

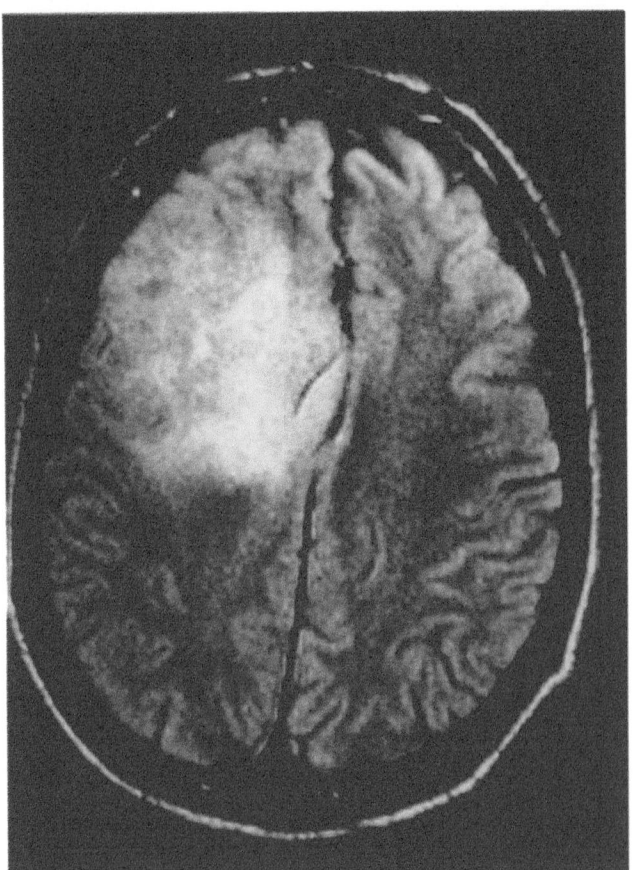

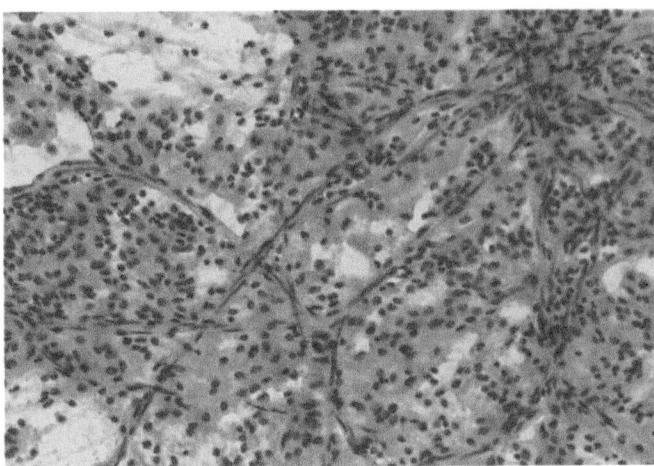

Figure 4.37 Oligodendroglioma, diffusely infiltrating, non-enhancing: (**a**) CT + C, (**b**) T1WI + C, (**c**) T2WI, (**d**) Giemsa × 200; CT shows subtle inhomogeneous hypodense alteration which is non-enhancing, with focal mineralization (a, arrow). The lesion is T1 grey-matter isointense, with weak focal enhancement (b, arrows); associated circumscribed hypointensity might be mineralization. T2 weighted image shows generalized ground-glass-type hyperintensity, maximal in white matter (c). Smear (d) shows typical cytology and branching capillary vasculature

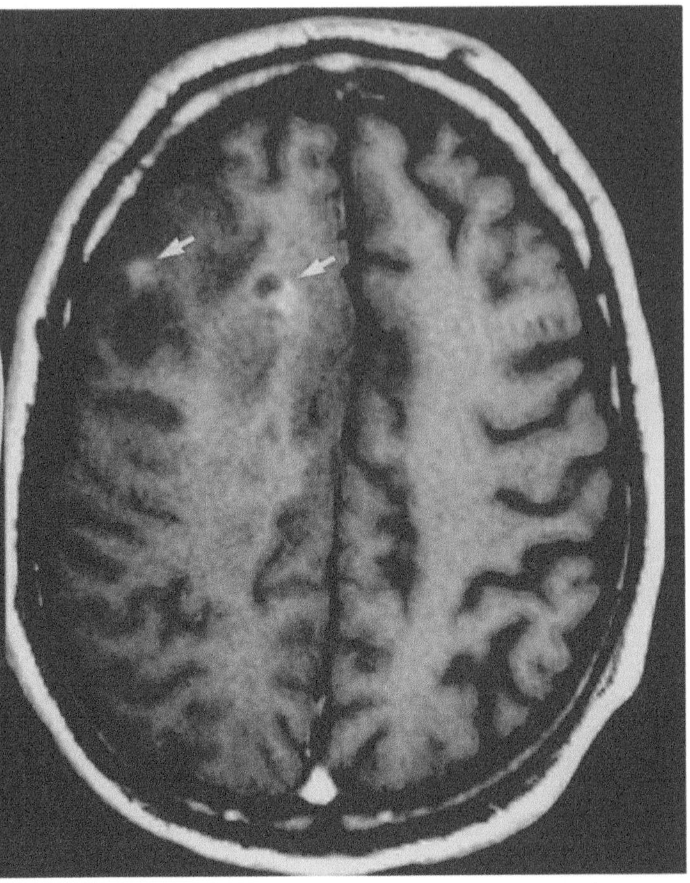

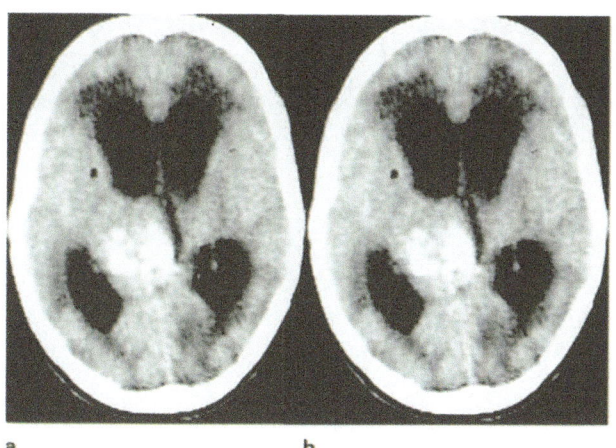
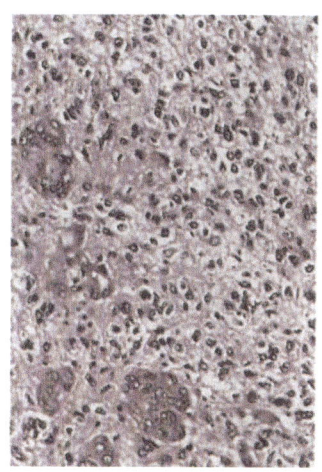
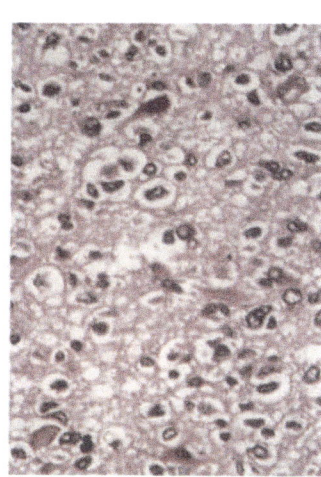

Figure 4.38 Oligodendroglioma, diencephalic, enhancing: (a) CT, (b) CT + C, (c) HE ×200/×400; brain isodense, heavily mineralized, strongly enhancing mass (a,b). Needle biopsy showed some evidence of glomeruloid vascular proliferation (c, left), in an otherwise typical oligodendroglioma (c, right), with calcospherites (see also **Figure 4.39** from a similar case)

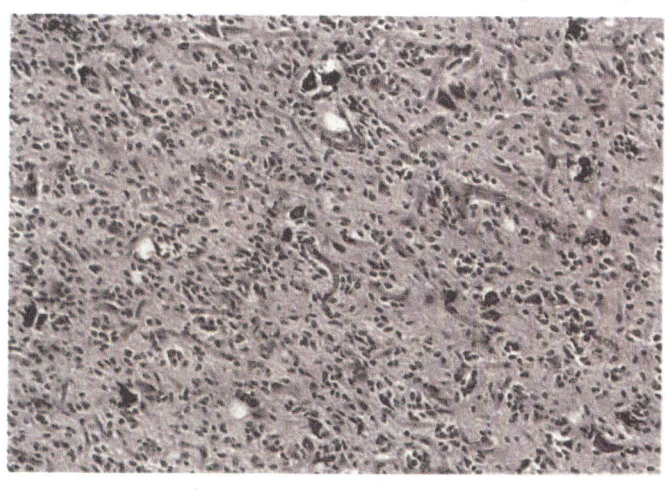
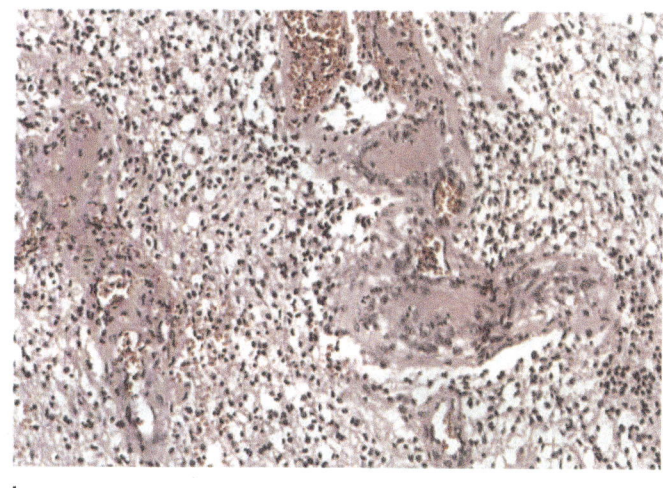

Figure 4.39 Oligodendroglioma, enhancing: (a,b) HE ×200; histology typical diffusely infiltrating tumour with mineralization (possibly of neurones) (a), and more solid tumour with abnormal vessels of the type seen in more malignant glioma (b), presumed to be responsible for enhancement. However, the tumour does not show other conventional criteria of malignancy

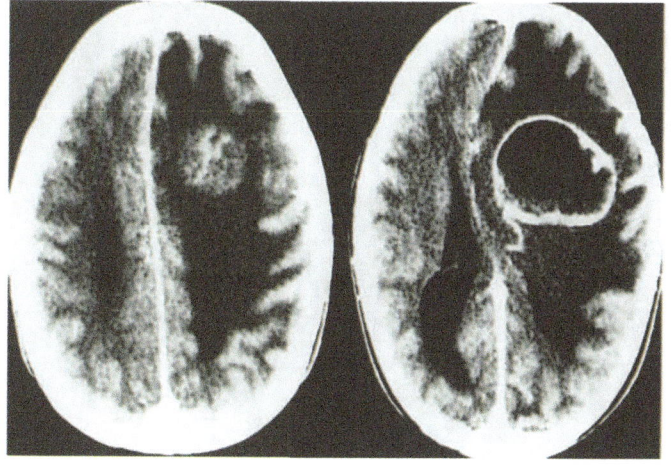
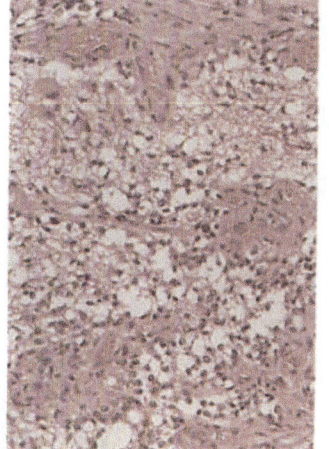
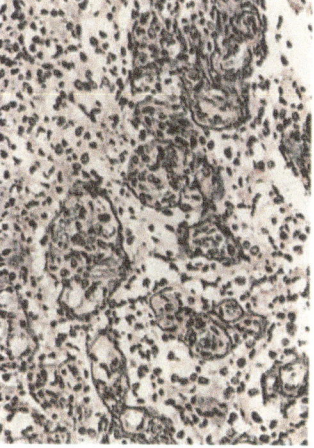

Figure 4.40 Oligo-astroblastoma, centrum and convexity: male, 10 years; (a,b) CT + C, (c) HE/Retic ×200, (d) (*overleaf*) HE/GFAP ×200; large circumscribed ring lesion extending to the convexity, with strongly enhancing wall and homogeneous, hypodense non-enhancing contents, possibly cystic. Histology shows tumour to be dimorphic, including oligodendroglioma with proliferative vasculature (c), and astroblastoma with capillary-type vessels (d). The precise site of samples in relation to the scan morphology is unfortunately not known. Necrosis, however, was not seen in the samples examined. (Histology reviewed by Prof SR VandenBerg, University of Virginia)

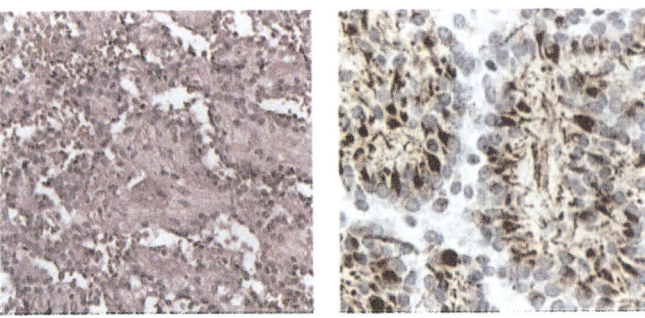

Figure 4.40(d)

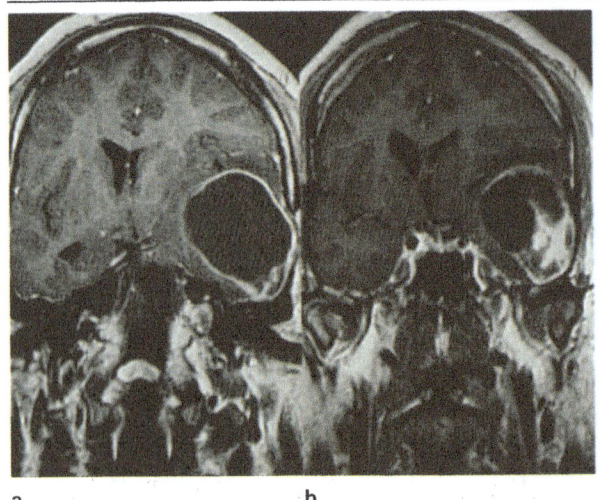

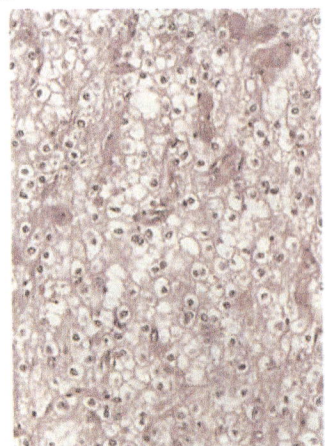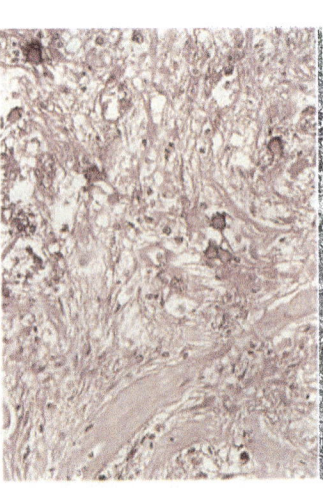

a   b   c

Figure 4.41 Oligodendroglioma-pilocytic astrocytoma, temporal lobe: male, 32 years, 8-year history of epilepsy; (**a,b**) T1WI + C, (**c**) HE ×200; solid/cystic peripherally enhancing cerebromeningeal tumour (the solid component was T2 hyperintense, but could not be differentiated from cyst on T2 sequences). Tumour cell populations form distinct areas, astrocytic component possessing more obviously abnormal vessels and calcosherites (c, right). Conventional histological features of malignancy were absent in the samples examined

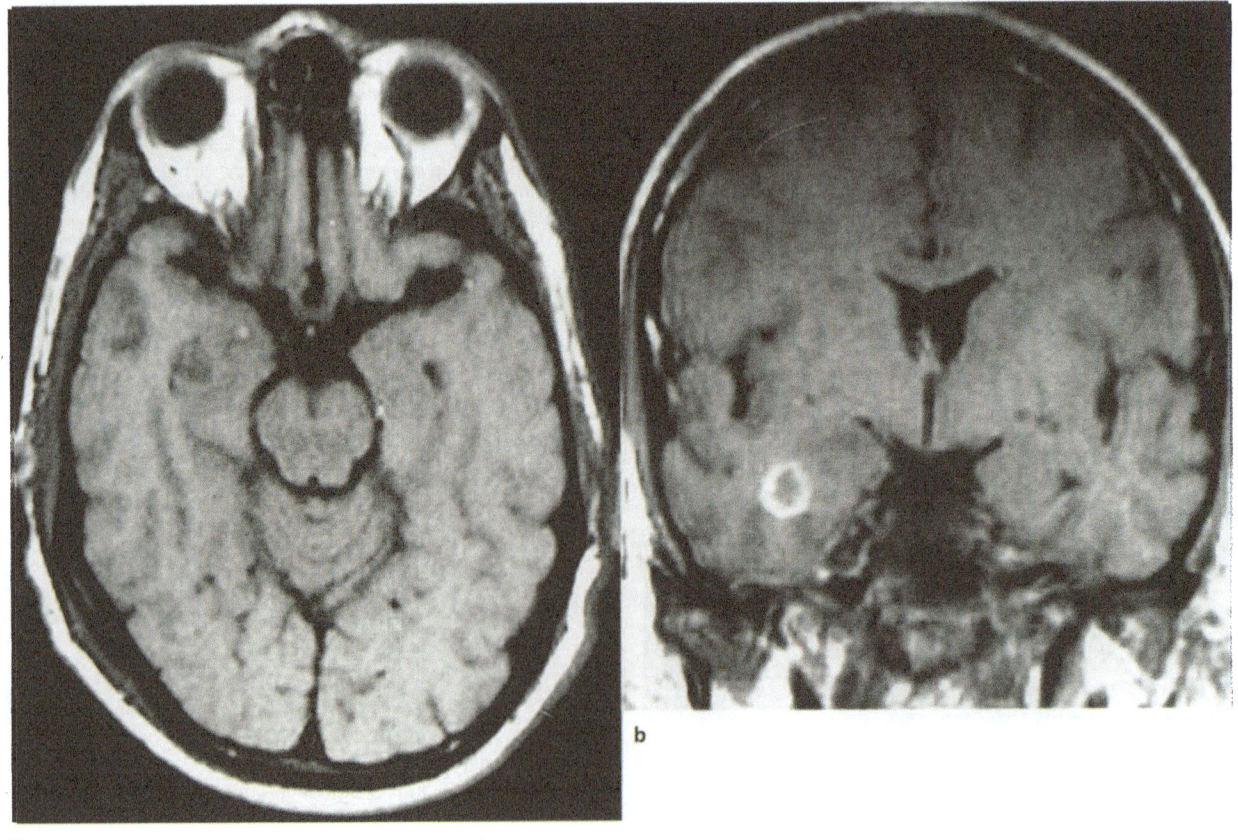

a   b

Figure 4.42 (*legend opposite*)

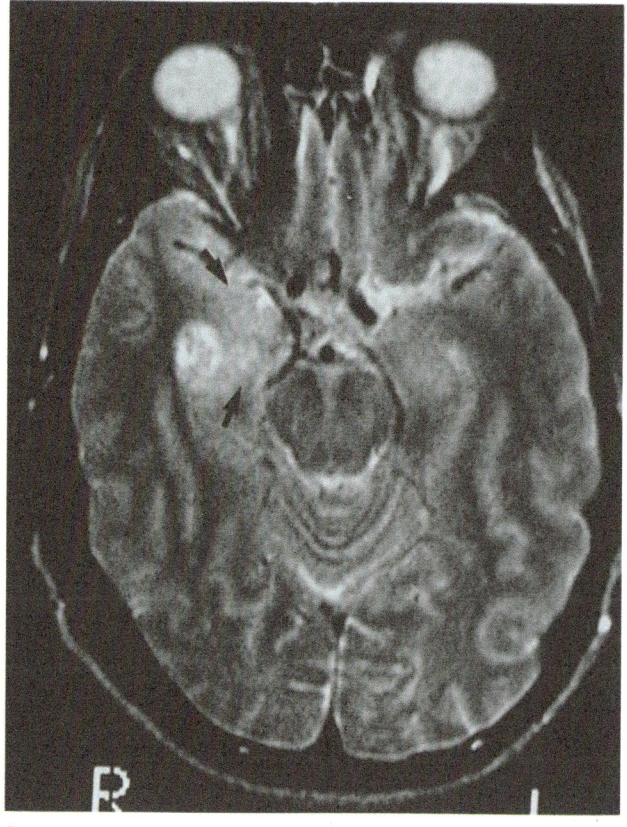

c

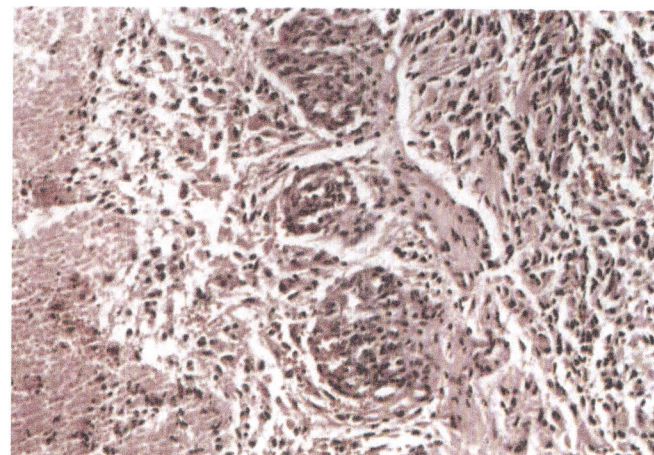

d

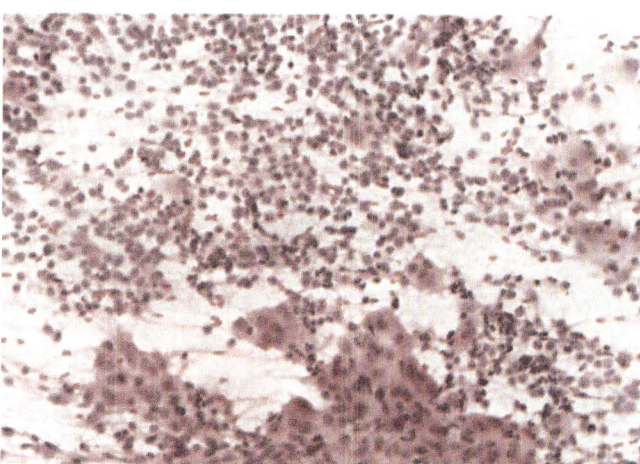

e

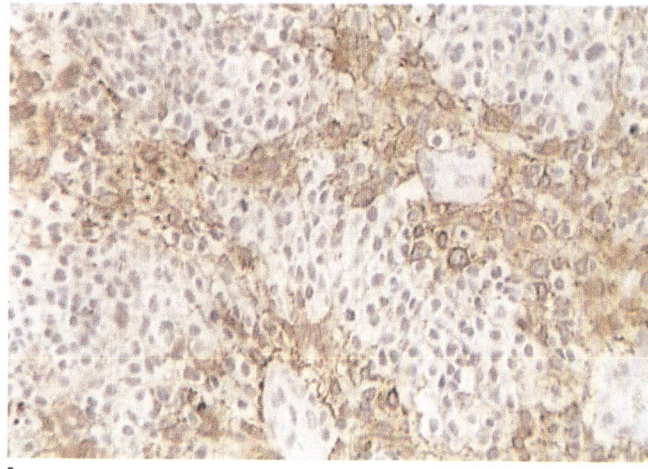

f

Figure 4.42 Oligodendroglioma-malignant astrocytoma, hippocampus: male, 50 years; (**a**) T1WI, (**b**) coronal T1WI + C, (**c**) T2WI, (**d**) HE × 200, (**e**) HE × 400, (**f**) GFAP × 400; images show a focal T1 hypointense (a), T2 inhomogeneous lesion (c), exhibiting ring enhancement, with central hypointensity (b). Medially the parahippocampal gyrus is expanded and slightly T2 hyperintense (c, arrows). At operation the focal lesion was grey/haemorrhagic and is assumed to represent the vascular and necrotic tissue shown in (d). Biopsy from the expanded hippocampus shows admixed oligoastrocytoma (e,f)

Table 4.1

Non-enhancing glioma
Fibrillary/protoplasmic astrocytoma
Cytologically anaplastic astrocytoma
Gliomatosis
Diffusely infiltrating oligodendroglioma

Enhancing glioma
I.   Homogeneous
   (a)   Circumscribed, diffuse
        pilocytic astrocytoma
        SEGC astrocytoma
        'cerebromeningeal' gliomas
   (b)   Incomplete
        gemistocytic astrocytoma
        ependymoma
        some 'cerebromeningeal' gliomas
        some mixed gliomas

II.   Inhomogeneous
        Malignant astrocytoma–glioblastoma
        Malignant glioma
        Mixed glioma

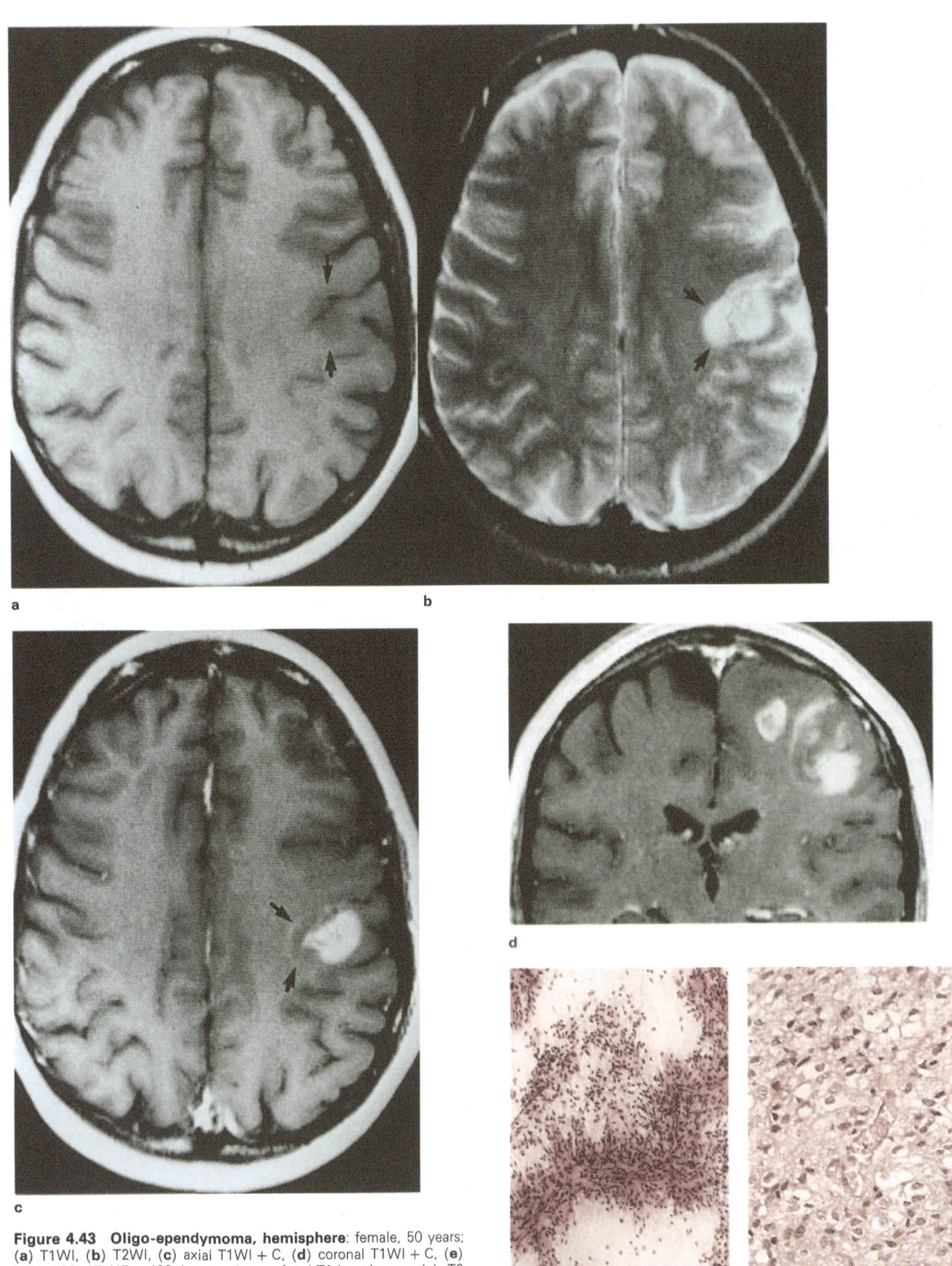

Figure 4.43 Oligo-ependymoma, hemisphere: female, 50 years; (**a**) T1WI, (**b**) T2WI, (**c**) axial T1WI + C, (**d**) coronal T1WI + C, (**e**) HE ×100, (**f**) HE ×400; images show a focal T1 hypointense (a), T2 hyperintense lesion (b); note non-enhancing component (b,c, arrows). Enhancement is also discontinuous on coronal views (d). The more prominently vascularized ependymal tissue (e) is likely to be responsible for the enhancement (compare vascularity with that of oligodendrogliomatous component (f). (See also discussion on enhancement patterns)

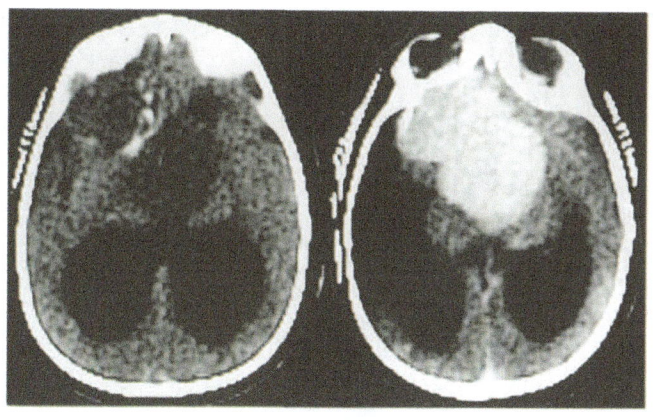

a

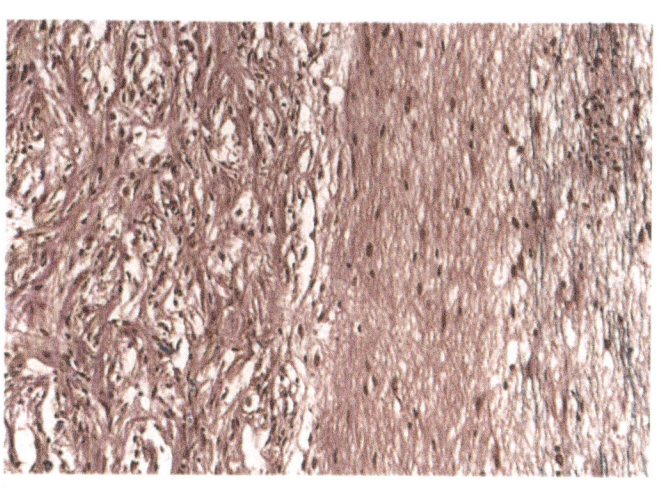

b

Figure 4.44 Pilocytic astrocytoma, juvenile, hypothalamic, with frontal extension: (**a**) CT/CT + C, (**b**) HELB × 200; early-generation CT scan shows lobulated hypodense, strongly and diffusely enhancing tumour. At operation anterior component appeared to be extraparenchymal. Histology shows characteristic JPA (note capillary spaces with counterstained red cells), with a sharp tumour–brain interface; the intervening cellular band is considered to be reactive gliosis

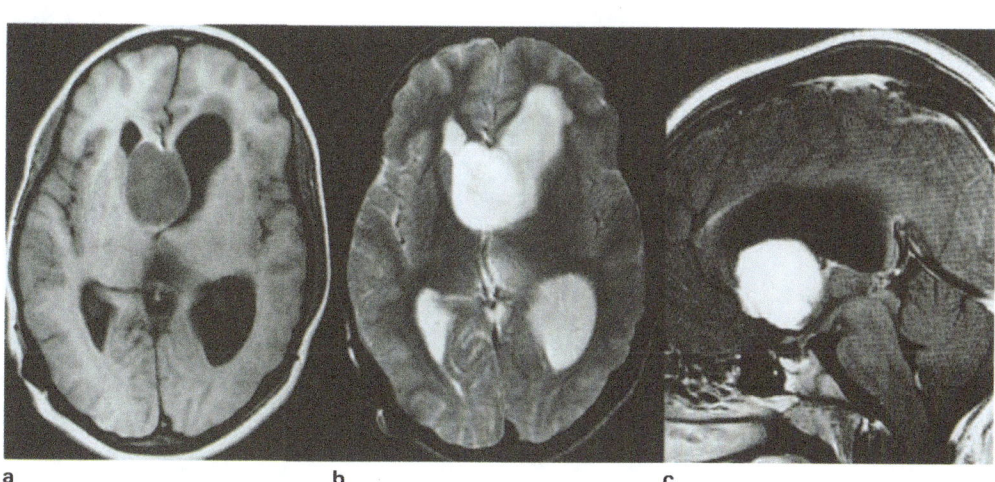

a   b   c

Figure 4.45 Pilocytic astrocytoma, juvenile, hypothalamic: (a) T1WI, (b) T2WI, (c) sagittal T1WI + C; images display the characteristic features of T1 hypointensity relative to cortex, marked T2 hyperintensity almost CSF isointense, and diffuse strong enhancement. Lesion appears to have grown within the septum. Histology was characteristic

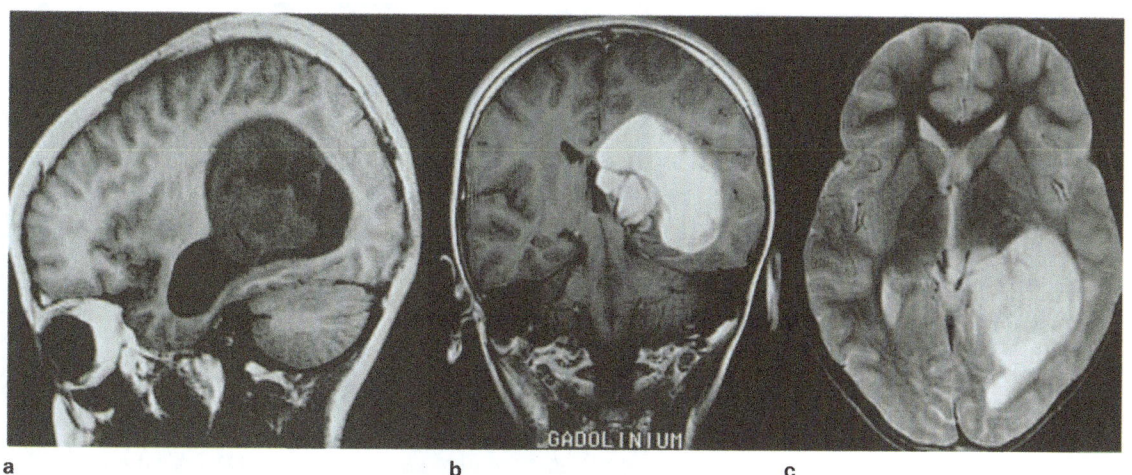

a   b   c

Figure 4.46 Pilocytic astrocytoma, juvenile, hemispheric/intraventricular: (a) T1WI, (b) T1WI + C, (c) T2WI, (d) (*overleaf*) PTAH and GFAP × 200; MR shows large circumscribed predominantly intraventricular mass containing numerous cysts. T1 cortex hypointense, T2 hyperintense, strongly diffusely enhancing. (Compare with **Figure 4.72**, in which solid epithelial tissue is T2 brain isointense.) Histology showed characteristic coarse fibrils with variously sized thin wall vessels. (Dr C Sinclair-Smith, Red Cross Children's Hospital)

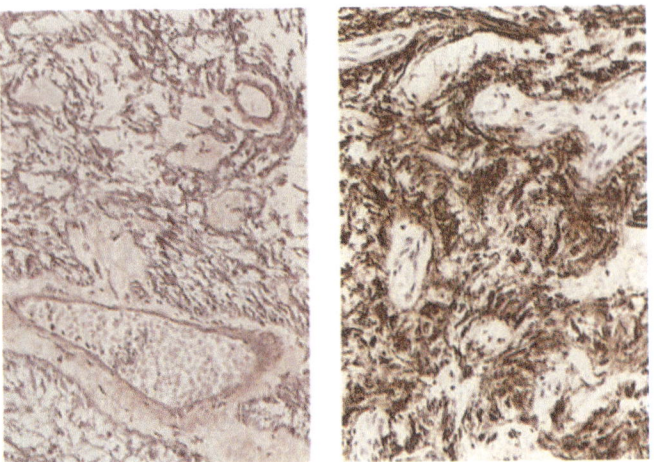

Figure 4.46(d)

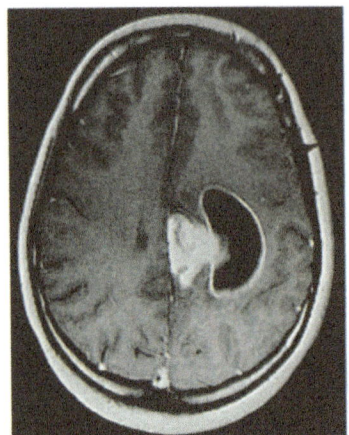

a

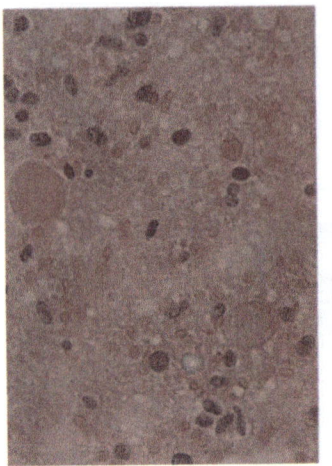
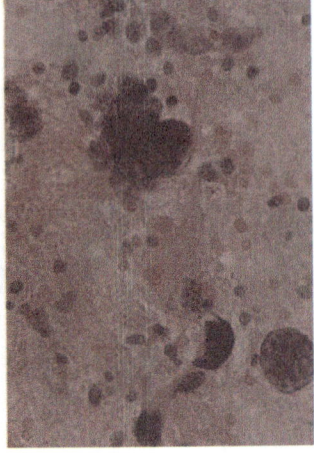

b

Figure 4.47 Pilocytic astrocytoma, juvenile, solid/cystic, hemisphere: (**a**) T1WI + C, (**b**) HE × 400; medial hemisphere, meningocerebral, strongly enhancing pilocytic astrocytoma with tumour/ parenchymal cyst. Enhancement of cyst wall suggests that it is neoplastic. In conjunction with these imaging features, widespread granular body formation and nuclear pleomorphism (b) are considered degenerative. (Dr RM Bowen, Groote Schuur Hospital)

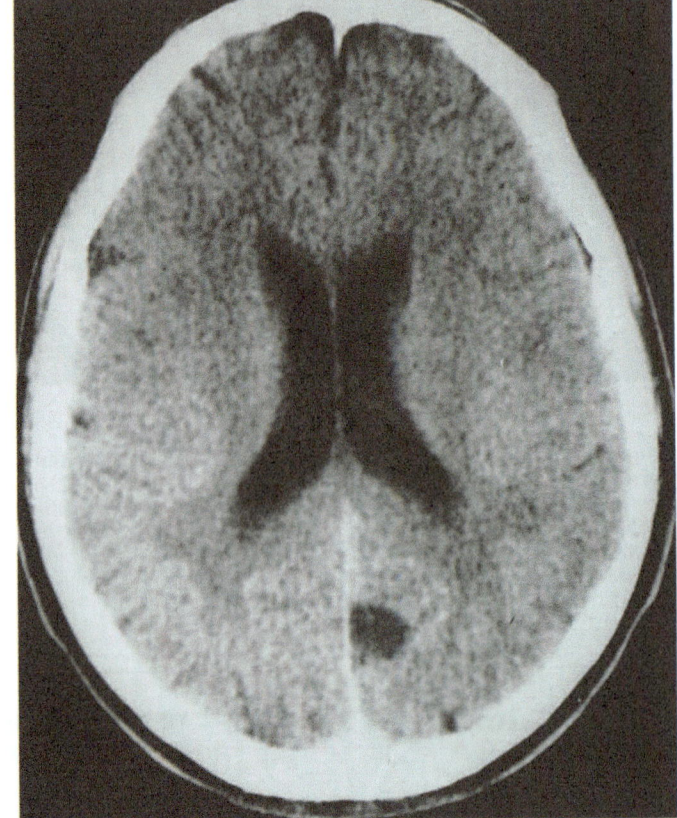

Figure 4.48(a)

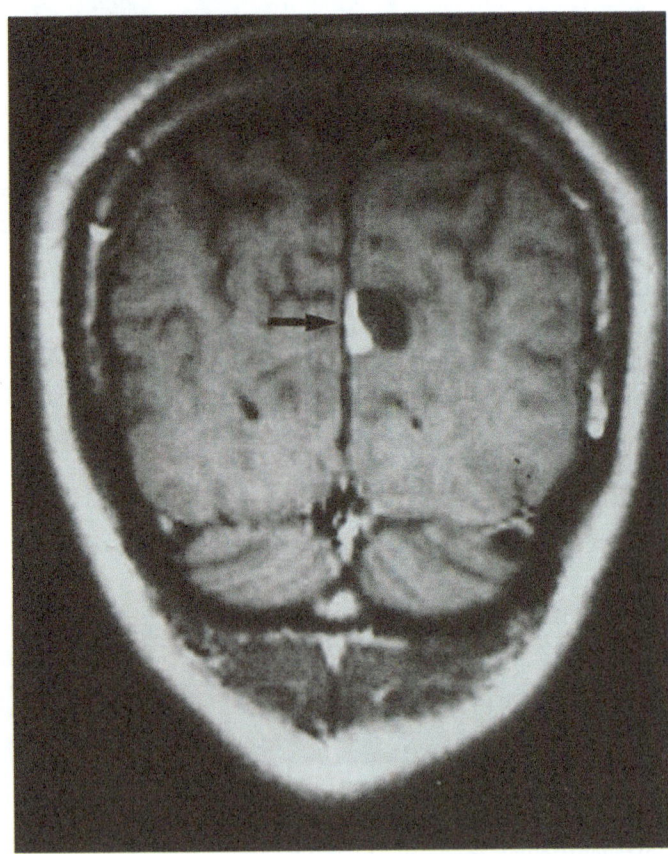

Figure 4.48(b)

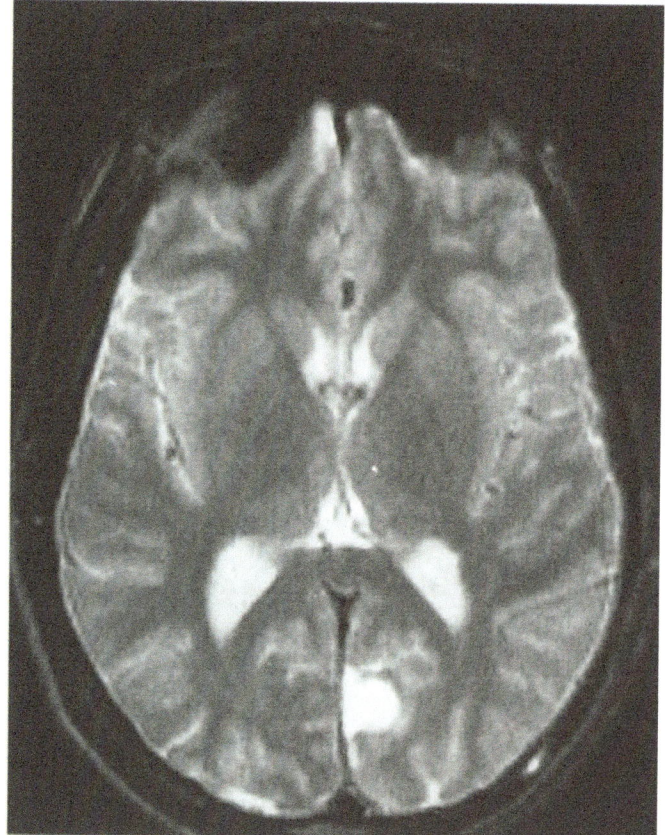

c

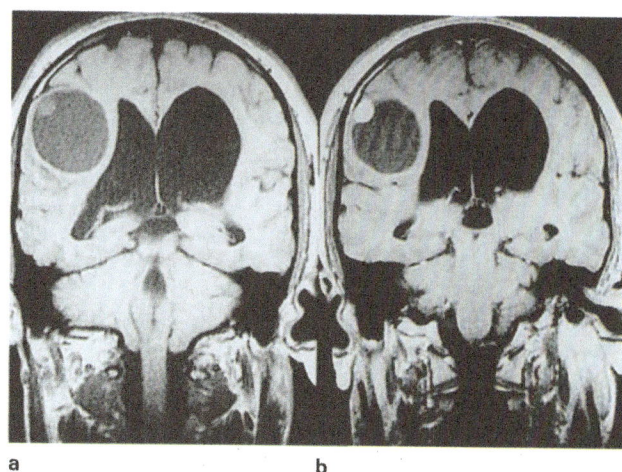

a b

Figure 4.49 Pilocytic astrocytoma, juvenile, hemispheric, cystic: (**a**) T1WI, (**b**) T1WI + C; large hemisphere cyst, with strongly enhancing cerebromeningeal nodule which was also T2 hyperintense. Histology was characteristic

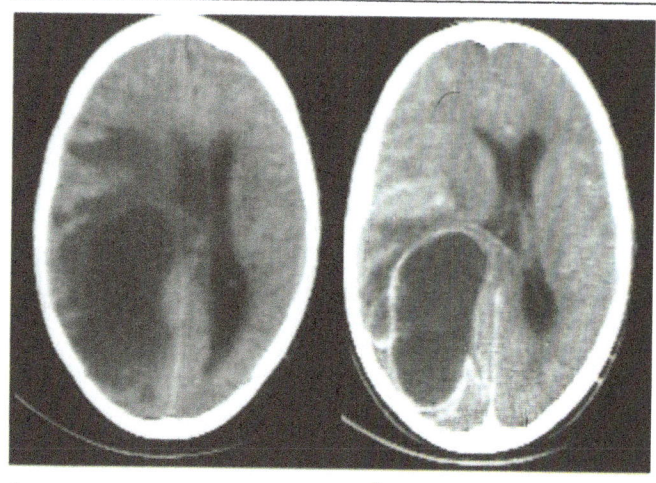

a b

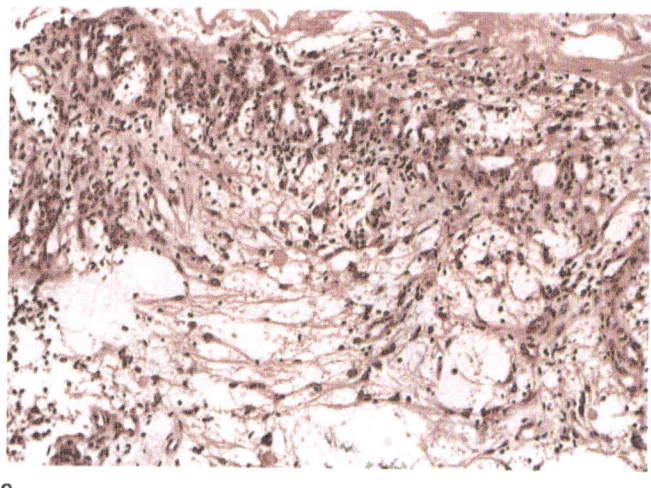

c

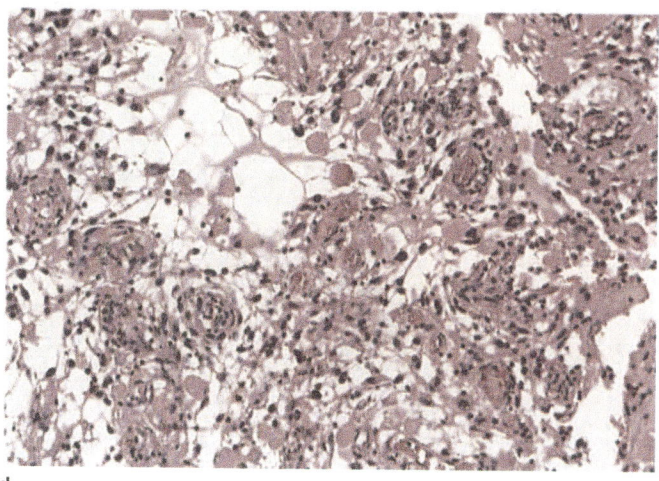

d

Figure 4.48 Pilocytic astrocytoma, juvenile, hemispheric, solid/cystic: (**a**) (*left*) CT + C, (**b**) (*left*) T1WI + C, (**c**) T2WI, (**d**) HE ×200; CT scan shows a small superficial occipital lobe cyst without apparent enhancement. Enhanced T1WI shows a strongly enhancing, superficial plaque of tissue which at operation was found to be subpial, and was easily excised. T2 sequence shows the tumour tissue to be CSF isointense. (Compare with **Figure 4.47** where cyst wall is also enhancing.) Histology shows features of a pilocytic astrocytoma with degenerative change, and large numbers of granular bodies (d)

Figure 4.50 Pilocytic astrocytoma, juvenile, hemispheric, cystic: (**a**) CT, (**b**) CT + C, (**c**) HE ×200; CT scan shows an exceptionally large apparently cystic mass, occupying entire occipital lobe, contents denser than CSF and a thin incomplete rim of enhancement. Typical tumour morphology gives way to progressive, spongiotic degeneration. Vessels are numerous and thin-walled, with foci of marked endothelial proliferation (c)

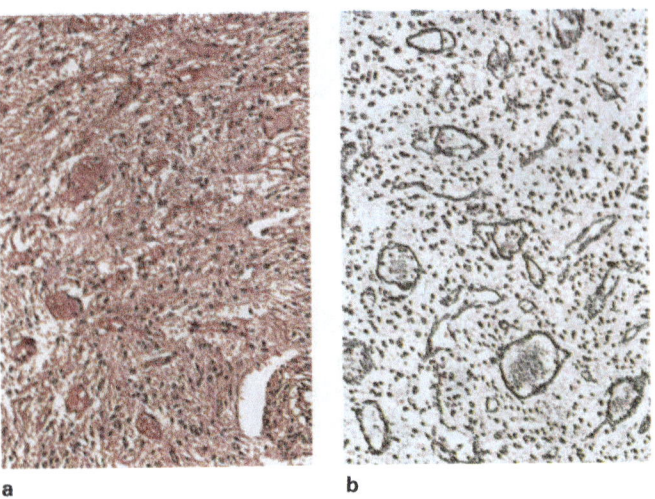

a   b

Figure 4.51   Pilocytic astrocytoma, juvenile, temporal lobe: (a)
HE × 200, (b) reticulin × 200; characteristic profuse, evenly dispersed
angioarchitecture responsible for homogeneous enhancement

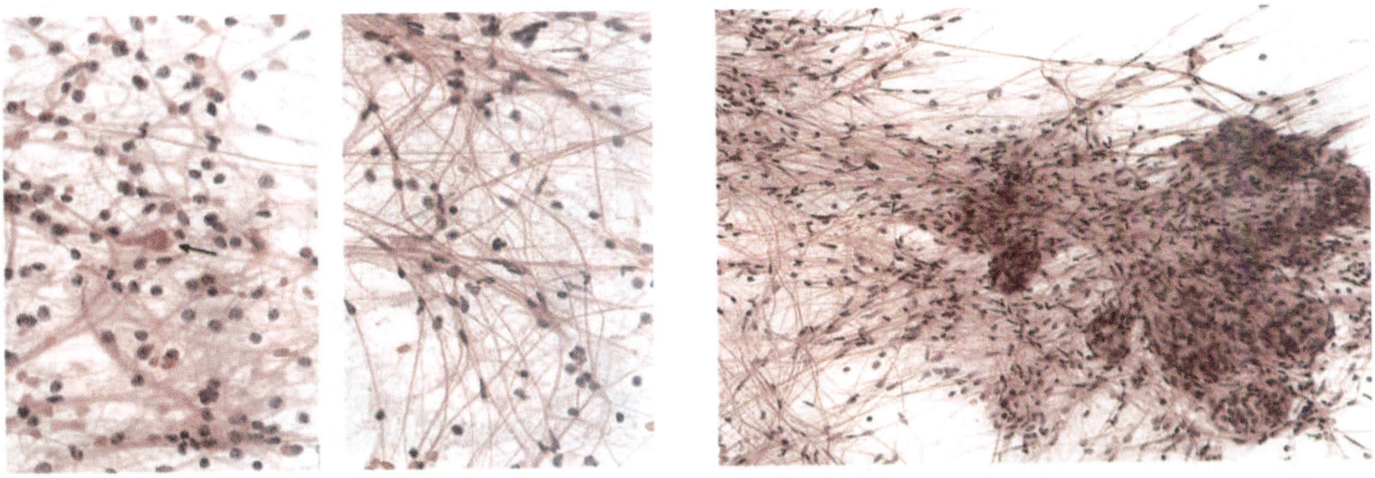

a   b

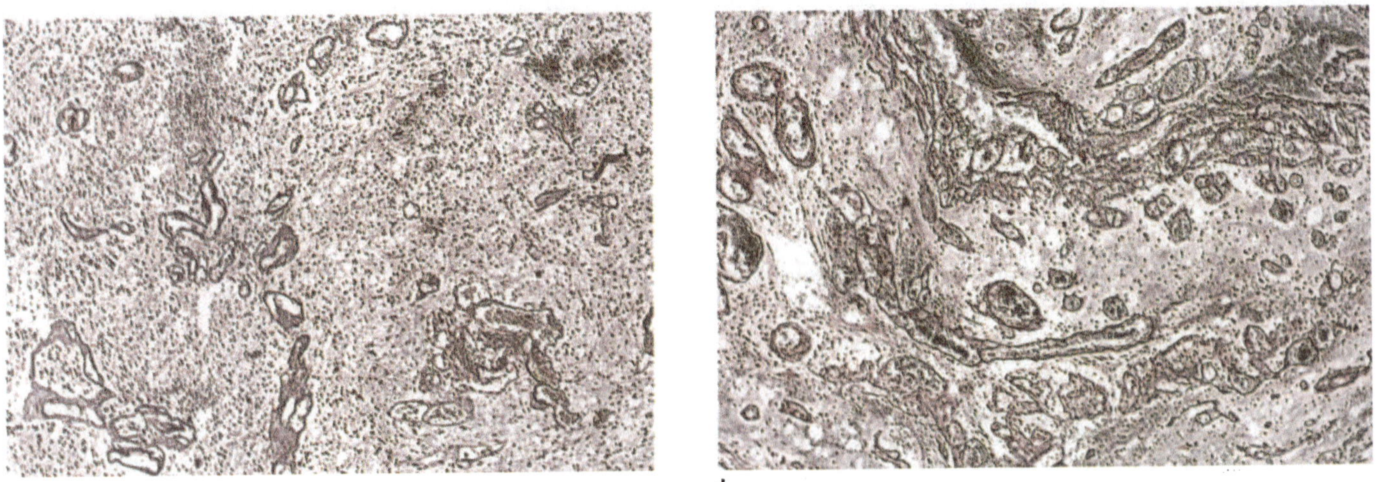

c   d

**Figure 4.52   Pilocytic astrocytoma, juvenile, hemispheric, cys-
tic**: (a) HE × 400, (b) HE × 200, (c,d) reticulin × 100; Smears (a,b)
illustrate characteristic fibrillated astrocytes with Rosenthal fibre

formation and hyperplastic blood vessels (b). Cyst wall (d) is densely
vascularized, compared with stroma (c), presumably due to compaction

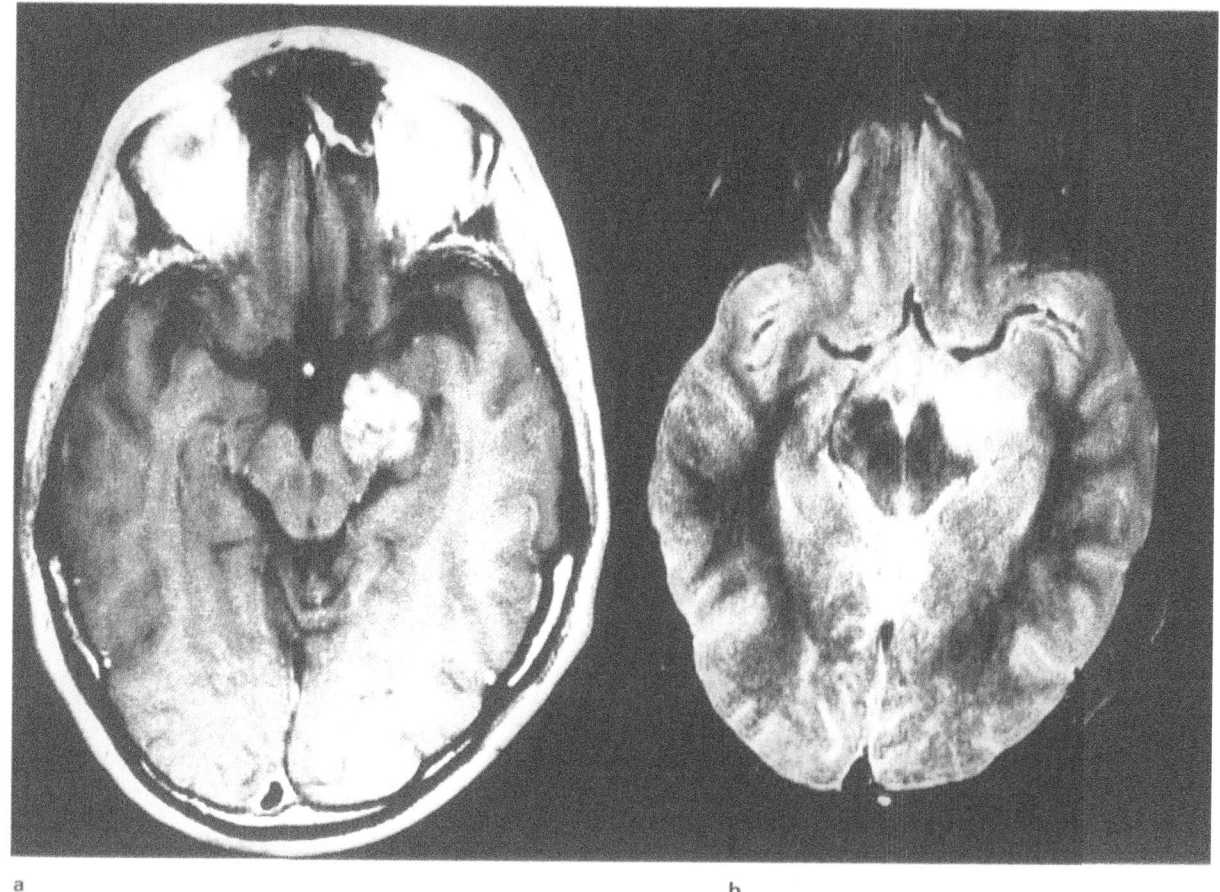

a

b

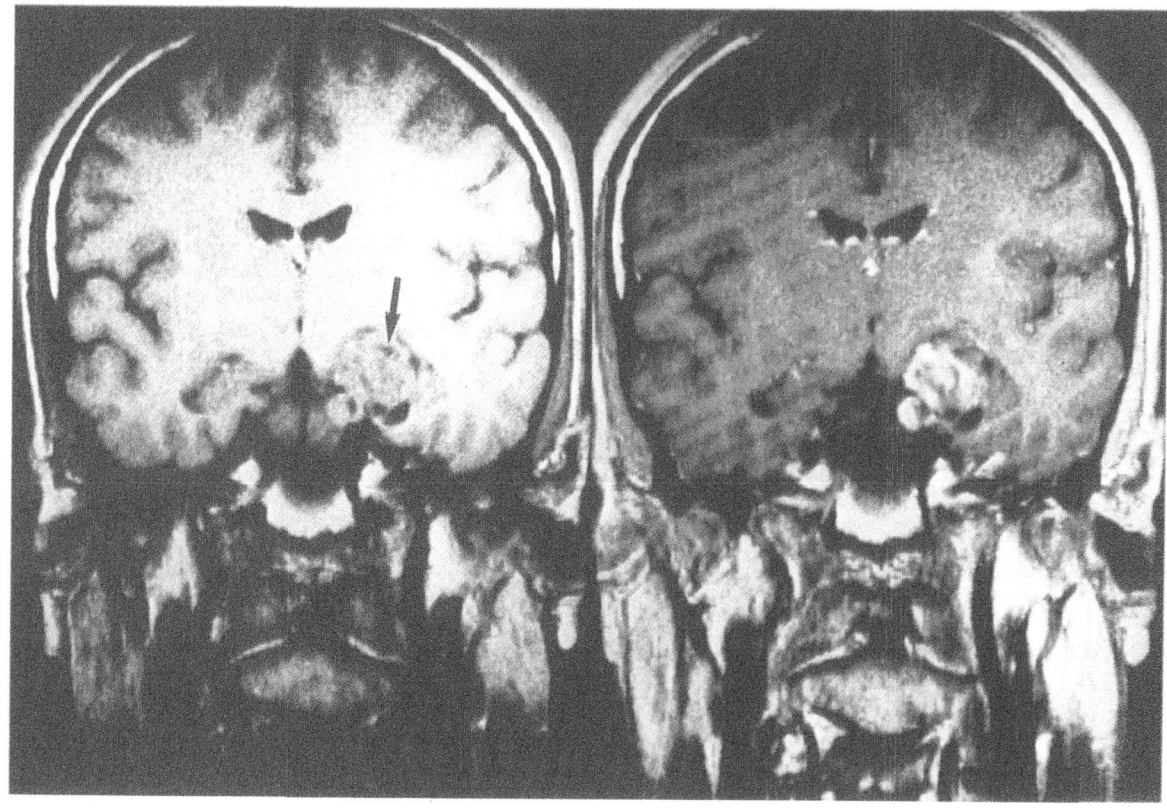

c

d

Figure 4.53 (*legend overleaf*)

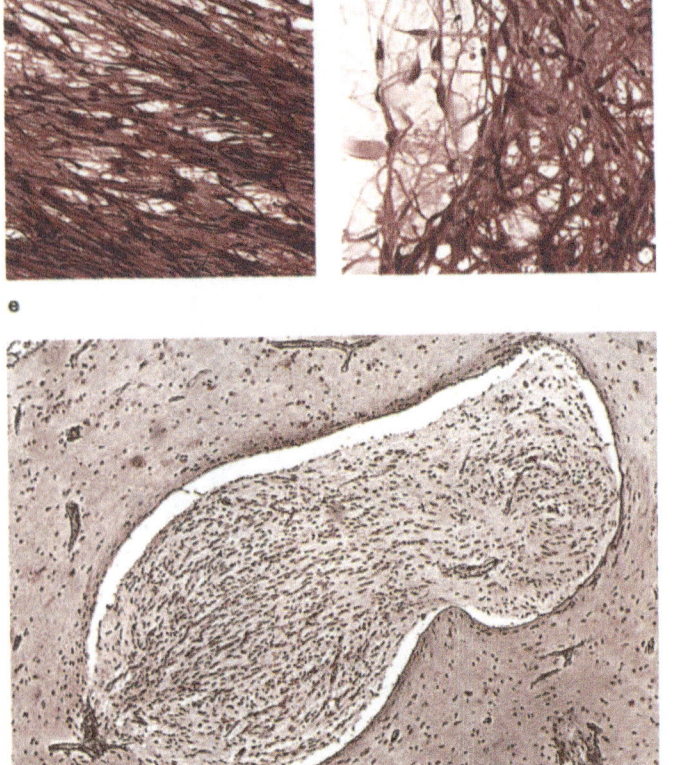

e

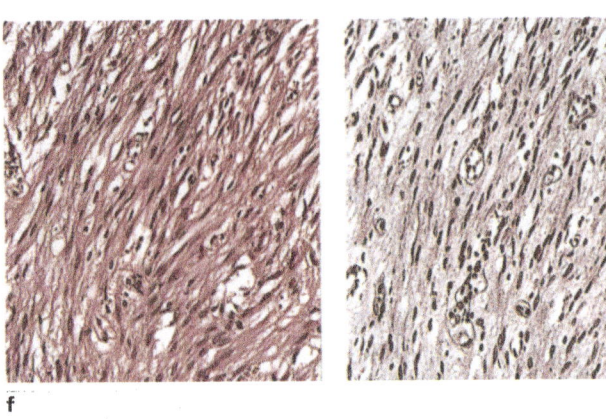

f

Figure 4.53 Pilocytic astrocytoma, adult, medial temporal lobe: (**a**) axial T1WI + C, (**b**) axial T2WI, (**c**) coronal T1WI, (**d**) coronal T1WI + C, (**e**) HE × 200, (**f**) HE/Retic × 100, (**g**) Retic × 40; tumour is strikingly meningeal in its topography, with a sharp profile and diffuse enhancement; hypointense foci (arrow) are cysts. Smear preparation (e) and paraffin section (f, left), show compact arrangement of fibrillated astrocytes, and capillary vasculature (f, right), with surrounding perivascular infiltration of brain (g)

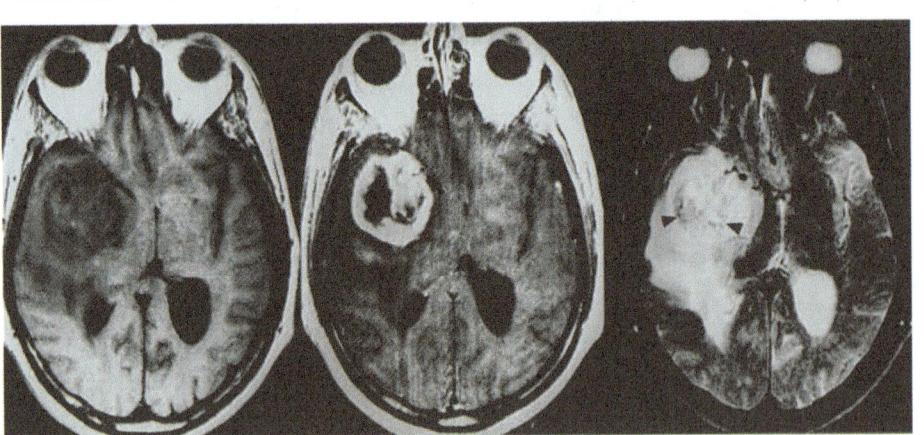

g

Figure 4.54 Pilocytic astrocytoma, adult, malignant: (**a**) T1WI, (**b**) T1WI + C, (**c**) T2WI, (**d**) HE × 100, (**e**) HE/reticulin × 200; tumour is cerebromeningeal and circumscribed. The untidy ring-form of enhancement (b) is also demarcated internally by a relatively T2 hypointense border (c, arrows), shown histologically (d) to consist of acute coagulative necrosis with evidence of anaplasia in the adjacent viable tissue. Morphology of perivascular invasion (e) is distinctive

a   b   c

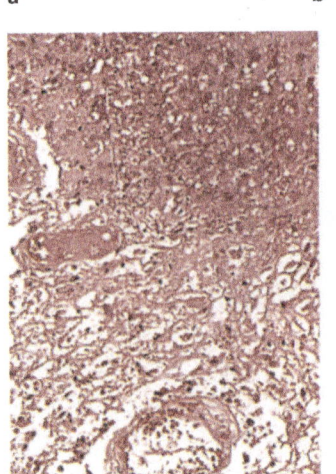
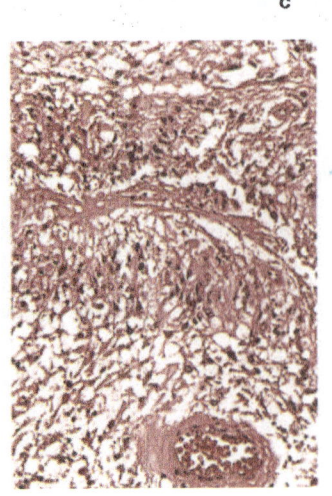
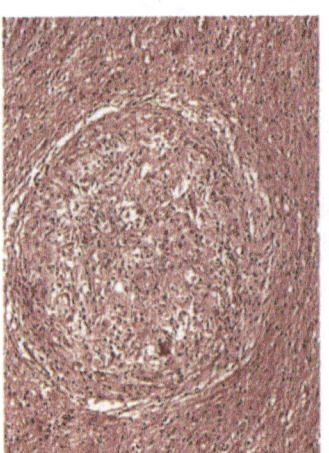
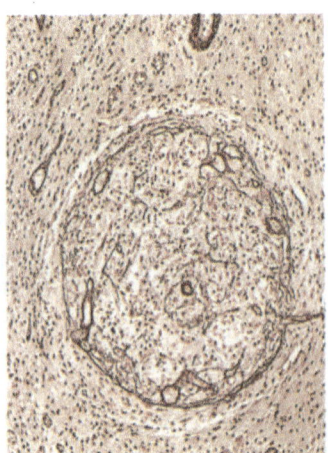

d   e

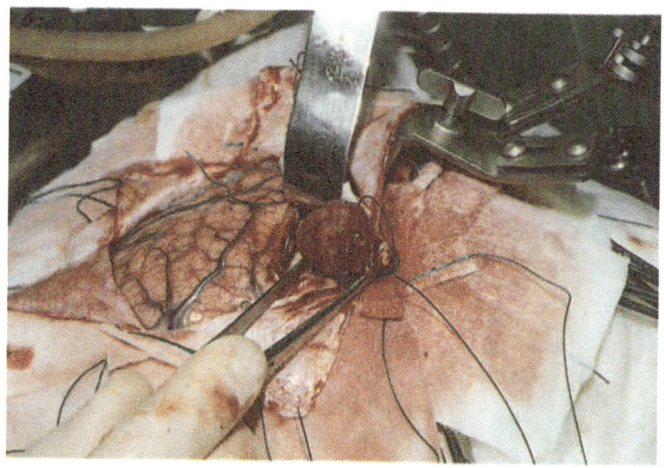

a

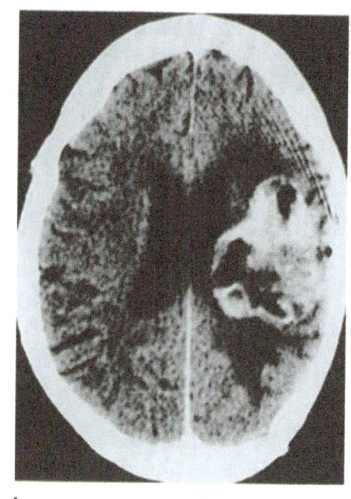

b

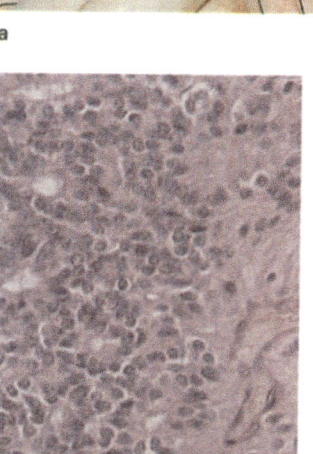 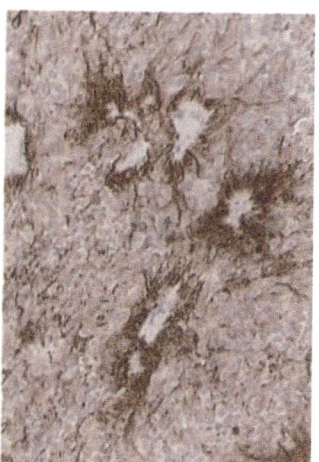

c

Figure 4.55 Ependymoma, cystic, hemisphere: male 21 years; (**a**) operative specimen, (**b**) CT + C, (**c**) HE × 400/GFAP × 200; tumour commenced as a cystic lesion with an enhancing nodule at age 10 years; initial operative specimen shows delivery of nodule from within cyst. Has recurred three times over a period of a decade, and current image shows a lobulated, solid/cystic, strongly but inhomogeneously enhancing mass, still at the site of the original lesion (b). Histology of well-differentiated ependymoma (c, left) has remained constant; GFAP emphasizes abundant capillary type vasculature (c, right)

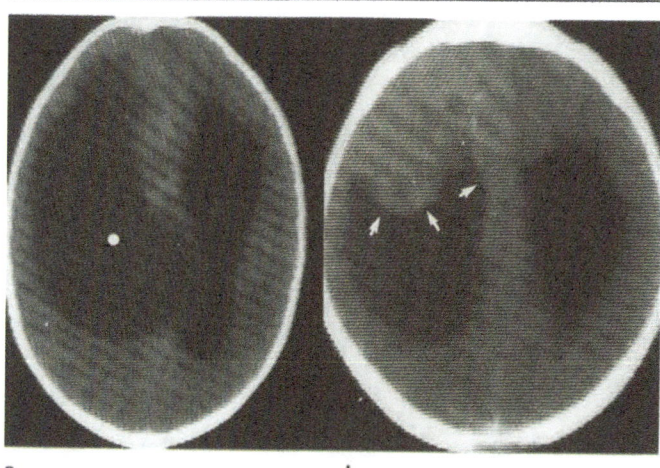

a   b

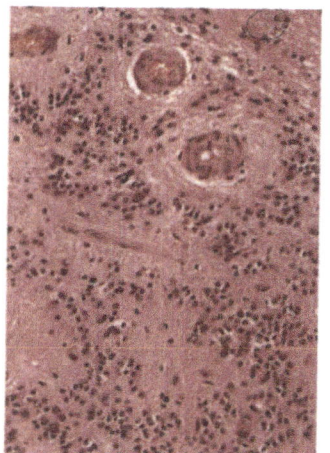 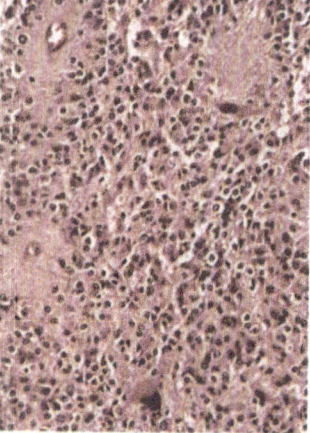

c

Figure 4.56 Ependymoma, anaplastic, cystic, hemisphere, male, 3 years; (**a,b**) CT + C, (**c**) HE × 200; giant intracerebral and intraventricular cyst (CSF hyperdense, white dot—compare with adjacent dilated ventricle), with a large, lobulated, inhomogeneously enhancing, nodular solid component (b, arrows), extending into the parenchyma. Histology shows characteristic perivascular nuclear-free zones of ependymoma (c, left), with considerable nuclear anaplasia but no necrosis (c, right). Note vasculature of more anaplastic tissue remains unchanged

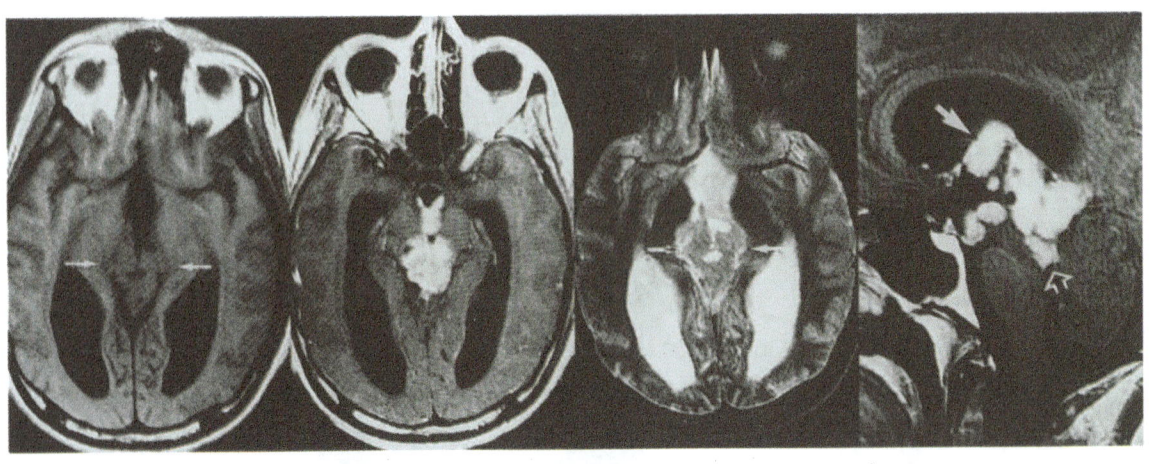

a b c d

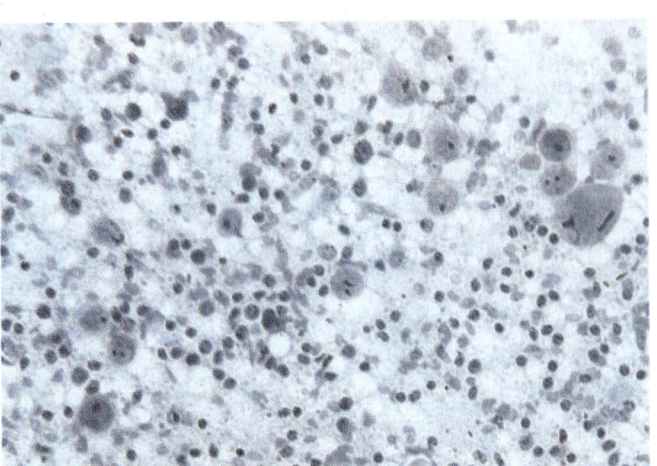

e

Figure 4.57 Germinoma, pineal: male, 19 years; (**a**) T1WI, (**b**) T1WI + C, (**c**) T2WI, (**d**) sagittal T1WI + C, (**e**) Tol blue × 400; images show a lobulated T1/T2 grey-matter isointense, strongly enhancing mass (a–c). Lesion is centred on the pineal region but shows extension into third ventricle (d, closed arrow) and aqueduct (d, open arrow). Smear preparation shows an admixture of large nucleolated and smaller lymphocyte-like cells, typical of germinoma (e). One year follow-up scan after radiotherapy showed complete disappearance of tumour, although midbrain tectum was pathologically T2 hyperintense (spongiosis)

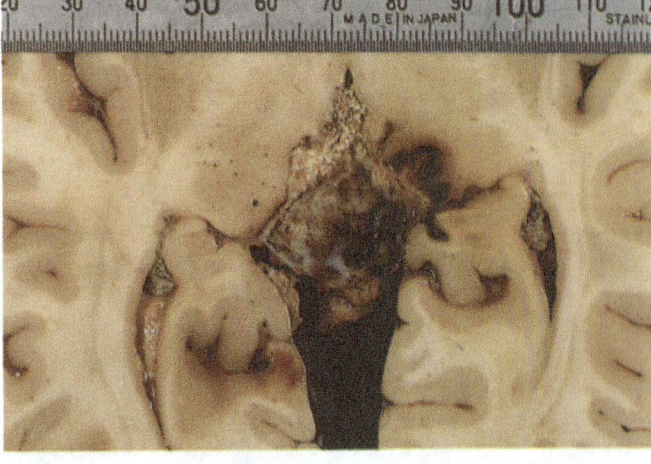

b

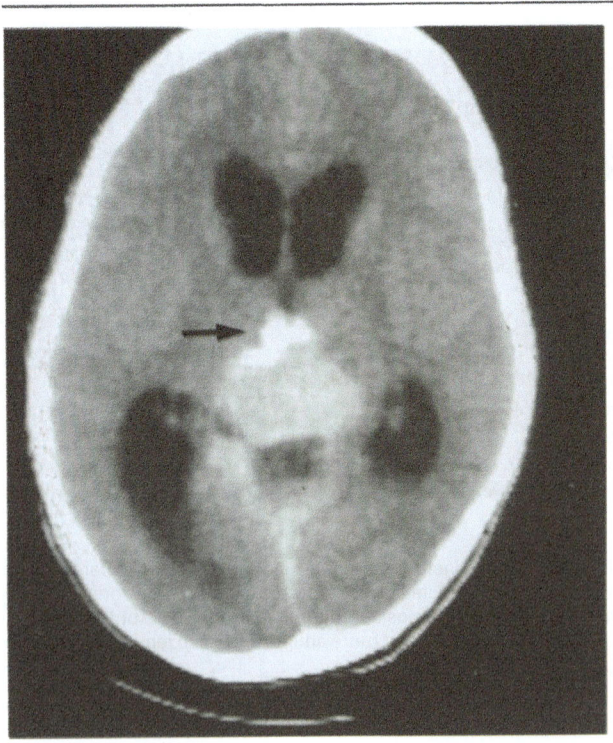

a

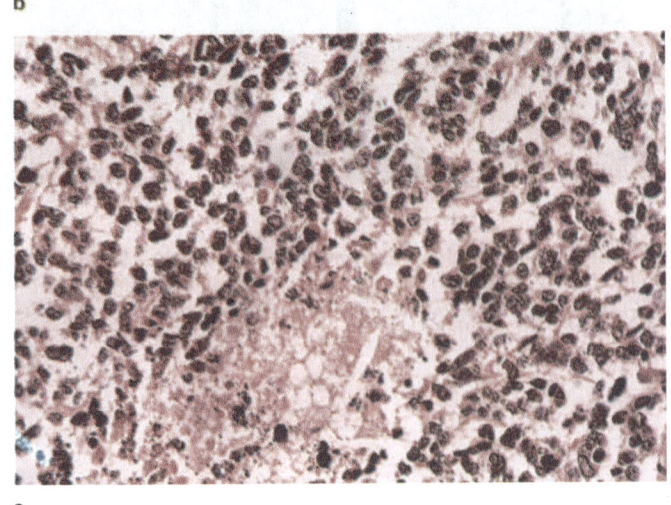

c

Figure 4.58 Pineoblastoma: female, 20 years; (**a**) CT + C, (**b**) fixed brain, (**c**) HE × 400; image shows an enhancing pineal region mass, with cystic and mineral inhomogeneity (arrow). Post-therapy autopsy specimen shows pseudo-encapsulation (haemorrhage is surgical) (b). Histology shows undifferentiated small-cell tumour with focal necrosis (c)

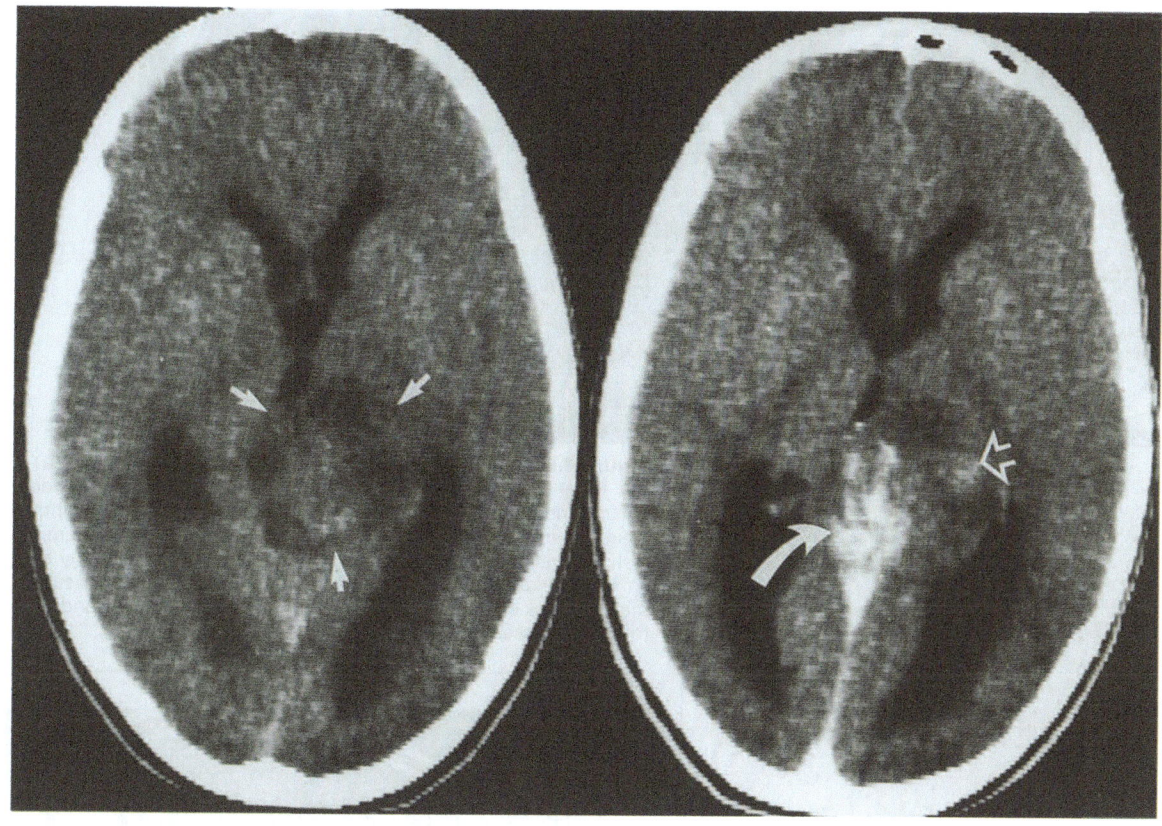

a   b

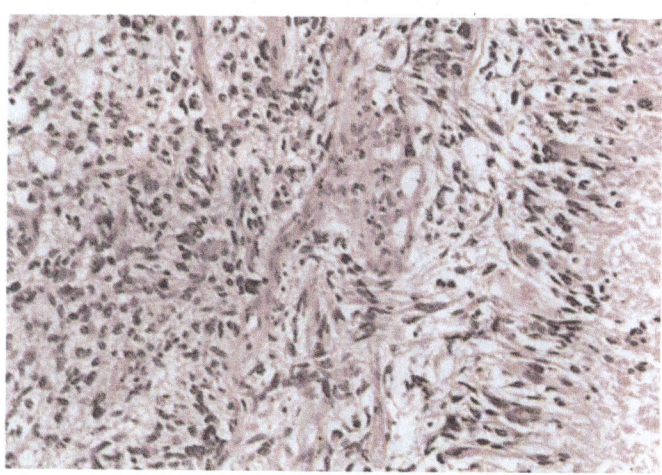

c

Figure 4.59 Glioma, pineal/diencephalic region: female, 15 years; (**a**) CT, (**b**) CT + C, (**c**) HE ×200; images show tumour to be circumscribed and mainly hypodense (a, arrows); strong central linear enhancement is probably venous (b, curved arrow), while weak inhomogeneous enhancement (b, open arrow) is consistent with the biopsy demonstration of malignant glioma-type glomeruloid vascular proliferation and necrosis (c)

4.7. HYPOTHALAMIC MASSES

The principal neoplasms of the region are extraparenchymal, including craniopharyngioma (section 5.2) and pituitary macroadenoma (section 5.3b). Juvenile pilocytic astrocytoma (section 5.4) is the most significant intrinsic tumour, originating from the chiasm or hypothalamus proper, characterized by T2 hyperintensity with strong enhancement (Figure 4.44). These combined features allow distinction from fibrillary astrocytoma and hamartoma, and also the very rare germinoma (Figure 4.57) and granular cell myoblastoma[58], both of which are brain isodense and isointense at short and long TR.

4.8. PINEAL REGION MASSES

Neoplasms at this site are said to constitute less than 1% of intracranial lesions in adults, but from 3% to 8% in children, of which germinoma is easily the commonest, as well as offering the additional diagnostic clue of intraventricular seeding (Figure 4.57). Attempts to correlate CT and microscopic morphology have not been successful, since all usually enhance, and many are mineralized (Figure 4.58). Both germinoma and pineal cell-derived tumours are of intermediate intensity at short and long TR, consistent with their known packing density at ultrastructural level, with fluid and mineral-type inhomogeneity[59,60]; overall hypodensity or T2 hyperintensity is more suggestive of glioma (Figure 4.59)[61]. Although MR has the advantage of displaying topography much more accurately (Figure 4.60), it is not specific, and as therapy is tailored to tumour type, histology is regarded as essential[62]. Because of the difficulty in approaching the pineal region surgically, specimens are usually small rongeur bites, often haemorrhagic, and diagnosis may depend mainly on cytological preparations. Figure 4.61 illustrates a tumour with unexpected histology.

Asymptomatic or benign pineal cysts, of the order of 10 mm diameter, are a not-infrequent incidental finding with contemporary imaging, exhibiting both peripheral and delayed enhancement[63]. Larger, symptomatic cysts are shown on MR to induce tectal compression and aqueduct stenosis (Figure 4.62)[64]. Despite the presence of pineal parenchyma present in the cyst wall, pineocytoma with this morphology is unlikely.

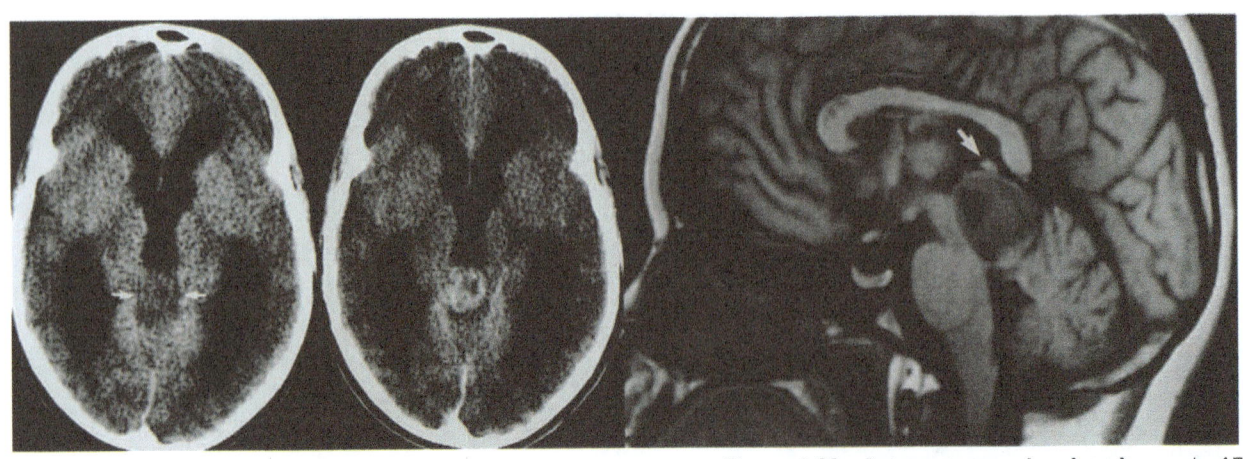

a   b   c

Figure 4.60 Astrocytoma, pineal region: male, 17 years; (**a**) CT, (**b**) CT + C, (**c**) T1WI, (**d**) HE ×200; images show a hypodense, circumscribed pineal region mass (a, arrows); however, sagittal T1 weighted image shows the lesion to arise from midbrain tectum, with distinct anatomically normal pineal gland (c, arrow). Histology shows an unremarkable fibrillated astrocytoma; sparse vasculature suggests that the weak enhancement on CT (b) is probably spurious and related to normal vessels of Galenic cistern

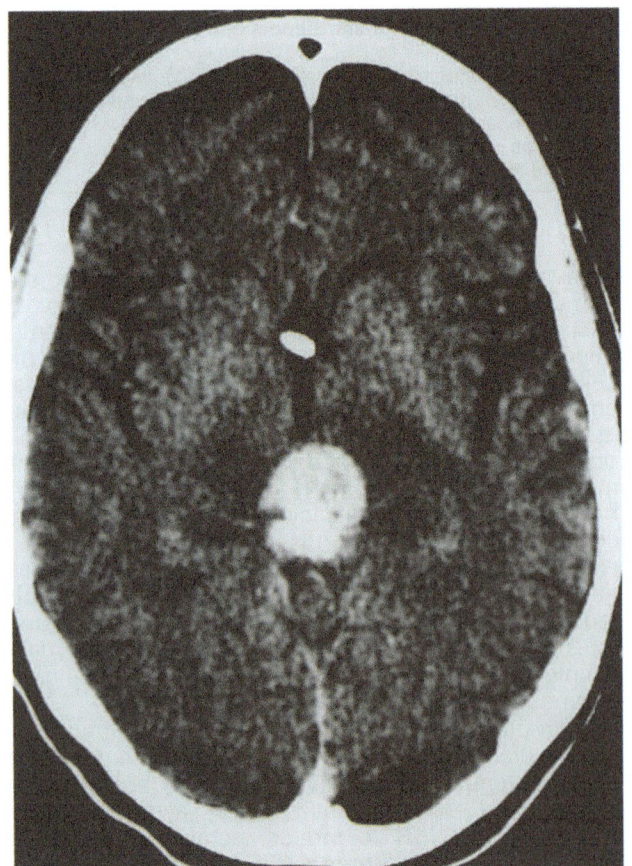

d

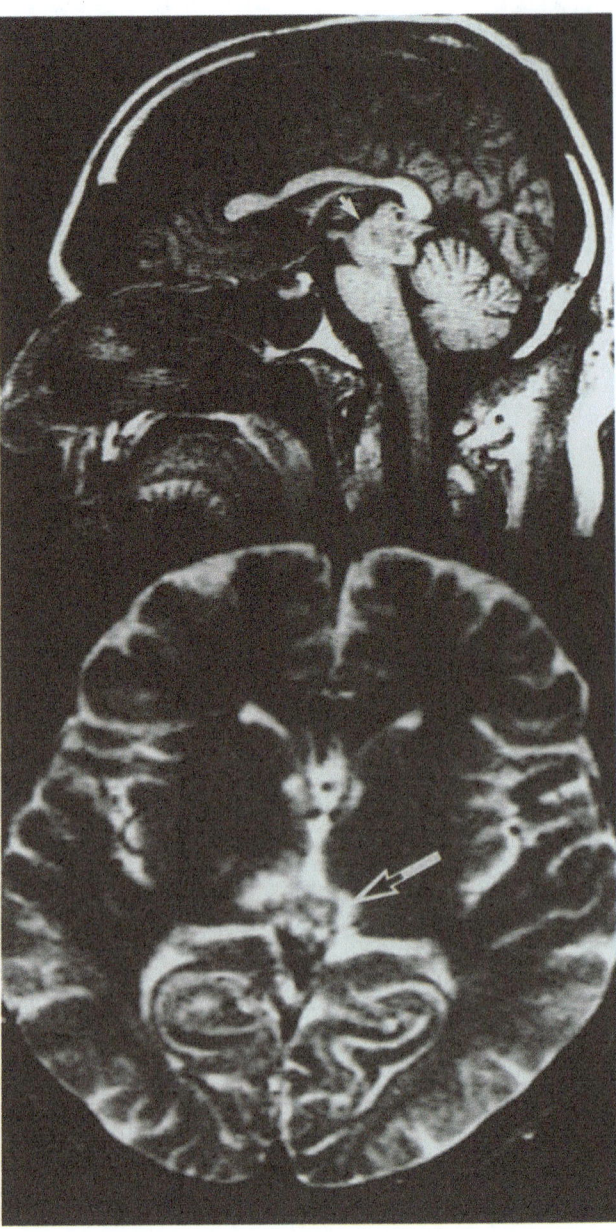

b

c

a   **Figure 4.61** (*legend opposite*)

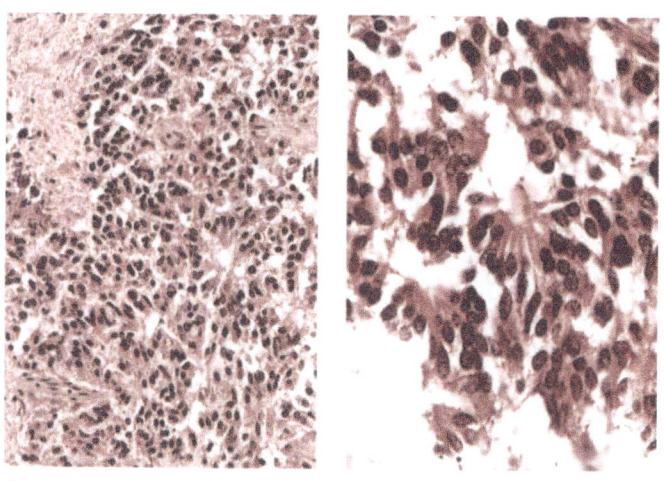

d

Figure 4.61 **Pineoblastoma**: male, 75 years; (**a**) CT + C, (**b**) T1WI, (**c**) T2WI, (**d**) HE × 200/× 400; images show a circumscribed, strongly enhancing pineal region mass with surrounding tissue hypodensity (a). The lesion is T1/T2 isointense – compare with signal intensity of adjacent pons and cerebellum (b); (slight inhomogeneity may be biopsy-related). Histology shows a cellular malignant tumour with necrosis (d, left), and fleurette-like structures (d, right). Tissue for ultrastructural examination was not available and the histological diagnosis was strongly influenced by the imaging features, isointensity in particular

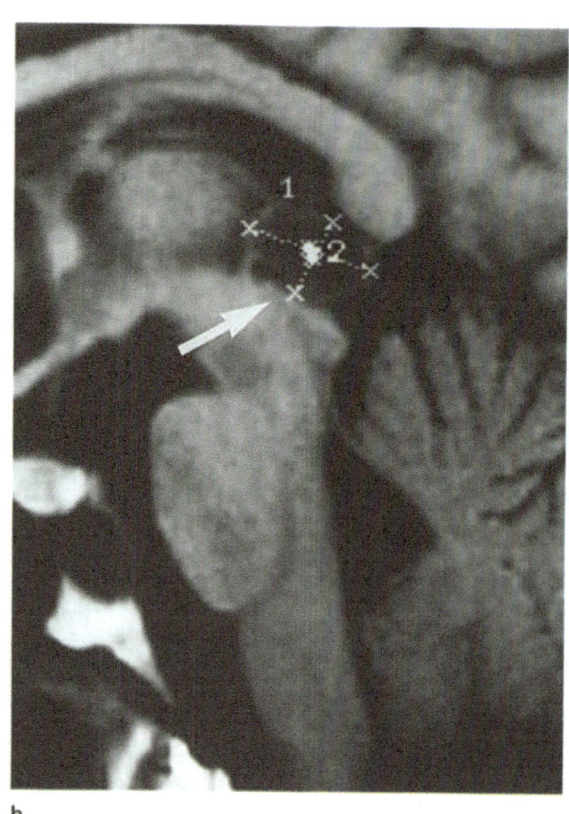

b

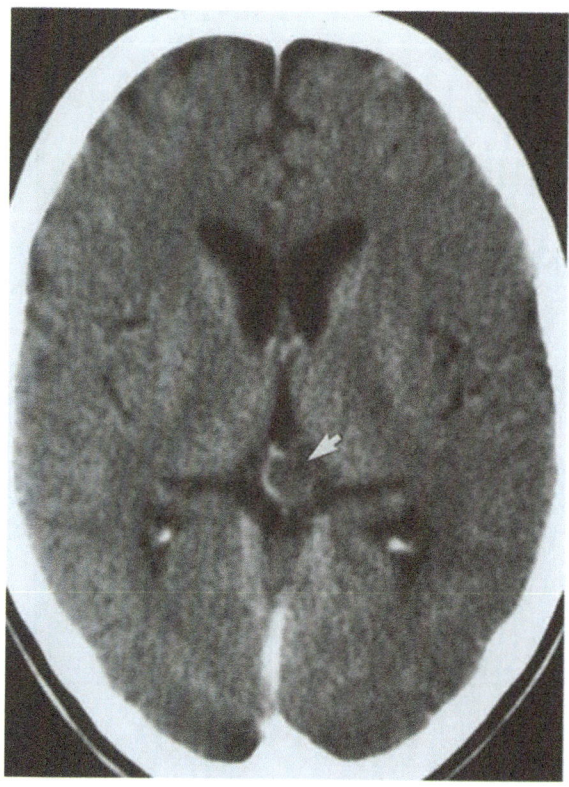

a

Figure 4.62 **Cyst, pineal**: (**a**) CT + C, (**b**) T1WI, (**c**) HE × 200/400, (**d**) HE × 200/NF × 400; female, 22 years, childhood hydrocephalus, shunted; lesion size and profile are typical of asymptomatic pineal cyst; however, isodense contents (a, arrow) and tectal–aqueductal compression (b, arrow) are unusual. Biopsy showed normal pineal parenchyma with no obvious cyst lining in the sample (c,d)

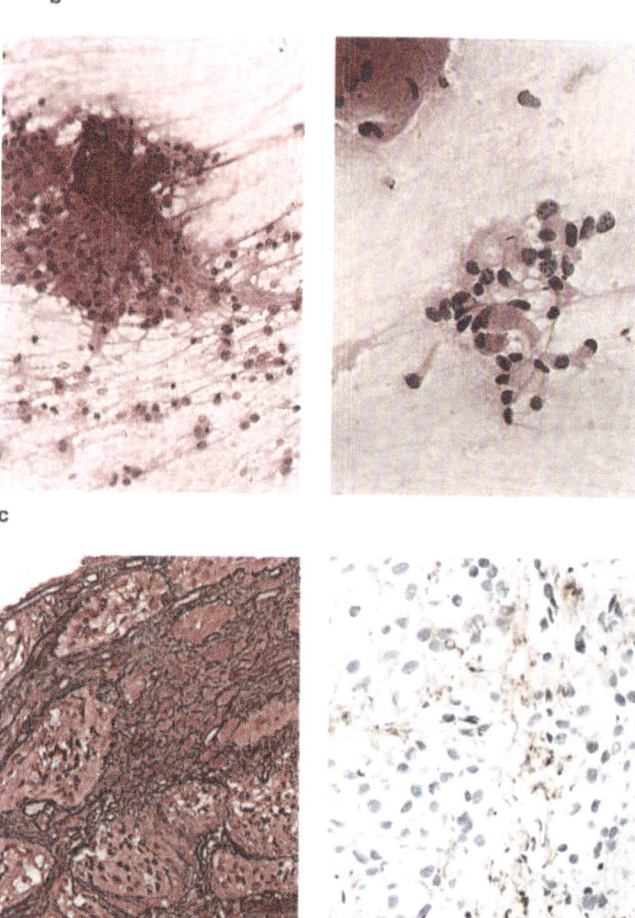

c

d

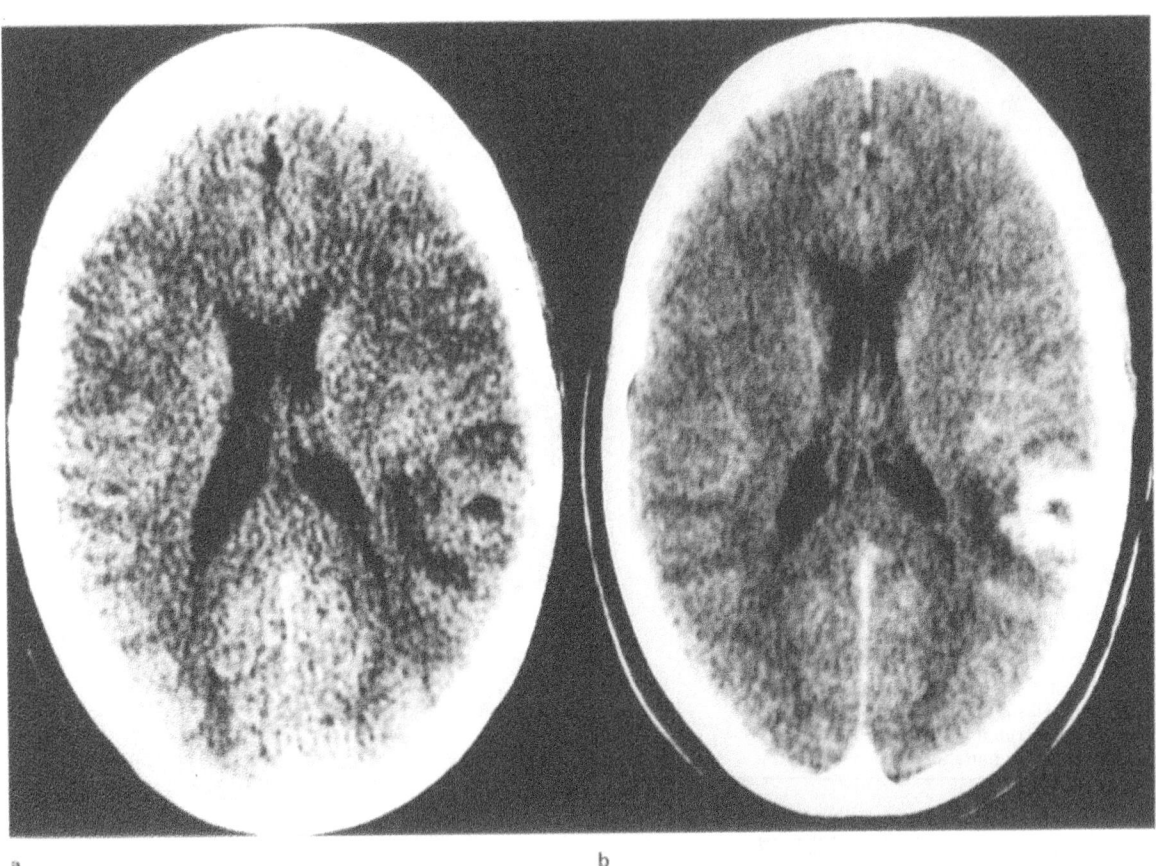

a   b

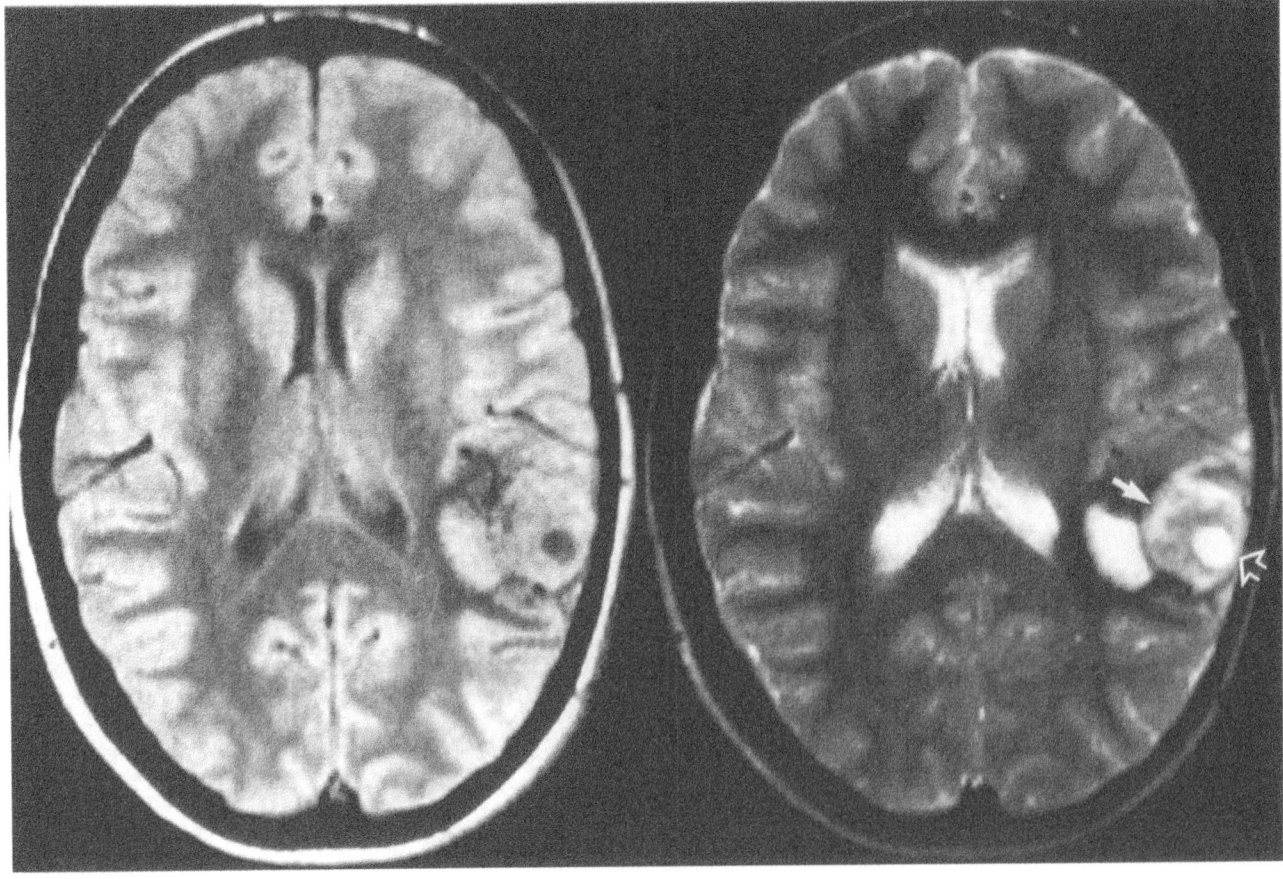

c   d

Figure 4.63 (*legend opposite*)

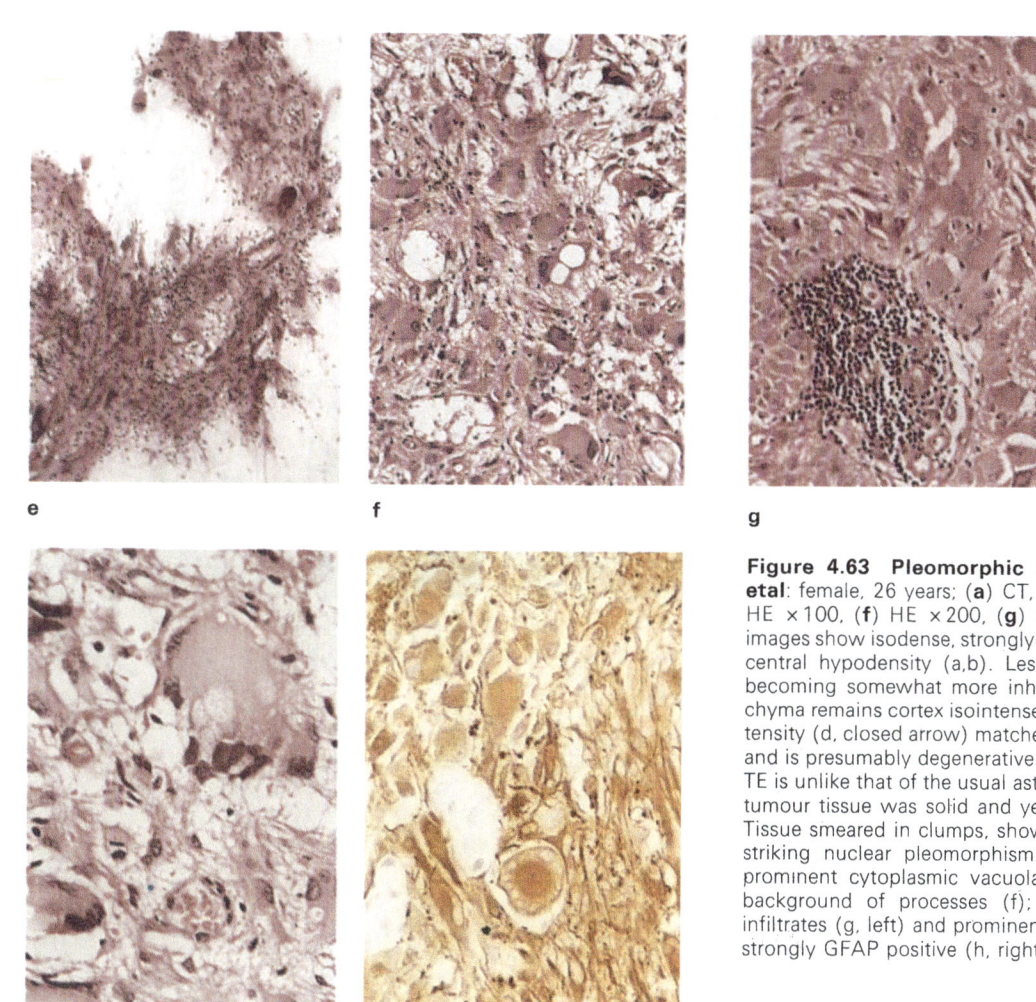

e   f   g

Figure 4.63 Pleomorphic xanthoastroctyoma, temporoparietal: female, 26 years; (**a**) CT, (**b**) CT + C, (**c**) PDWI, (**d**) T2WI, (**e**) HE ×100, (**f**) HE ×200, (**g**) HE/Retic ×200, (**h**) HE/GFAP ×400; images show isodense, strongly enhancing cerebromeningeal mass with central hypodensity (a,b). Lesion is cortex isointense at PDWI (c), becoming somewhat more inhomogeneous, although tumour parenchyma remains cortex isointense at long TE (d). (Peripheral T2 hyperintensity (d, closed arrow) matches that of cyst (d, open arrow) and CSF, and is presumably degenerative.) The pattern of signal intensity at long TE is unlike that of the usual astrocytoma or glioblastoma. At operation tumour tissue was solid and yellowish, without evidence of necrosis. Tissue smeared in clumps, showing sparsely fibrillated cells exhibiting striking nuclear pleomorphism (e); fixed tissue reveals in addition prominent cytoplasmic vacuolation, multinucleate giant cells and a background of processes (f); other features included lymphocytic infiltrates (g, left) and prominent reticulin (g, right); tumour cells were strongly GFAP positive (h, right)

h

4.9. CEREBROMENINGEAL NEUROEPITHELIAL TUMOURS

Just as the concept of intra- versus extra-axial location is a standard point of diagnostic departure so, we think, is the designation of a primary neoplasm which is intrinsic to both parenchyma and meninges. The concept serves to identify a group of distinctively circumscribed, hemispheric tumours typically affecting younger subjects, of relatively benign biological behaviour, and which invariably require extensive tissue sampling together with special diagnostic techniques (special stains, immunohistochemistry, ultrastructure) for proper evaluation. Probably the first tumour of the genre to attract attention was the brainstem gliofibroma[65,66], noted by both radiologists and neurosurgeons to be exophytic, strongly enhancing and biologically benign (Figures 6.29 and 6.30). Supratentorial masses possessing similar characteristics include pleomorphic xanthoastrocytoma and the infantile desmoplastic astrocytoma–ganglioglioma group.

4.9a. Pleomorphic xanthoastroctyoma[67]

The temporal lobe appears to be a preferred site, although the tumour can occur elsewhere, presenting on CT as an isodense, enhancing mass sometimes resembling a meningioma[68]. Probably because of desmoplasia, T2 hyperintensity is less than usual for astrocytomas, with cellular lipidization also a theoretical consideration. These

effects are counteracted focally by micro- and macrocyst formation (Figure 4.63). Significant mitotic activity and necrosis should not be present, but the periphery of the tumour may resemble an infiltrating fibrillary astrocytoma, and recurrence (Figures 4.64 and 4.65) and malignant change[69] have been reported.

4.9b. Desmoplastic infantile glioma[70]

Included in this category are desmoplastic cerebral astrocytoma[71] (syn.: superficial cerebral astrocytoma attached to dura)[72] and desmoplastic infantile ganglioglioma[73]. These rare infantile tumours are notable for their large cystic components (Figure 4.66); usually frontoparietal, superficial and strongly enhancing, they exhibit a spectrum of morphologies ranging from GFAP-positive, spindle-shaped cells (resembling fibroblasts) to variably admixed, neuroepithelial cells, showing astrocytic and neuronal differentiation (primitive and ganglionic) of assumed histogenetic kinship. Reticulin, abundant throughout the tumour stroma, is associated with obliteration of the subarachnoid space, giving the impression of a mesenchymal tumour, frequently with dural adhesion. Density and signal intensities similar to brain parenchyma are to be expected[74], whilst enhancement is consistent with vascularity which is angiomatoid. Neither mitoses nor significant necrosis are a feature, and the prognosis is favourable.

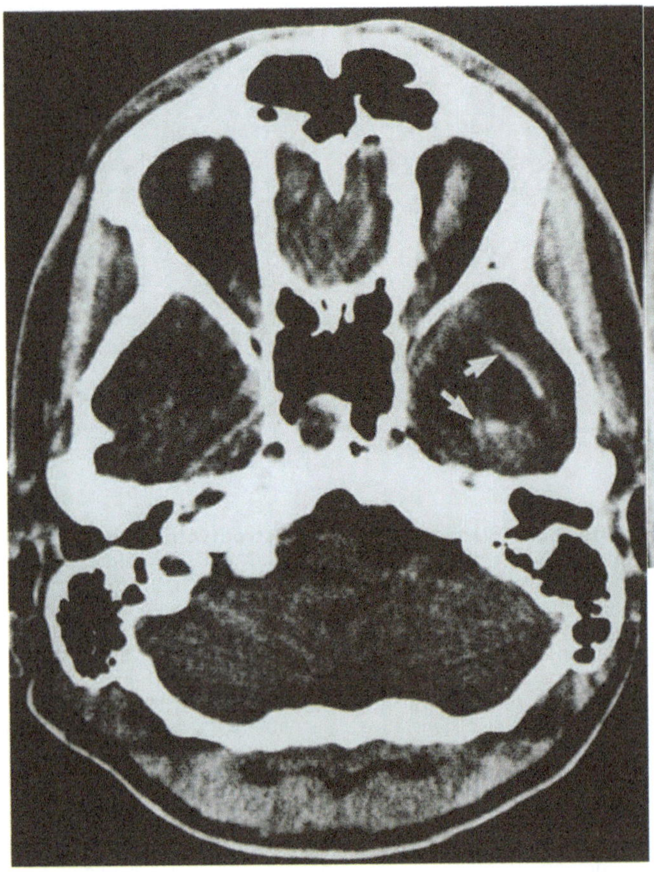

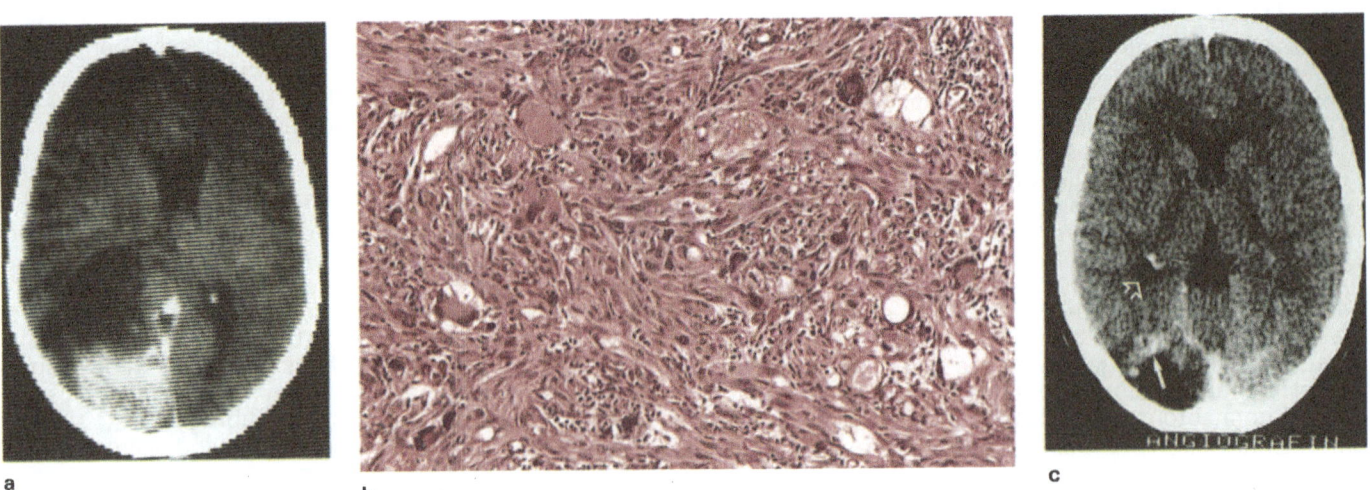

Figure 4.64 Pleomorphic xanthoastrocytoma, temporal: male, 23 years; (**a**) CT + C, (**b**) T1WI + C, (**c**) GFAP × 400; images show a cerebromeningeal, hypodense lesion with discontinuous ring-like enhancement (a, arrows). Postoperative follow-up MR shows superficial meningocerebral enhancement (b, arrows), with atrophic alteration of temporal lobe. At reoperation tumour tissue was visualized to be restricted to lobectomy site and dura. The histological appearances were virtually identical to those illustrated in **Figure 4.63**, except for less striking GFAP positivity (c)

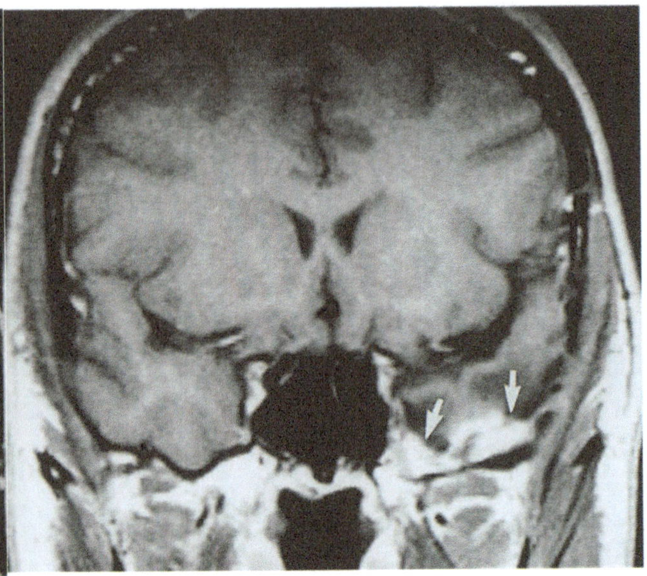

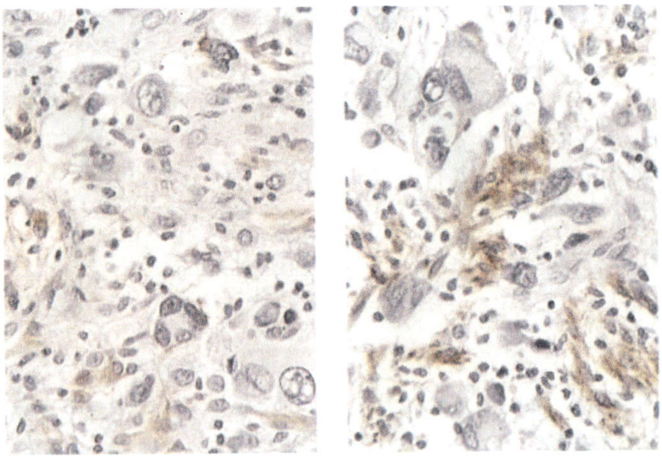

Figure 4.65 Pleomorphic xanthoastrocytoma, occipital: female, 24 years; (**a**) CT + C, (**b**) HE × 200, (**c**) CT + C, (**d**) HE × 400, (**e**) CT + C, (**f**) HE × 400/× 200; initial scan shows an occipital, cerebromeningeal (isodense), strongly enhancing mass with a large adjacent cyst (a). Biopsy revealed a typical pleomorphic xanthoastrocytoma (b). One year follow-up scan shows an occipital lobe cyst with patchy enhancement of adjacent parenchyma (c, arrow); note dilatation of posterior horn (c, open arrow), signifying absence of mass effect.

Biopsy of enhancing tissue shows sheets of lipidized astrocytes; corner of field may show incipient necrosis, but overall morphology was considered unchanged (d). Third scan, 9 months later, shows cyst space to be replaced by enhancing tumour tissue (e, arrow); changes in adjacent occipital lobe are considered atrophic (including white-matter hypodensity and dilated posterior horn). Pleomorphism is still apparent but lipidization is less obvious (f, left); dural involvement appears more cellular and desmoplastic (f, right)

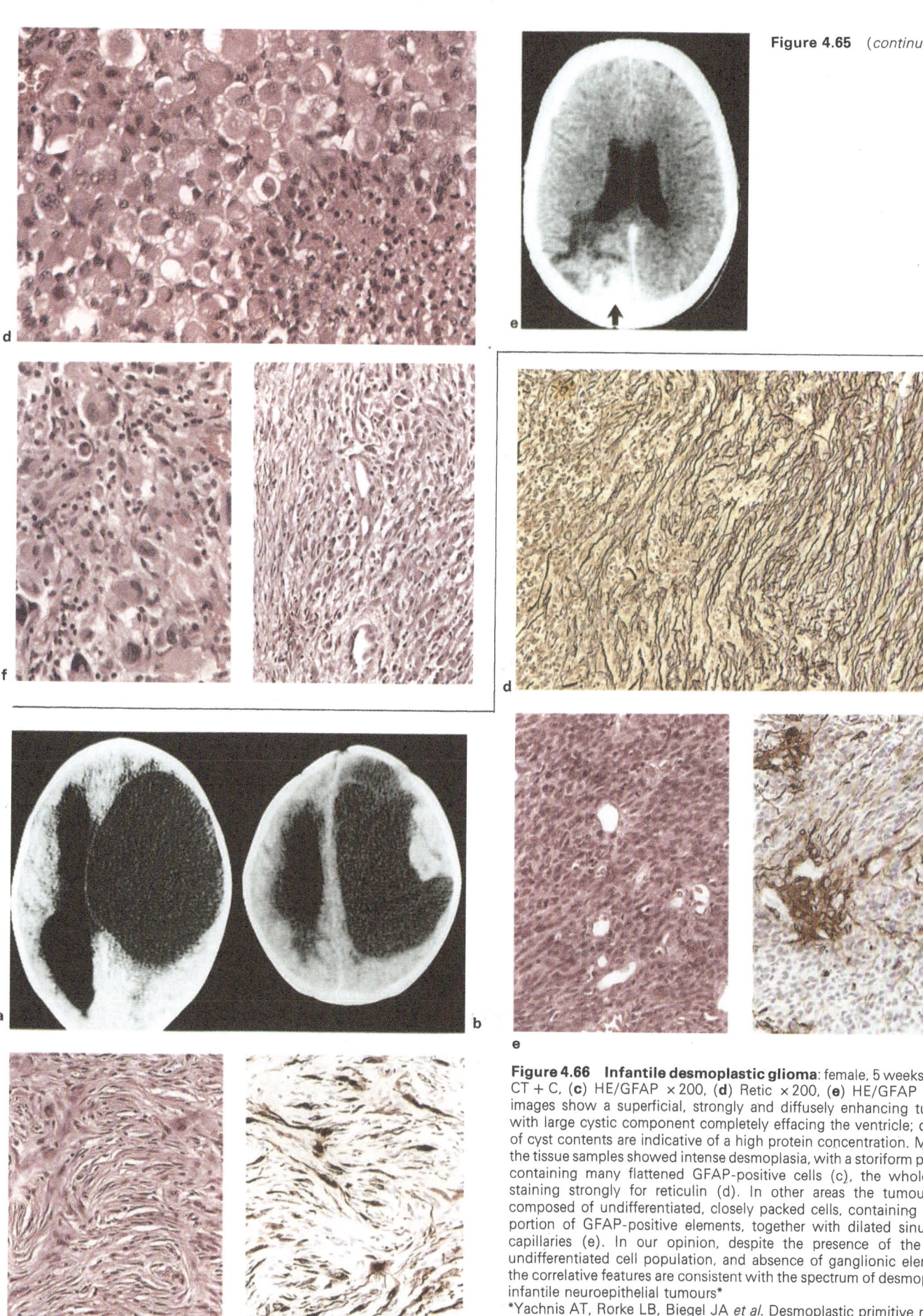

Figure 4.65 (*continued*)

Figure 4.66 Infantile desmoplastic glioma: female, 5 weeks. (**a,b**) CT + C, (**c**) HE/GFAP ×200, (**d**) Retic ×200, (**e**) HE/GFAP ×200; images show a superficial, strongly and diffusely enhancing tumour, with large cystic component completely effacing the ventricle; density of cyst contents are indicative of a high protein concentration. Most of the tissue samples showed intense desmoplasia, with a storiform pattern, containing many flattened GFAP-positive cells (c), the whole field staining strongly for reticulin (d). In other areas the tumour was composed of undifferentiated, closely packed cells, containing a proportion of GFAP-positive elements, together with dilated sinusoidal capillaries (e). In our opinion, despite the presence of the small undifferentiated cell population, and absence of ganglionic elements, the correlative features are consistent with the spectrum of desmoplastic infantile neuroepithelial tumours*

*Yachnis AT, Rorke LB, Biegel JA *et al*. Desmoplastic primitive neuroectodermal tumor with divergent differentiation. Broadening the spectrum of desmoplastic infantile neuroepithelial tumors. Am J Surg Pathol. 1992;16(10):998–1006.

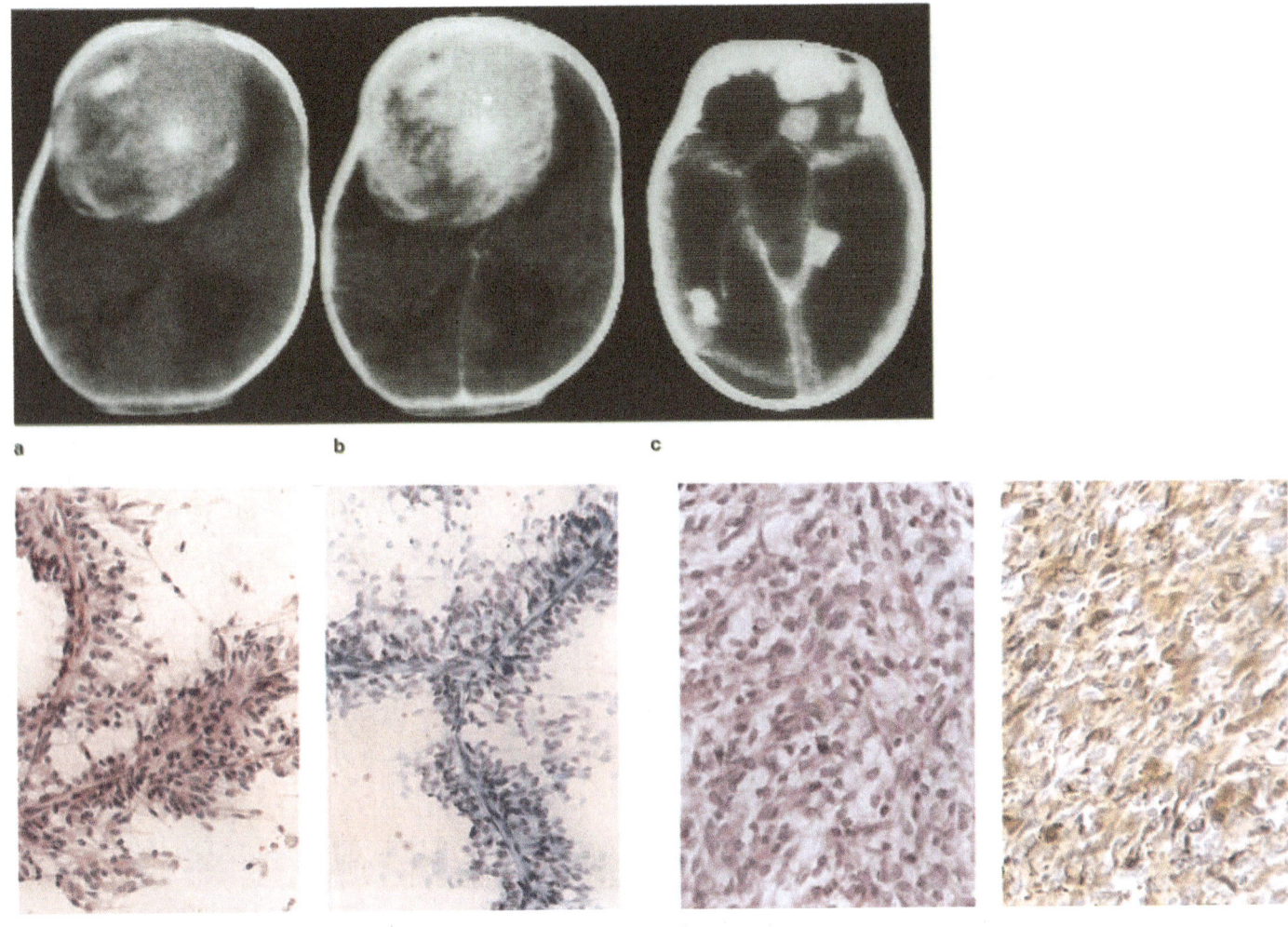

a   b   c

d   e

Figure 4.67   Glioma, giant, infantile: (**a**) CT, (**b,c**) CT + C, (**d**)
HE/Tol blue ×200, (**e**) HE/GFAP ×400; female, 1 month; images
show a large, hyperdense (a), strongly enhancing mass (b), noted at
surgery to be mainly 'extraparenchymal'. Smear preparation shows
sparsely fibrillated cells adherent to capillary-type vessels (d), found to
be intensely GFAP-positive (e). The tumour has a dense capillary
angioarchitecture consistent with the finding of strong enhancement.
All the features of this neoplasm are unusual and the diagnosis of glioma
is based solely on the immunohistochemistry. In particular the pattern
of enhancement is the opposite of what might be expected of a malignant
astrocytoma or glioblastoma. Six-month follow-up scan shows multiple,
discrete homogeneously enhancing lesions (c)

4.9c.   Other 'gliomas' involving the surface of the brain

Apart from previously discussed cerebromeningeal, mixed
gliomas (section 4.6e), our material includes a type
of infantile, cerebromeningeal, cellular GFAP-positive
glioma which was exceptionally large, circumscribed and
homogeneously enhancing, composed of cells which do
not conform to the usual astrocytic genotype, and lacking
evidence of desmoplasia. The collective features of size,
diffuse enhancement and absence of necrosis suggest a
distinctive, relatively benign growth (Figure 4.67).

4.10.   (LATERAL) VENTRICULAR MASSES

Most intraventricular masses can now be distinguished
on MR according to paraventricular, septal, choroid
plexus and juxtasellar origin, with age and such factors
as phakomatotic stigmata being crucial collateral data[75].
Although practically every type of primary (Figure 4.68)
or secondary neoplasm has been described within the
ventricles, true residents are limited to ependymoma–
subependymoma, subependymal glomerate or giant cell
astrocytoma (SEGCA), central neurocytoma and choroid
plexus papilloma/carcinoma. As a pathological principle
the unrestricted growth which the CSF space initially
affords these neoplasms, results in a non-specifically
lobulated and circumscribed profile (Figure 4.72). Distinguishing features generally comply with the combined
attributes of cytoplasmic volume, cell junctions, extracellular space, neovasculature, mineralization, etc., with
enhancement or its absence providing a broad basis for
categorization (Table 4.2, page 123).

4.10a.   Ependymoma and subependymoma

For general discussion on ependymomas see section 6.7a,
hemispheric ependymoma, section 4.6f, and subependymoma (SE), section 6.7a.

In contrast with its restricted intraventricular topography within the posterior fossa, supratentorial ependymoma (Figure 4.55) usually exhibits unequivocal intraparenchymal growth[76], even in the presence of

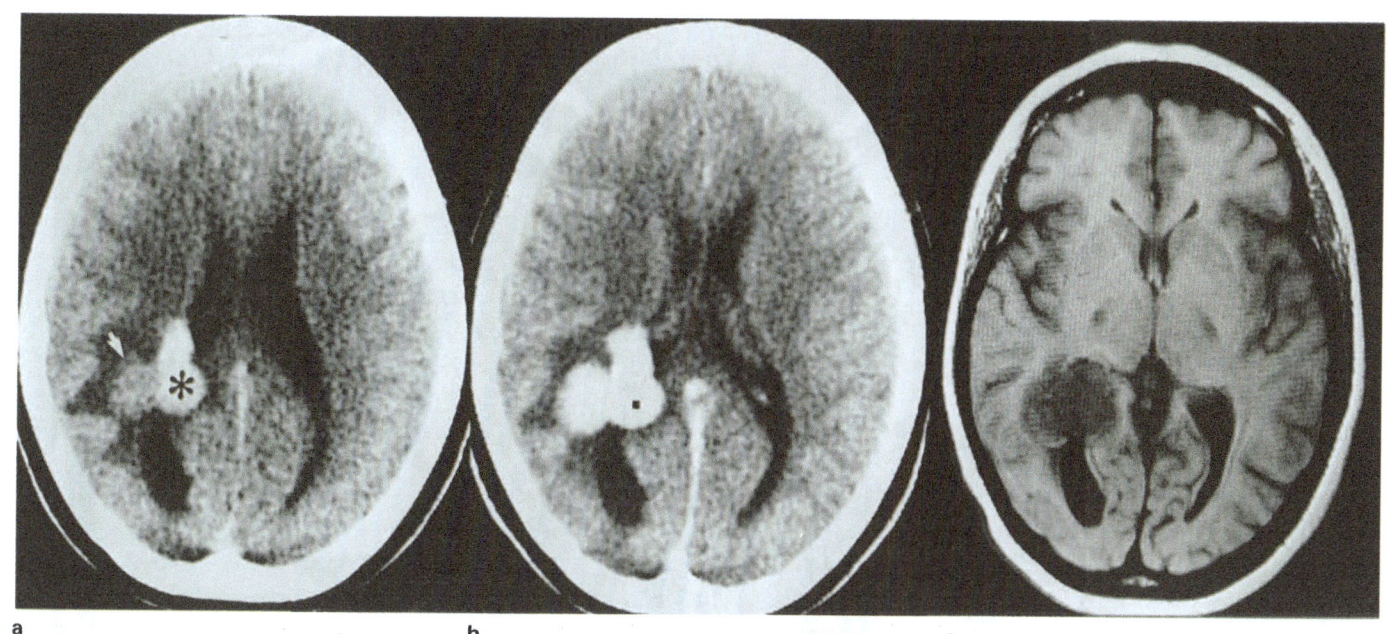

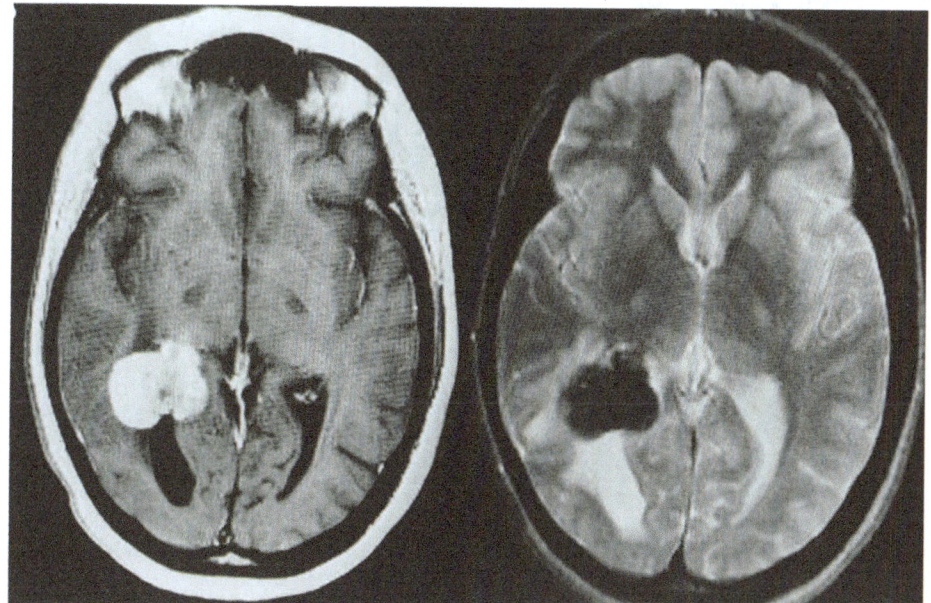

Figure 4.68 Meningioma, fibroblastic, intraventricular: (**a**) CT, (**b**) CT + C, (**c**) T1WI, (**d**) T1WI + C, (**e**) T2WI, (**f**) HE/VG ×200; lesion has cortex isodense, intraparenchymal (a, arrow) and hyperdense, intraventricular components (a, asterisk), both of which show strong diffuse enhancement (b). MR shows intraventricular component to be relatively inhomogeneous before and after contrast (c,d), but entire lesion is exceptionally hypointense on T2 weighted image. Unusual features, besides topography, include parenchymal involvement and CT hyperdensity/T2 hypointensity; latter cannot be explained solely by the presence of dense collagen (f), and the presence of some form of mineral is assumed despite negative von Kossa stain

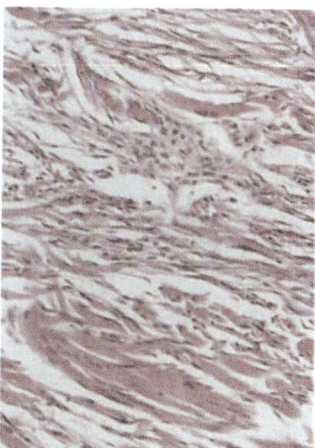

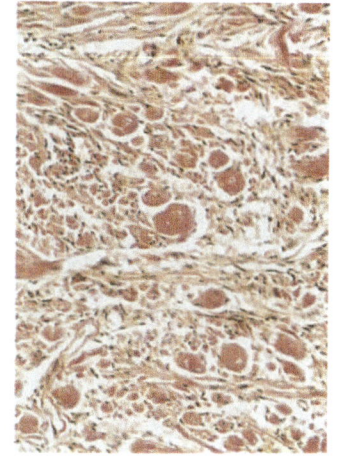

intraventricular extension. However, purely intraventricular lesions are illustrated[77], being central, lobulated, T2 hyperintense, and diffusely or incompletely enhancing.

The apparently unresolved question as to whether SE enhances or not[75] ought to be answered by the microscopic morphology, in which vessels are notably sparse. The strong central enhancement illustrated in Figure 4.69 is due to an unusual vascular glomerate, lacking interspersed tumour cells and presumed to be degenerative. The surrounding rim of subependyoma tissue is non-enhancing.

4.10b. Subependymal giant cell astrocytoma[78]

Best known in the context of tuberous sclerosis, SGCA can occur as an isolated lesion, having imaging characteristics of juvenile (dimorphic) pilocytic astrocytoma, but prone to mineralization. High spin (proton) density component is assumed to be interstitial water, whilst florid (angiomatous)[79] vasculature, including dilated, thin-walled channels, is consistent with typically strong enhancement (Figures 4.70 and 4.71).

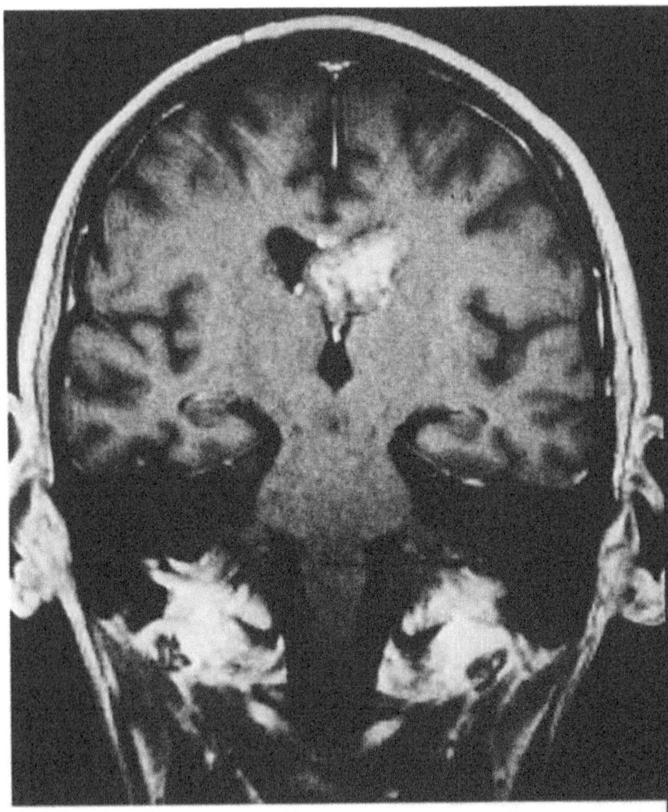

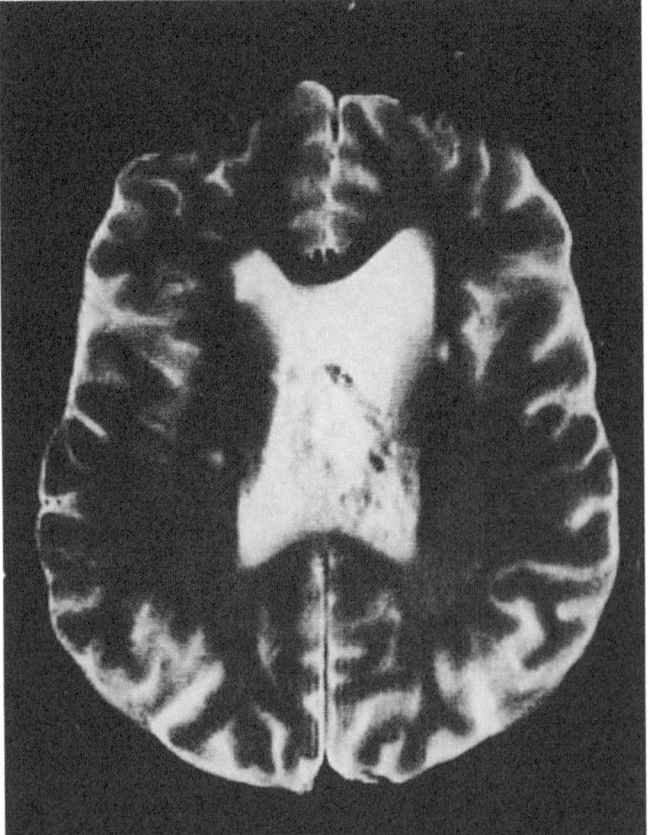

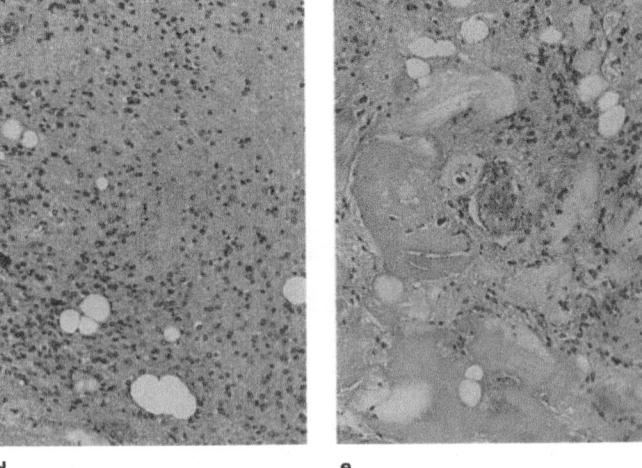

Figure 4.69 Subependymoma, lateral ventricle: male, 60 years; (**a**) T1WI + C, (**b**) PDWI, (**c**) T2WI, (**d,e**) HE × 200; enhanced T1 image shows an intraventricular mass, with brain isointense rim and strong central enhancement (a); tumour, which appears to be arising from ventricular wall, is homogeneously hyperintense on PDWI (b), but rim becomes inhomogeneously hypointense at long TR/TE (c). Histology shows morphology typical of subependymoma (d), but with unusual, extensive vascular hyalinization (e), considered to represent the interior of the mass (enhancing portion). Tumour also contains microcysts and haemosiderin

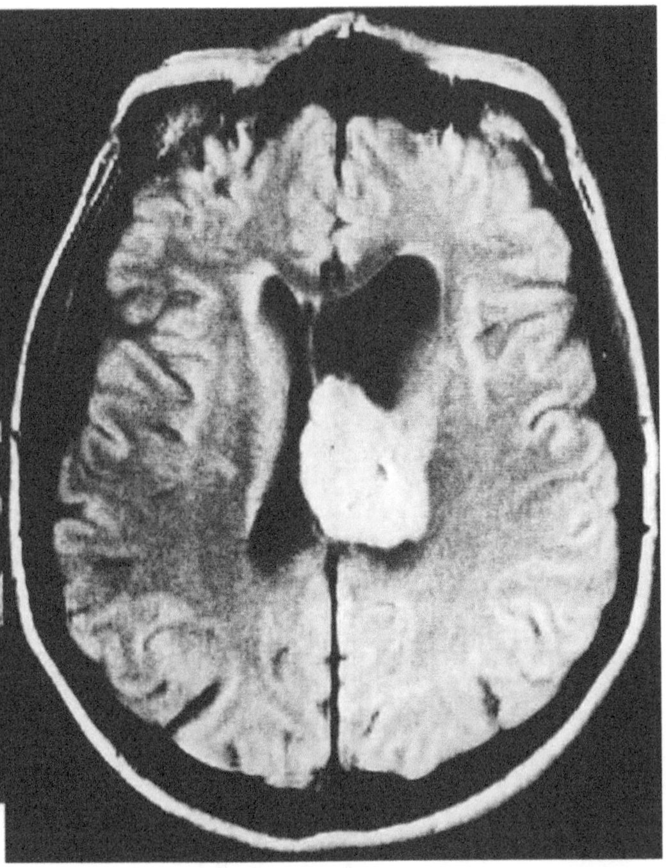

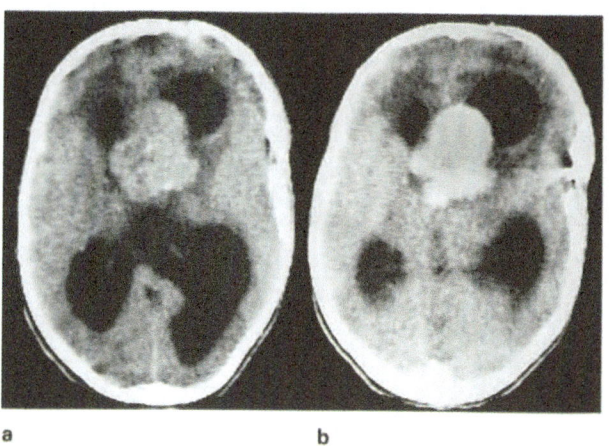

a   b

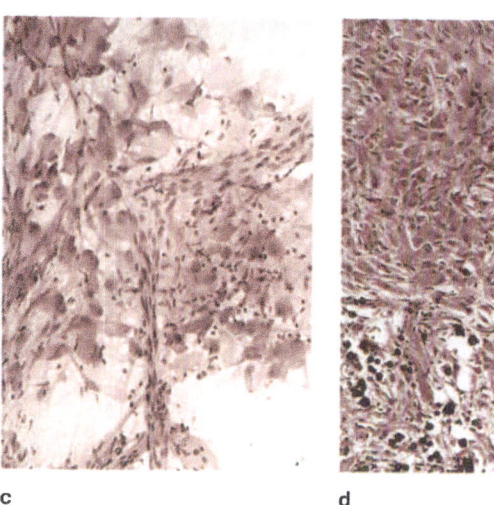

c   d

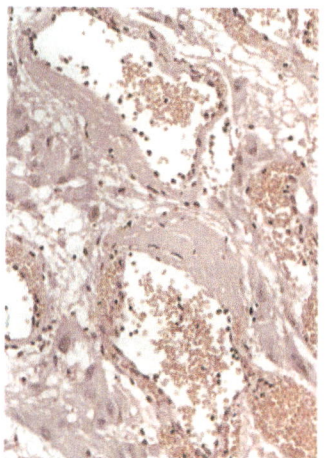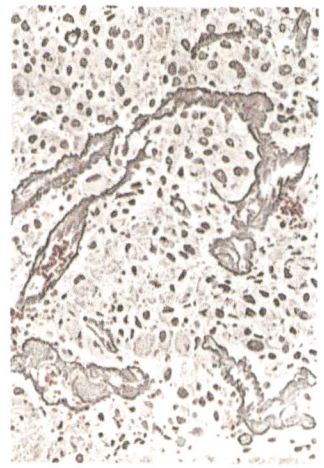

e

Figure 4.70 **Subependymal giant-cell astrocytoma**: (a) CT, (b) CT + C, (c,d) HE ×200, (e) HE/Retic ×200; sharply circumscribed hyperdense intraventricular mass which enhances diffusely. Morphology is characteristic, including giant cells (c), mineralization (d) and vasculature (e)

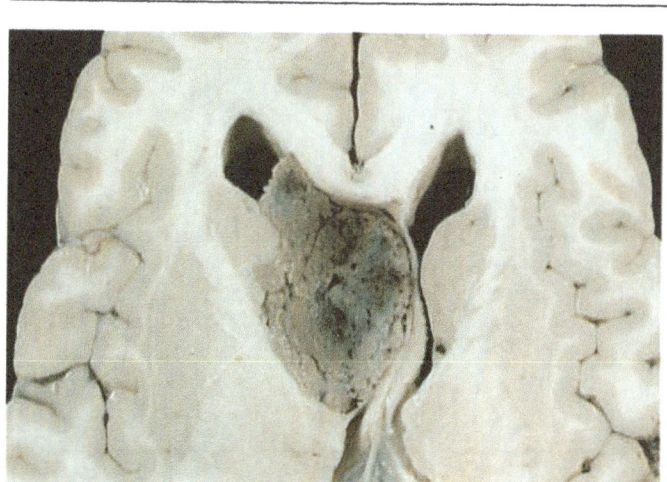

a

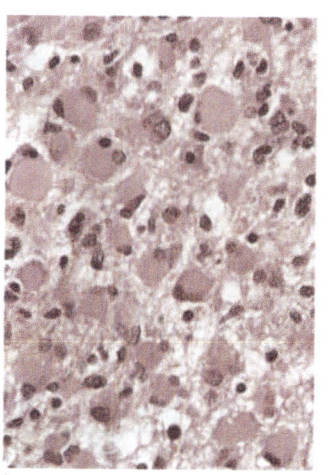

b

Figure 4.71 **Subependymal giant cell astrocytoma**: (a) fixed brain, (b) HE ×400; tumour is composed of numerous tiny lobules with some intervening areas of cystic degeneration (see coarse lobulation visible in **Figure 4.70a**). Histology compares appearance of gemistocytes (b, left) and giant astrocytes (b, right)

Table 4.2

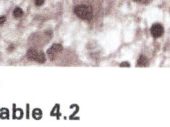

	Long TR parenchymal signal	Contrast	Signal void
Epithelial	Iso	+ +	Vascular
Neural	Iso	+	Mineral
Glial			
ependymoma	Hyper	+ / −	—
subependymoma	Hyper	− / +	—
giant cell astrocytoma	Hyper	+ +	Mineral
juvenile pilocytic astrocytoma	Hyper	+ +	—
fibrillary astrocytoma	Hyper	—	—

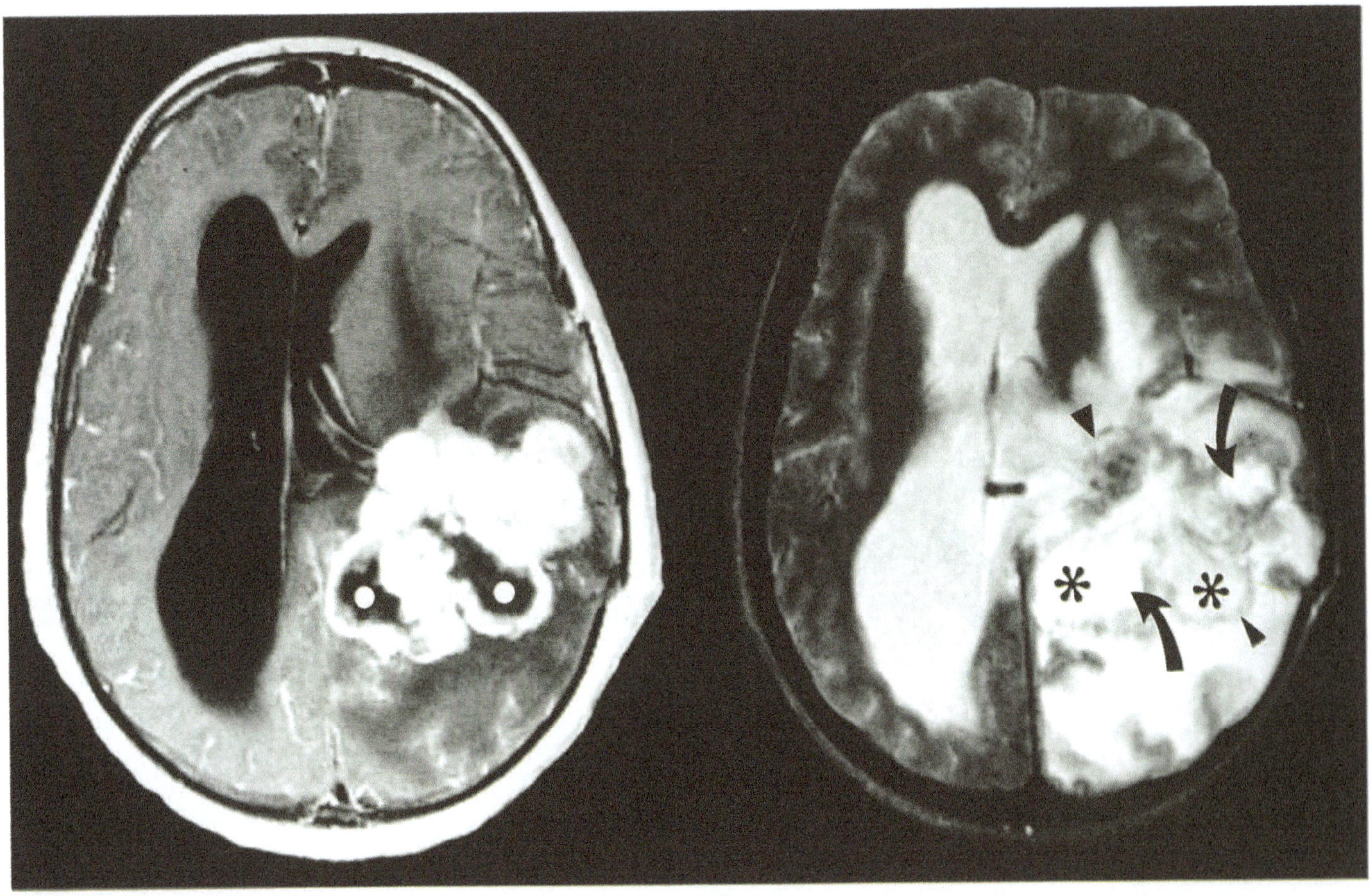

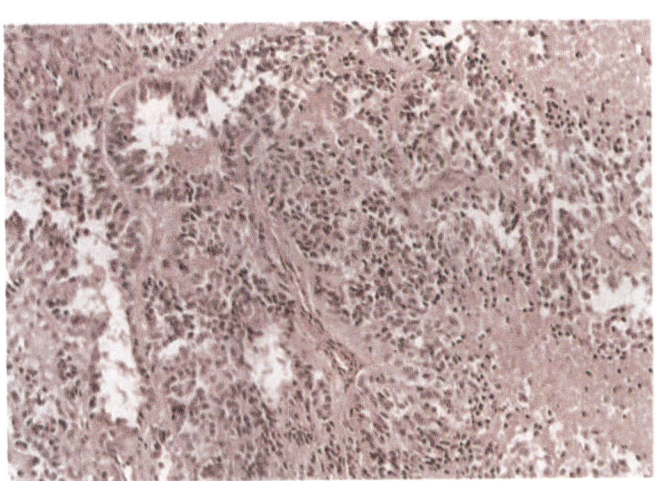

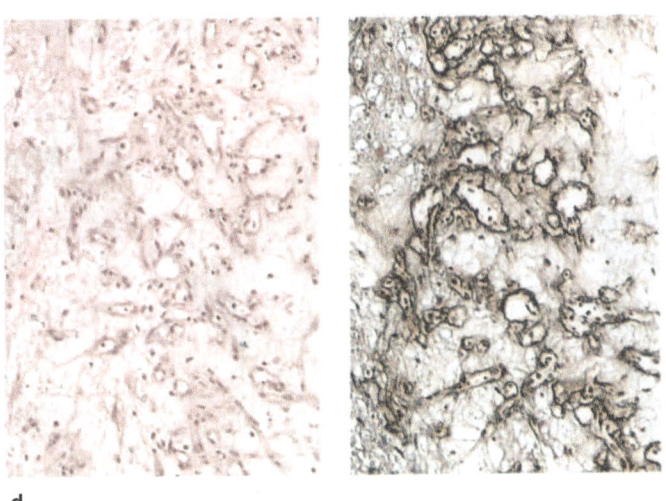

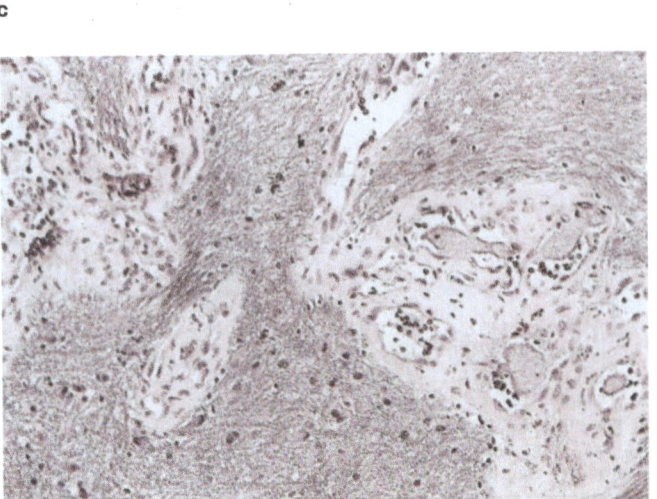

Figure 4.72 Choroid plexus carcinoma: male, 14 years; (**a**) T1WI + C, (**b**) T2WI, (**c**) HE ×200, (**d**) HE/Retic ×200, (**e**) PTAH ×200; images show a large, solid/cystic, lobulated tumour probably arising within the posterior horn of the lateral ventricle. At long TR, tumour rim becomes relatively hypointense (b, arrow-heads), corresponding to papillary carcinoma (c). Note that the cystic (a, dots) and solid interior components of the lesion, become almost indistinguishable at long TR/TE (b); foci of hyperintensity (b, curved arrows), with same signal intensity as cysts (b, asterisks), are myxomatous, vascularized stroma (d, left). Tumour brain interface shows unusual admixture of vascularized and gliotic tissue (e). Carcinoma cells were GFAP, S100, EMA, keratin, HCG and alpha-fetoprotein-negative

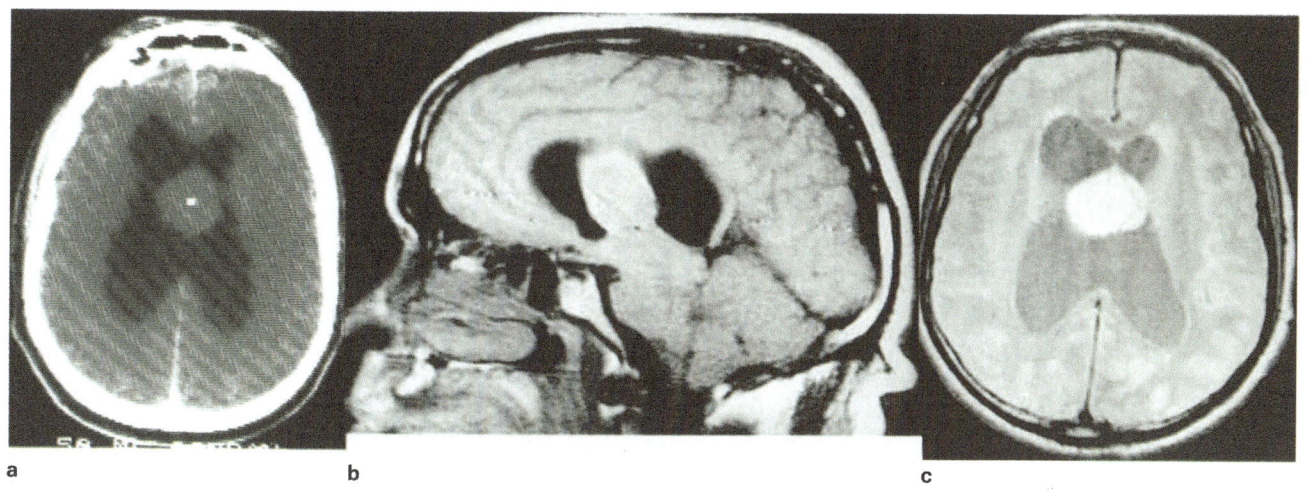

a   b   c

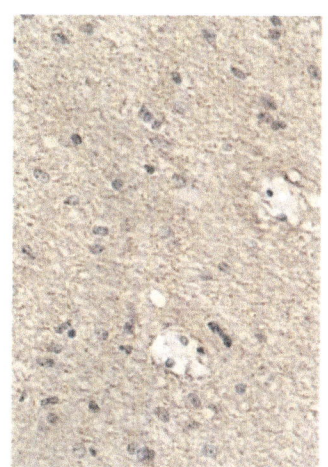

Figure 4.73 Astrocytoma, fibrillary, septal: male, 44 years; (a) CT + C, (b) T1WI, (c) PDWI, (d) PTAH/GFAP ×400, (e) EM ×10000; images show a circumscribed, isodense, non-enhancing septal mass (a), which is T1 isointense/PD hyperintense. Histologically tumour is composed of sparse nuclei embedded in a dense GFAP-positive fibrillar stroma, which also contains occasional capillaries (d,e). Hyperintensity at long TR does not accord with isodensity/T1 isointensity, or EM evidence of relatively restricted interstitial space (e). Distended processes (e, asterisk) may account for T2 hyperintensity. Note organelles (open arrows) and intermediate filament aggregates (closed arrows)

d

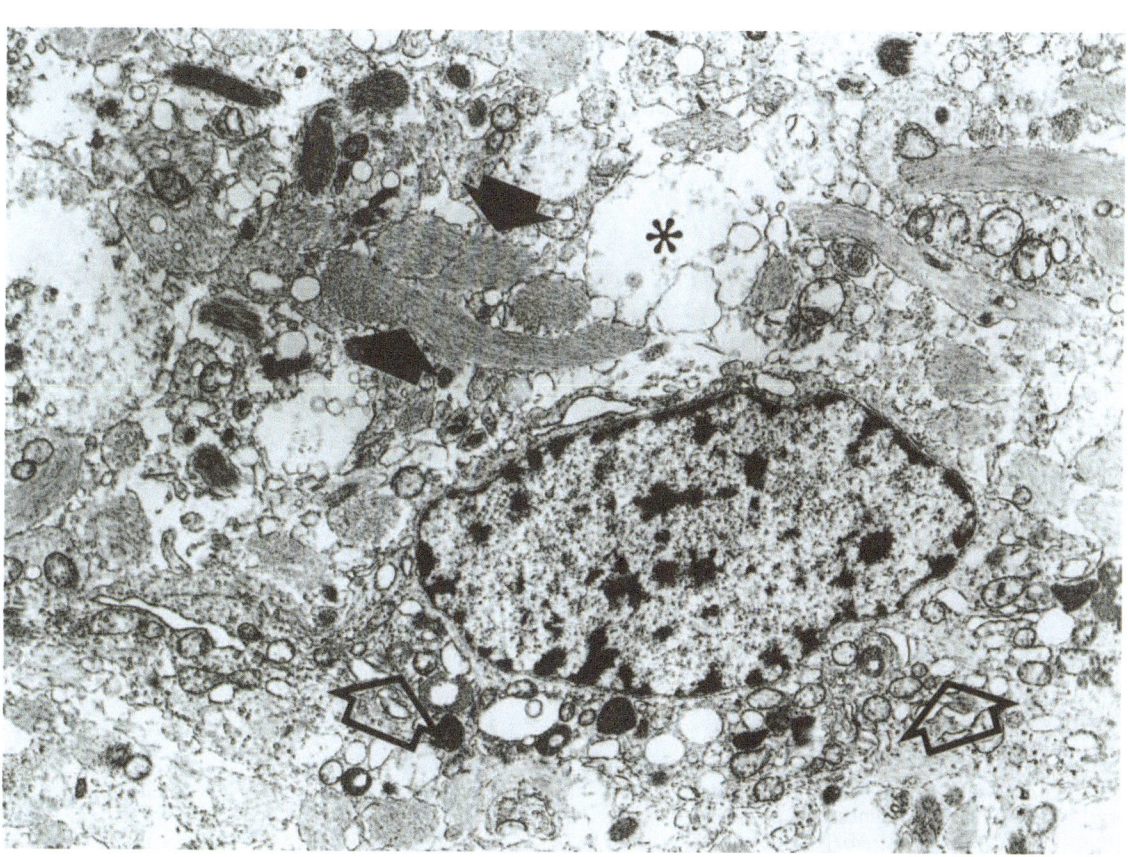

e

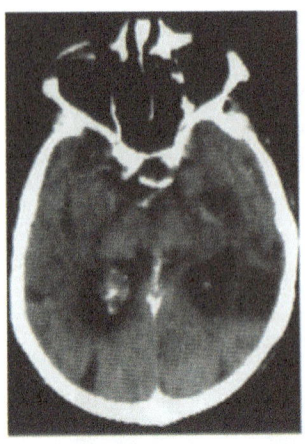

a

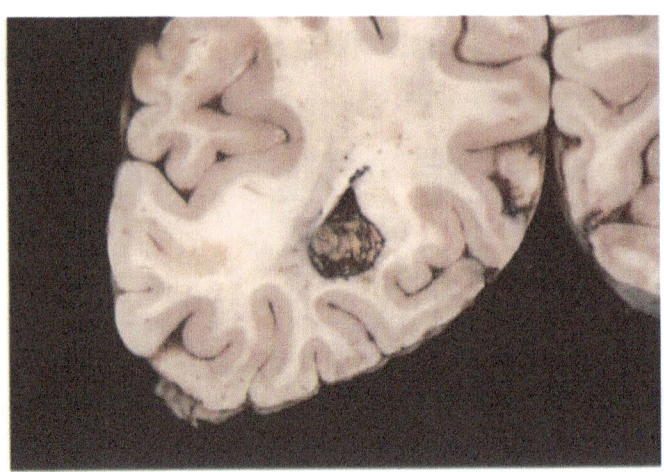

b

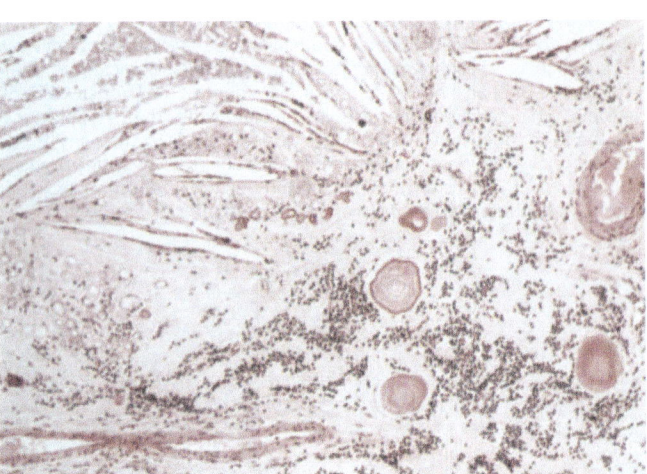

c

Figure 4.74 Xanthogranuloma, choroid plexus: male, 60 years; (a) CT + C, (b) fixed brain slice, (c) HE ×100; dilated ventricle is occupied by an inhomogeneously enhancing mass (a), corresponding to the typically variegated choroid plexus xanthoma shown in the fixed specimen (b). Histology shows hyalinized choroid plexus stroma containing psammomatous bodies, mineral deposits and cholesterol crystal clefts; note normal-looking vessels (all separate cases)

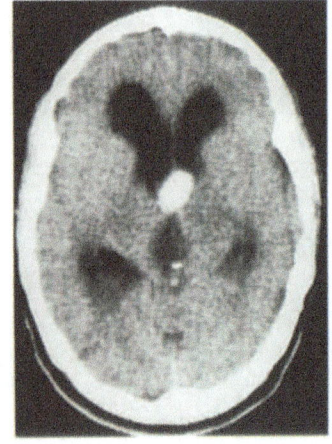

a

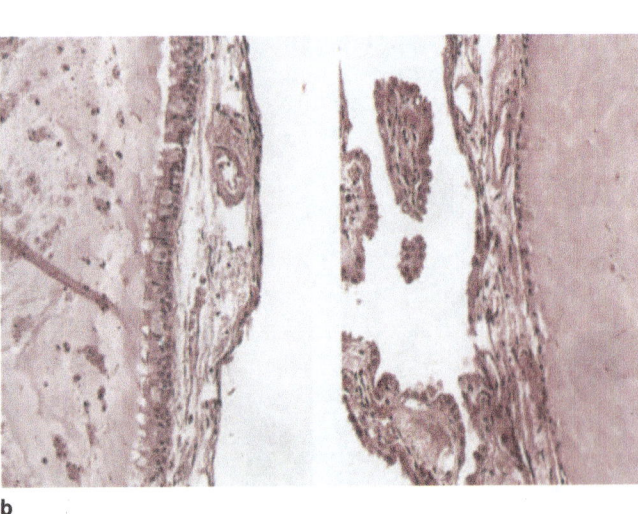

b

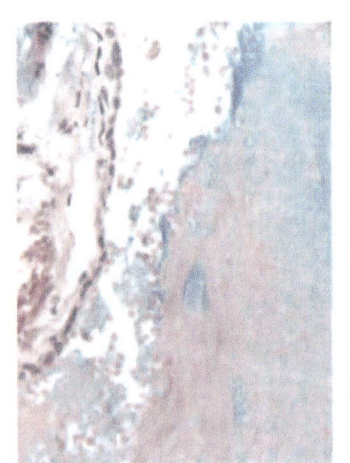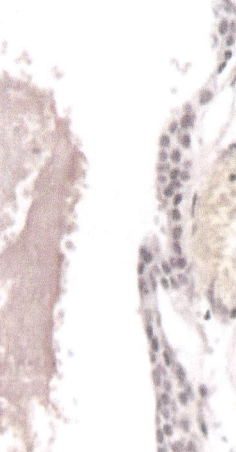

c

Figure 4.75 Colloid cyst, 3rd ventricle: (a) CT, (b) HE ×400, (c) AB/PAS and mucin ×400; CT hyperdense anterior 3rd ventricle mass. Operative cyst lined by secretory epithelium which becomes flattened columnar in areas. Note external vascularized tissue, presumably derived from choroid. Contents consist of degenerate cell outlines, recognizable red blood cells and mixture of mucin-positive and AB/PAS-positive material (c)

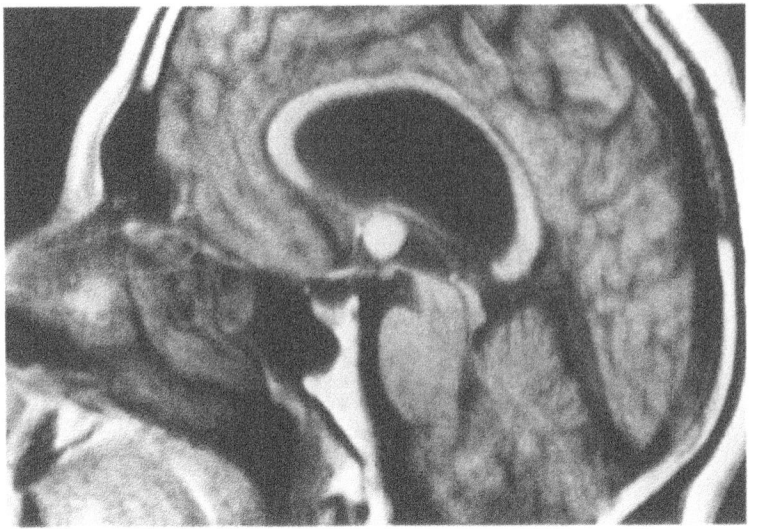

a

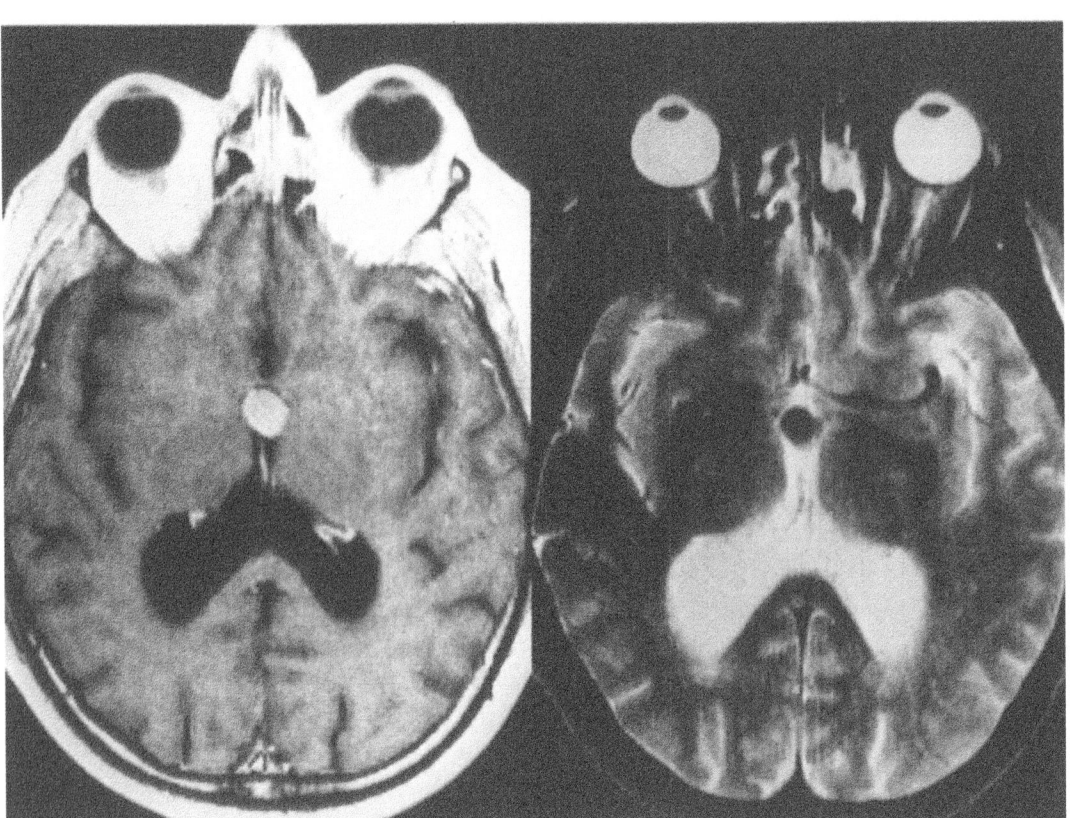

b   c

Figure 4.76 Colloid cyst, 3rd ventricle: (a) sagittal T1WI, (b) axial T1WI + C, (c) T2WI; sequences show the lesion to be moderately T1 hyperintense (compare with signal of adjacent corpus callosum) and slightly brighter after contrast (b). T2WI shows marked signal shortening

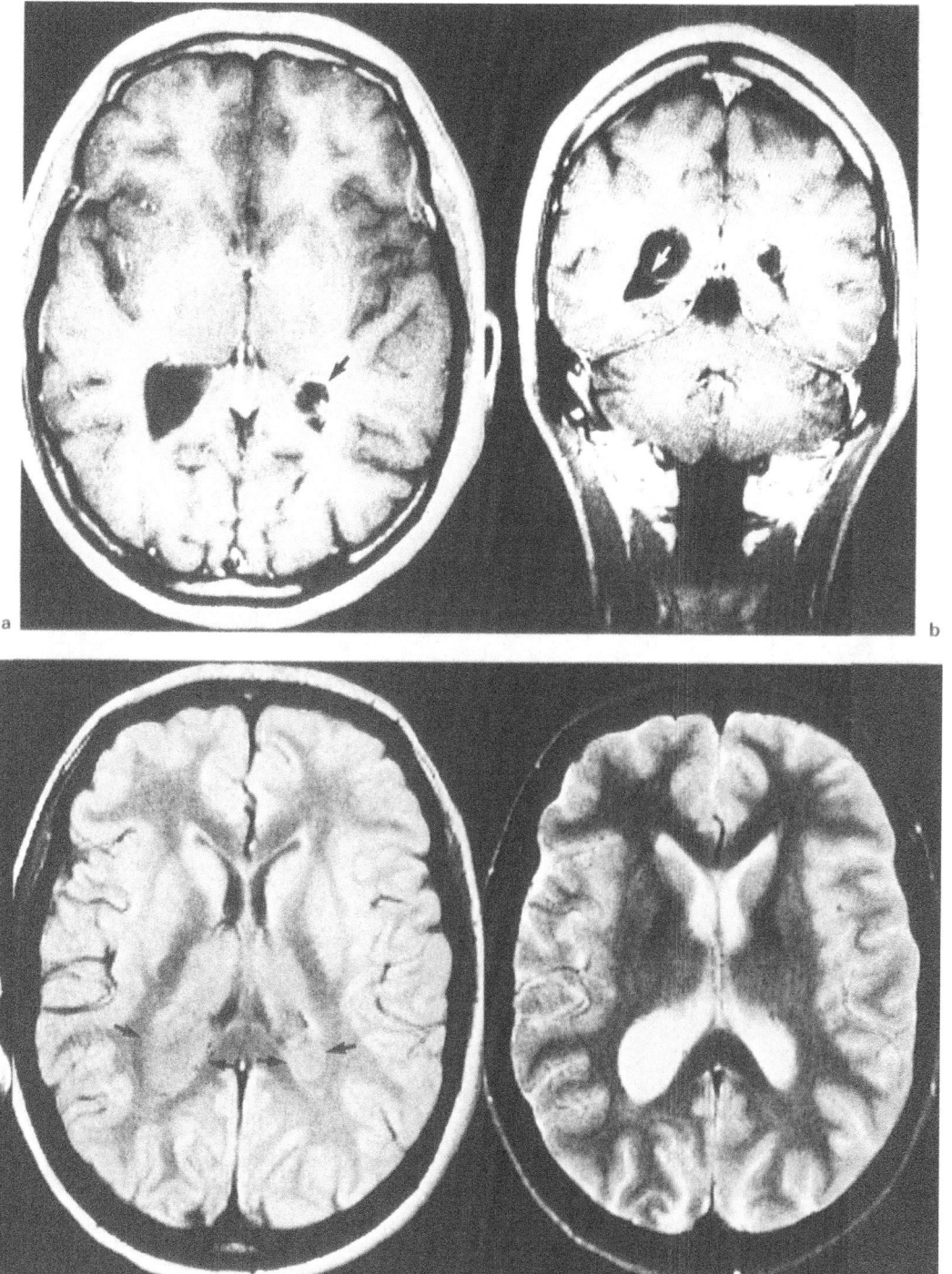

Figure 4.77 Cyst, choroidal, trigone region: female, 44 years; (**a,b**) T1WI + C, (**c**) PDWI, (**d**) T2WI; posterior horns are occupied by cysts, one of which shows rim enhancement (a, arrow), presumably choroid plexus. Intraventricular part of larger cyst wall is visible on coronal view (b, arrow). Contents of both cysts are hyperintense relative to CSF (c, arrows), becoming CSF isointense (hence invisible) at long TR (d). (CT scan showed trigone dilatation only. Histological specimen consisted purely of choroid plexus.) Dr J Lotz, City Park Hospital

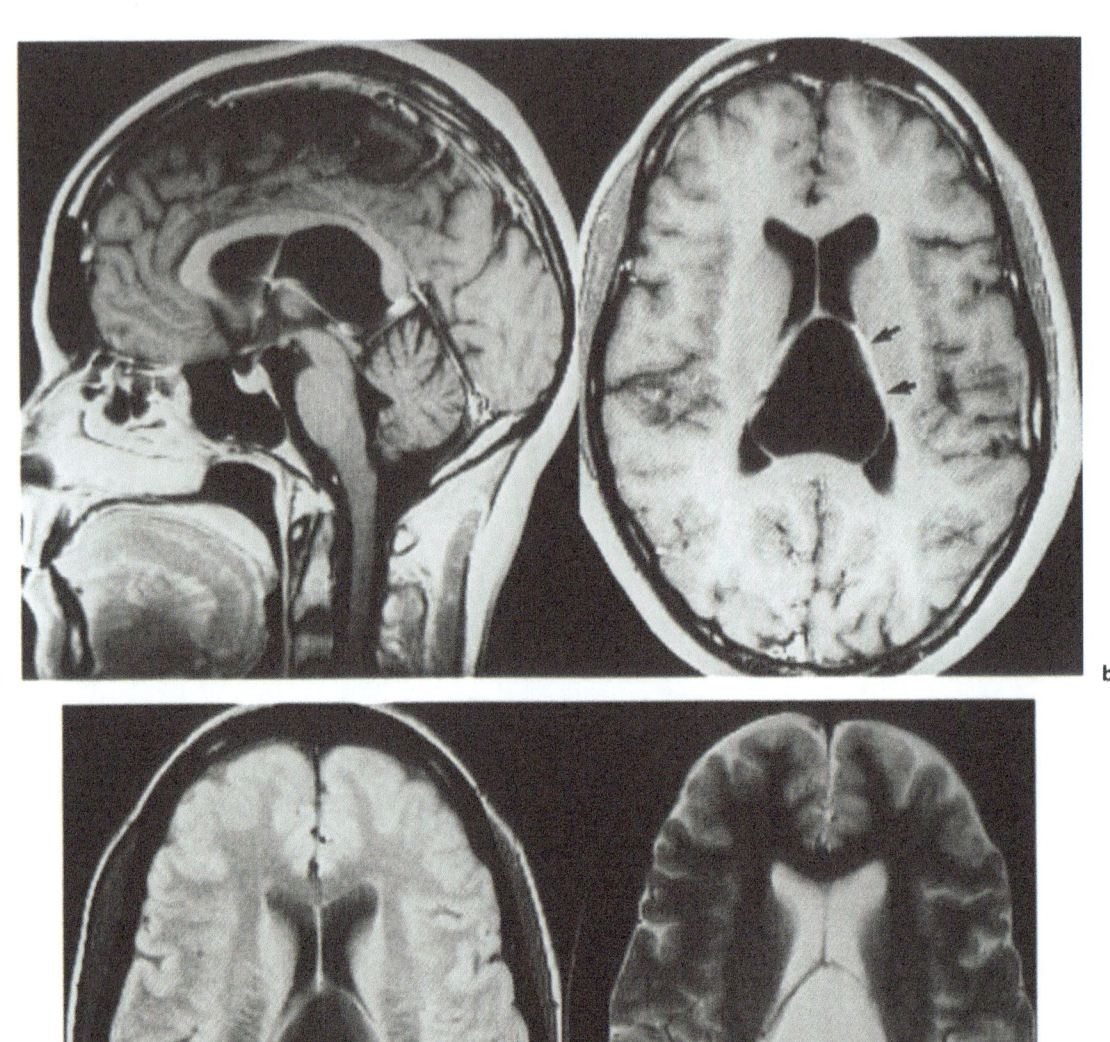

Figure 4.78 Cyst, neuroepithelial, intraventricular: (a) sagittal T1WI + C, (b) axial T1WI + C, (c) PDWI, (d) T2WI; a cyst, whose topography conforms to the tela choroidea, has CSF isointense contents on all sequences. Lateral linear enhancement is choroid plexus (b, arrows). Although the cyst has some features of a mass, including deformation of corpus callosum and pineal region, there is no evidence of CSF obstruction

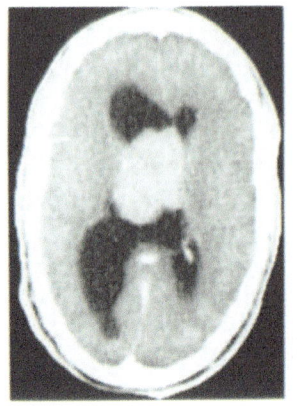
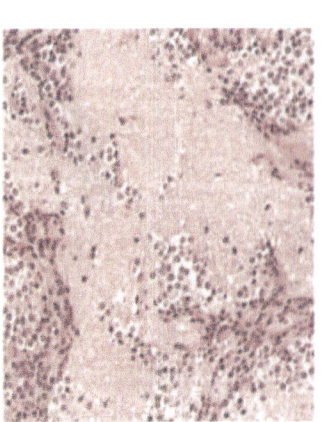
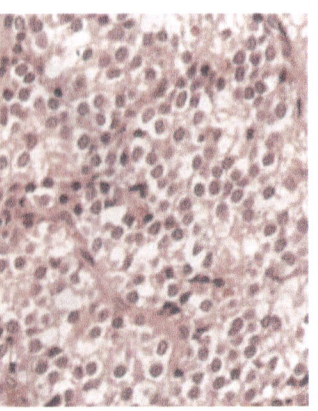

Figure 4.79 Neurocytoma, intraventricular: male, 31 years; (a) CT + C, (b) HE ×200/×400; image shows an intraventricular, strongly enhancing tumour (brain isodense). The tumour is composed of oligodendroglial-like cells (b, right), with islands of neuropil-like stroma (b, left). (GFAP stain was negative)

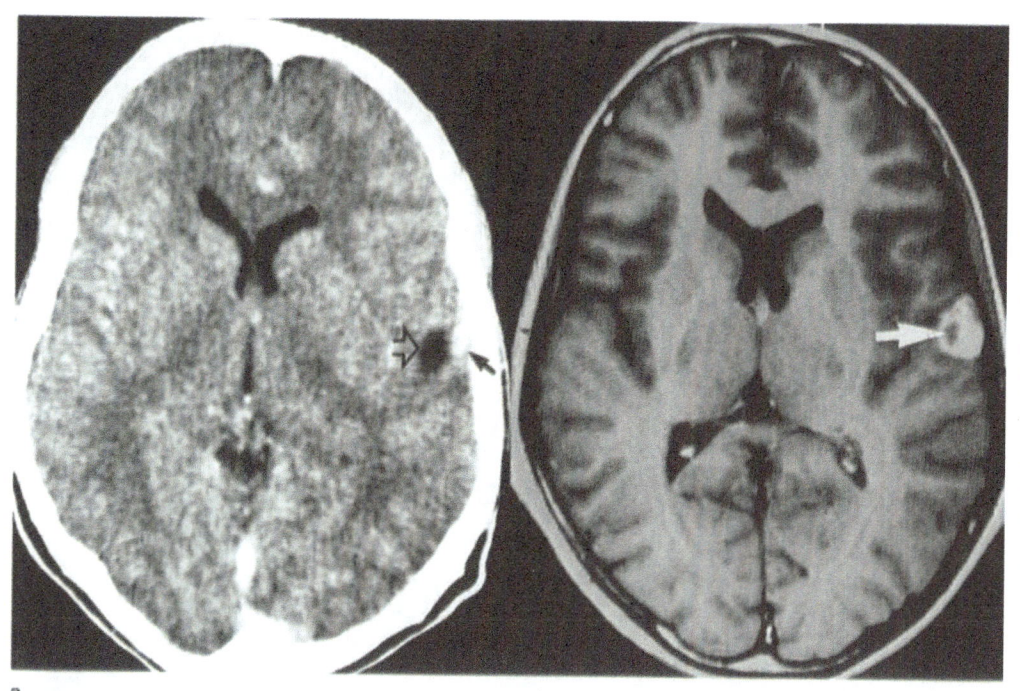

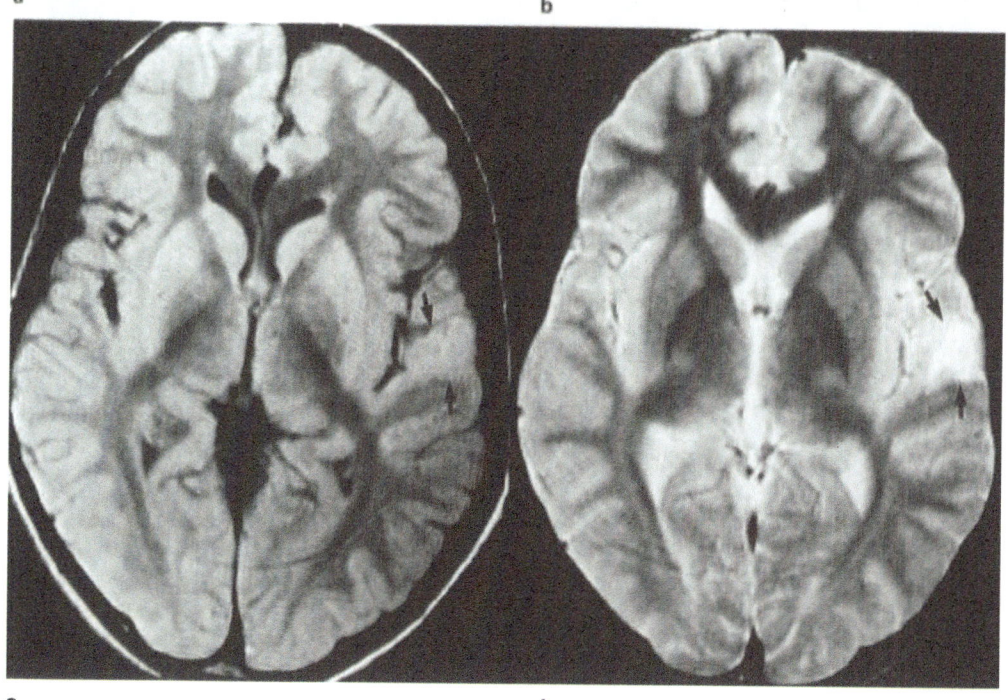

Figure 4.80 Ganglioglioma: male, 7 years; (**a**) CT + C, (**b**) T1WI + C, (**c**) PDWI, (**d**) T2WI, (**e**) HE ×200, (**f**) Palmgren ×400, (**g**) Retic ×200; lesion is mainly hypodense on CT, with focal, superficial enhancement (a, arrow), which becomes much more diffuse on MR (b). T1 (image not shown) and proton density isointensity (c), and enhancement are against fibrillary astrocytoma. Histology shows a characteristic blend of neuronal perikarya and processes, with interspersed astrocytic cells (e); extensive capillary angioarchitecture (g) explains enhancement (nonenhancing hypodense/T1 hypointense nidus could be explained by uniform astrocyma tissue). The glial component (whether pure or mixed) must be responsible for T2 hyperintensity (d). Silver stain confirms the presence of plentiful black-staining neuritic processes (f). Dr D Le Roux, East London

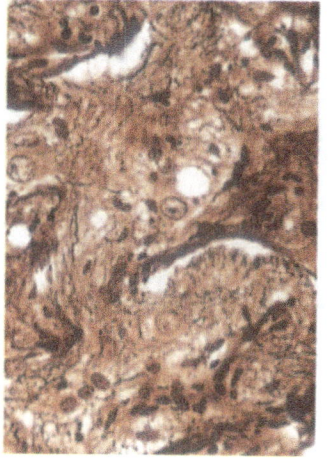

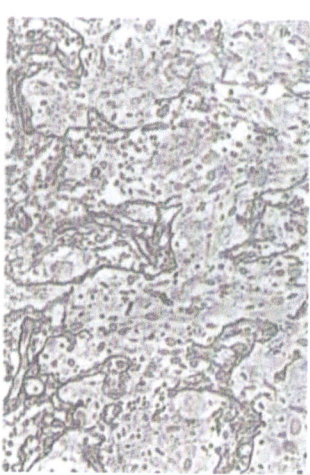

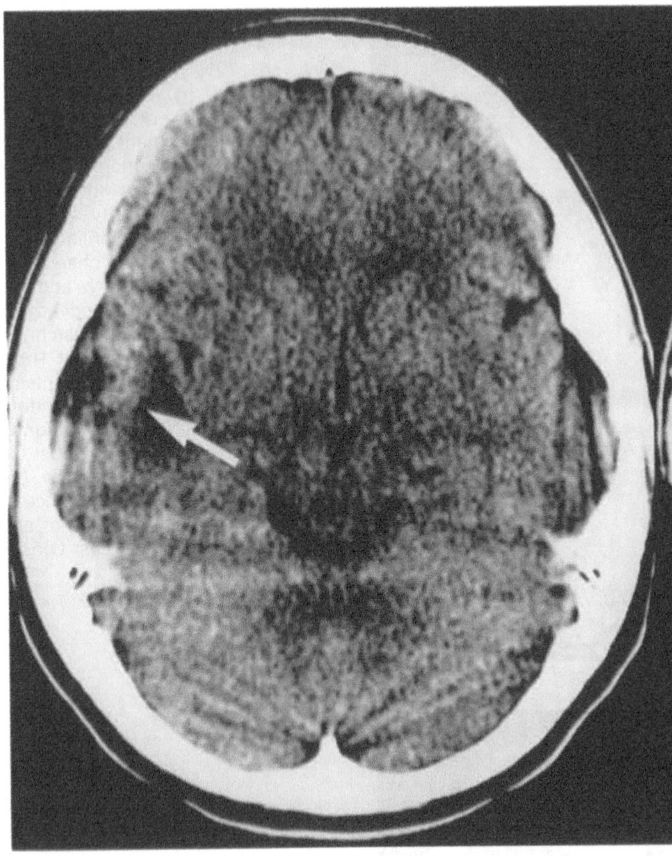

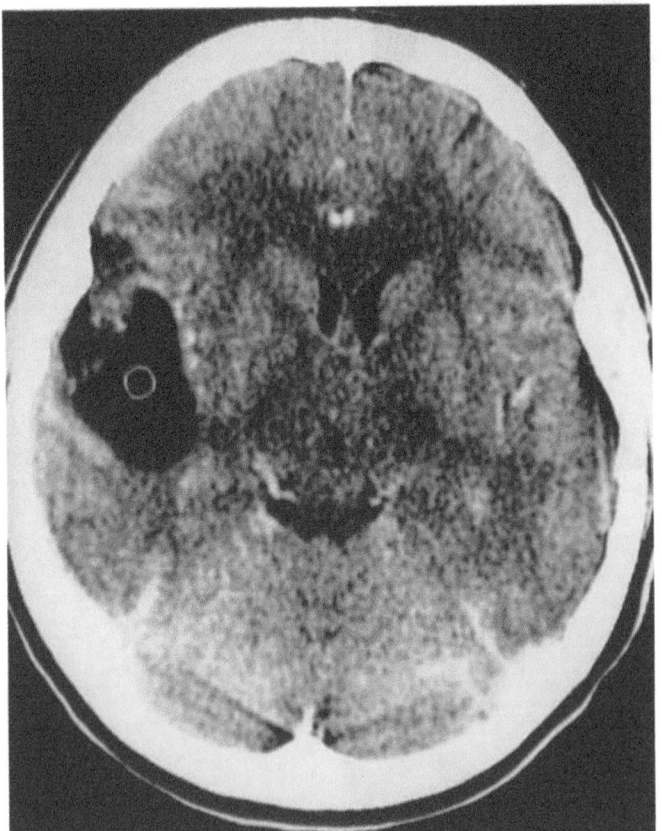

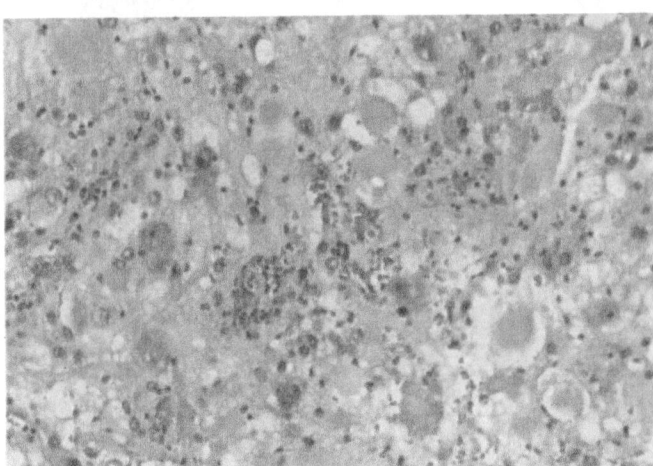

Figure 4.81 Gangliocytoma: female, 23 years; (**a**) CT, (**b,c**) CT + C, (**d**) HE × 200; hypo/isodense cerebromeningeal mass, with patchy enhancement (a,b, arrows) and large, non-enhancing adjacent cyst, artefactually hypodense (c). The tumour is composed of sheets of large ganglion-like cells, with numerous interspersed granular bodies, presumably of degenerate pathogenesis (d). The significance of the widespread vacuolation is not known, but could affect the MR image. (Tumour cells were GFAP-negative)

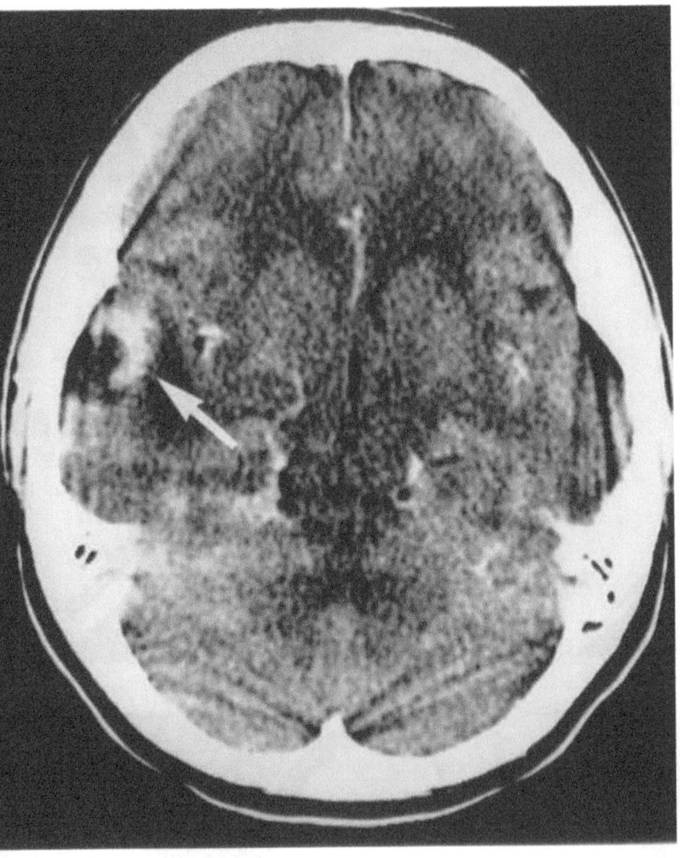

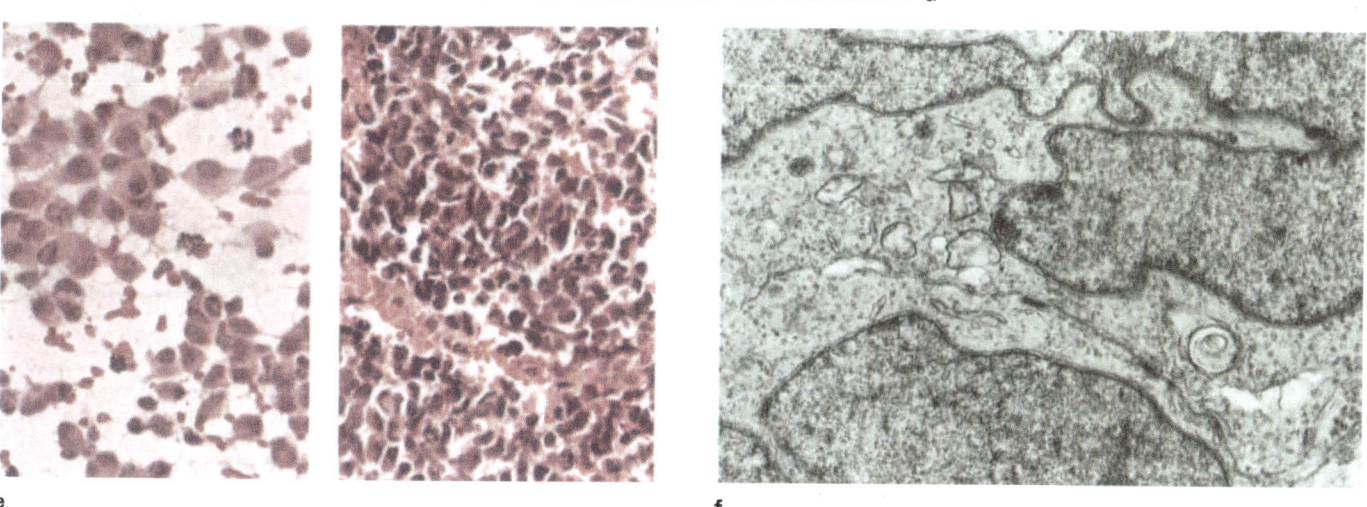

Figure 4.82 PNET, hemispheric: male, 12 years; (**a**) CT + C, (**b**) T1WI, (**c**) PDWI, (**d**) T2WI, (**e**) HE ×400, (**f**) EM ×27 000; strongly enhancing cerebromeningeal mass (a), which is cortex isointense on all sequences (b–d). Increasingly hyperintense foci at long TR represent cystic degeneration (arrows), presumed to occur on the same basis as illustrated in Figure 6.42. Cytology and paraffin section shows a cellular tumour, composed of monomorphic, small cells, with high nuclear/cytoplasmic ratio (e); ultrastructurally the tumour cells are nondescript, with occasional junctions and negligible intercellular space (f), correlating well with cortical isointensity. The pathogenesis of enhancement is unexplained

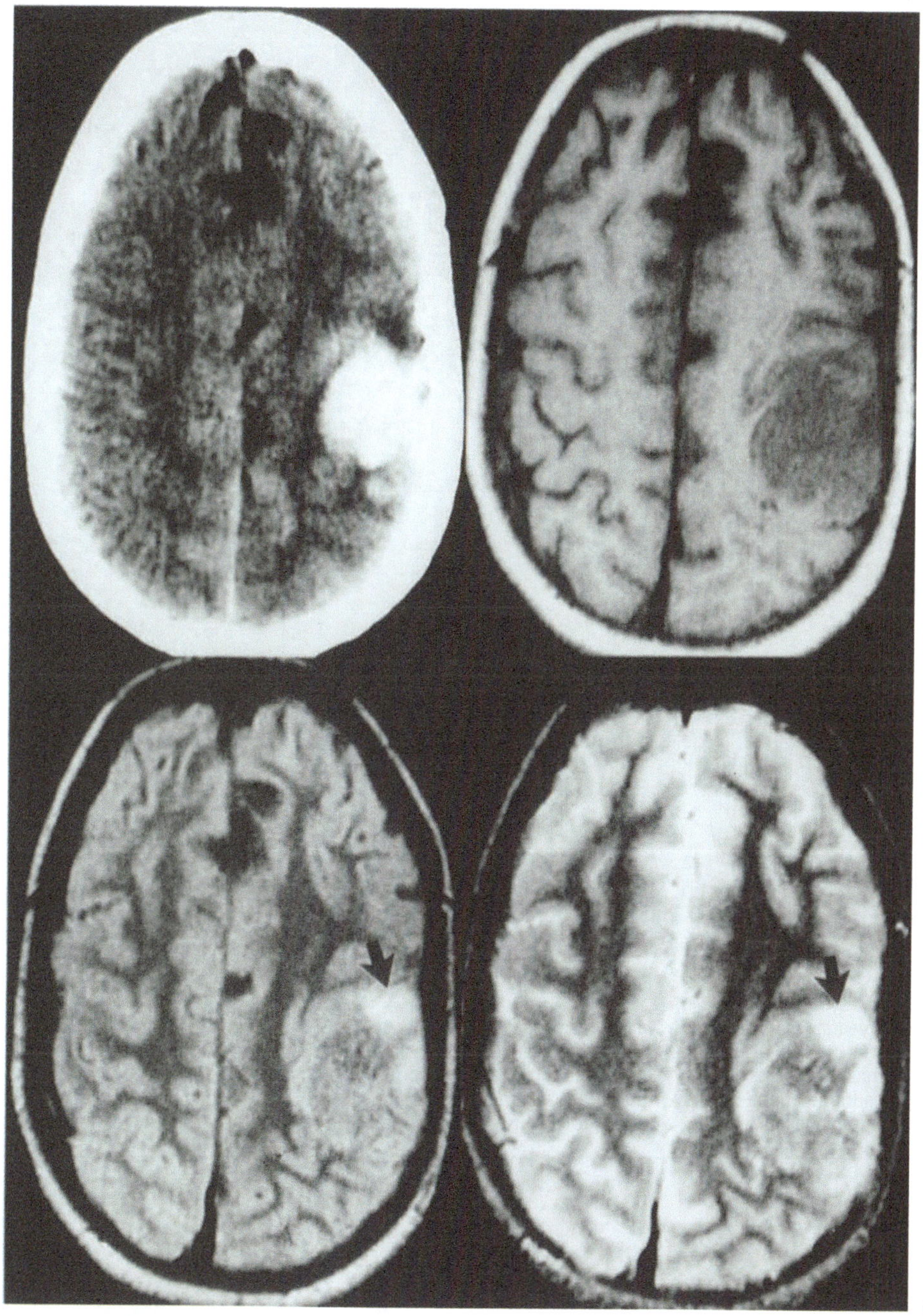

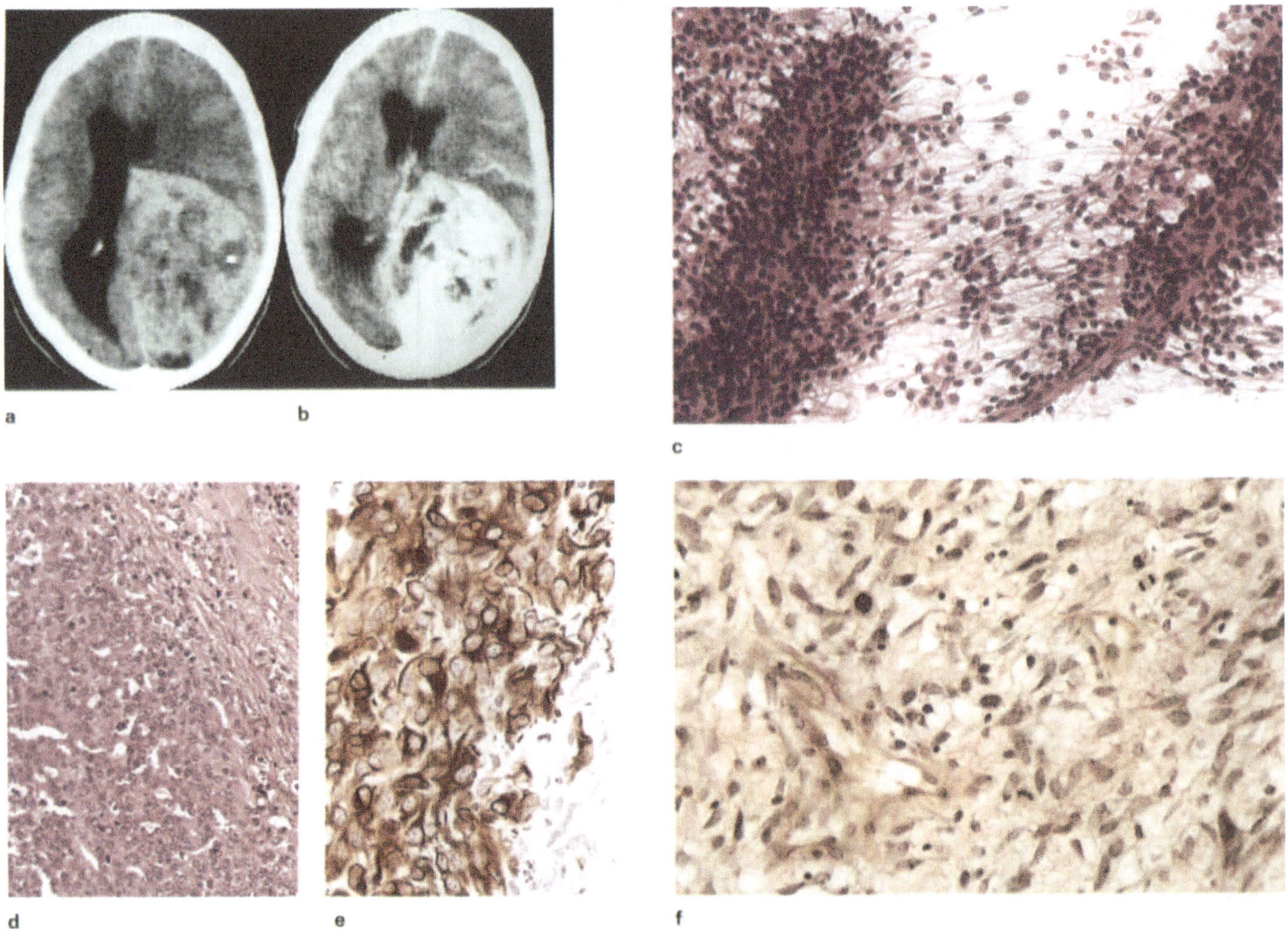

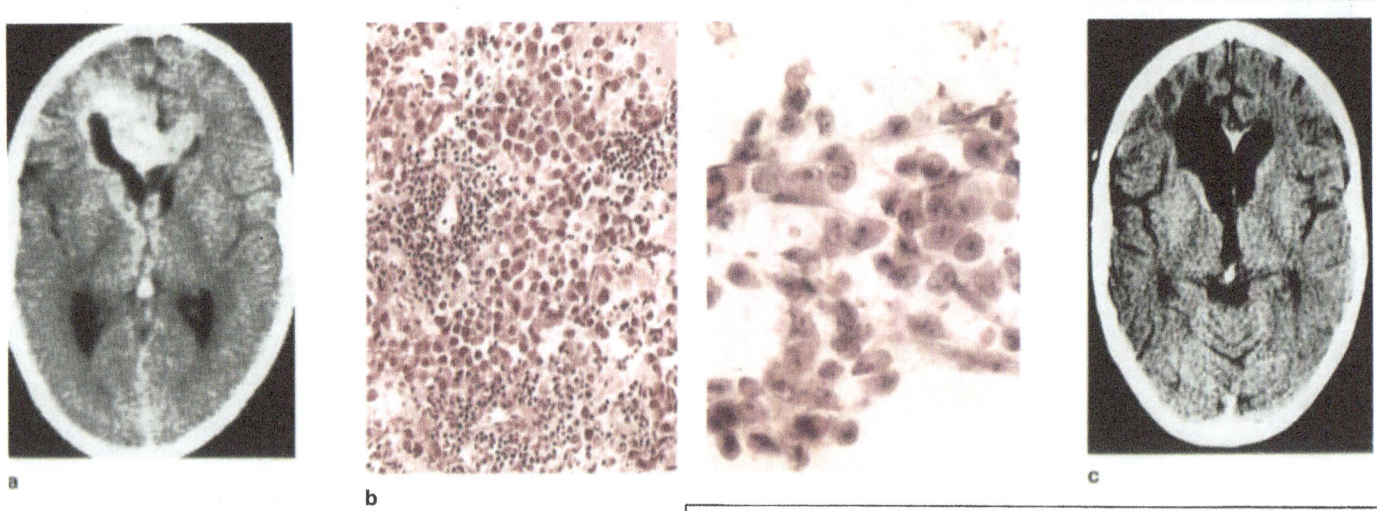

Figure 4.83 Gliosarcoma, occipital: female, 28 years; (**a**) CT, (**b**) CT + C, (**c,d**) HE × 200, (**e**) GFAP × 400, (**f**) VG × 400; a large inhomogeneous, hyperdense, cerebromeningeal mass replaces the occipital lobe (a), showing strong, but irregular enhancement (b). Perivascular, fibrillated cells present in smear are suggestive of a glial neoplasm (c). Histologically the tumour consists of discrete foci of monomorphic, GFAP-positive cells (left, d,e), with intervening neoplastic mesenchymal tissue containing many mitoses (e, right and f); note focal necrosis and haemorrhage (d, right), presumably accounting for inhomogeneity. Both components of the neoplasm are well vascularized

Figure 4.84 Germinoma, corpus callosum and periventricular tissue: male, 11 years; (**a**) CT + C, (**b**) HE × 200/× 400, (**c**) CT; initial scan shows expansion and enhancement of the anterior corpus callosum and periventricular tissues of an abnormally shaped right anterior horn. Morphological features of tumour cells with large vesicular nuclei and interspersed islands of lymphocyte-like cells are suggestive of germinoma (b). Post-radiotherapy follow-up study 1 year later shows complete disappearance of tumour with parenchymal atrophy and focal mineralization (c). Enhancement characteristics and response to therapy support the presumptive histological diagnosis of germinoma.

Figure 4.85 (*opposite*) **Desmoplastic, osseous/meningocerebral, primitive neuroepithelial tumour with divergent differentiation**: female, 1 year; (**a–c**) CT + C, (**d**) HE × 100/× 200, (**e**) HE × 200, (**f**) HE × 100, (**g**) GFAP × 200, (**h**) HE × 200, (**i**) HE × 40; images show osseous component of lesion which is both lytic (a, asterisk) and mineralizing (b, asterisk), as well as diffusely enhancing (b, open arrows and c); cystic intraventricular component (e, asterisk) is in direct continuity. Intraparenchymal component of lesion includes small-cell/PNET-type morphology (d, left), (*continued opposite*)

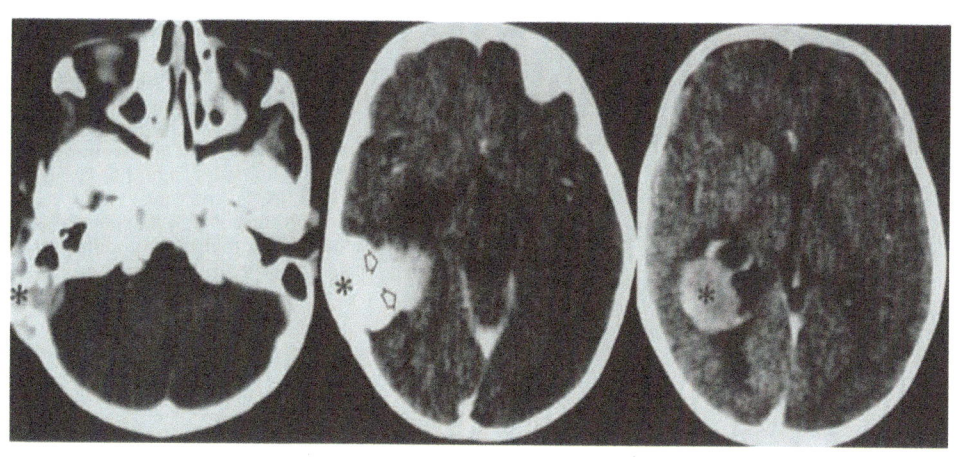

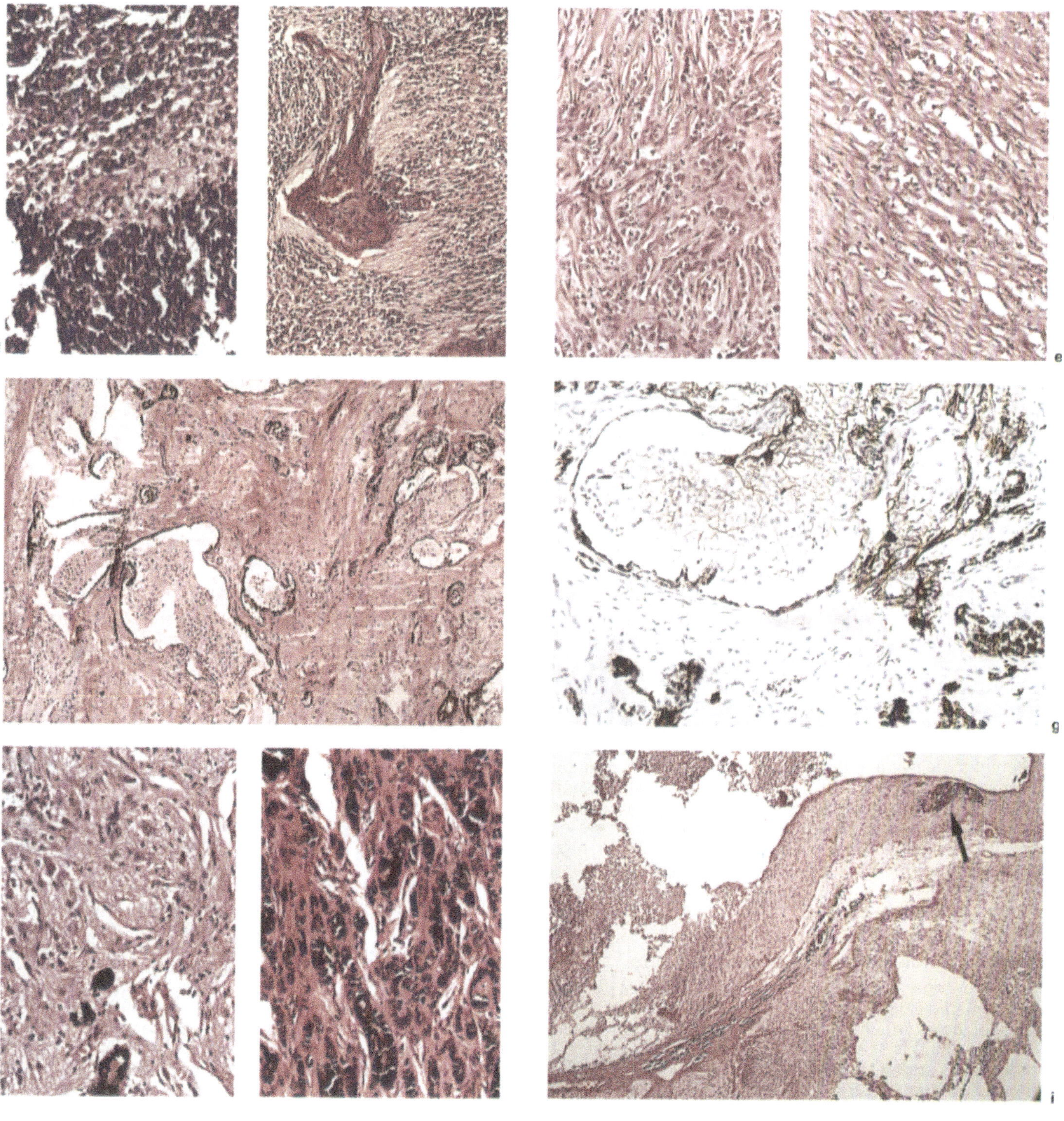

a b c

Figure 4.85 (*continued*) with ependymal differentiation and prominent vasculature (d, right), becoming desmoplastic superficially (e). Osseous/meningeal component shows islands of neuropil, lying within melanotic-neuroepithelial lined spaces (f). Elsewhere these components include well-differentiated ganglioglioma (h, left), and collections of melanotic, neuroepithelial cells (h, right). Cysts are partly lined by neoplastic ependyma, with germinal matrix-like aggregates (i, arrow).

d e

f g

h i

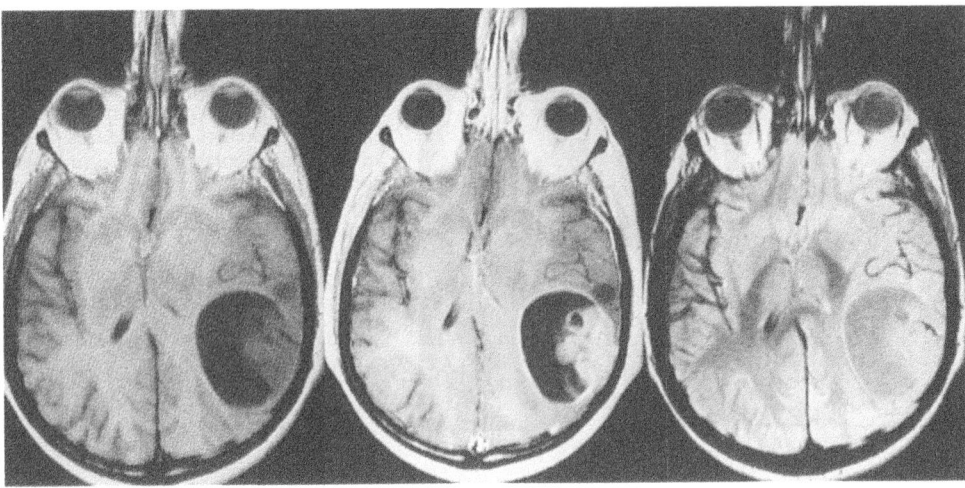

Figure 4.86   Metastatic disease, carcinoma, solid/cystic: (a) T1WI, (b) T1WI + C, (c) PDWI; solid cystic lesion, solid part appearing as a lobulated T1/T2 isointense tissue, which enhances strongly (characteristic of epithelial as opposed to most glial tumours; morphology is less specific). Note that cyst wall is also enhancing, presumably neoplastic tissue. Histology was that of an undifferentiated carcinoma

a   b   c

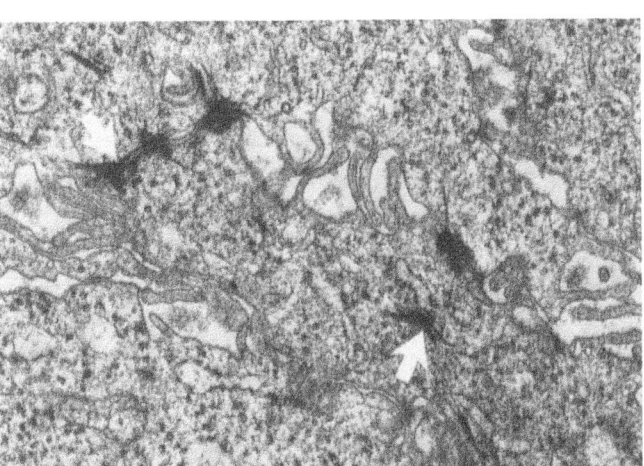

Figure 4.87   Metastatic squamous carcinoma: illustrates desmosomes and tonofilaments (arrows), ultrastructural features responsible for parenchymal isodensity and isointensity. EM ×16 000

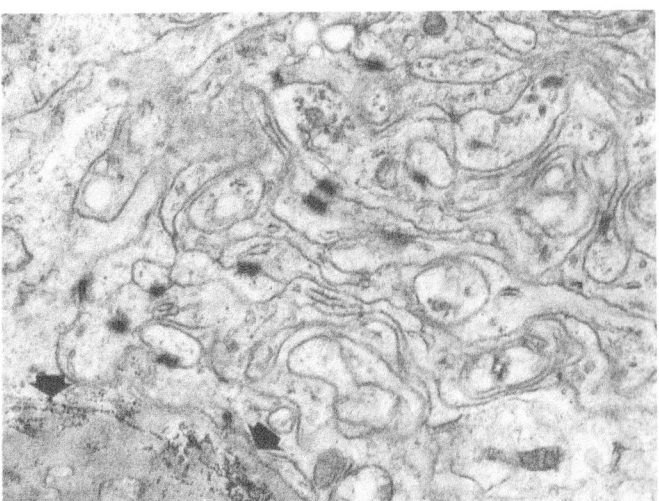

Figure 4.88   Meningioma: the paradigm of a tumour containing no interstitial space; field is packed with interdigitating processes, with numerous junctions. Electron-dense material (arrows) is basal lamina. EM ×11 000

4.11c.   Gliosarcoma[105]

CT has confirmed the gross pathological findings of a usually large, superficial neoplasm, inhomogeneously brain-hyperdense with strong enhancement[106] (Figure 4.83). The features are consistent with the dimorphic nature of the tumour, said to be usually a mixture of astrocytic glioma and fibrosarcoma, these two neoplastic elements being responsible for vascular and reticulin proliferation respectively[107]. The glial component may be relatively well differentiated, and is presumably responsible for reported T2 hyperintensity[108]. Neoplastic mesenchymal tissue, which makes intraoperative smear preparation very difficult, may also rarely give rise to cartilage and osteoid, and is likely to decrease attenuation and induce signal shortening.

4.11d.   'Unclassifiable' primary tumours

It is the experience of every neuropathologist to have encountered a number of presumptively primary intracranial neoplasms which, for a variety of reasons, defy precise classification. If the imaging features and response to therapy are added to the morphology, further insights are usually gained (Figures 4.84 and 4.85).

4.12.   METASTATIC DISEASE

Metastatic spread to the nervous system displays strong anatomical systematization, in that lesions tend to be located within and confined to the parenchyma, the CSF spaces (Figure 3.38), and the subdural space independently; rarer sites include the choroid plexus and cranial nerve roots. Although the trophic factors determining them are uncertain (see comment below), the consistency of these forms of growth provides a natural clinical, imaging and pathological approach. The following discussion deals specifically with parenchymal or cerebromeningeal metastases; subarachnoid spread (meningeal carcinomatosis) and dural involvement are described in section 3.5a.

Intracerebral metastases are usually imaged prospectively, against the syndrome of known malignancy, and their presence merely confirms the diagnosis. The particular clinical problem centres on an individual presenting with a primary neurological disturbance, in whom CT or MR demonstrates a solitary, often 'cystic', enhancing lesion which requires to be distinguished from primary neoplasia and other focal, enhancing lesions (Figure 4.86). From the imaging literature it appears that the extremely variable density and signal intensity of parenchymal metastases allow only three precepts: namely, that

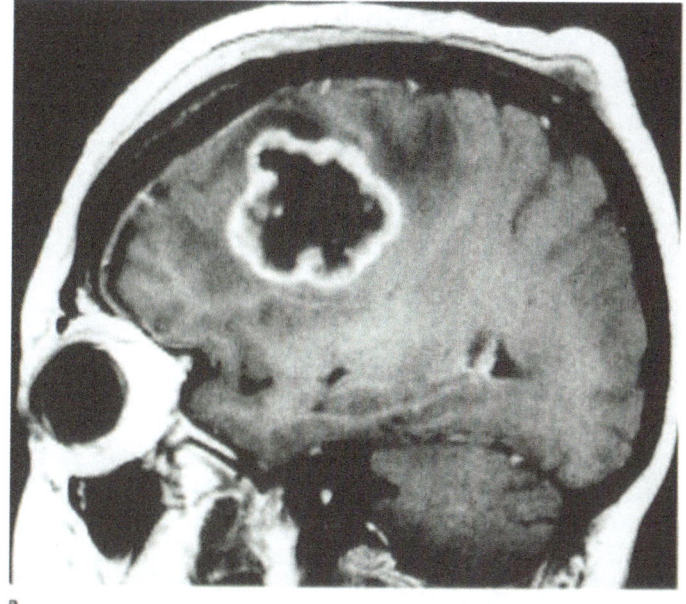

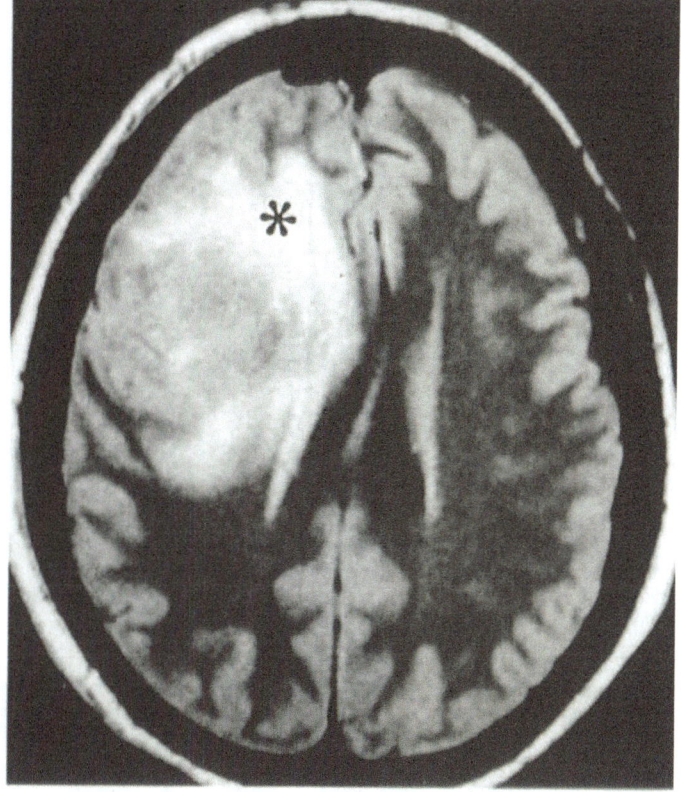

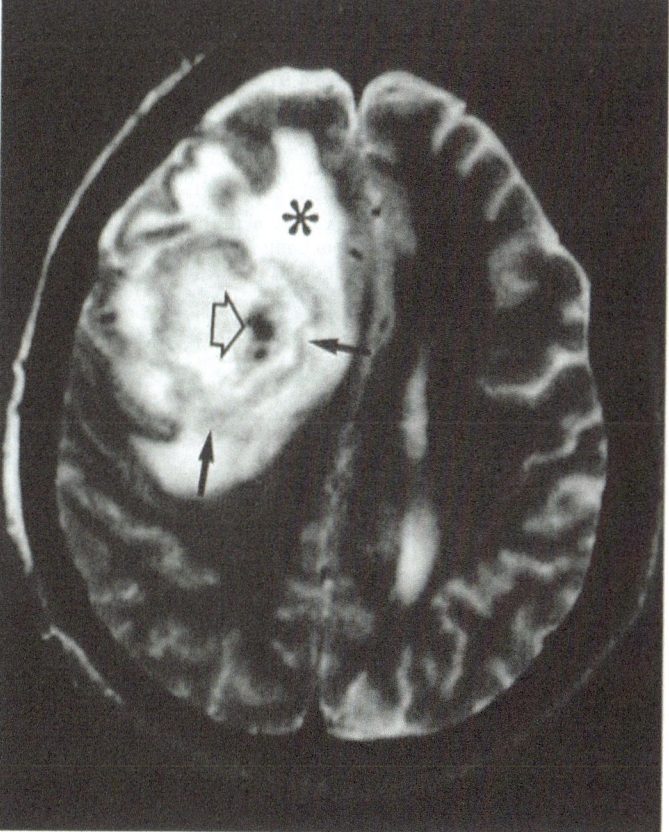

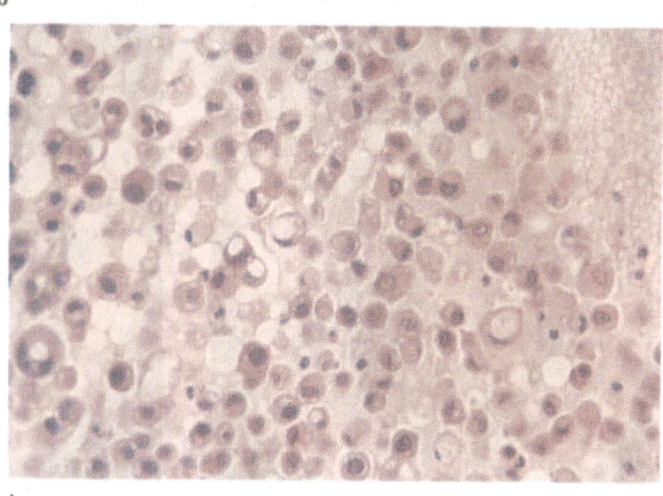

Figure 4.89 Metastatic disease, adenocarcinoma, cystic: (**a**) T1WI + C, (**b**) PDWI, (**c**) T2WI, (**d**) HE × 400; lesion has a sharply circumscribed crenated, enhancing edge, with inhomogeneously hypointense contents (a), which become moderately hyperintense at long TR, compared with surrounding vasogenic oedema (asterisk, b,c). Wall at long TR is cortex isointense (c, arrows); focal hypointensity (c, open arrow) is assumed to be post-needling haemorrhage. At operation liquid aspirate was thought to be pus, although wall morphology, lesion site and clinical picture were against inflammatory mass. Smear preparation shows sheets of neoplastic cells, including signet-ring forms (d)

relaxation times are generally prolonged, the surrounding brain is oedematous, and enhancement of tumour tissue is the rule[109–111]. Our belief, as will have been stated repeatedly in this text, is that in the case of cells having a filamentous cytosol and desmosomes (Figure 4.87) and lacking cytoplasmic storage (i.e. low cellular proton density), the single most important signal relaxation determinant will be the interstitial space. Accordingly, aggregates of cells, whether epithelial or meningothelial (Figure 4.88), will tend to approximate the normal density and signal intensity of grey matter. Conversely, the most important factors initiating signal prolongation (and CT hypodensity) in such tissues, is likely to be degeneration, necrosis and microcystic change. Thus 'healthy' neoplastic epithelial tissue is most easily seen at long TR, when it appears more or less cerebral cortex-isointense and is therefore delineated externally by oedematous brain parenchyma, and sometimes internally by T2-hyperintense necrosis or cyst formation. At short TR, solid, metastatic tumour tissue is usually indistinguishable from

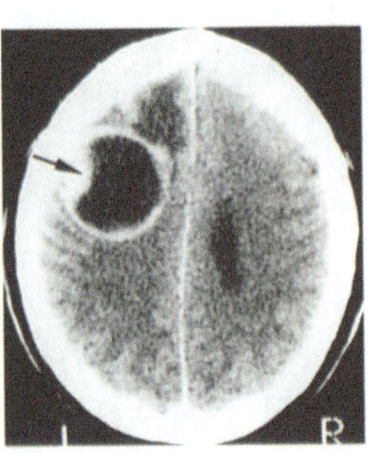
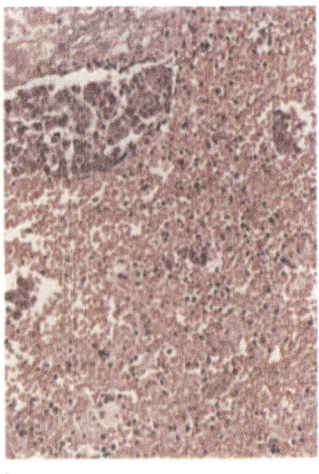
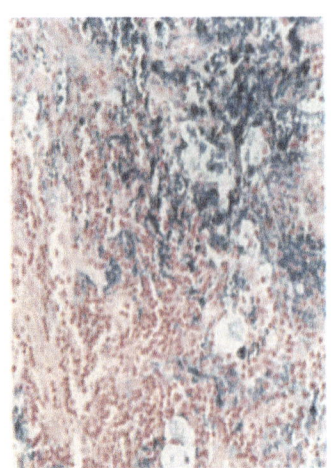

Figure 4.90   Metastatic disease, carcinoma, haemorrhagic: (a) CT + C, (**b**) HE/Perl's ×200; hyperdense ring lesion, with nodular component (arrow) and hypodense contents. Density of tumour tissue was identical prior to contrast administration, presumably due to the effects of haemorrhage (b), including heavy iron deposition

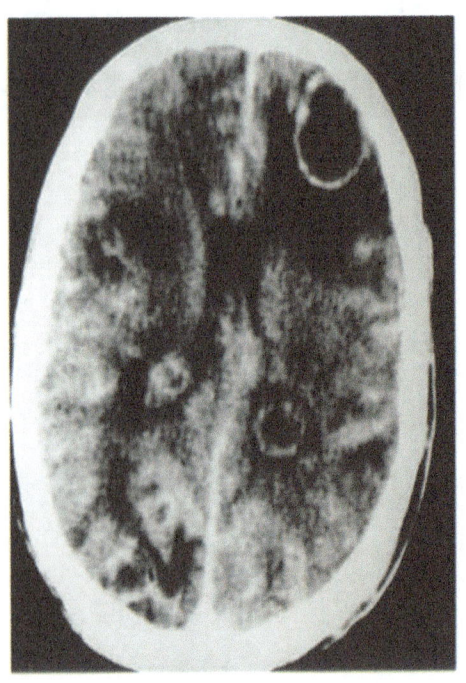
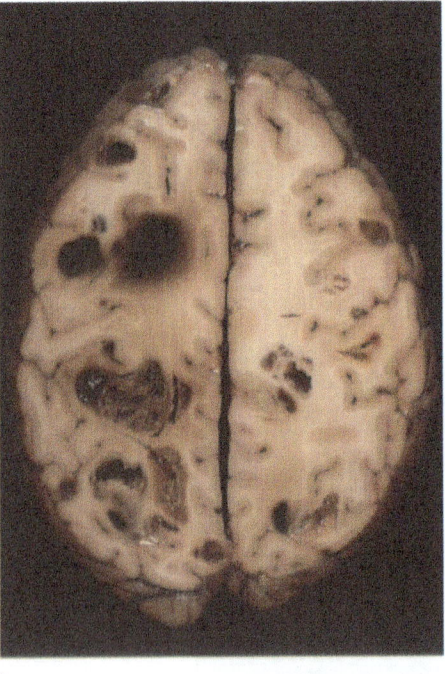

Figure 4.91   Metastatic disease, hepatoma, boundary zone distribution: (a) CT + C, (**b**) fixed brain slice; multiple, centrally hypodense, ring-enhancing lesions distributed in the arterial boundary zones of both hemispheres (a). At autopsy lesions were visible on the brain surface; most deposits are centrally necrotic, with evidence of old and recent haemorrhage (b)

brain, but almost invariably displays strong enhancement, so that morphology is always defined with respect to contrast administration.

Typical lesions are diffusely enhancing (order of 15 mm), i.e. 'solid'; or peripherally enhancing (order of 20 mm or more), with or without tissue nodules, and hypodense-T1 hypointense/T2 hyperintense contents (Figures 4.86, 4.89 and 4.90). Sometimes the topography of multiple lesions is typically in the arterial boundary zones (Figure 4.91). Histological correlates include a richly vascularized tumour stroma which is sharply delineated from brain parenchyma because of the absence of interstitial or perivascular infiltration (Figure 6.56). With the exception of heavily pigmented melanoma cells the nature of the metastatic tissue itself has no specificity in terms of density or signal intensity, and the images of metastases frequently share features of glioma or granuloma (Figure 4.92).

Even in very small lesions, foci of coagulative necrosis are usually present, becoming progressive centrally, mainly as a function of tumour size, and distinguishable from viable tissue only after contrast administration (Figure 4.93). T2 hyperintensity accompanies liquefaction or cystic degeneration, whilst T1 hypointensity is dependent on a decline in protein content. It appears that, no matter how extensive necrosis may be, a rim of tumour always survives to provide some enhancement.

With brain isointensity as the paradigm for neoplastic epithelial tissue, the pathological basis of signal inhomogeneity can be easily appreciated, including secretion, patchy necrosis, desmoplasia, old or recent haemorrhage, and mineralization, the last being possibly more common in squamous lesions[112]. Metastases which are regularly grossly haemorrhagic include choriocarcinoma (Figure 4.94), renal cell carcinoma and melanoma, although MR often fails to corroborate blood-induced CT hyperdensity.

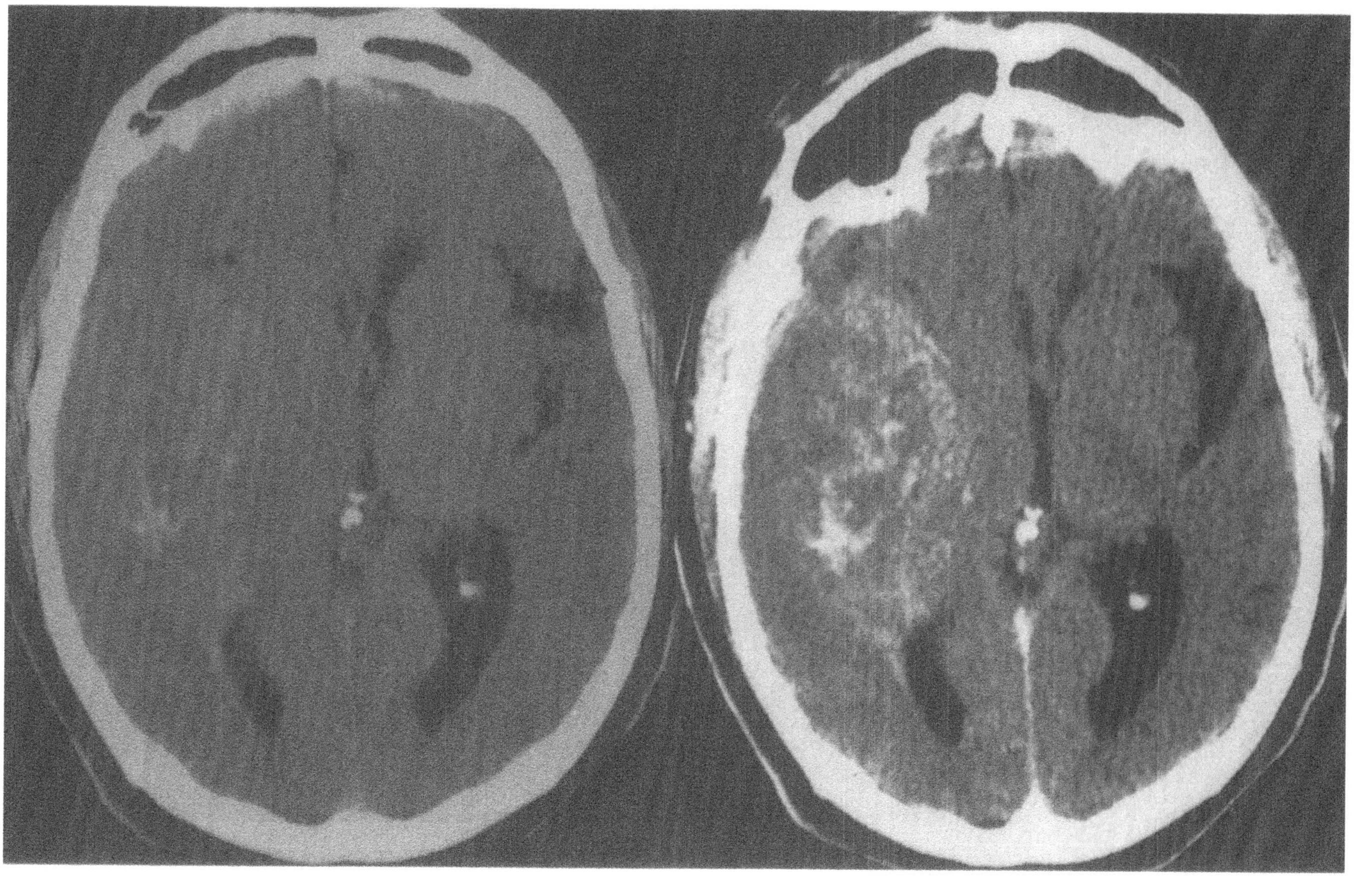

a

b

Figure 4.92 Metastatic disease, undifferentiated carcinoma: (**a**) CT, (**b**) CT + C; ill-defined, iso/hyperdense, inhomogeneously enhancing mass whose morphology, hyperdensity apart, is suggestive of a primary malignant glial neoplasm. However, biopsy revealed an undifferentiated carcinoma which, in view of subsequent chest X-ray, submental and cervical lymphadenopathy, is probably of lung origin

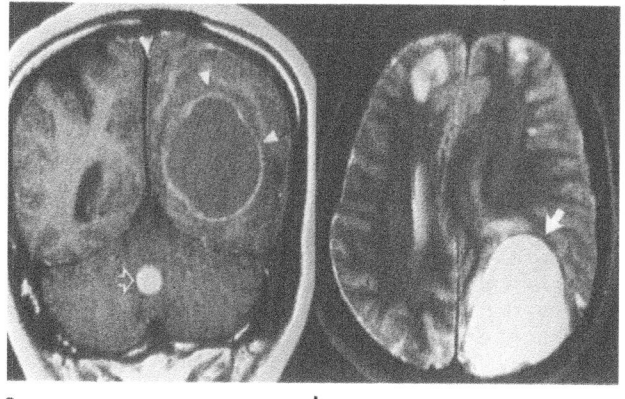

a   b

Figure 4.93 Metastatic disease, adenocarcinoma, cystic: (**a**) T1WI + C, (**b**) T2WI; giant occipital cyst with thin evenly enhancing wall (a, arrow-heads); smaller lesion in cerebellum is solid and diffusely enhancing (open arrow). Contents of cyst are cortex isointense on T1, but are strongly T2 hyperintense, suggestive of high protein concentration. Note distinct rim of signal shortening (b, arrow), consistent with the histology of a mucin-secreting adenocarcinoma (see text). Frontal lobe hyperintense foci (b) are indicative of the presence of additional, smaller lesions. (Dr A Bok, Panorama Hospital)

In the same way, macroscopic melanotic tumours frequently fail to display T1 shortening (Figure 4.95). A sharp tumour–brain interface and central necrosis are logically absent in lymphoma, exhibiting, as it normally does, both perivascular and interstitial growth (Figure 4.98). Mucin secretion is assumed to be the cause of marked T2 signal shortening (T2 hypointensity), without necessarily affecting the T1 signal intensity (Figure 6.56).

For the neuropathologist, diagnostic requirements usually fall into two main categories: confirmation of the nature of a metastasis which is being excised because it is solitary and accessible; and the identification of a mass which could, on both clinical and imaging grounds, be primary or secondary. From the discussion above, such a lesion will invariably be inhomogeneous, solid-cystic, with some ring or linear enhancement and, cytological experience apart, the success of the biopsy procedure is related to certain technical factors which are discussed in section 1.5. The sharp plasmalemmae, cell clumping and complete lack of fibrillation (Figure 4.96) so characteristic of metastatic carcinoma, are to be found only in the enhancing component of the tumour; although this is self-evident, surgeons performing needle biopsy without stereotactic equipment are prone to aspirate abnormally soft tissue and even cyst fluid, which is usually cytologically unsatisfactory (but not always) (Figure 4.89). At this hospital, cytospin of cyst fluid is not practised routinely, and it is our opinion that larger cystic lesions exhibiting marked variation in wall thickness should always be submitted to open biopsy.

In absolute figures, carcinoma of the lung, followed by malignant melanoma and breast carcinoma, are the most frequent primary sites of brain metastases. Of interest is the finding of various workers that malignant melanoma tends to metastasize to the frontal and temporal lobes, breast carcinoma to the cerebellum and basal ganglia,

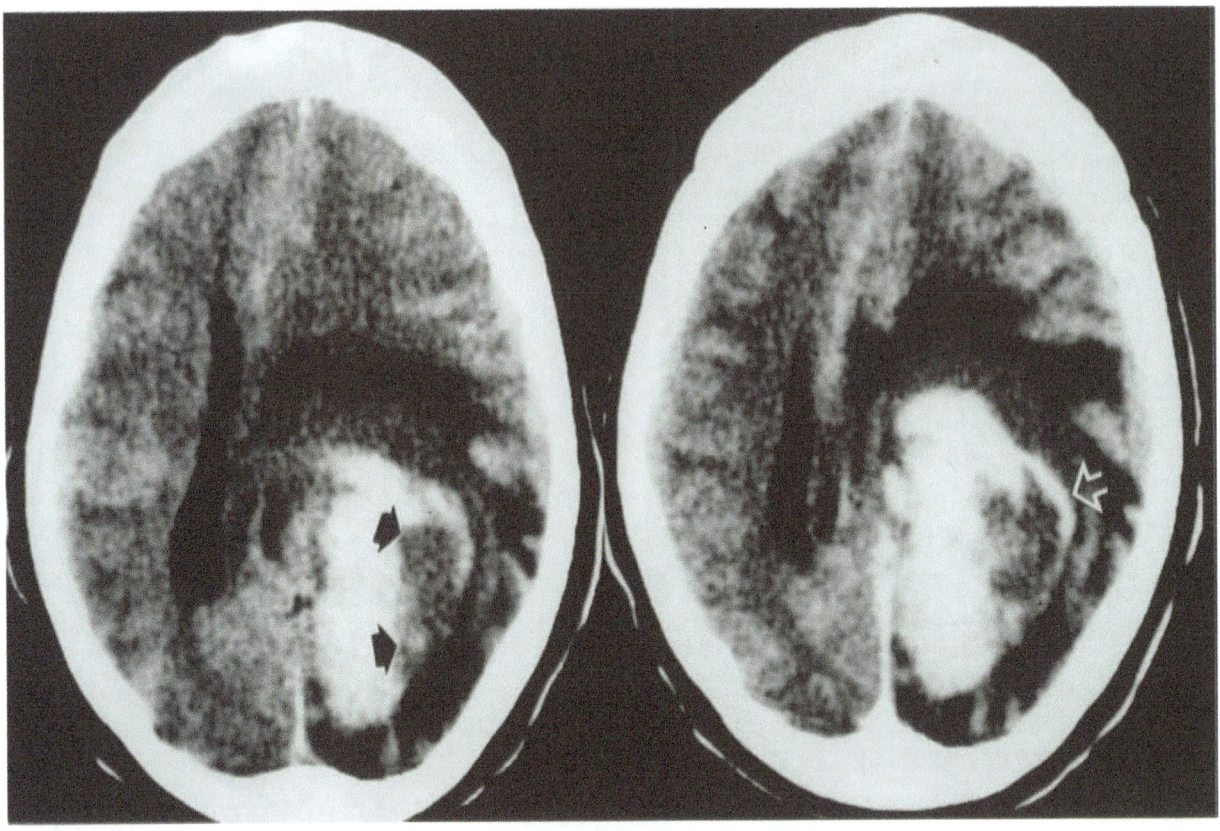

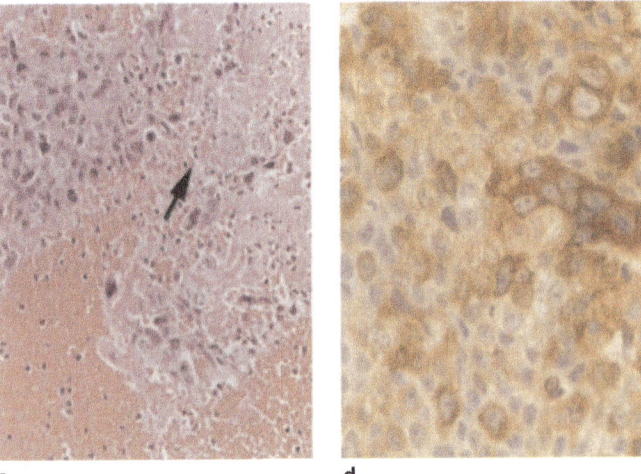

Figure 4.94 Metastatic disease, choriocarcinoma: female, 29 years; (**a**) CT, (**b**) CT + C, (**c**) HE ×200, (**d**) HCG ×400; occipital hyperdense mass with partially contained isodense component (a, arrows); lesion brightens perceptibly after contrast administration, particularly rim (b, open arrow). Operative specimen was mainly clotted blood, and isodense tissue on scan is assumed to be consistent with solid, but largely necrotic tumour (c, arrow). Viable tumour cells show strong, brown-staining, HCG positivity (d)

large-cell carcinoma of the lung to the occipital lobe and squamous-cell carcinoma of the lung to the cerebellum[113], these tendencies possibly being related to regional differences in endothelial cell surface properties *vis-à-vis* metastasizing cells.

4.13. LYMPHOMA (see also section 2.6e)

The incidence of primary CNS lymphoma, already increased in immunocompromised individuals, has on this account been predicted to become the commonest primary brain neoplasm[114]. Imaging features, despite some unusual variants, tend to be rather typical, including location in the deep grey matter, corpus callosum and ventricular walls, where bilateral spread is particularly characteristic[115] (Figures 4.97 and 4.98). Hordes of neoplastic round cells with a high nuclear–cytoplasmic ratio but lacking intercellular attachments (Figure 4.99), combine with local interstitial space widening to confer intermediate density and signal alteration to the mass lesion, delineated on the long TR images by surrounding vasogenic oedema[116]. Strong, usually homogeneous enhancement results from vascular proliferation and damage (Figure 4.100), and multifocal lesions with these features are characteristic (Figure 4.101) illustrating, by comparison, the diagnostic difficulty which arises with immunodeficiency syndrome-related central necrosis[117,118] (Figure 4.102).

Most cases of CNS lymphoma are intermediate or high-grade B cell type[119–121], and although T cell[122], primary Hodgkin's[123] and Burkitt's lymphoma[124] are documented, there are no reported distinguishing imaging features[125]. Angiotropic lymphoma (malignant angioendotheliosis) is associated with multifocal, angiopathic ischaemic necrosis[126].

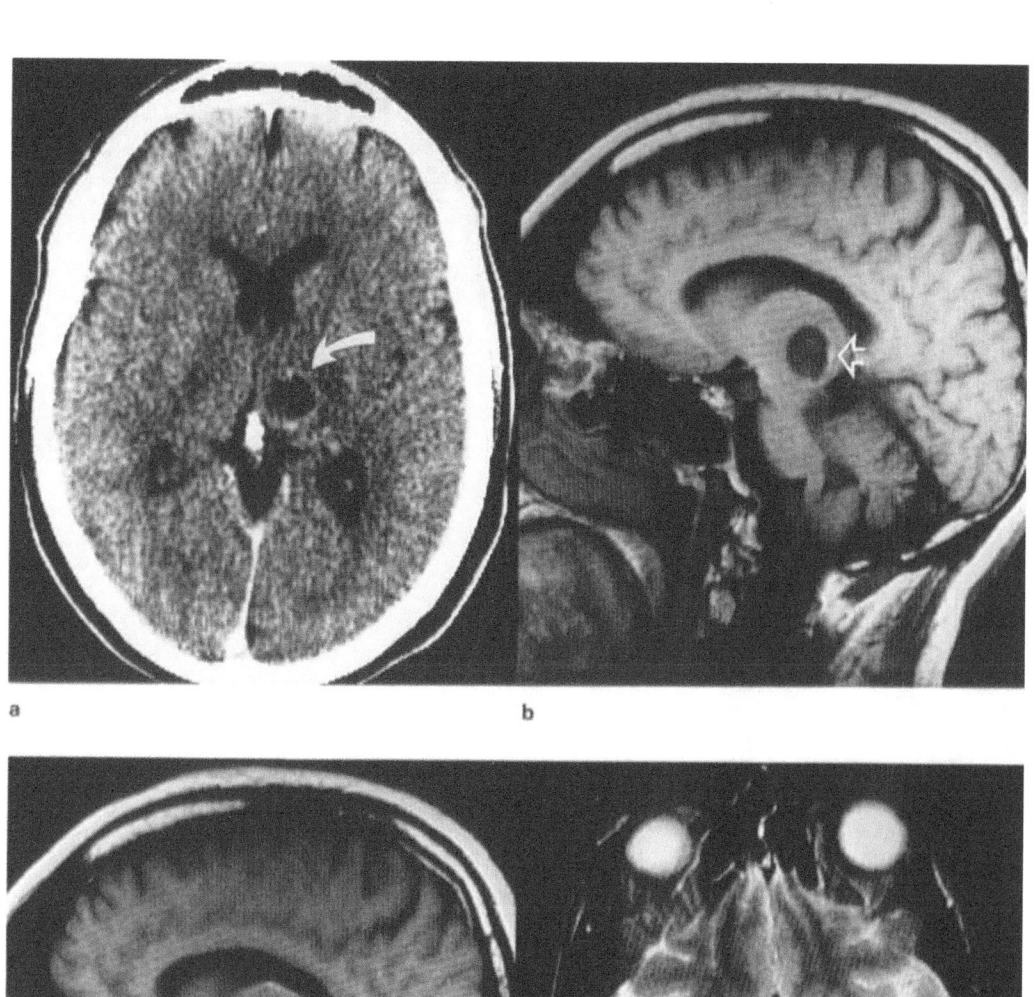

a   b

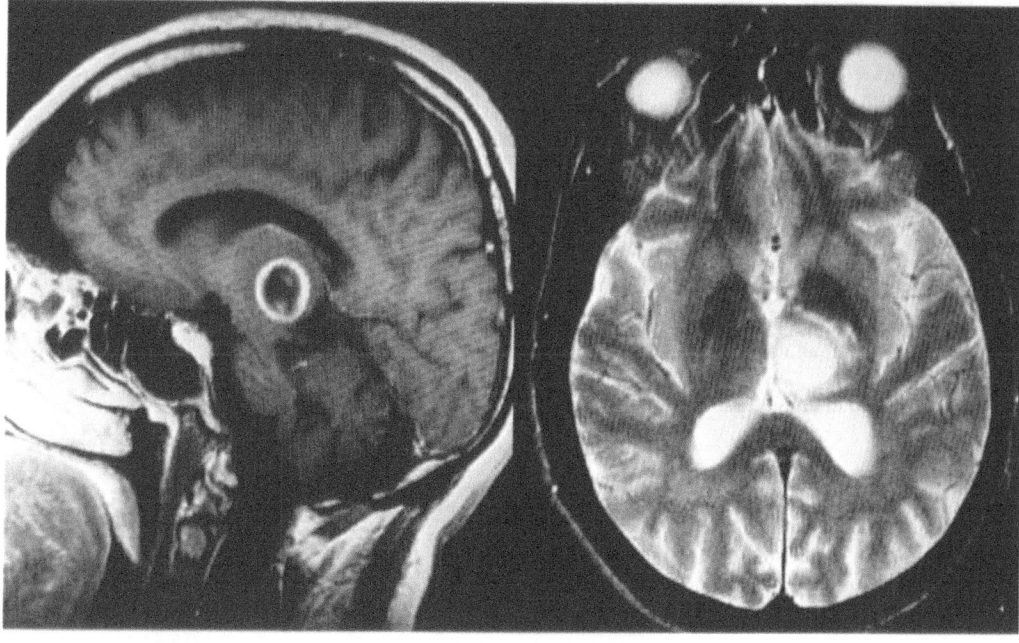

c   d

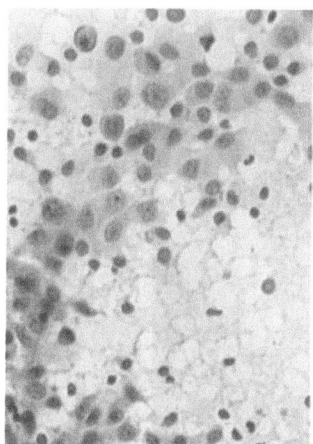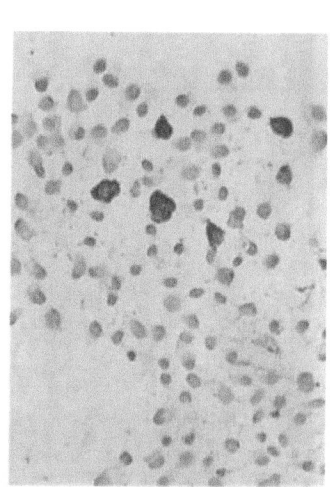

Figure 4.95 Metastatic disease, melanoma: (**a**) CT + C, (**b**) sagittal T1WI, (**c**) T1WI + C, (**d**) T2WI, (**e**) HE/melanin × 400; 'cystic' diencephalic lesion, with faint rim enhancement (a, arrow). Lesion is hypointense on T1 weighted images, with subtle rim hyperintensity (b, open arrow) and strong peripheral enhancement (c); contents are almost CSF isointense at long TR (d). At operation tumour was both haemorrhagic and melanotic, so that lack of signal shortening, on both accounts, is paradoxical and unexplained. Cytology shows sheets of cells having large nuclei and abundant cytoplasm; melanin was easily identified (e)

e

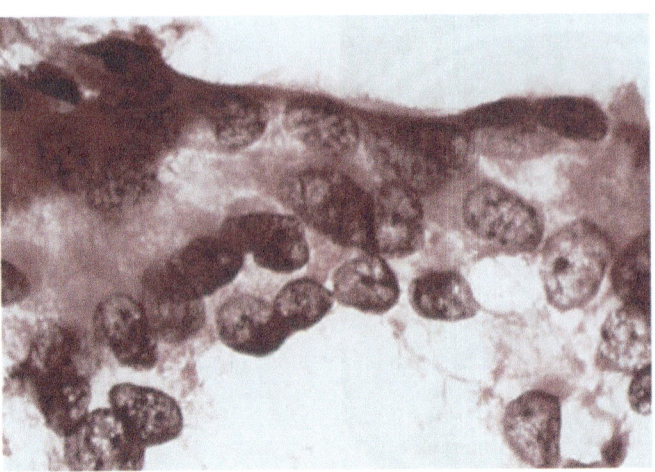

Figure 4.96 Metastatic disease: illustrates characteristic smearing of carcinoma cells. HE × 400

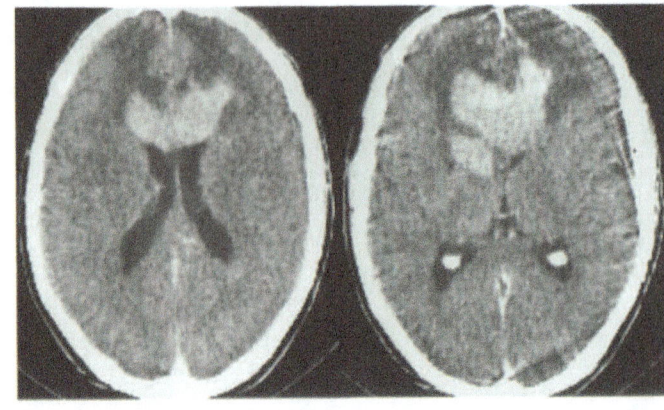

a

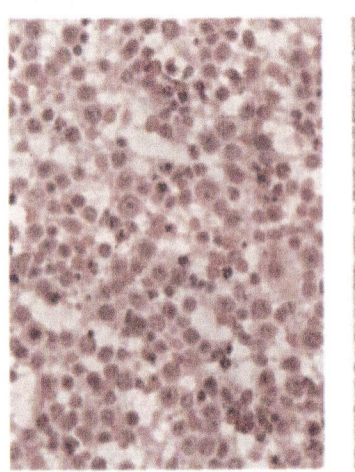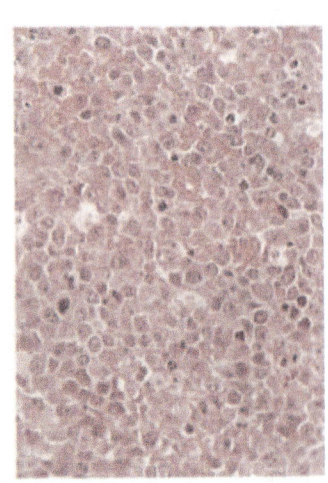

b

Figure 4.97 Lymphoma, primary, callosal: male, 56 years; (**a**) CT + C, (**b**) HE × 400; bilateral symmetrical, anterior corpus callosum, strongly enhancing tumour, growing into the anterior horns. Comparative smear/paraffin section shows typical features of lymphoma (b)

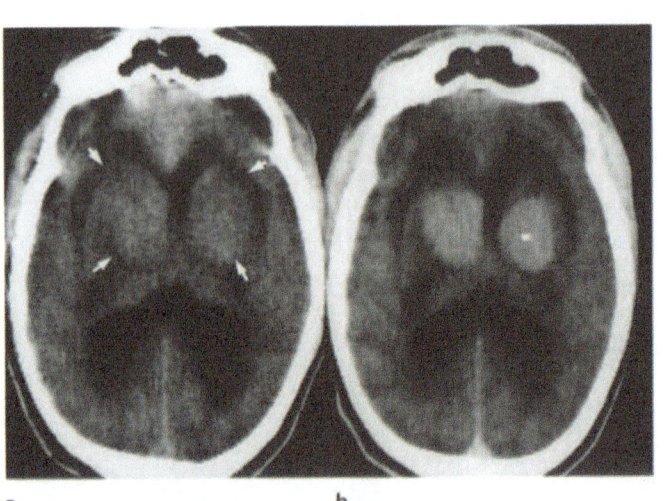

a   b

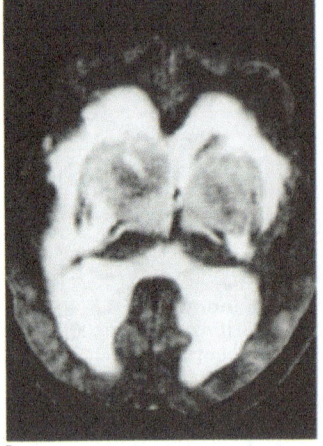

c

Figure 4.98 Lymphoma, metastatic, deep grey: male, 50 years, known systemic lymphoma, on treatment; (**a**) CT, (**b**) CT + C, (**c**) T2WI, (**d**) fixed brain slice; bilateral symmetrical isodense expansion of deep grey matter (a, arrows), with weak homogeneous enhancement (b). At long TR lesion is cortex isointense, being delineated by surrounding oedema and CSF hyperintensity. (The symmetrical involvement of deep grey (d), is more typical of primary lymphoma, raising the possibility that this patient has developed another primary tumour)

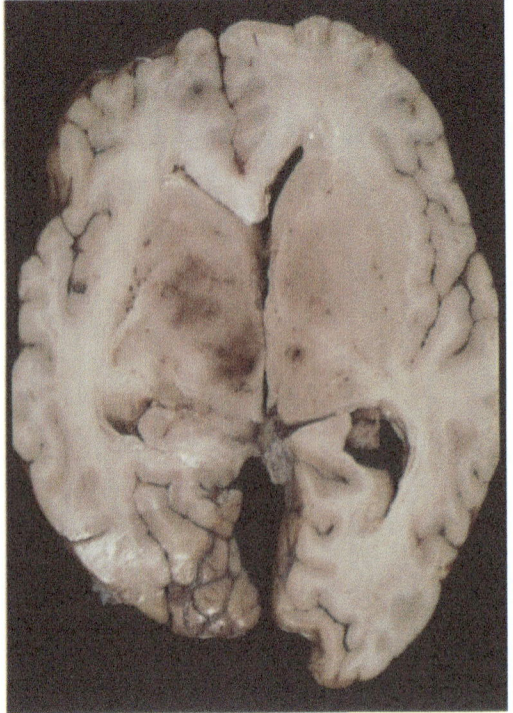

d

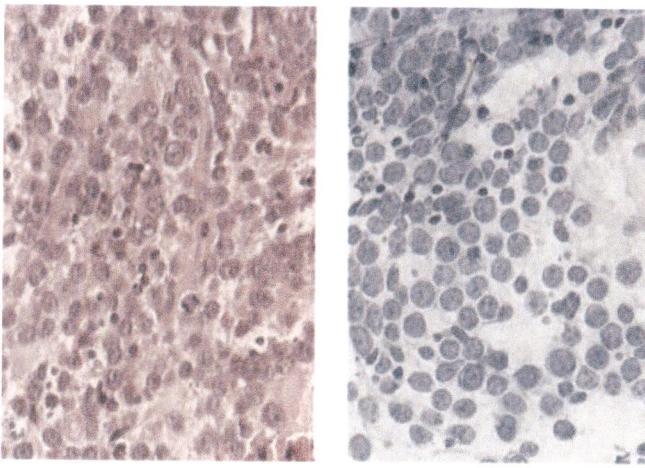

Figure 4.99   B cell lymphoma: immunoblastic PCNSL composed of large cells with prominent nucleoli. Note the even spread of cells and lack of intercellular junctions. HE/Tol blue ×400

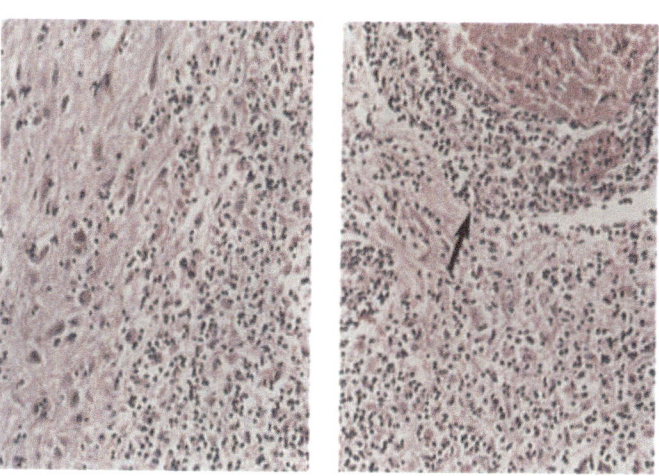

a

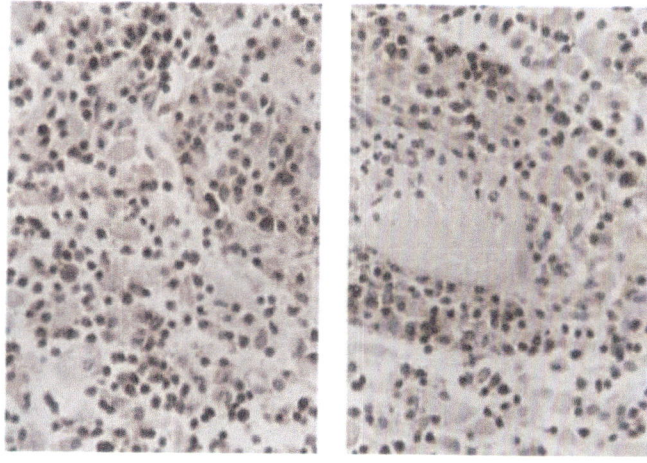

b

Figure 4.100   T cell lymphoma: (**a**) HE ×100, (**b**) UCHL1; typical densely cellular parenchymal and vascular infiltration (a, arrow), by variably sized round and angulated lymphocytes, exhibiting immuno-histochemical staining with the pan T cell monoclonal antibody UCHL1 (b)

REFERENCES

1. Pozzati E, Guiliani G, Gaist G et al. Chronic expanding hematoma. J Neurosurg. 1986;65:611–14.
2. Destian S, Sze G, Krol G et al. MR imaging of haemorrhagic intracranial neoplasms. AJNR. 1988;9:1115–22.
3. Bell BA, Kendall BE, Symon L. Angiographically occult arteriovenous malformations of the brain. J Neurol Neurosurg Psychiatry. 1978;41:1057–64.
4. Lobato RD, Peres C, Rivas JJ, Cordobes F. Clinical, radiological and pathological spectrum of angiographically occult intracranial vascular malformations. J Neurosurg. 1988;68:518–31.
5. Sigal R, Krief O, Houtteville JP. Occult cerebrovascular malformations: follow-up with MR imaging. Radiology. 1990;176:815–19.
6. Russell DS, Rubinstein LJ. Pathology of tumours of the nervous system, 5th edn. London: Edward Arnold; 1989:727–46.
7. Rigamonti D, Johnson PC, Spetzler RF et al. Cavernous malformations and capillary telangiectasia: a spectrum within a single pathological entity. Neurosurgery. 1991;28:60–4.
8. Chandler WF, Farhat SM, Pauli FJ. Intrathalamic epidermoid tumor: case report. J Neurosurg. 1975;43:614–17.
9. Markwalder TM, Zimmerman A. Intracerebral ciliated epithelial cyst. Surg Neurol. 1979;11:195–8.
10. Nakasu Y, Handa J, Watanabe K. Progressive neurological deficits with benign intracerebral cysts. J Neurosurg. 1986;65:706–9.
11. Wilkins RH, Burger PC. Benign intraparenchymal brain cysts without an epithelial lining. J Neurosurg. 1988;68:378–82.
12. Lotz J, Hewlett RH, Alheit B et al. Neurocysticercosis: correlative pathomorphology and MR imaging. Neuroradiology. 1988;30:35–41.
13. Zimmerman RD, Weingarten K. Neuroimaging of cerebral abscesses. Neuroimaging Clin N Am. 1991;1:1–16.
14. Enzmann DR, Britt RH, Placone R. Staging of human brain abscess by computed tomography. Radiology. 1983;146:703–8.
15. Whelan MA, Hilel SK. Computed tomography as a guide in the diagnosis and follow-up of brain abscesses. Radiology. 1980;135:663–71.
16. Haimes AB, Zimmerman RD, Morgello S et al. MR imaging of brain abscesses. AJNR. 1989;10:279–91.
17. Shuper A, Levitsky HI, Cornblath DR. Earlier invasive CNS aspergillosis. Neuroradiology. 1991;33:183–5.
18. McDonald WI, Miller DH, Barnes D. The pathological evolution of multiple sclerosis. Neuropathol Appl Neurobiol. 1992;18:319–34.
19. Otsuka SI, Nakatsu S, Matsumoto S et al. Multiple sclerosis simulating brain tumor on CT. JCAT. 1989;13:674–8.
20. McDonald WI, Miller DH, Barnes D. The pathological evolution of multiple sclerosis. Neuropathol Appl Neurobiol. 1992;18:319–34.
21. Nesbit GM, Forbes GS, Scheithauer BW et al. Multiple sclerosis: histopathologic correlation and MR and/or CT correlation in 37 cases at biopsy and 3 cases at autopsy. Radiology. 1991;180:467–74.
22. Russell DS, Rubinstein LJ. Pathology of tumours of the nervous system, 5th edn. London: Edward Arnold; 1989:92–5.
23. Giuffre R. Biological aspects of brain tumours in infancy and childhood. Child's Nerv Syst. 1989;5:55–9.

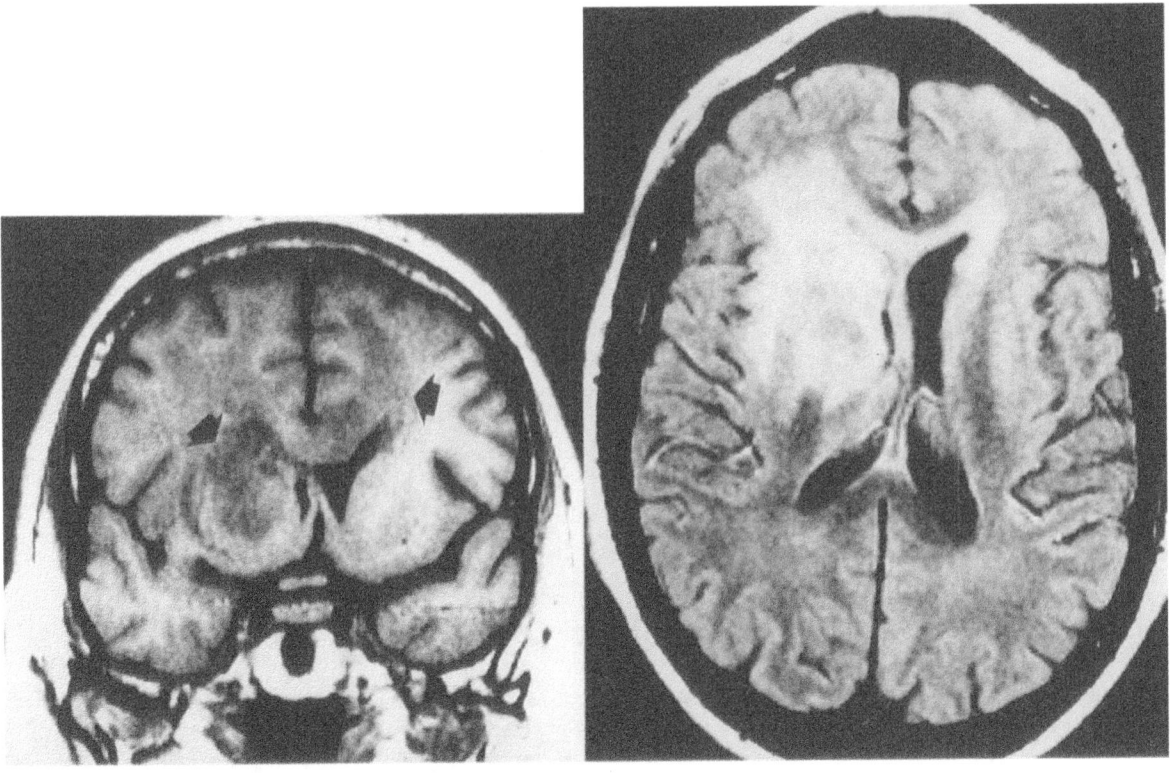

a
b

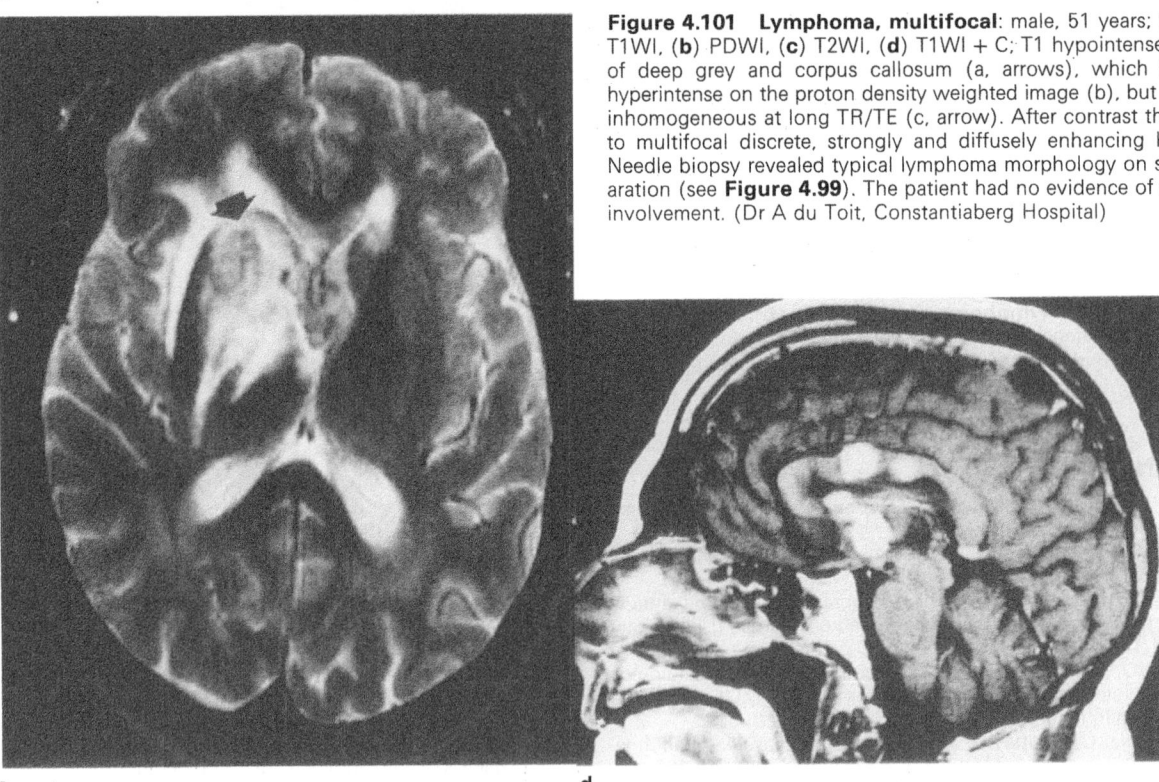

Figure 4.101 Lymphoma, multifocal: male, 51 years; (**a**) coronal T1WI, (**b**) PDWI, (**c**) T2WI, (**d**) T1WI + C; T1 hypointense expansion of deep grey and corpus callosum (a, arrows), which is diffusely hyperintense on the proton density weighted image (b), but much more inhomogeneous at long TR/TE (c, arrow). After contrast these resolve to multifocal discrete, strongly and diffusely enhancing lesions (d). Needle biopsy revealed typical lymphoma morphology on smear preparation (see **Figure 4.99**). The patient had no evidence of extracranial involvement. (Dr A du Toit, Constantiaberg Hospital)

c
d

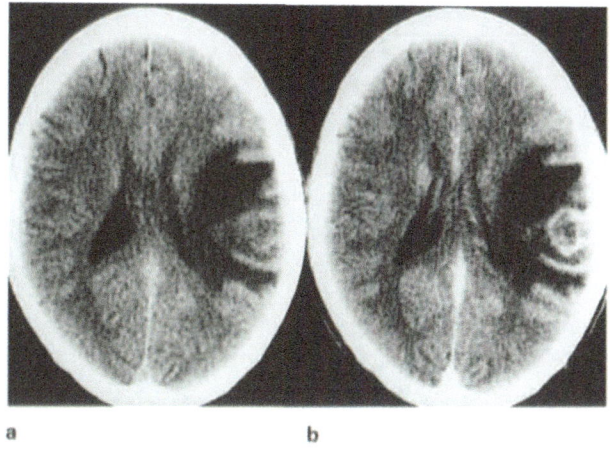

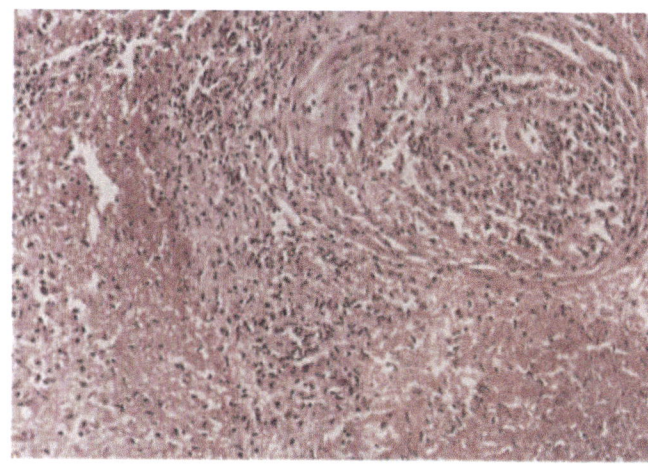

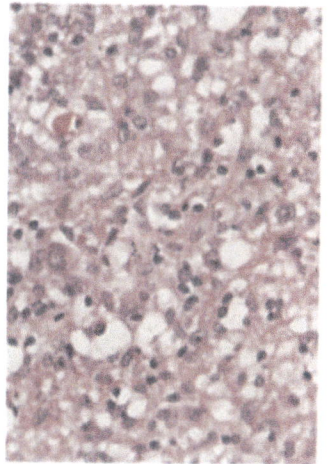
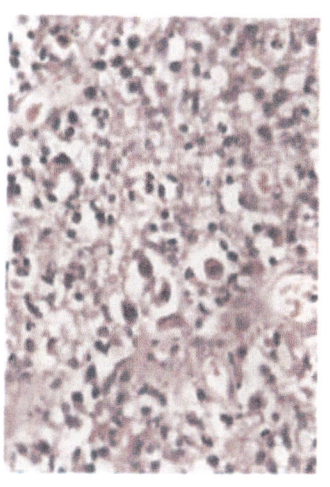
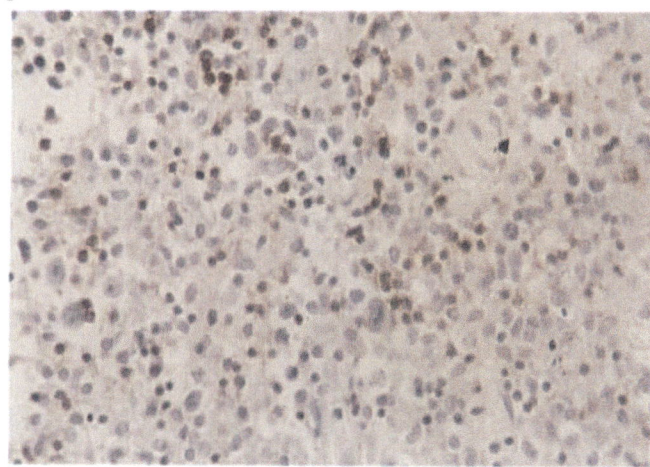

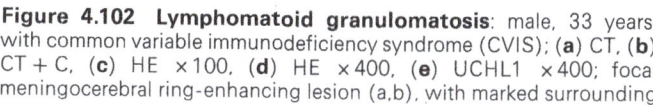

Figure 4.102 Lymphomatoid granulomatosis: male, 33 years, with common variable immunodeficiency syndrome (CVIS); (**a**) CT, (**b**) CT + C, (**c**) HE ×100, (**d**) HE ×400, (**e**) UCHL1 ×400; focal meningocerebral ring-enhancing lesion (a,b), with marked surrounding oedema. Features are not specific, but brain isodensity favours coagulative necrosis. Histology shows angiocentric/angionecrotic (c), polymorphic lymphoreticular infiltrate (d), with atypical neoplastic cells staining with UCHL1 (e)

24. Kadota RP, Allen JB, Hartman GA, Spruce WE. Brain tumours in children. J Pediatr. 1989;4(1):511–19.
25. Scott EW, Mickle JP. Pediatric diencephalic gliomas – a review of 18 cases. Pediatr Neurosci. 1987;13:225–32.
26. Packer RJ, Sutton LN, Rosenstock JG et al. Pineal region tumors of childhood. Pediatrics. 1984;74:97–102.
27. Albright AL, Price RA, Guthkelch AN. Brainstem gliomas of children. A clinicopathological study. Cancer. 1983;52:2313–19.
28. Mantravadi RVP, Phatak R, Bellur S et al. Brain stem gliomas: an autopsy study of 25 cases. Cancer. 1982;49:1294–6.
29. Littman P, Jarret P, Bilanuik LT et al. Pediatric brain stem gliomas. Cancer. 1980;45:2787–92.
30. Freeman AI. Introduction. Cancer (suppl). 1985;56:1743–4.
31. Nelson JS, Tsukada Y, Schoenfeld D et al. Necrosis as a prognostic criterion in malignant supratentorial, astrocytic gliomas. Cancer. 1983;52:550–4.
32. Atlas SW. Adult supratentorial tumors. Semin Roentgenol. 1990;25:130–54.
33. Dean BL, Drayer BP, Bird CR et al. Gliomas: classification with MR imaging. Radiology. 1990;174:411–15.
34. Bernstein JJ, Laws ER, Levine KV et al. C6 glioma–astrocytoma cell and fetal astrocyte migration into artificial basement membrane: a permissive substrate for neuronal tumours but not fetal astrocytes. Neurosurgery. 1991;28(5):652–7.
35. Gado MH, Phelps ME, Coleman RE. An extravascular component of contrast enhancement in cranial computed tomography. Part I: The tissue–blood ratio of contrast enhancement. Radiology. 1975;117:589–93.
36. Gado MH, Phelps ME, Coleman RE. An extravascular component of contrast enhancement in cranial computed tomography. Part II: contrast enhancement and the blood–tissue barrier. Radiology. 1975;117:595–7.
37. Long DM. Capillary ultrastructure and the blood–brain barrier in human malignant brain tumours. J Neurosurg. 1970;32:127–44.
38. Lee YY, Van Tassel P, Bruner JM et al. Juvenile pilocytic astrocytomas: CT & MR characteristics. AJNR. 1989;10:363–70.
39. Miki H, Hirano A. Electron microscopic studies of optic nerve glioma in an 18 month old child. Am J Ophthalmol. 1975;79:589.
40. Hirano A, Matsui T. Vascular structures in brain tumours. Hum Pathol. 1975;6(5):611–21.
41. Weller RO, Foy M, Cox S. The development and ultrastructure of the microvasculature in malignant gliomas. Neuropathol Appl Neurobiol. 1977;3:307–22.
42. Burger PC, Vogel FS, Green SB, Strike TA. Glioblastoma multiforme and anaplastic astrocytoma. Pathologic criteria and prognostic implications. Cancer. 1985;56:1106–11.
43. Leeds NE, Elkin CM, Zimmerman RD. Gliomas of the brain. Semin Roentgenol. 1984;19:27–43.
44. Abe H, Hasegawa H, Kobayashi Y et al. A gemistocytic astrocytoma demonstrated high intensity on MR images. Neuroradiology. 1990;32:166–7.
45. Earnest F, Kelly PJ, Scheithauer BW et al. Cerebral astrocytomas: histopathologic correlation of MR and CT contrast enhancement with stereotactic biopsy. Radiology. 1988;166:823–7.
46. Dumas-Duport C, Scheithauer BW, Kelly PJ. A histologic and cytologic method for the spatial definition of gliomas. Mayo Clin Proc. 1987;62:435–49.
47. Vonovakos D, Marcu H, Hacker H. Oligodendrogliomas: CT patterns with emphasis on features of malignancy. JCAT. 1979;3:783–8.
48. Lee Y-Y, Van Tassel P. Intracranial oligodendrogliomas: imaging findings in 35 untreated cases. AJNR. 1989;10:119–27.
49. Russel DS, Rubinstein LJ. Pathology of tumours of the nervous system, 5th edn. London: Edward Arnold, 1989:182–6.
50. Ludwig CL, Smith MT, Godfrey AD, Armbrustmacher VW. A clinicopathologic study of 323 patients with oligodendroglioma. Ann Neurol. 1986;19:15–21.

The suprasellar cistern is limited below by the hypophysis, dorsum sellae and cavernous sinus, and above by the floor of the third ventricle. It is bounded anteriorly by the sphenoid jugum and clinoids, on each side by the medial temporal lobes, and posteriorly by the cerebral peduncles, at which point the suprasellar, ambient and prepontine cisterns are continuous. Its principal contents include the infundibulum, optic nerves and chiasm, the internal carotid–circle vessels, and arachnoid tissue. Usually, the space is referred to as suprasellar by neurosurgeons, and para- or juxtasellar by radiologists. Most texts give a list of lesions which can occur in this region[1,2], but for practical purposes the large majority of masses originate from the floor, mainly pituitary adenoma or craniopharyngioma, or a related cyst. Lesions from other structures, such as optic nerve and hypothalamic glioma, infundibular and vascular masses, are rare, and although granulomatous inflammation regularly affects the leptomeninges at this site, isolated inflammatory and parasitic masses are also very uncommon.

The process of identifying the origin and relationships of a suprasellar mass has been transformed by contrast MR, and nowadays the principal diagnostic problems are concerned with the nature and implications of cyst formation and tissue enhancement, in which regard patient age exerts a particularly strong bias. Whether or not a clearly intrasellar component can be demonstrated, symptomatic cysts are by definition supra- or juxtasellar, to the extent that clinical presentation is of visual failure, endocrine disturbance or CSF obstruction. Correlative imaging and pathological studies have shown that neither peripheral enhancement (or its absence), nor fluid signal characteristics are specific; rather that different combinations of these features tend to shift the balance of probabilities, and because a cyst may be neoplastic, a tissue diagnosis is usually necessary. A degree of non-specificity also affects solid-cystic lesions.

Surgical exposure for a suprasellar mass is usually via a subtemporal approach with use of the operating microscope, affording the pathologist exquisitely detailed visualization of abnormal structures. In many instances adhesions render complete excision impossible, so that tissue samples are always very small and thus difficult to orientate and liable to trauma. Cyst fluid, now of considerable correlative importance, has to be collected by needle aspiration.

5.1. PRIMARY CYSTS

Primary cysts of assumed developmental origin are discussed more fully in section 3.1. All have been described in the suprasellar region. The histogenesis of type II craniopharyngioma is an unresolved problem (see below).

5.1a. Epidermoid cyst

The imaging features and pathology of epidermoid cyst are presented in section 6.1b, suprasellar location being characteristic though less common (Figure 5.1). The natural history of epidermoidoma elsewhere, of progressive elaboration of flaky keratin without complication, suggests that this lesion does not give rise to the occasional suprasellar cyst whose contents are either 'machine oil' or buttery amorphous debris in type[3]; these the writers assume to be craniopharyngiomas, probably type I (see below).

5.1b. Arachnoid and neuroepithelial cysts

Symptomatic distension of the suprasellar cistern sometimes occurs as a result of CSF obstruction by Liliequist's membrane, constituting a type of arachnoid pouch[4,5]. Sagittal views are required to demonstrate continuity between the suprasellar and propontine cisterns (Figure 5.2). Neuroepithelial cyst at this site may be indistinguishable (Figure 5.3).

5.1c. Rathke's cleft cyst

In occurrence this is the rarest of suprasellar cysts, almost always having an intrasellar component and usually asymptomatic. Cyst lining, most characteristic as ciliated columnar type, is also variable, including goblet, cuboidal and squamous cells[6,7]. Contents may range from hypo- to hyperintense[8], including corresponding T2 hypointensity (Figure 5.4), more or less consistent with their macroscopic appearance, and enhancement is absent.

5.2. CRANIOPHARYNGIOMA

Craniopharyngiomas are generally solid/cystic lesions, in which the cystic component usually predominates (Figures 5.5 and 5.6). Not uncommonly, the tumour is entirely cystic (Figure 5.7), complicating the diagnosis (see below). Adamantinomatous tissue (Figure 5.8), which characterizes the childhood lesion (type I craniopharyngioma), is often absent from the adult tumour (type II), which is instead composed of papillary stratified squamous epithelium devoid of keratin, and may include intracytoplasmic mucin (goblet cells) and ciliated cells[9]; this tissue, in our opinion, is reminiscent of upper respiratory tract epithelium (Figure 5.9).

Solid tumour tissue exhibits expected T1 cortex isointensity (Figure 5.6), whilst moderate T2 hyperintensity[10] is probably explained by the formation of microcysts, an alteration of adamantinomatous tissue and/or degeneration of the stroma[11], apparent in almost every low-power field (Figure 5.8). The precise source of enhancement in craniopharyngioma, often poor or patchy, is unclear; some tumours are a complex of neoplastic and vascularized connective tissue (Figure 5.8), whilst others abut directly onto adjacent, infolded, vascularized gliotic neural parenchyma (Figure 5.10), these morphological variations being difficult to correlate in biopsy material. In the case illustrated in Figure 5.11, biopsy fragments from the edge of the tumour show the vasculature to be mainly within the surrounding reactive glial tissue.

Nodular keratin (Figure 5.8), said to be pathognomonic of type I craniopharyngioma[12], and easily recognizable in smear preparations (Figure 5.12), provides a nidus for mineralization (Figure 5.8) and also initiates the process of ulceration, granulomatous response, exudation and haemorrhage (Figure 5.6). Based on such pathogenesis the nature of cyst fluid is bound to be very variable,

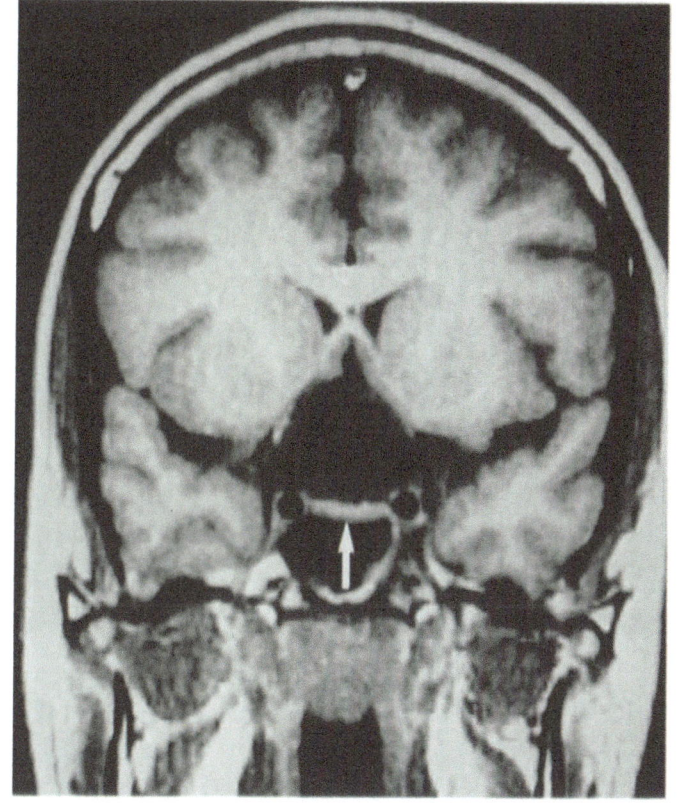

a

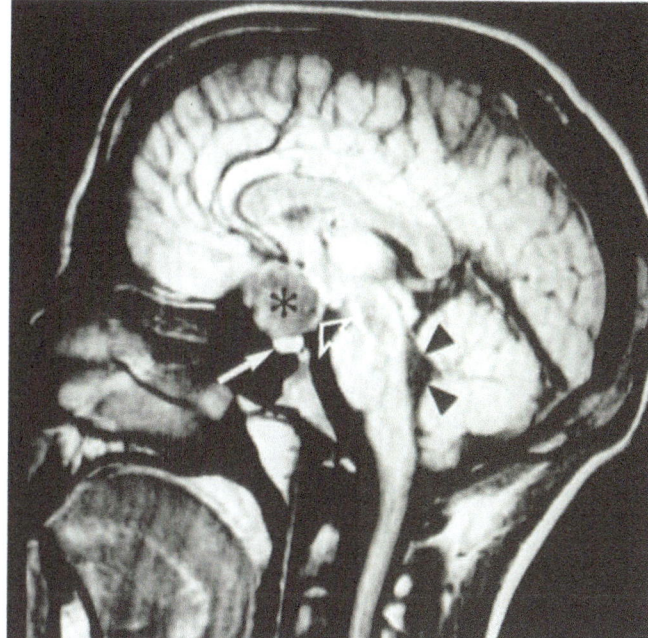

b

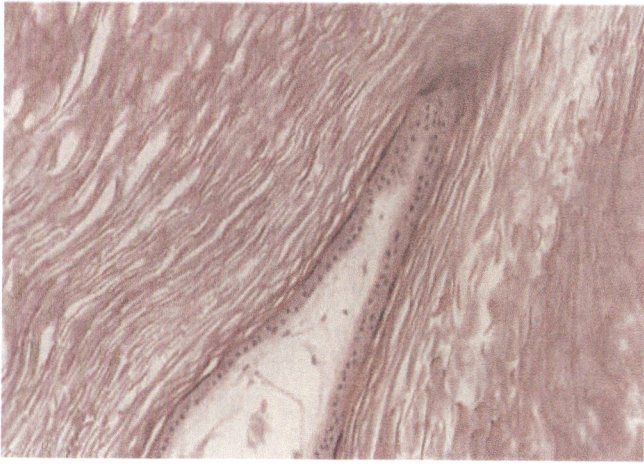

d

c

Figure 5.1   Epidermoidoma, suprasellar: female, 17 years; lifelong history of visual disturbance and onset of recent headache; (**a**) coronal T1WI, (**b**) sagittal PDWI, (**c**) sagittal T2WI, (**d**) HE × 200; images show a lobulated, non-enhancing suprasellar cyst compressing the pituitary gland (a–c, arrows) and extending upwards to displace the optic chiasm (b, open arrow) and anterior 3rd ventricle. No capsule obvious, and contents are inhomogeneous T1 hypointense–T2 hyperintense (dry/flaky keratin – d). Parenchyma of the gland is clearly differentiated on the T2 images (c). Note intermediate signal intensity of cyst contents (b, asterisk), compared with the signal from 4th ventricle CSF (arrow-heads

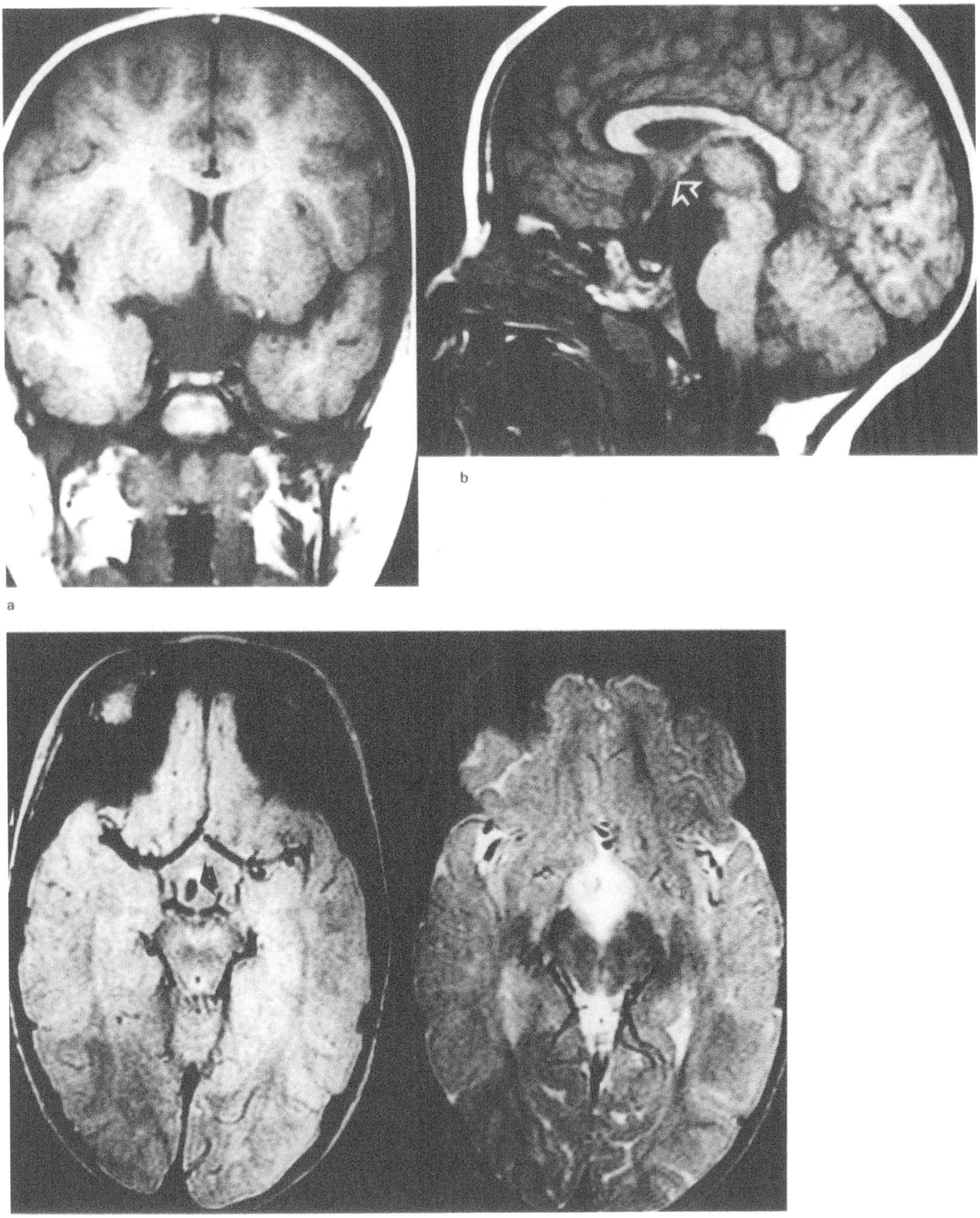

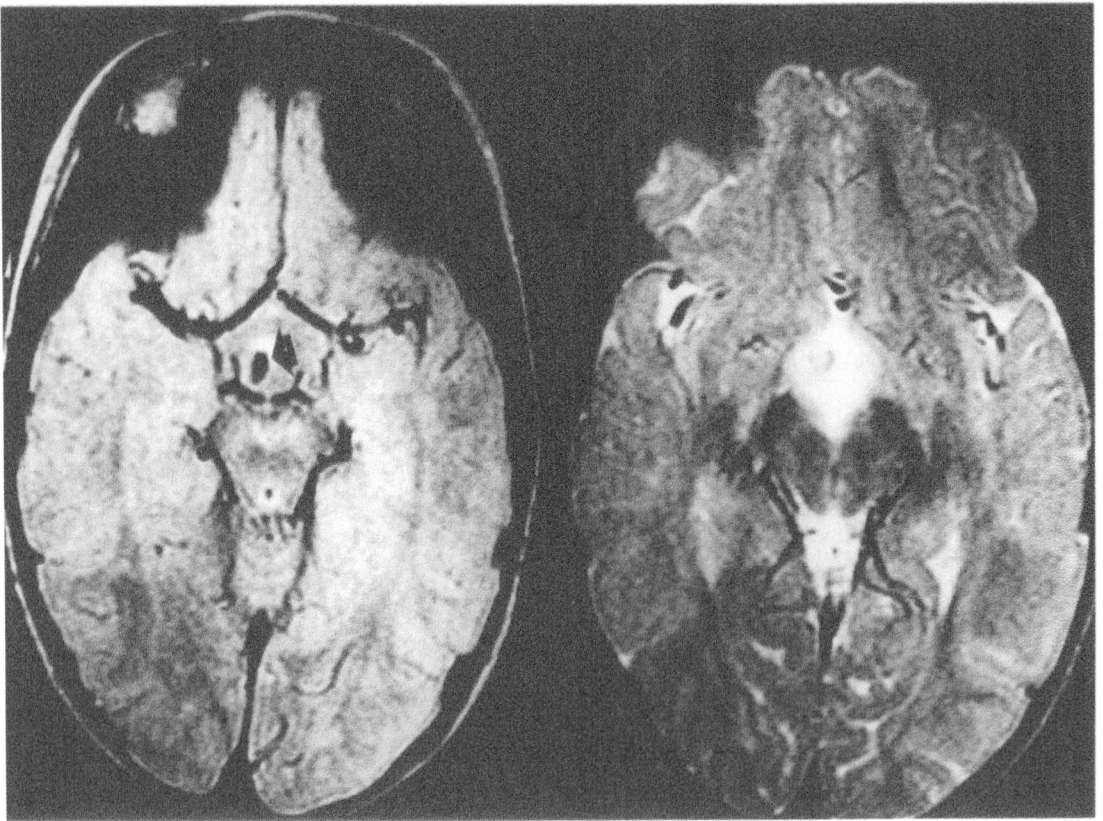

Figure 5.2 Arachnoid cyst, suprasellar: (**a**) coronal T1WI, (**b**) sagittal T1WI, (**c**) axial PDWI, (**d**) axial T2WI; suprasellar space is expanded but anatomical structures are still identifiable, including floor of V3 (b, arrow). Cyst contents are CSF isointense on T1 and T2W images, but paradoxically hyperintense with flow void (c, arrow) on PDWI, presumably due to turbulence

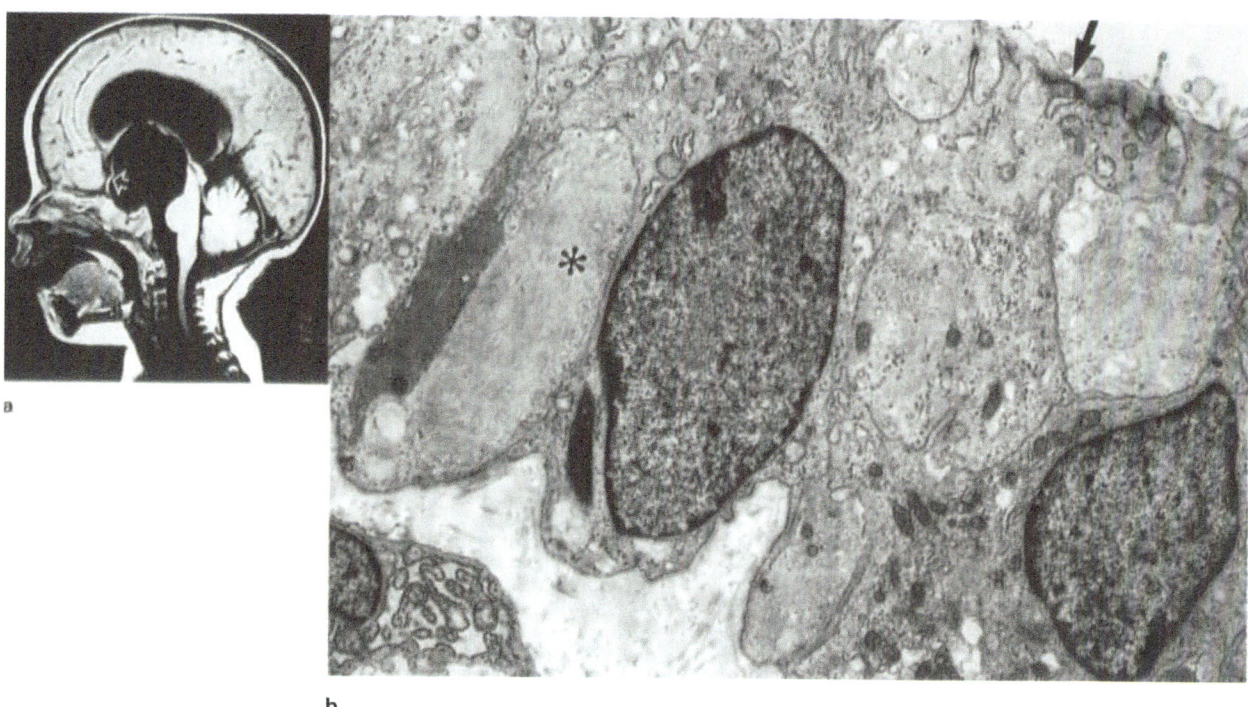

a

b

Figure 5.3 Neuroepithelial cyst, suprasellar: infant, 1 week, hydrocephalus; (**a**) sagittal T1WI, (**b**) EM ×9300; image shows cystic effacement of the suprasellar cistern and the 3rd ventricle; linear structure anteriorly (open arrow) is probably the chiasm; EM of cyst wall shows intracytoplasmic filaments (asterisk), complex junctions (arrow) and microvilli, features suggestive of neuroepithelium, and therefore of probable intracerebral/intraventricular origin. (Drs R Melvill and C Sinclair-Smith, Constantiaberg and Red Cross Children's Hospital)

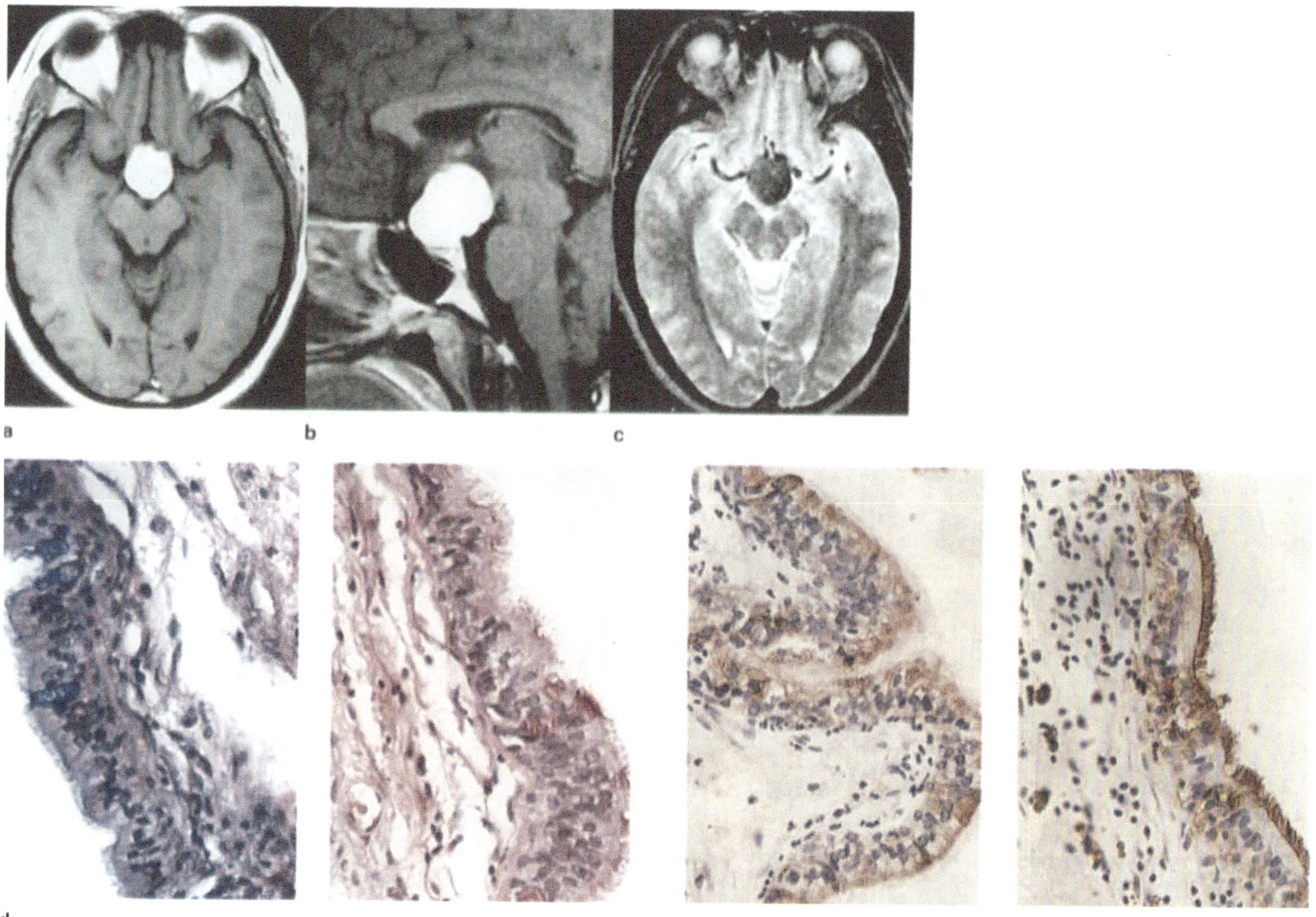

a   b   c

d   e

Figure 5.4 (*legend overleaf*)

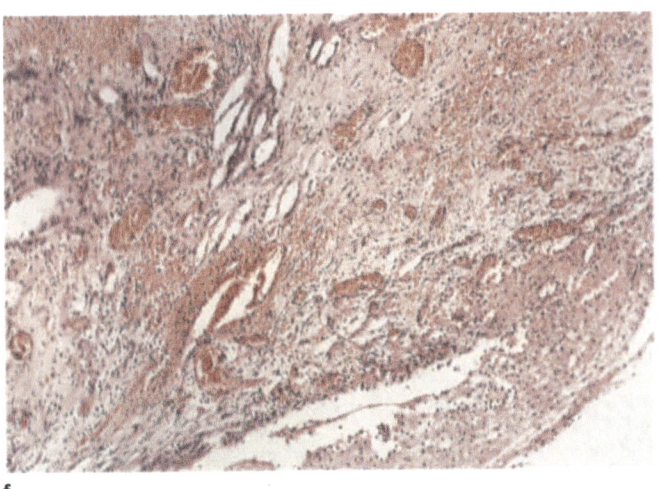

f

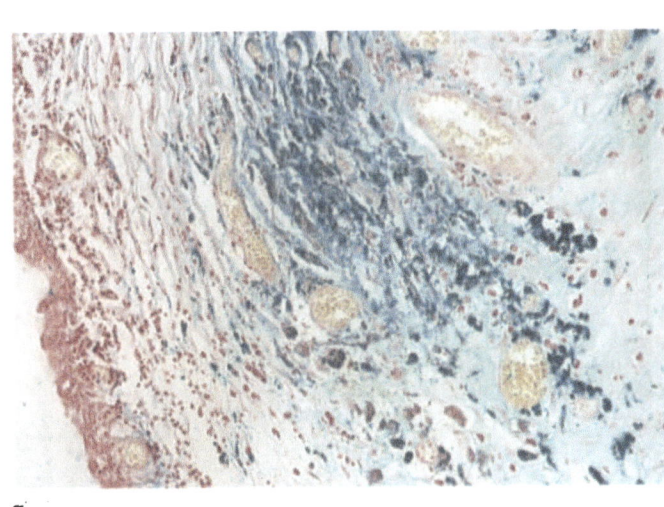

g

Figure 5.4   Rathke's cleft cyst, suprasellar: (**a**) T1WI, (**b**) sagittal T1WI, (**c**) T21WI, (**d**) APAS/mucin ×400, (**e**) EMA/CEA ×400, (**f**) HE ×100, (**g**) Perl's ×200; images show cyst contents to be uniformly T1 hyperintense (a,b), T2 hypointense (c); signal and morphology combine to suggest a suprasellar cyst with high protein concentration, rather than lipoma. At operation cyst aspirate was deep brown and coagulated spontaneously. Histology reveals a pseudostratified columnar epithelium with goblet cells (d); note cytoplasmic and membrane distribution of EMA and CEA, respectively (e); in areas the lining is elevated by organizing haemorrhage (f,g), with exudate overlying ulcerated cyst lining

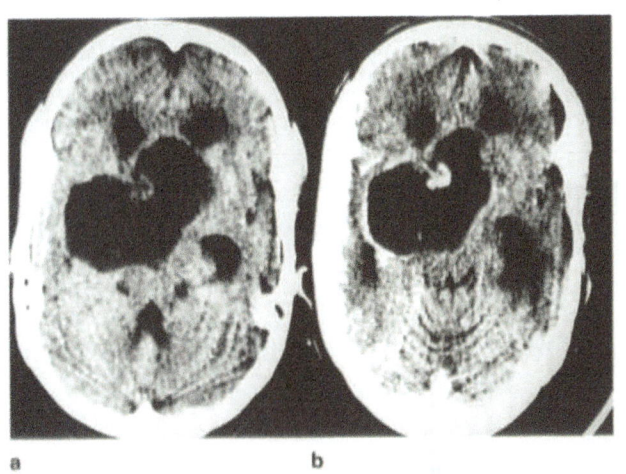

a   b

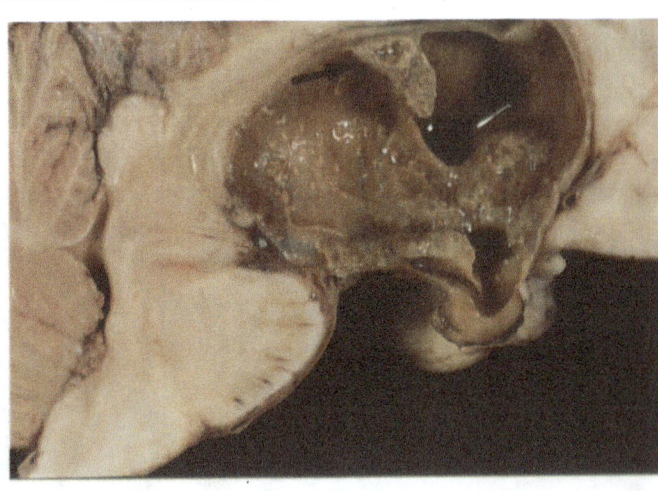

c

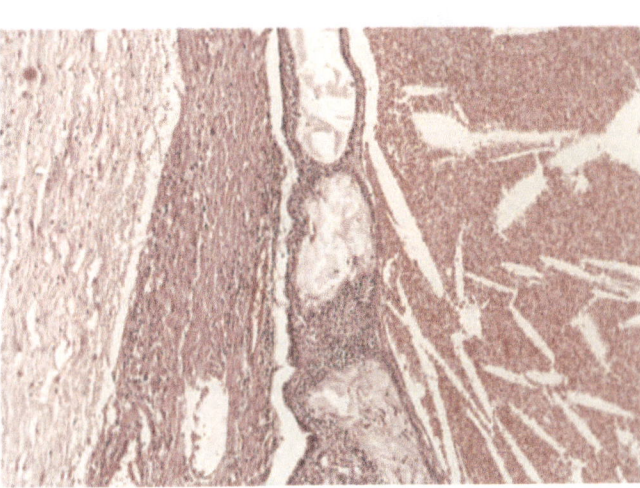

d

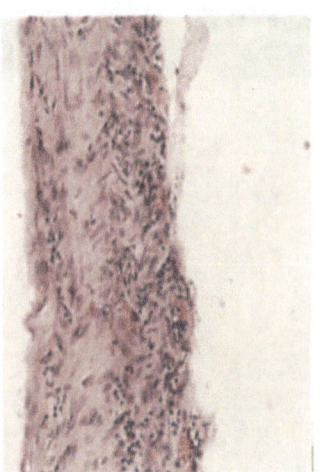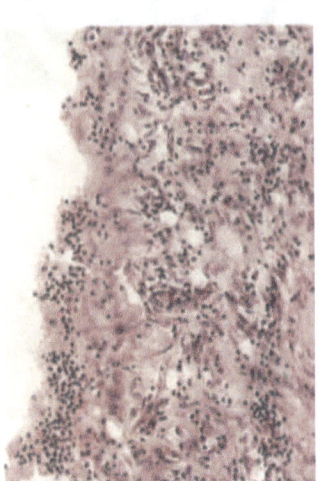

e

Figure 5.5   Craniopharyngioma, haemorrhagic cystic with enhancing nodule: (**a**) CT, (**b**) CT + C, (**c**) fixed specimen, (**d**) HE ×100, (**e**) HE ×100/×200, (**f**) (*opposite*) HE ×100/×200; images show irregular parasellar cyst with inhomogeneous CSF hyperdense contents (a), and patchy enhancement of wall and central nodule (corresponding to tissue shown in fixed specimen (c, arrow). Cyst contents which were haemorrhagic (motor oil) are a composite of blood, fibrin, cholesterol crystals and inflammatory exudate including macrophages (d). The wall consists of adamantinomatous tissue and vascularized connective tissue (d), the former focally ulcerated (e). Adjacent brain is gliotic and spongiotic. Sample from enhancing nodule illustrates nature of tumour vascularity (f)

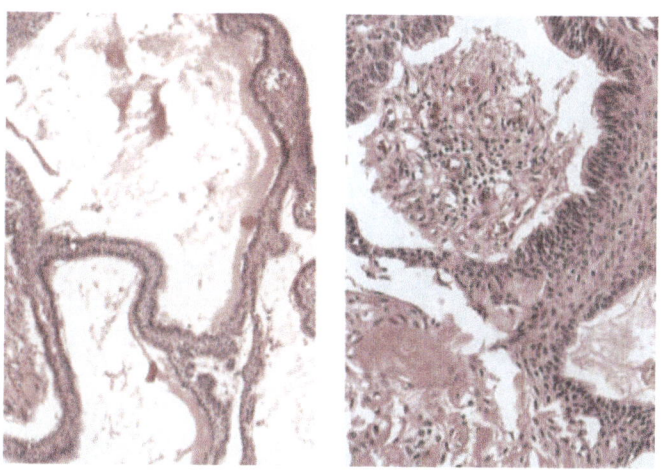

Figure 5.5(f)

Figure 5.6 (*below*) **Craniopharyngioma, cystic with enhancing nodule and ossification**: (**a**) T1WI, (**b**) T1WI + C, (**c**) HE × 40, (**d**) HE × 200; images show a large suprasellar–intraventricular cyst, with slightly inhomogeneous contents, hyperintense relative to CSF. Enhancement is confined to the central nodular component. Signal void (arrow) reflects ossification (d) (see also **Figure 5.7**). Fresh and organizing focal haemorrhage (c), found in surgical specimen, is not apparent on the scan

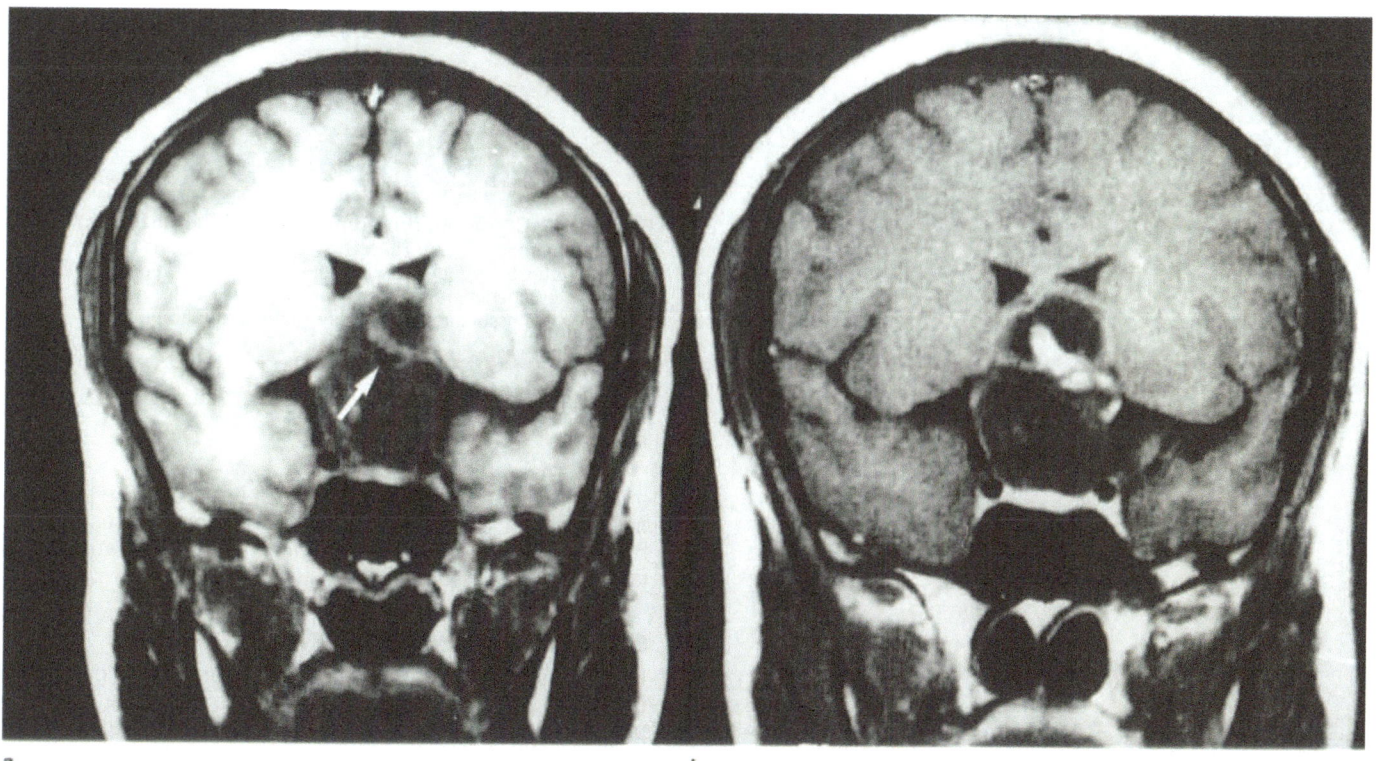

a   b

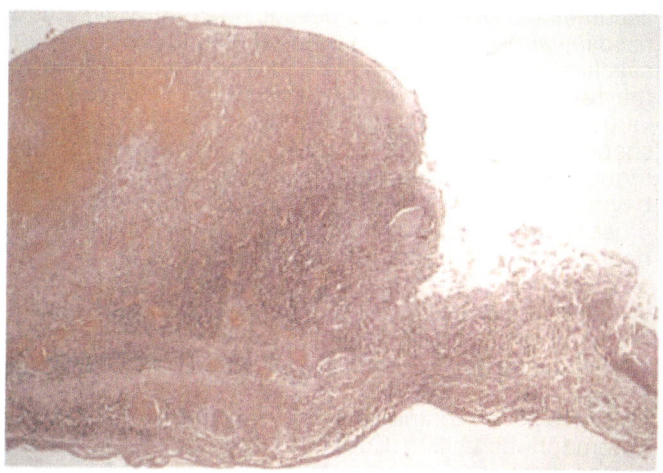

c

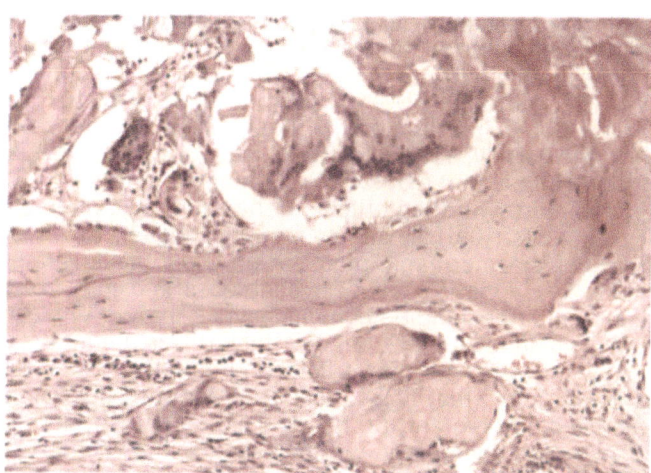

d

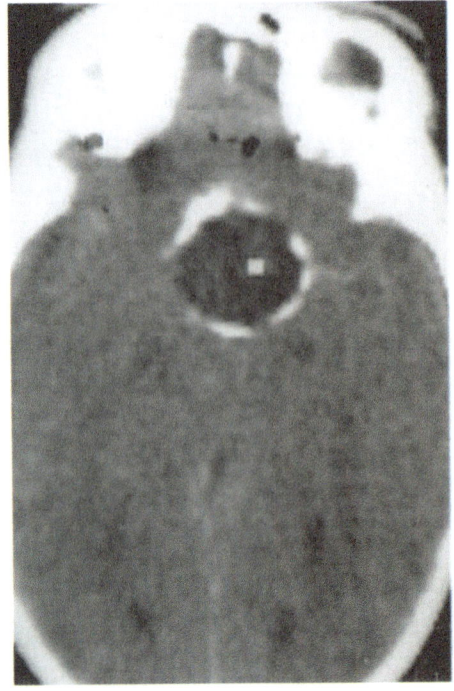

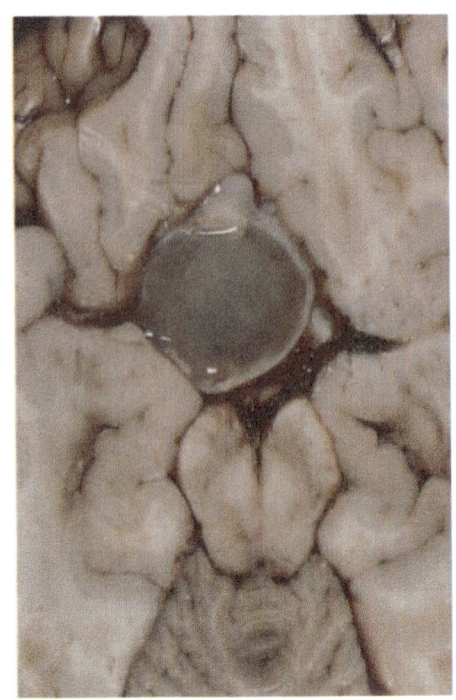

a   b

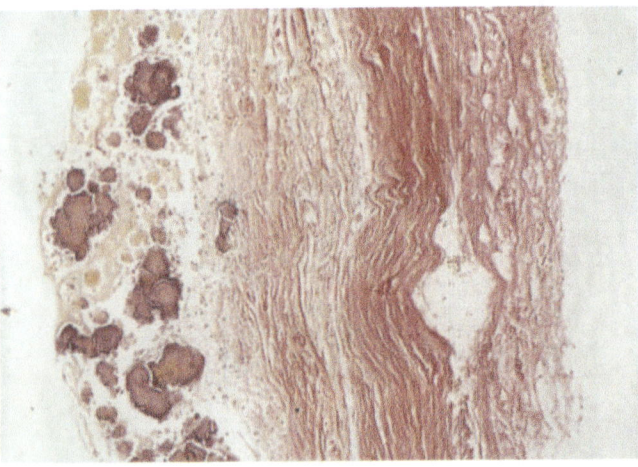

c

Figure 5.7   Craniopharyngioma, cystic, mineralized: (**a**) CT + C, (**b**) fixed brain specimen, (**c**) VG ×100; CT shows cyst, in brain-dead patient, with CSF-hyperdense contents and mineralized wall. Note cyst fluid in fixed specimen is almost transparent (b). Heavy mineralization of cyst wall is associated with loss of identifiable tumour (c)

including protein, macrophages, cholesterol crystals, red blood cells and debris (Figure 5.13), so that signal intensity at short TR may be expected to be equally variable, although always hyperintense relative to CSF (Figures 5.6, 5.8 and 5.9). 'Motor-oil' fluid often, but not exclusively, found in type I craniopharyngioma, is assumed to impart marked T1 shortening[10] (Figure 5.13), in common with the contents of haemorrhagic retention cyst (section 2.5): it should be remembered, however, that non-haemorrhagic proteinaceous fluid as illustrated in Figure 5.7 may also be T1 hyperintense, and conversely, some craniopharyngiomas contain typical brown, cholesterol-rich fluid which does not have the hyperintensity expected of haemorrhagic fluid (Figure 5.8). (Cyst fluid analyses show that T1 shortening, although a function of methaemoglobin and protein concentration, is independent of the concentration of cholesterol or triglycerides[13].) The lesion shown in Figure 5.14 lacks an identifiable lining and the contents are inspissated, so that the diagnosis rests on the presence of nodular keratin. We have found that this substance (nodular keratin) will not stain with the polyclonal antibody which marks the 56

and 64 kDa molecular weight cytokeratins in the epithelial cells of both type I craniopharyngioma (Figures 5.8 and 5.13) and epidermoidoma, and the flaky keratin of the latter (Figure 2.10).

5.3.   PITUITARY ADENOMA

It appears that the concept of a functioning tumour within the adenohypophysis, and therefore invisible with the prevailing techniques of the day (plain films and cysternography), owes its origins to the paper published by Hardy[14]. The extensive imaging literature on adenomas accumulated over the past decade, now so well summarized in various texts[15,16], has entrenched the morphological classification of microadenomas and macroadenomas, the former being arbitrarily defined as not exceeding a vertical height of 10 mm, besides having a variety of shapes and sites within the adenohypophysis and usually inducing some deformity of the infundibulum. Once beyond the confines of the sella, meso- and macroadenomas are accepted as having a wide range of morphology, density and signal intensity.

Somewhat contemporaneously, laboratory techniques in electron microscopy and immunohistochemistry combined to oust the tinctorial classifications of adenomas by demonstrating the functional diversity of stain-homogeneous populations (e.g. acidophils) as well as the presence of membrane-bound electron-dense granules in chromophobe cells[17]. Current endocrine practice, which places great reliance on imaging, has limited the role of diagnostic neuropathology in the management of pituitary tumours to those cases of macroadenomas which are either inducing visual failure, or tumours of either group which do not respond to medical treatment.

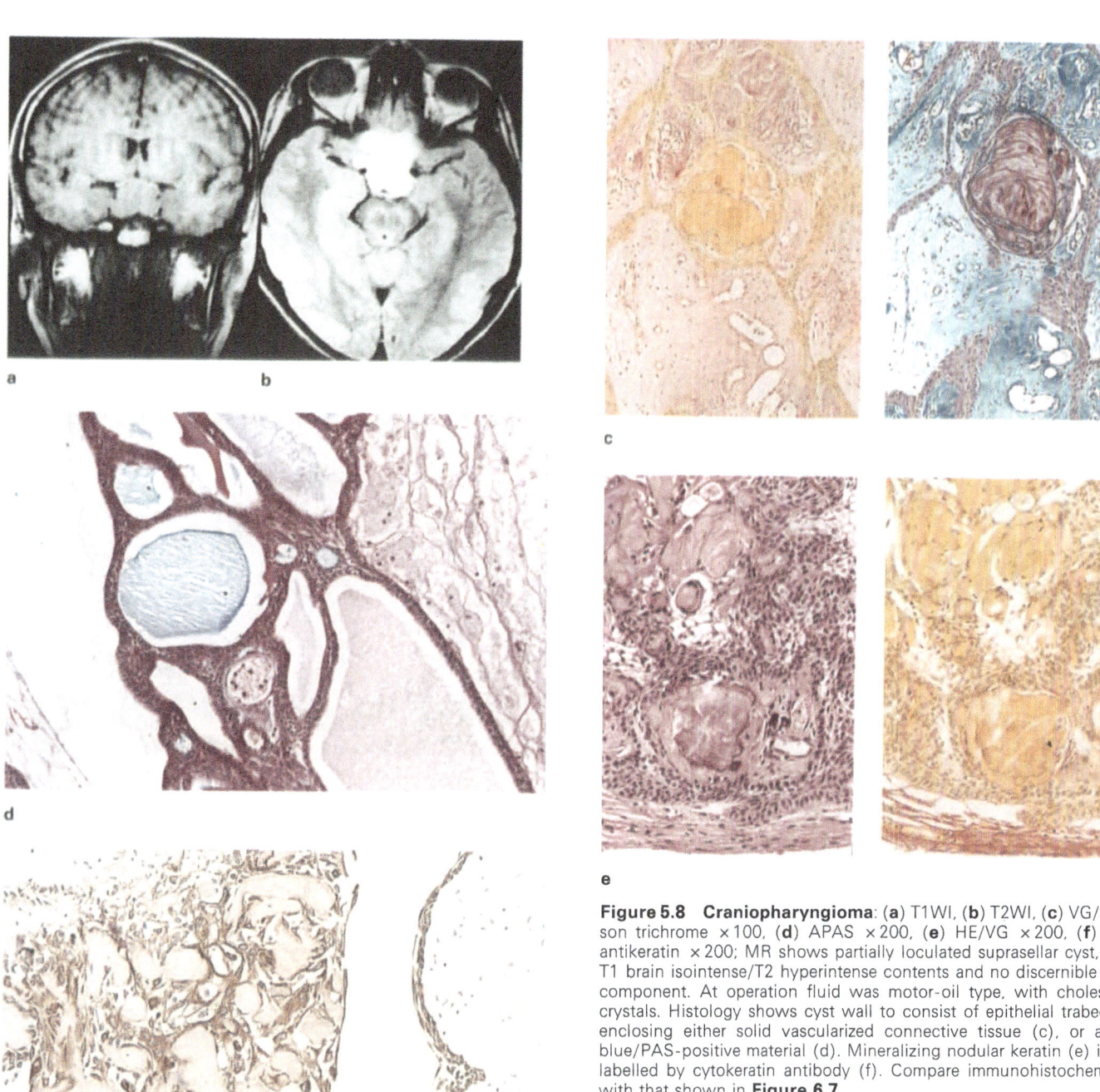

Figure 5.8 Craniopharyngioma: (**a**) T1WI, (**b**) T2WI, (**c**) VG/Masson trichrome × 100, (**d**) APAS × 200, (**e**) HE/VG × 200, (**f**) PAP antikeratin × 200; MR shows partially loculated suprasellar cyst, with T1 brain isointense/T2 hyperintense contents and no discernible solid component. At operation fluid was motor-oil type, with cholesterol crystals. Histology shows cyst wall to consist of epithelial trabeculae enclosing either solid vascularized connective tissue (c), or alcian blue/PAS-positive material (d). Mineralizing nodular keratin (e) is not labelled by cytokeratin antibody (f). Compare immunohistochemistry with that shown in **Figure 6.7**

In the case of surgically treated microadenomas, the majority of which are prolactin-secreting, clinical–endocrine data provide a presumptive functional diagnosis to the extent that many neurosurgeons are satisfied to suck out the contents of the affected lobe, without attempting to obtain pathological verification. This unfortunate attitude is likely to deprive many pathologists of the chance to witness, with the operating microscope, the striking, even pathognomonic, fluidity of adenoma tissue as it is tapped through the floor of the sella; at the same time the difficulty in obtaining samples from these small tumours for routine examination is one reason why their imaging features are not fully explained.

5.3a. Microadenoma

The majority of these small tumours are relatively hypointense compared with the normal signal of the anterior pituitary on T1 weighted images (Figures 5.15 and 5.16), and are also refractory to enhancement with contrast agents such as gadolinium[18], characteristics which are considered diagnostic. Nevertheless, the distinction between normal and abnormal tissue on MR has been

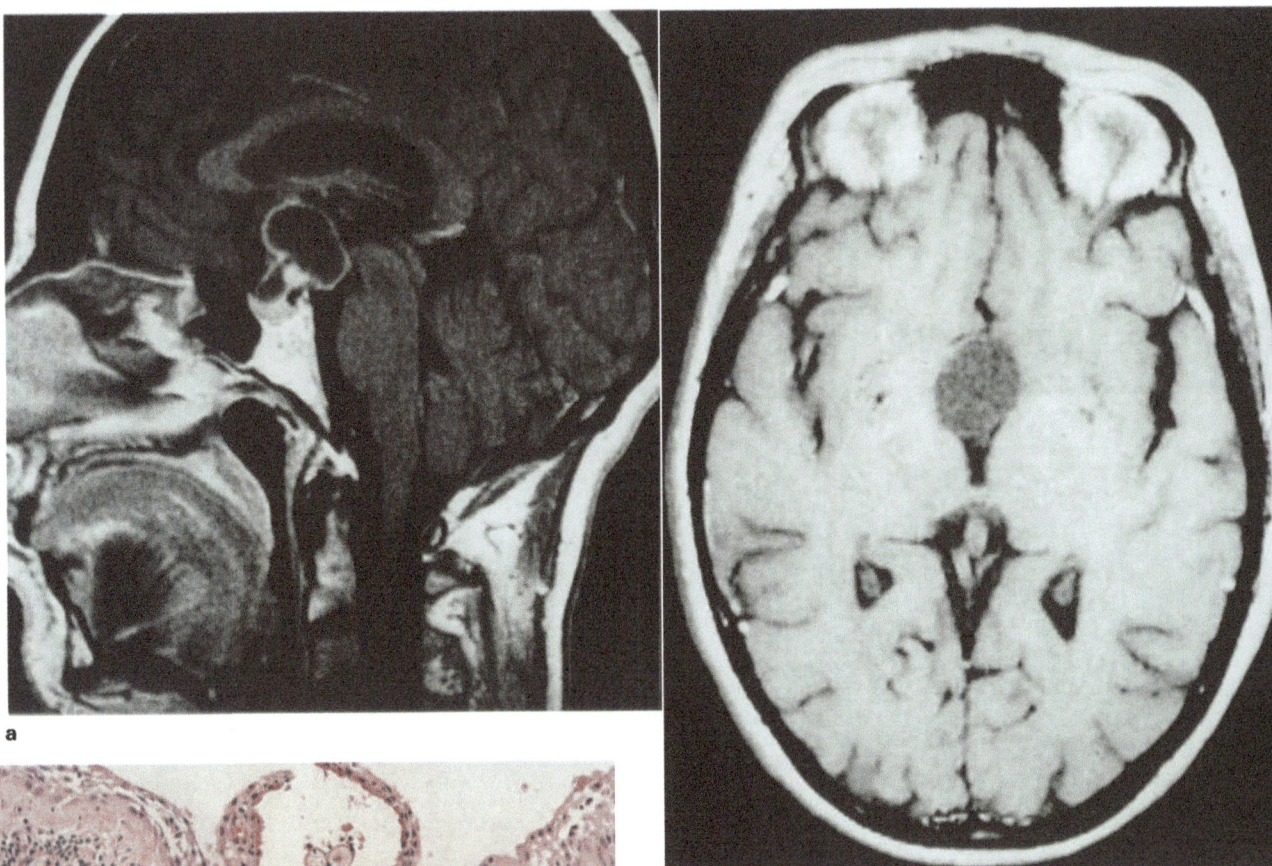

Figure 5.9 Craniopharyngioma type II: female, 50 years; (**a**) sagittal T1WI + C, (**b**) PDWI, (**c**) PAS ×200; intra- and suprasellar cystic lesion with enhancing rim and nodule. Contents are CSF mildly hyperintense on T1W and PDW images, consistent with high protein contents. At surgery clear yellowish fluid aspirated. Histology shows lining to consist of a mixed epithelium (squamous/columnar), with secretory activity, having a thick hyalinized basement membrane. Adjacent brain shows prominent blood vessels and an inflammatory infiltrate

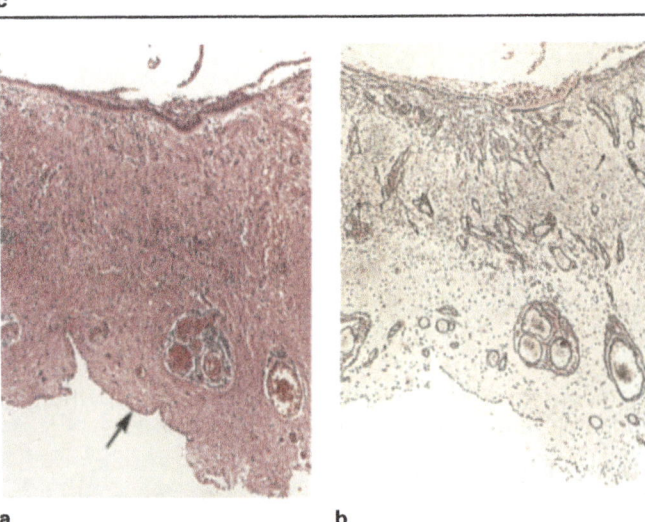

Figure 5.10 Craniopharyngioma, cystic, enhancing wall: (**a**) HE ×100, (**b**) Retic ×100; morphology illustrates the cyst wall to consist predominantly of vascularized gliotic neural parenchyma, having an attenuated epithelial lining. Note ependyma opposite (arrow). Cholesterol concentration was 5.07 mmol/l

pithily described as 'oftentimes subtle'[15], a warning which merits the attention of pathologists. Both the structural basis for hypointensity at short TR and differential enhancement, can only be surmised, at present. The magnetic susceptibilities of secretory granules seem to be excluded on the grounds that functionally different tumours may look identical[15]. Lobular and vascular architecture, on the other hand, are strikingly different, comparing normal and abnormal tissue, with hypertrophy and hyperplasia of cell aggregates (Figures 5.17 and 5.18), relative diminution of vessels per tissue unit, and proliferation and degeneration of sinusoidal reticulin (Figure 5.24) constituting typical features of neoplasia. However these factors may apply to the usual image, it would still be necessary to explain why some tumours are gland isointense or even enhancing, whilst the effect on signal intensity of organelles, filaments and amyloid (Figure 5.22) which contribute to histopathological variants such as oncocytes and Crooke's hyaline, still needs to be assessed.

There seems no doubt that the paucity of reticulin in both micro- and macroadenomas explains the characteristic smearing texture of these tumours, with the formation of sheets of cells (Figure 5.19) and interspersed, stellate capillary fragments. By comparison, the normal gland

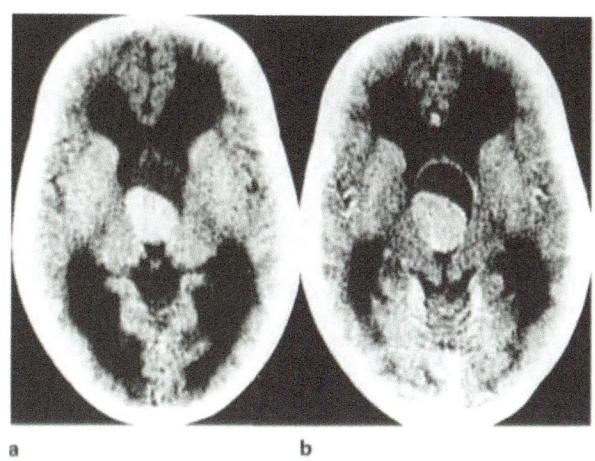

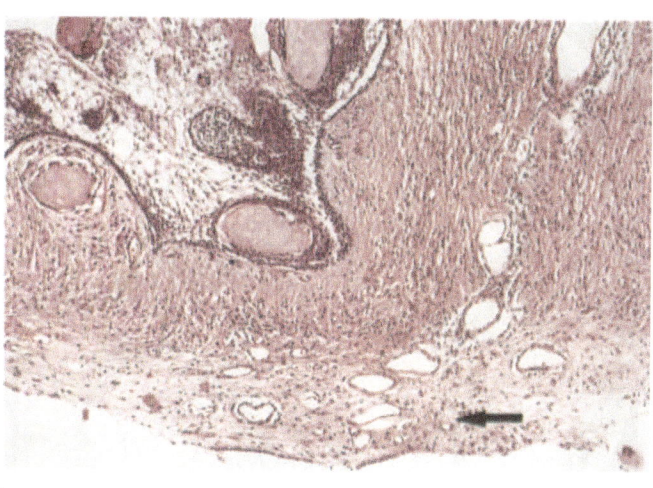

Figure 5.11 Craniopharyngioma, solid/cystic: (a) CT, (b) CT + C, (c) HE × 100; images show intraventricular solid/cystic mass; solid component of the tumour is brain hyperdense, non-enhancing. Enhancing cyst wall consists of focally mineralized adamantinomatous and dense adjacent gliovascular tissue (c). Subependymal parenchyma is also vascularized (c, arrow)

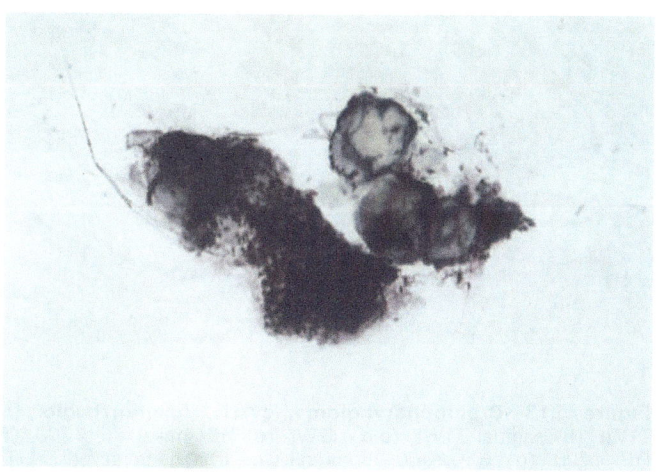

Figure 5.12 Craniopharyngioma: smear illustrating characteristic nodular keratin. Tol blue × 100

smears with difficulty (Figure 5.17) on account of its fibrous nature (Figure 5.20). Adenoma cells are round–oval, with some variation in size, with prominent nucleoli and crisp plasmalemmae which are liable to disruption of cytoplasm during the smear preparation (Figure 1.19).

5.3b. Macroadenoma

Although, by definition, a macroadenoma needs only to exceed the bounds of the sella, endocrine silence (or patient ignorance) often ensures gross enlargement until optic pathway deformity declares itself. Prior to this, haemorrhagic infarction is the presenting mechanism of macroadenomas. Neoplasms which displace the roof of the suprasellar cistern, often referred to as giant adenomas, have no adjacent adenohypophysis for comparison and are described as being approximately grey matter isointense at short TR (Figure 5.21), and diffusely hyperintense at long TR. T1 signal prolongation (Figure 5.25) is most easily explained in terms of cyst formation (Figure 5.23), but more subtle inhomogeneities are probably due to ischeamia and haemorrhage (Figure 5.24). T2 hyperintensity must reflect a plentiful, non-fibrillar cytosol, as is the case in chordoma.

Solid macroadenomas display rapid, moderate-to-strong enhancement (Figure 5.24) on both CT and MR, compared with intrasellar tumours (see above), a paradox since their morphology is not significantly different, and one which is emphasized by the fact that all large tumours behave this way, even when cystic degeneration leaves little stroma intact (Figures 5.22 and 5.25).

As used by an earlier generation of neurosurgeons[19], the term 'invasive adenoma' described the macroscopic appearance of lobulated tumour tissue growing up from the sella dura, sometimes penetrating this structure at more than one point (Figure 5.26). CT and MR have further defined invasion of neighbouring structures including the sphenoid sinus, nasopharynx (Figure 5.27) and cavernous sinus, and although there is no useful correlation between these growths and their cytological features[20], a possible functional relationship may exist, with prolactinomas exhibiting the highest incidence of invasion[21]. Macroadenoma encapsulation is probably meningeal-derived, since it is almost completely absent from the intraparenchymal component of the lesion (Figures 5.24 and 5.28).

5.3c. Hypophysitis

Though rare, autoimmune inflammatory expansion of the pituitary may mimic an adenoma in every way, including visual disturbance, CT and MR appearance[22], recent pregnancy being the most important clinical association. Histologically, clusters of parenchymal cells are widely separated by hordes of mature lymphocytes, the lesion being a pseudotumour. Non-infectious, non-caseating giant-cell granulomatous inflammation may be expected to have similar effects[23].

5.4. OTHER LESIONS

The systematic and exhaustive approach of Zimmerman[2] to lesions in and around the sella proves the variety of conditions which can affect the region, and for which a checklist is useful. Uncommon masses whose correlative features are presented elsewhere in this text, include meningioma[24] (Figure 5.29 and section 3.4a), chordoma

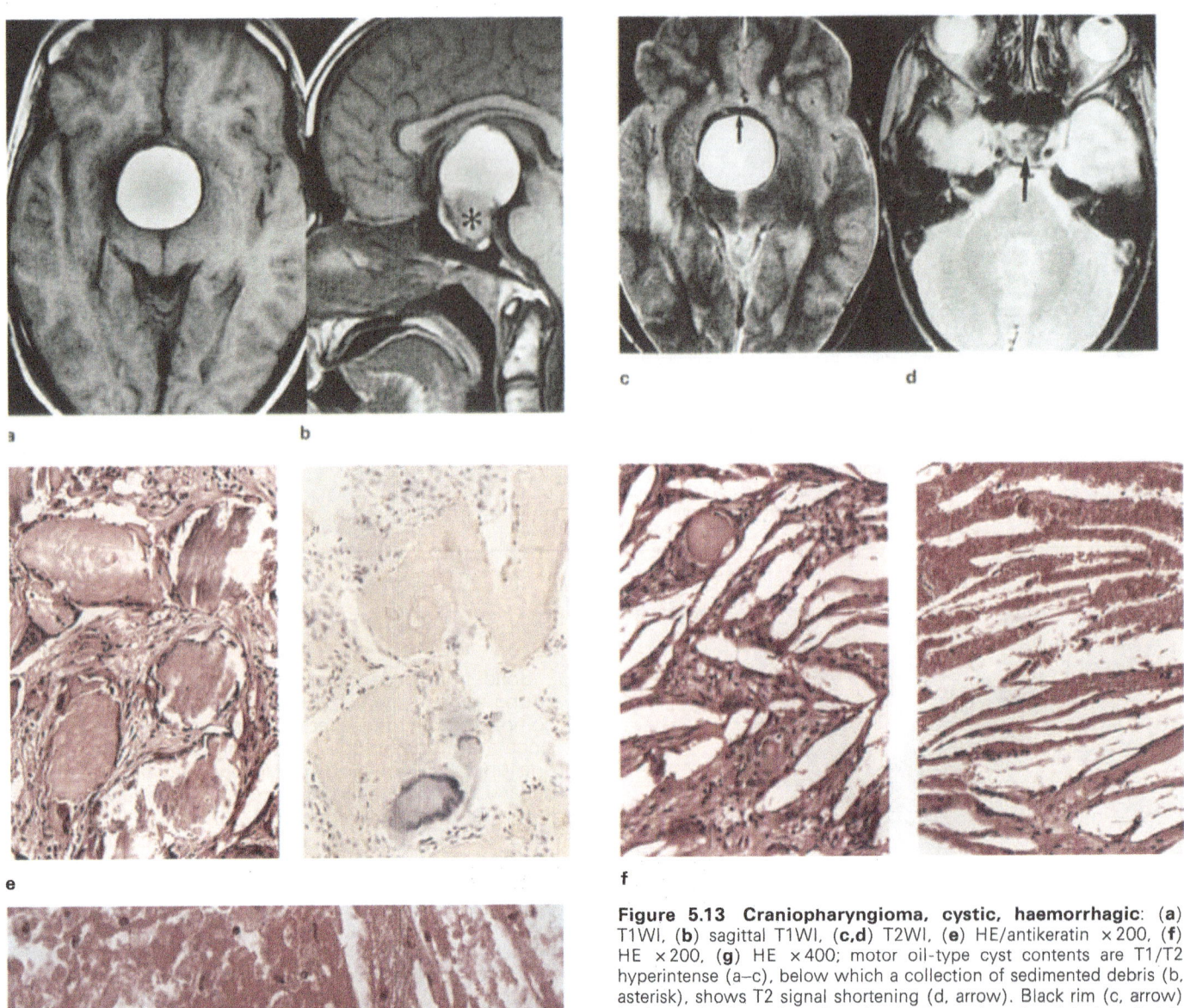

Figure 5.13 Craniopharyngioma, cystic, haemorrhagic: (**a**) T1WI, (**b**) sagittal T1WI, (**c,d**) T2WI, (**e**) HE/antikeratin ×200, (**f**) HE ×200, (**g**) HE ×400; motor oil-type cyst contents are T1/T2 hyperintense (a–c), below which a collection of sedimented debris (b, asterisk), shows T2 signal shortening (d, arrow). Black rim (c, arrow) is chemical shift artefact. Granular debris consists of nodular keratin (e), cholesterol crystals (f), blood and haemosiderophages (g). (Cholesterol concentration was 11.03 mmol/l – compare with **Figures 5.10** and **2.13**)

(Figure 5.30 and section 2.6f), germinoma (Figure 5.31), granuloma (section 3.2) and parasites (section 3.3). Resectable vascular masses such as cavernous haemangioma[25] (Figure 5.32) are possibly of increasing interest to the pathologist.

Despite not being amenable to complete resection, gliomas of the chiasm region (Figure 5.33) are usually subject to tissue diagnosis on account of histological and biological variability, non-specific imaging features and differing management schedules[26]. Pilocytic astrocytoma (sections 4.6f and 6.6a), may also involve or arise from the adjacent hypothalamus (Figure 5.34) and optic nerve (Figure 5.35). Although these have similar cytological characteristics, the former diffusely infiltrates the optic nerve, preserving its septation, whilst the latter is soft and gelatinous, containing sparse reticulin and therefore effectively reduced by aspiration (Figure 5.34). In older individuals, tumours of the optic nerve conform to anaplastic or malignant astrocytomas, diffusely infiltrating and appropriately non- or inhomogeneously enhancing (section 4.6c).

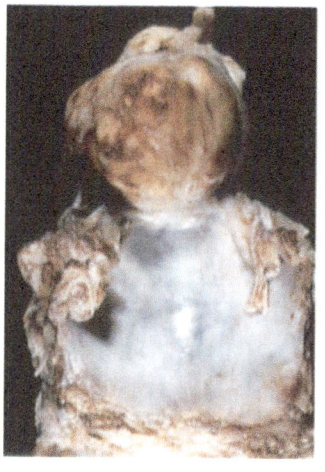
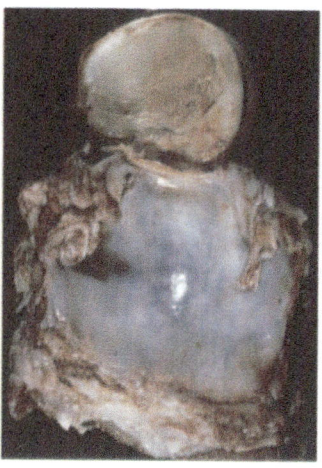

a

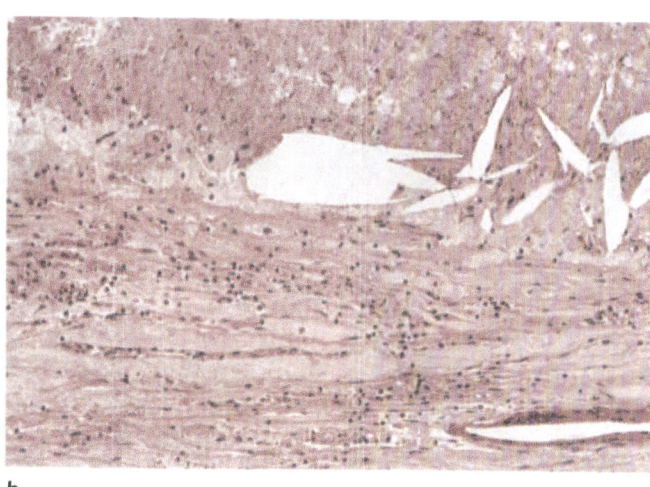

b

Figure 5.14 Craniopharyngioma: (**a**) fixed specimen, (**b**) HE × 200; fixed specimen shows clivus with suprasellar mass having a xanthomatous exterior and homogeneous inspissated contents, shown histologically (b) to consist of macrophages and cholesterol crystals. Epithelium of cyst lining could not be characterized but nodular keratin was present

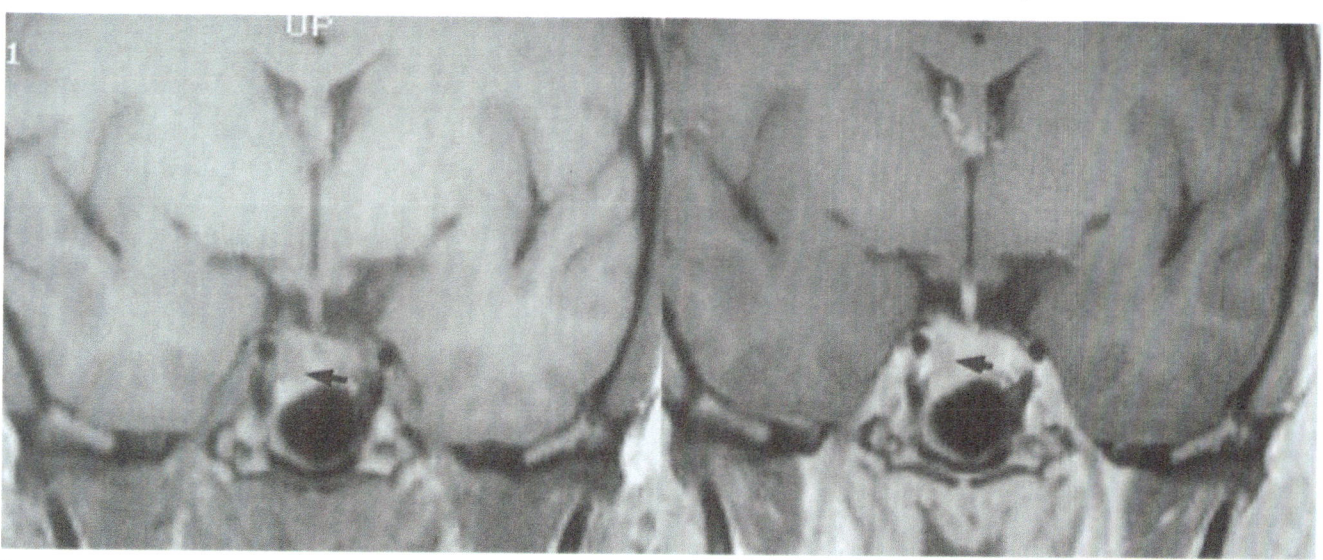

a

b

Figure 5.15 Microadenoma: female, 24 years; amenorrhoea/galac-torrhoea syndrome; (**a**) T1WI, (**b**) T1WI + C; expansion of right lobe of pituitary with focal hypointensity (arrows) is apparent before and after contrast. Lesion was not biopsied

Hamartomatous masses associated with endocrine disturbance, which project into the suprasellar space, have been excised with clinical improvement[27]. The profile of these small lesions is often characteristic (Figures 5.36 and 5.37), although grosser examples may fill the cistern[28]. As might be expected, the signal from hamartomatous tissue is generally T1 grey-matter isointense, but more importantly, also proton-density isointense[29], a point of differentiation from glioma; T2 hyperintensity could represent paucity of cells and myelin relative to normal brain (Figure 5.36). Operative specimens should always be fixed for light and electron microscopy.

REFERENCES

1. Osborn AG. MRI of the sellar/juxtasellar region. Part 1: intrasellar and suprasellar masses. MRI Decisions. 1990;4:21–30.

2. Zimmerman RA. Imaging of intrasellar, suprasellar and parasellar tumors. Semin Roentgenol. 1990;25:174–97.

3. Tampieri D, Melanson D, Ethier R. MR imaging of epidermoid cysts. AJNR. 1989;10:351–6.

4. Gentry LR, Smoker WR, Turski PA *et al.* Suprasellar arachnoid cysts. 1. CT recognition. AJNR. 1986;7:79–86.

5. Krawchenko J, Collins C. Pathology of an arachnoid cyst. J Neurosurg. 1979;50:224–8.

6. Shuangshoti S, Netsky MG, Nashold BS. Epithelial cysts related to sella turcica. Arch Pathol. 1970;90:444–50.

7. Yoshida J, Kobayashi T, Kageyama N *et al.* Symptomatic Rathke's cleft cyst: morphologic study with light and electron microscopy and tissue culture. J Neurosurg. 1977;47:451–8.

8. Kucharczyk W, Peck WW, Kelly WM *et al.* Rathke cleft cysts: CT, MR imaging and pathologic features. Radiology. 1987;165:491–5.

9. Burger PC, Scheithauer BW, Vogel FS. Surgical pathology of the nervous system and its coverings, 3rd edn. New York: Churchill Livingstone; 1991:546.

10. Pusey E, Kortman KE, Flannigan BD *et al.* MR of craniopharyngioma: tumor delineation and characterisation. AJNR. 1987;8:439–44.

11. Petito CK, DeGirolami U, Earle KM. Craniopharyngiomas: a clinical and pathological review. Cancer. 1976;37:1944–52.

12. Burger PC, Scheithauer BW, Vogel FS. Surgical pathology of the nervous system and its coverings, 3rd edn. New York: Churchill Livingstone; 1991:540.

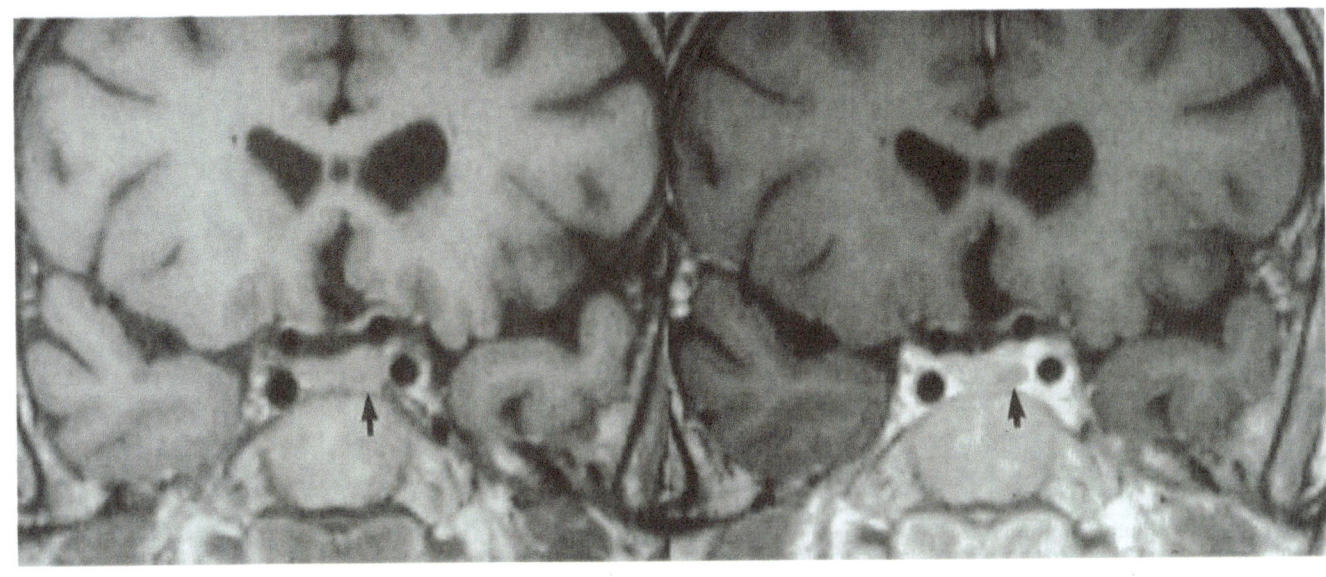

a   b

Figure 5.16   Microadenoma: male, 44 years; impotence and prolac-tinaemia; **(a)** T1WI, **(b)** T1WI + C; asymmetric expansion (a, arrow) of the pituitary with focal hypointensity that becomes apparent only after contrast (b, arrow). Lesion was not biopsied; responded to medical treatment. (Compare with **Figure 5.15**)

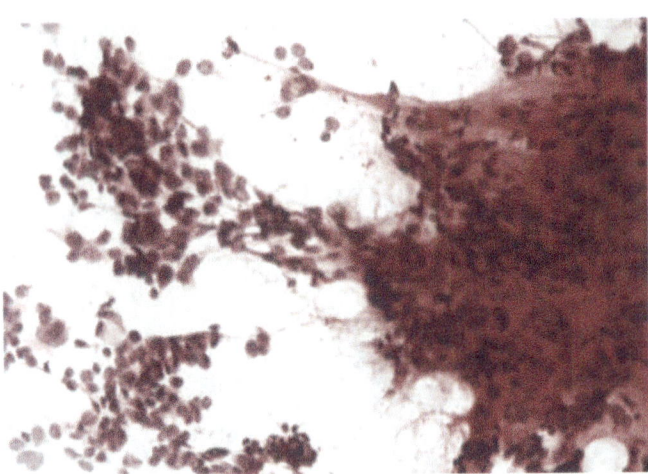

Figure 5.17   Microadenoma: illustrating dispersed tumour cells (left) and dense tissue of normal gland. HE × 400

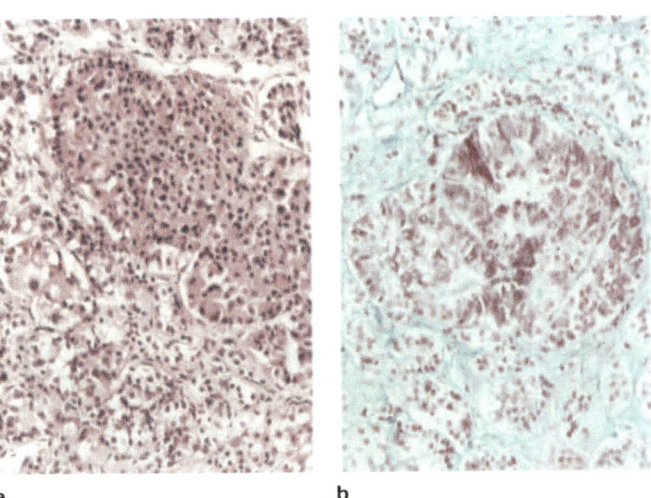

a   b

Figure 5.18   Microadenoma, Cushing's: **(a)** HE × 200, **(b)** OFG × 200; biopsy tissue shows a lobule of cells lacking normal stromal architecture (a), exhibiting PAS positivity (b)

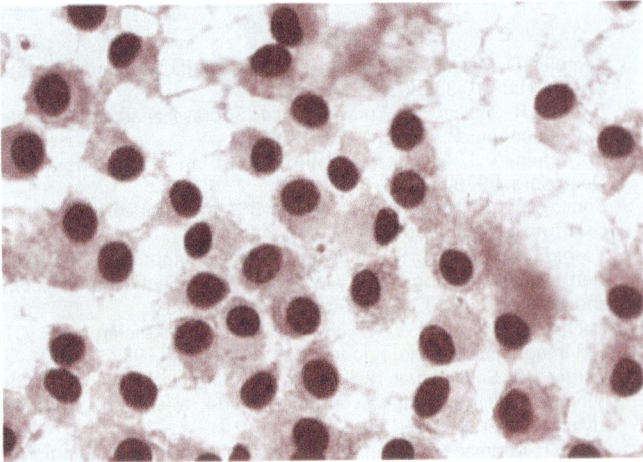

Figure 5.19   Macroadenoma: smear preparation illustrating even spread of adenoma cells; compare with **Figure 5.17**. HE × 400

13. Ahmadi J, Estian S, Apuzzo MLJ *et al*. Cystic fluid in craniopharyn-giomas: MR imaging and quantitative analysis. Radiology. 1992;182:783–5.

14. Hardy J. Transsphenoidal microsurgery of the normal and pathologic pituitary. Clin Neurosurg. 1969;16:185–217.

15. Kucharczyk W, Montanera WJ. The sella and parasellar region. In: Atlas SW, ed. Magnetic resonance imaging of the brain and spine. New York: Raven Press; 1991:625–67.

16. Huk WJ, Heindel W. Intracranial tumors: tumors of the pituitary. In: Huk WJ, Gademann G, Friedmann, eds. GMRI of central nervous system diseases. Berlin: Springer-Verlag; 1990:257–70.

17. Halmi NS, Duello T. 'Acidophil' pituitary tumors. A reappraisal with differential staining and immunocytochemical techniques. Arch Pathol Lab Med. 1976;100:346–51.

18. Newton D, Dillon W, Norman D *et al*. Gd-DTPA-enhanced imaging of pituitary adenomas. AJNR. 1989;10:949–54.

19. Jefferson G. Extrasellar extensions of pituitary adenoma. In: Selected papers. London: Pitman Medical; 1960:374–402.

20. Scheithauer BW. Surgical pathology of the pituitary: the adenomas. Pathol Annu. 1984;19(part II):267–329.

21. Scheithauer BW, Kovacs K, Laws ER *et al*. Pathology of invasive pituitary tumors with special reference to functional classification. J Neurosurg. 1986;65:733–44.

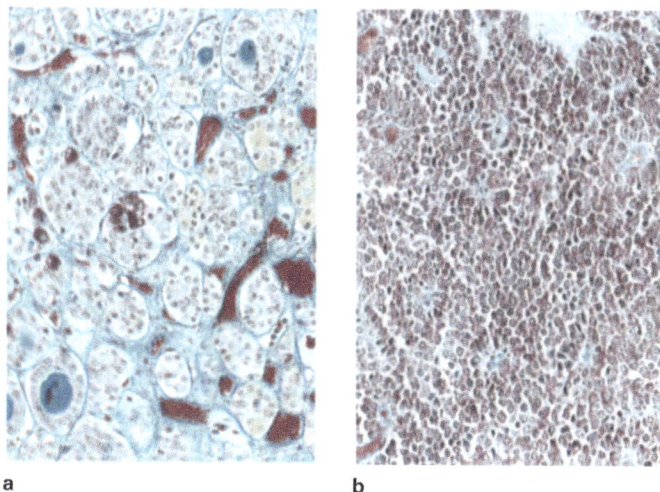

a   b

Figure 5.20 Macroadenoma, Cushing's: comparative sections from normal (**a**) and adenoma (**b**) illustrating complete loss of acinar architecture and sinusoidal blood vessels. OFG ×200

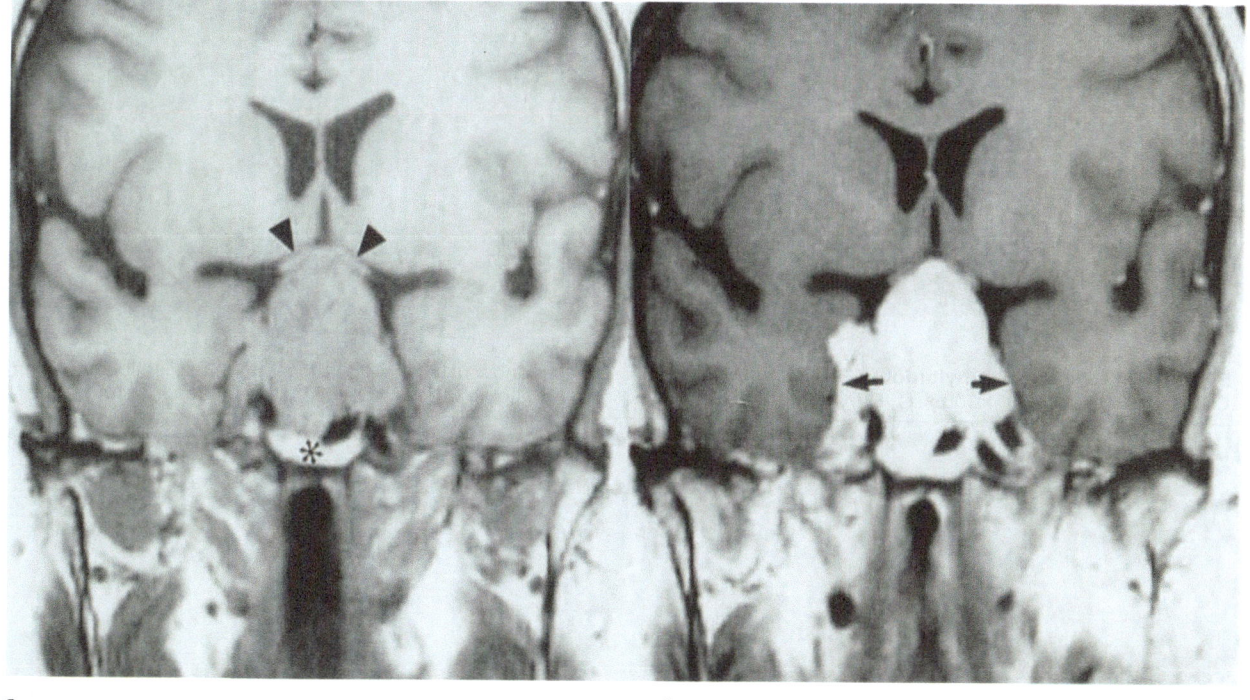

a   b

Figure 5.21 Macroadenoma with invasion: (**a**) T1WI, (**b**) T1WI + C; images show characteristic homogeneous brain isointensity and diffuse enhancement. Tumour has displaced the optic chiasm superiorly (a, arrow-heads) and also shows cavernous sinus invasion (b, arrows). Hyperintense structure inferiorly is sphenoid marrow (a, asterisk)

22. Levine SN, Benzel EC, Fowler MR *et al.* Lymphocytic hypophysitis: clinical, radiological and magnetic resonance imaging characterisation. Neurosurgery. 1988;22:937–41.
23. Talon CT, Duff TA. Giant cell granuloma involving the pituitary gland. J Neurosurg. 1980;50:584–7.
24. Castillo M, David PC, Ross WM *et al.* Meningioma of the optic nerves and chiasm. JCAT. 1989;13:679.
25. Tien R, Dillon WP. MR imaging of cavernous hemangioma of the optic chiasm. JCAT. 1989;13:1087–100.
26. Flickenger JC, Torres C, Deutsch M. Management of low grade gliomas of the optic nerve and chiasm. Cancer. 1988;61:635–42.
27. Benningfield SJ, Bonnici F, Cremin BJ. Magnetic resonance imaging of hypothalamic hamartomas. Br J Radiol. 1988;61:1177–80.
28. Hubbard AM, Egelhof JC. MR imaging of large hypothalamic hamartomas in two infants. AJNR. 1989;10:1277–8.
29. Boyko OB, Curnes JC, Oaks W. Hamartoma of the tuber cinereum: CT, MR and pathologic findings. AJNR. 1991;12:309–14.

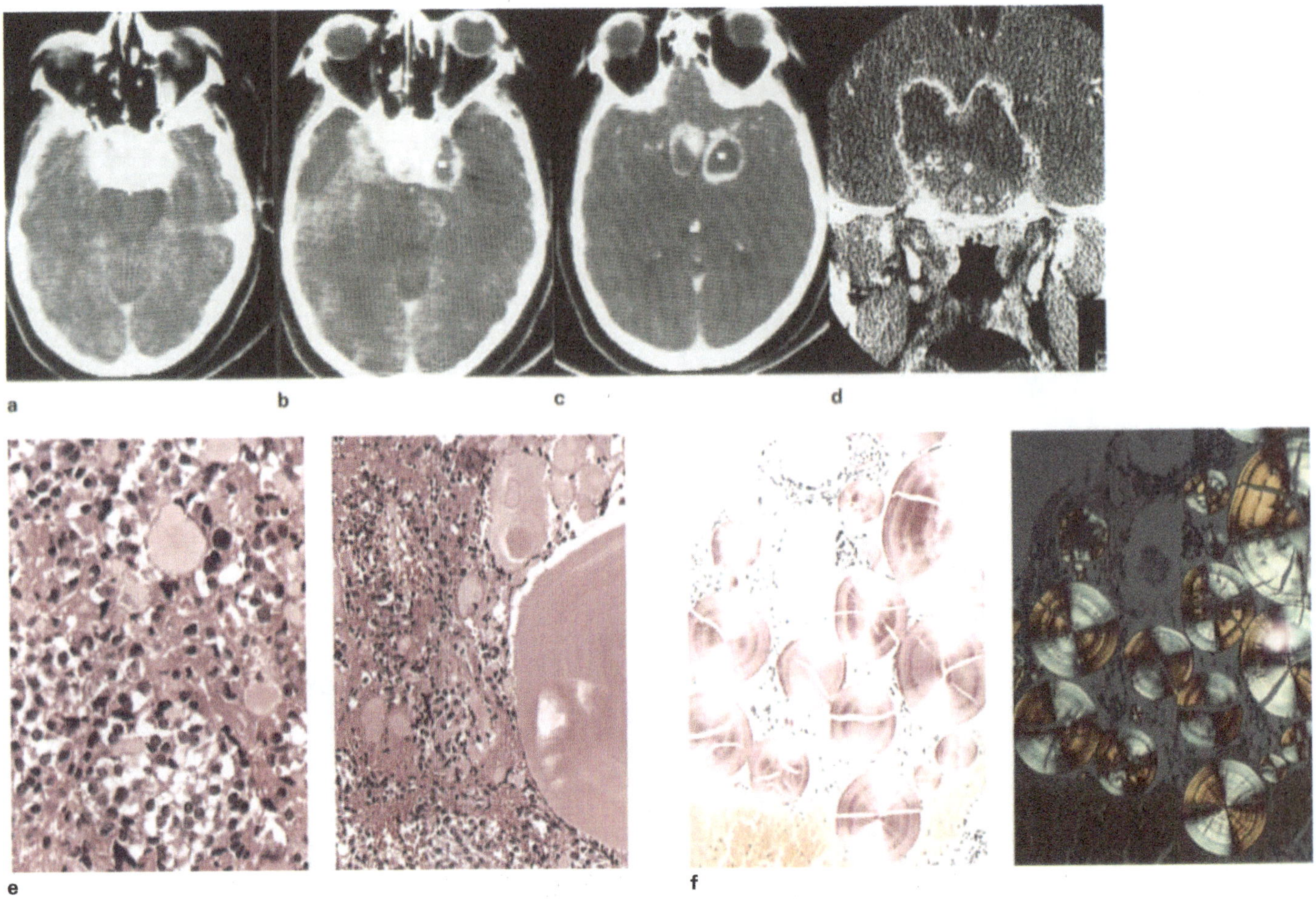

a   b   c   d

e

f

Figure 5.22 Giant adenoma, amyloidoma: (**a–c**) CT + C, (**d**) coronal CT + C, (**e**) HE ×200/×100, (**f**) CR/polarized CR ×40; images show mainly cystic lesion with unusual bilobed upward extension. Histology shows abundant amyloid deposition (e,f)

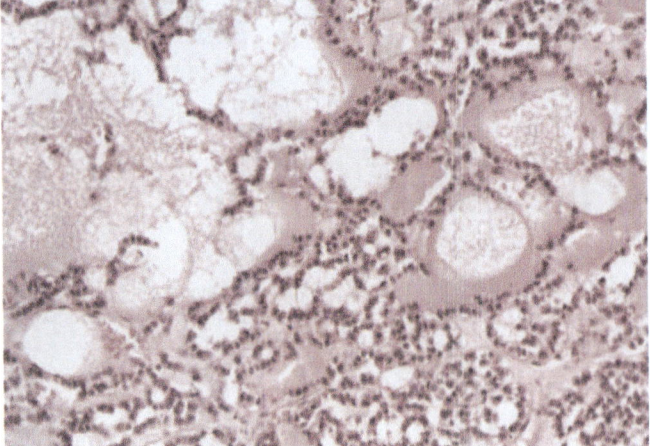

Figure 5.23 Adenoma, pituitary: illustrating cystic degeneration (see **Figure 5.25**); proteinaceous fluid is likely to induce T1 signal shortening relative to CSF. HE ×200

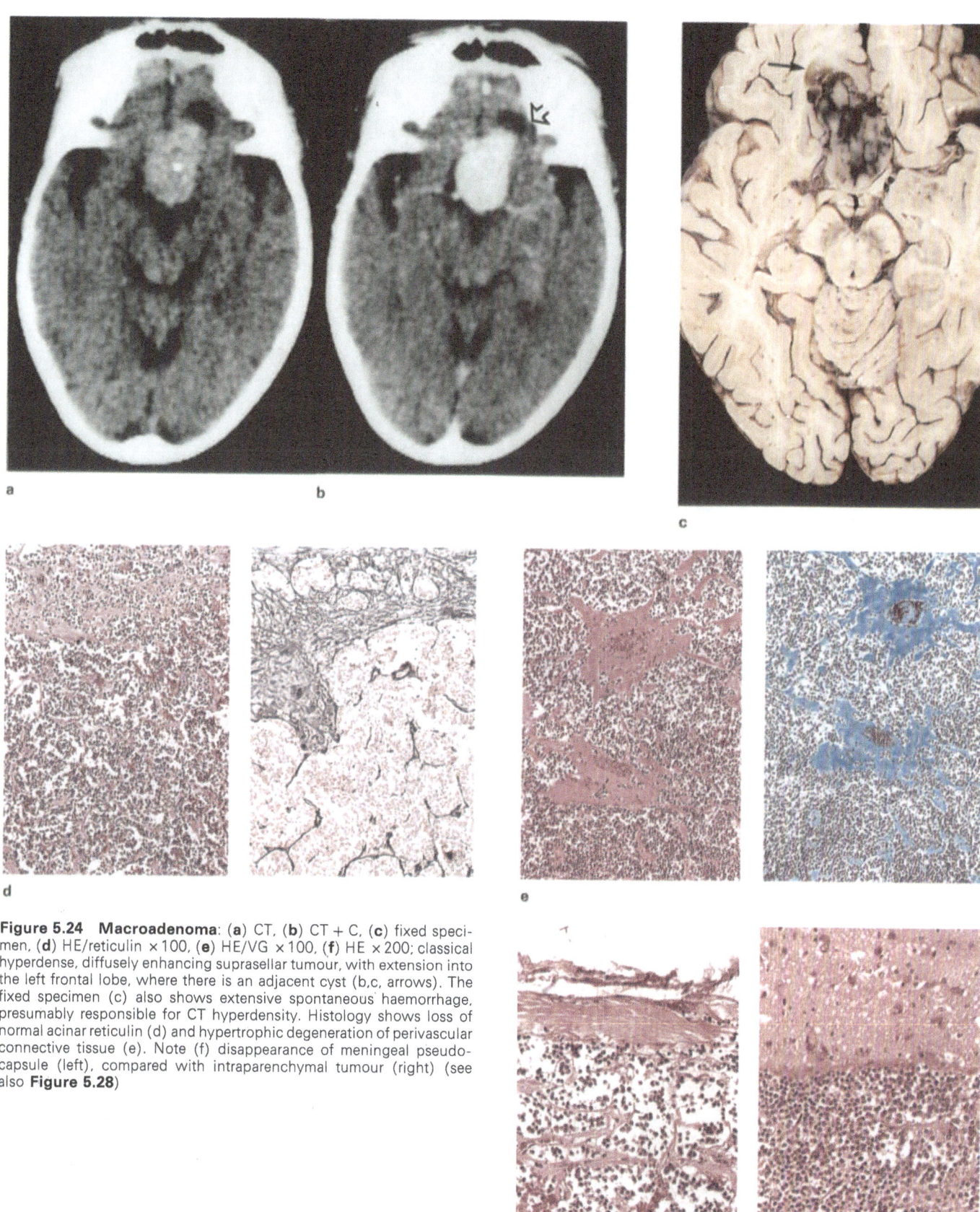

Figure 5.24 Macroadenoma: (**a**) CT, (**b**) CT + C, (**c**) fixed specimen, (**d**) HE/reticulin ×100, (**e**) HE/VG ×100, (**f**) HE ×200; classical hyperdense, diffusely enhancing suprasellar tumour, with extension into the left frontal lobe, where there is an adjacent cyst (b,c, arrows). The fixed specimen (c) also shows extensive spontaneous haemorrhage, presumably responsible for CT hyperdensity. Histology shows loss of normal acinar reticulin (d) and hypertrophic degeneration of perivascular connective tissue (e). Note (f) disappearance of meningeal pseudo-capsule (left), compared with intraparenchymal tumour (right) (see also **Figure 5.28**)

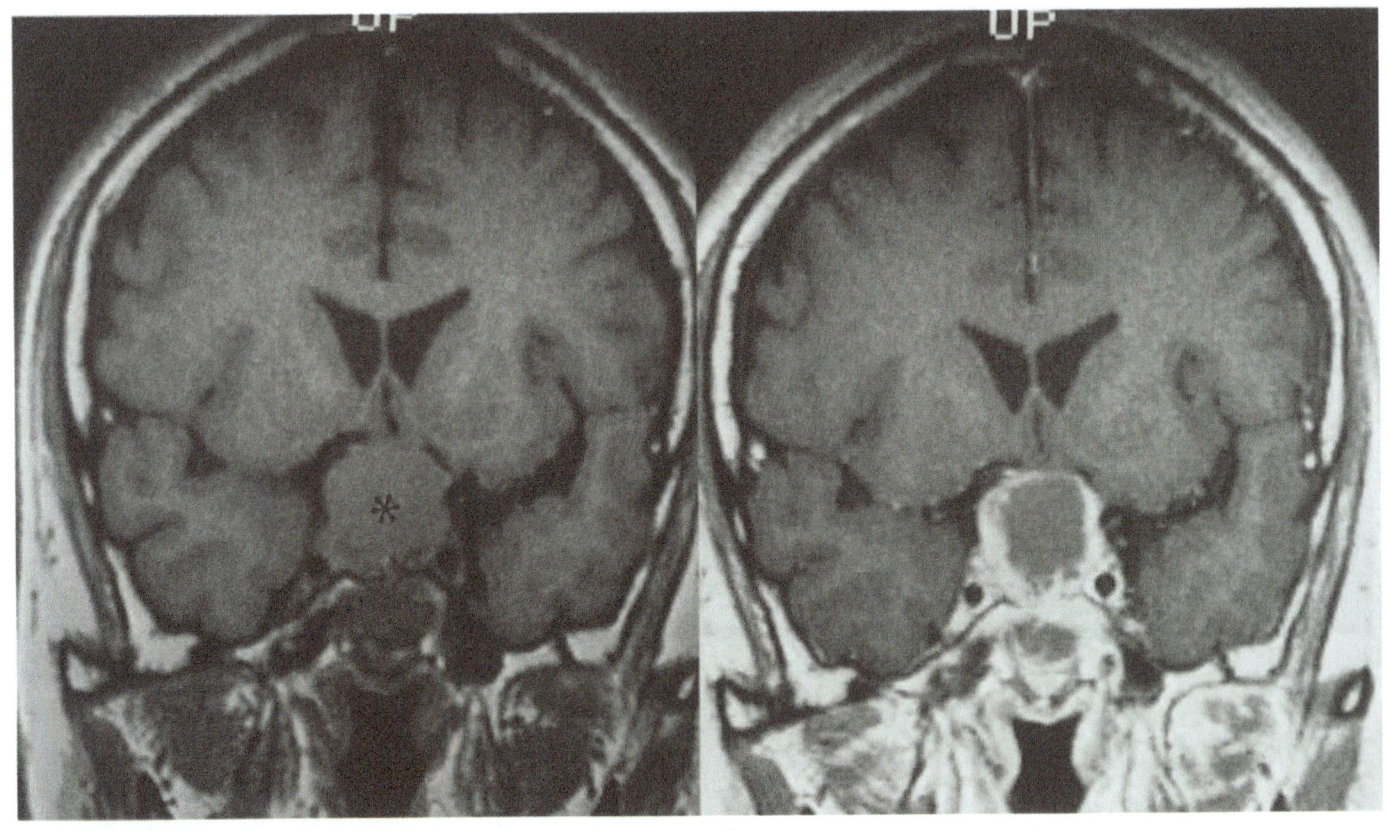

a

b

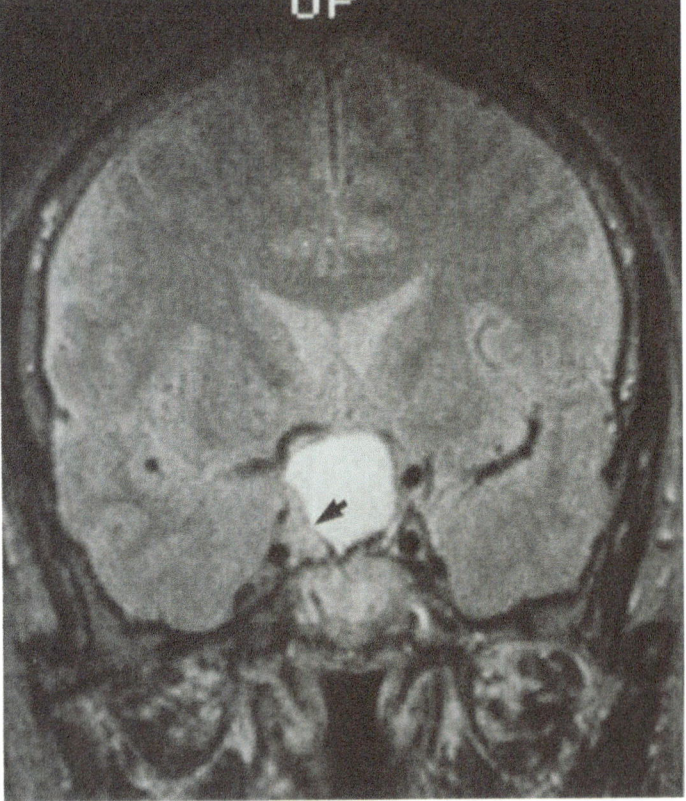

c

Figure 5.25   Macroadenoma, cystic: (**a**) T1WI, (**b**) T1WI + C, (**c**) T2WI; images illustrate uniform T1 brain/adenoma isointensity of cyst fluid before contrast (a, asterisk), and T2 hyperintensity (c), presumably due to protein content. Enhancement (b) and T2 cortex isointensity (c, arrows), of residual cystic tumour is characteristic

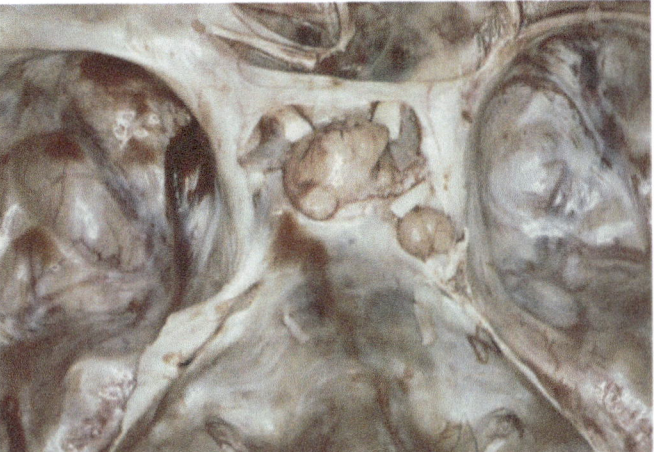

Figure 5.26   Macroadenoma, invasive: autopsy view of sella showing independent penetration of diaphragm and dura by adenoma

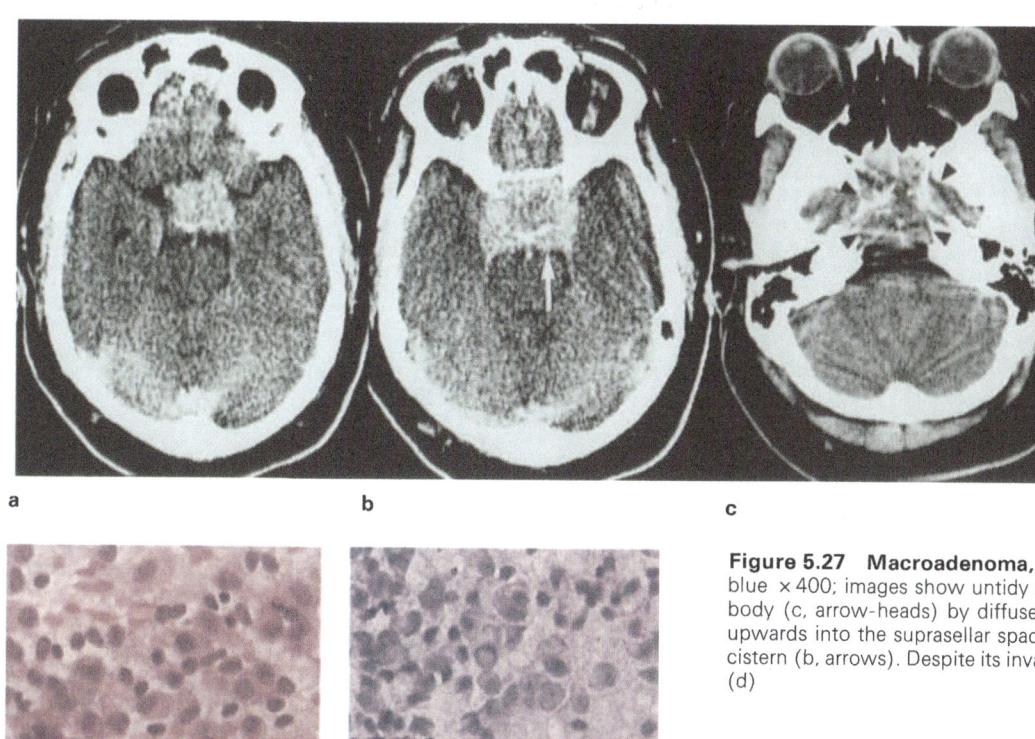

a   b   c

d

Figure 5.27 Macroadenoma, invasive: (**a–c**) CT + C, (**d**) HE/Tol blue × 400; images show untidy destruction of the sella and sphenoid body (c, arrow-heads) by diffusely enhancing tumour, which extends upwards into the suprasellar space and posteriorly into the prepontine cistern (b, arrows). Despite its invasive nature, cytology is unremarkable (d)

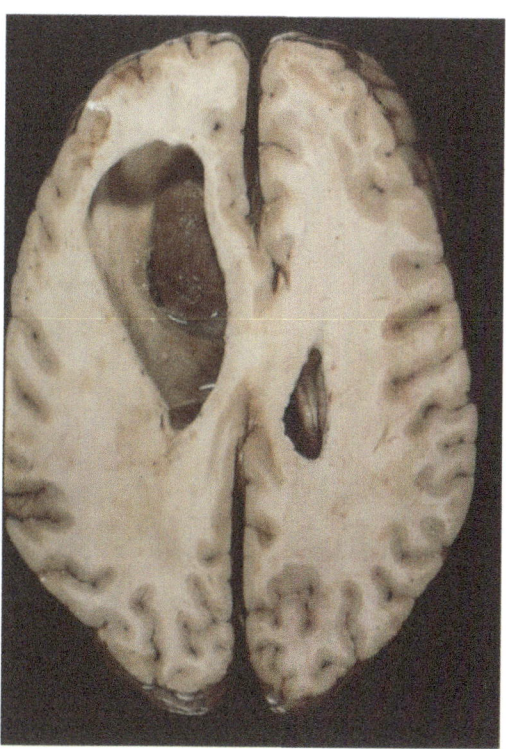

Figure 5.28 Giant adenoma, intraventricular: fixed brain specimen shows unencapsulated tumour projecting into the ventricle and partly covered by ependyma

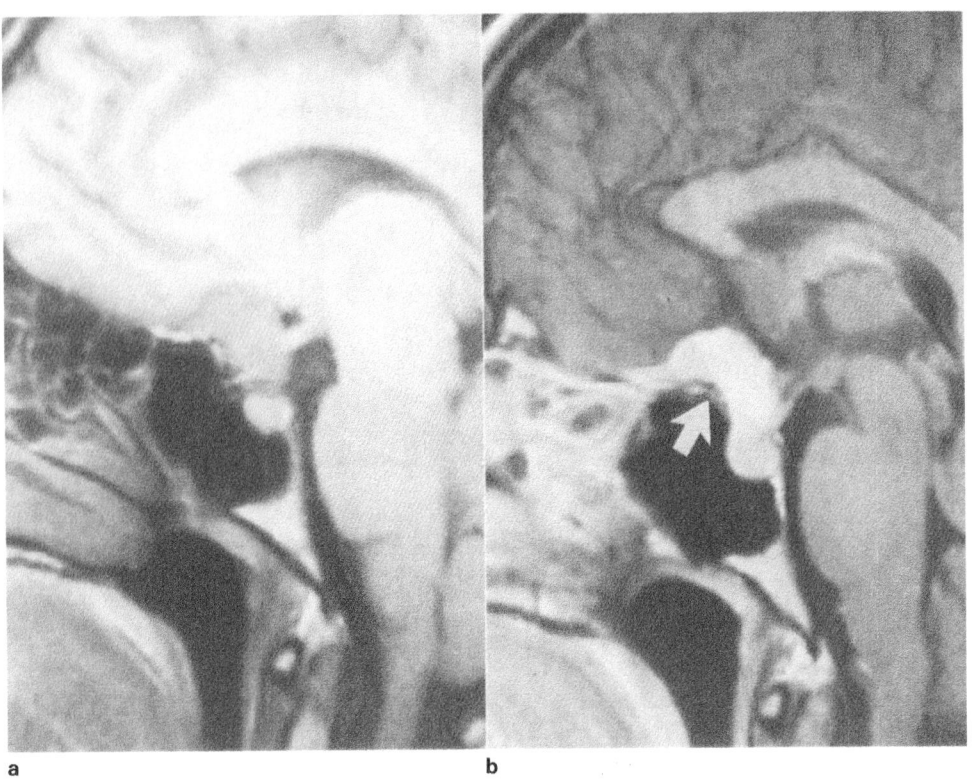

a   b

Figure 5.29   Meningioma, jugum: (**a**) T1WI, (**b**) T1WI + C; images show a cortex isointense diffusely enhancing mass lying above the sella and extending anteriorly over the jugum which is hyperostotic (arrow). Note distinct signal difference from hypophysis before and after contrast

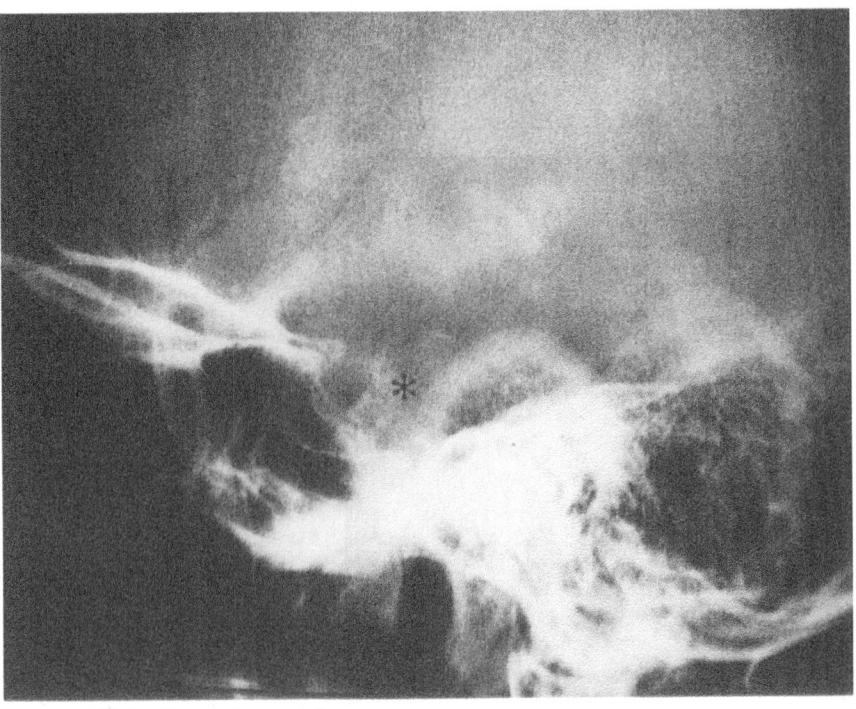

Figure 5.30(a)   (*legend opposite*)

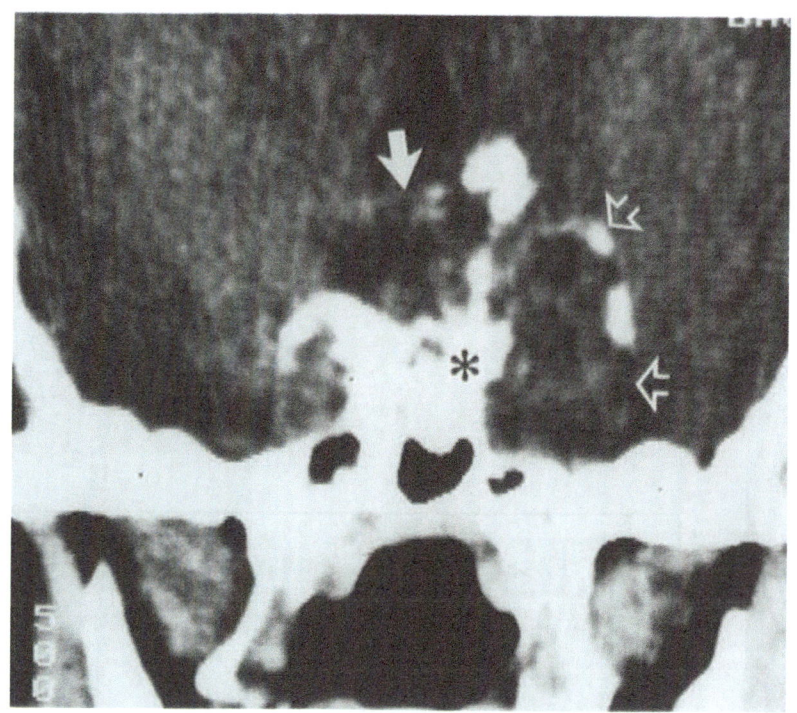

b

Figure 5.30   Chordoma, supra- and juxtasellar: (a) skull x-ray, (b) coronal CT, (c) CT + C, (d) HE/Tol blue ×400, (e) HE ×200; partially mineralized tumour erodes dorsum sellae (a,b, asterisks), extends into cavernous sinus/temporal lobe (b, open arrows), suprasellar space and 3rd ventricle (b, closed arrow). The lesion is inhomogeneous, weakly enhancing (c). Cytology is characteristic (e); histology confirms ossification (f). Case illustrates supra- and juxtasellar extension of a predominantly clival tumour, which is unlike craniopharyngioma. (Compare this lesion with the erosive adenoma illustrated in **Figure 5.27**)

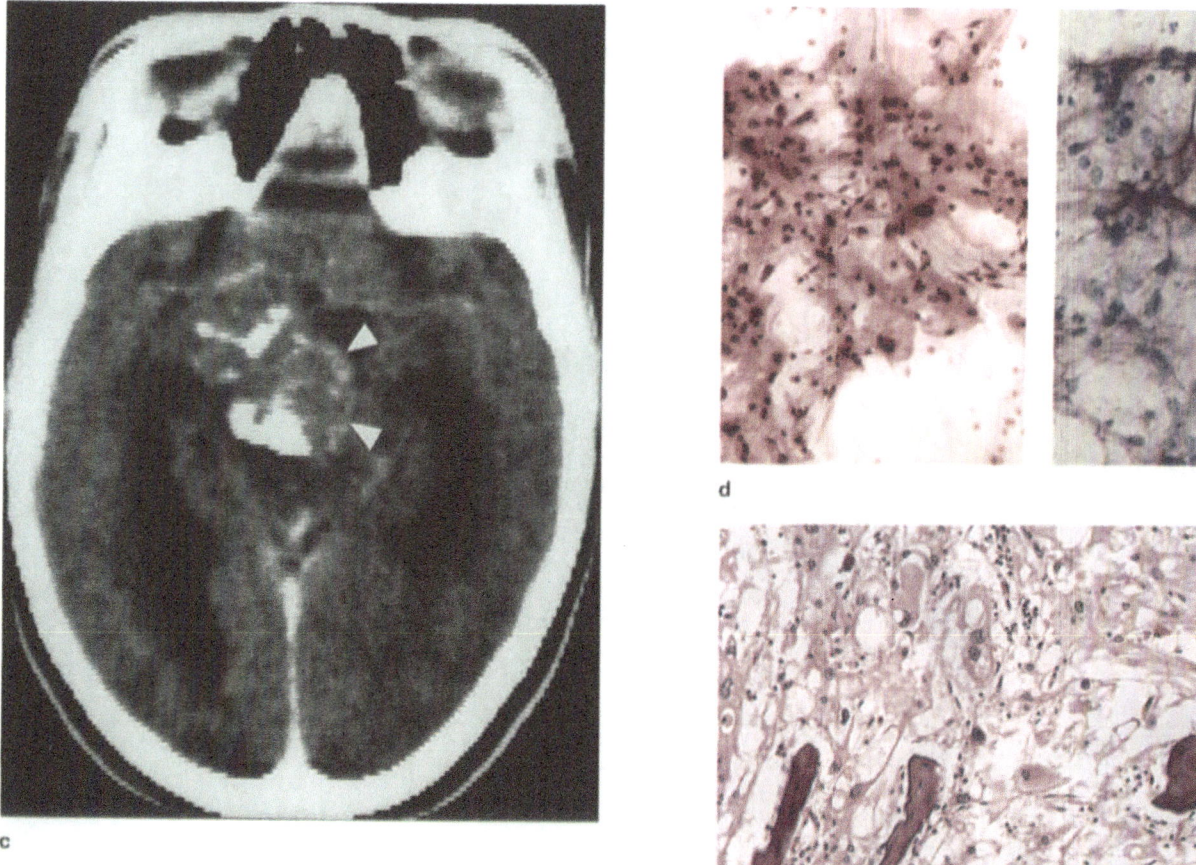

c

d

e

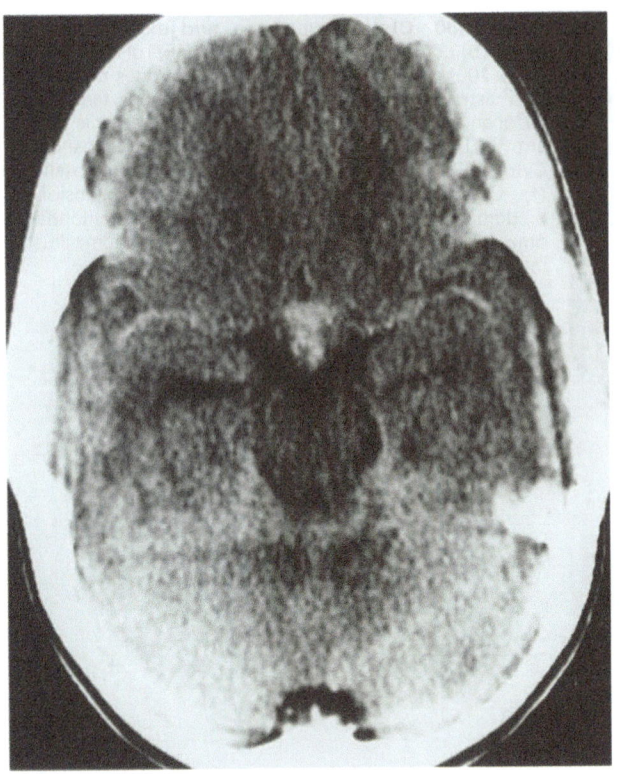

a

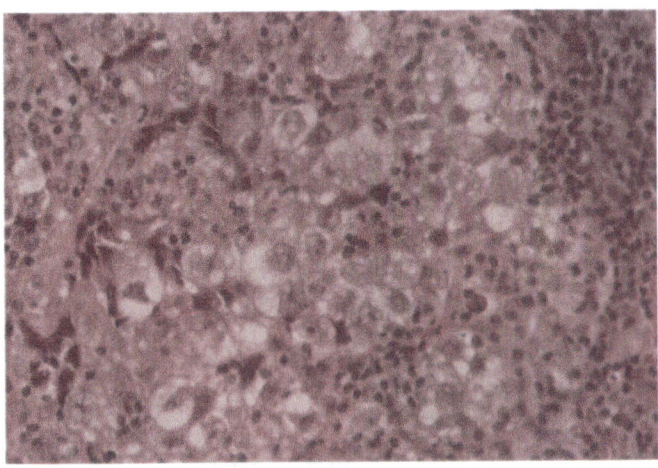

b

Figure 5.31 Germinoma, hypothalamus/infundibulum: (a) CT + C, (b) HE × 400; image shows ill-defined central enhancing mass obliterating the inferior part of the 3rd ventricle. Expansion of the pituitary stalk was observed at surgery. Histology shows characteristic large vacuolated cells with prominent nucleoli and admixed lymphocytic component

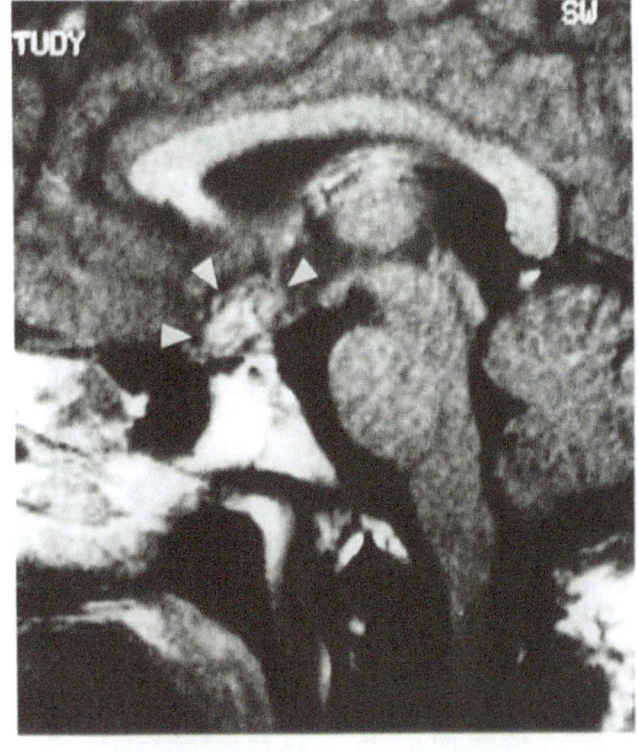

b

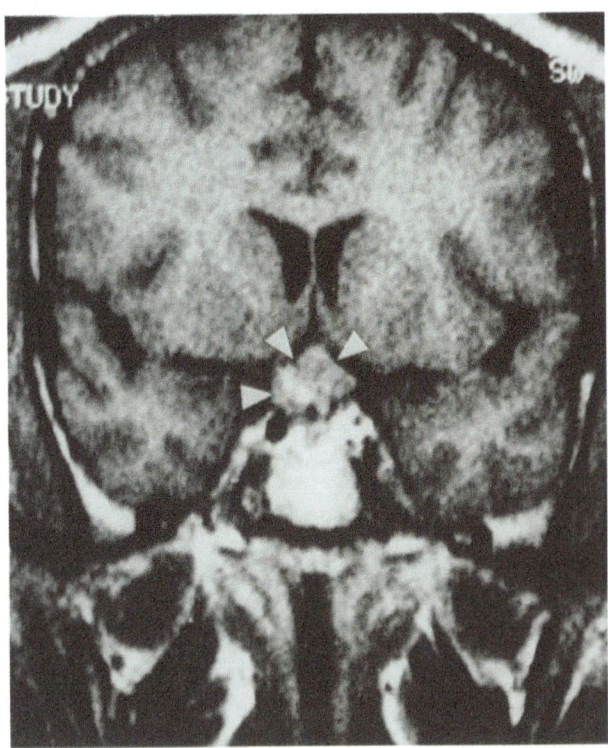

a

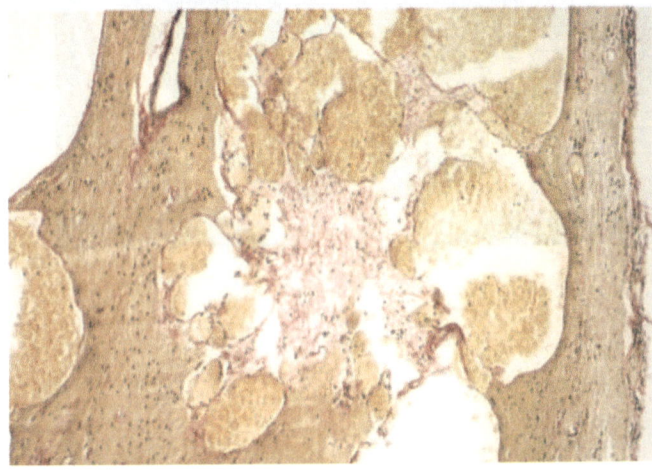

c

Figure 5.32 Angioma, optic nerve: (a) coronal T1WI + C, (b) sagittal T1WI + C, (c) VG × 100; images show T1 inhomogeneous, patchily enhancing suprasellar mass with loss of chiasmatic detail (arrows). Histology shows numerous dilated vascular spaces with gliotic intervening neural tissue and focal collagen proliferation

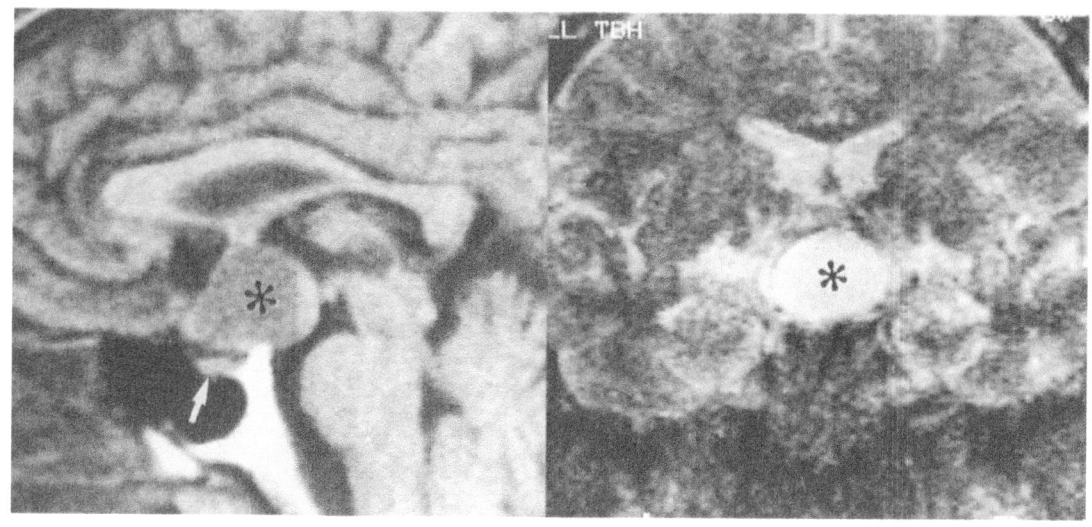

a   b

Figure 5.33 Optic chiasm glioma: (**a**) sagittal T1WI, (**b**) coronal T2WI; images show a suprasellar mass (asterisk) which is characteristically homogeneously T1 hypointense/T2 hyperintense. Pituitary (a, arrow) is clearly seen. Mass at surgery was confined to the optic chiasm; this, together with the imaging features, was considered diagnostic of astrocytoma

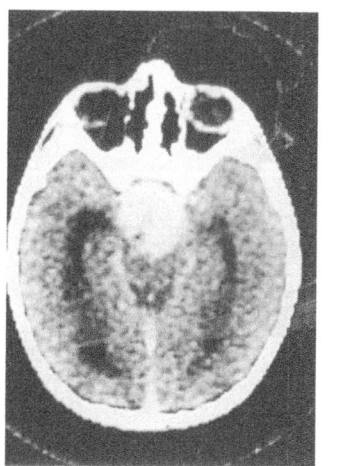
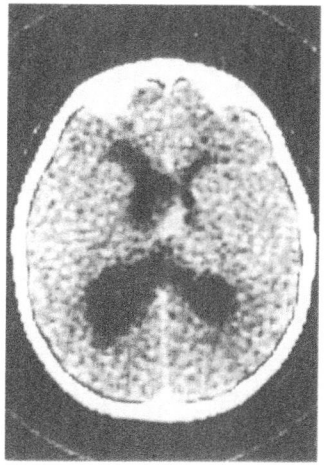

Figure 5.34 Pilocytic astrocytoma, juvenile, hypothalamic/chiasmatic: male, 3 years; first-generation scanner shows a circumscribed diffusely enhancing mass which was considered to be suprasellar; however, age and imaging features make JPA the most likely lesion. Histology was characteristic

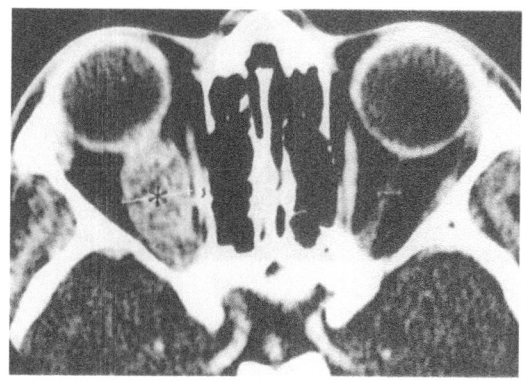

a

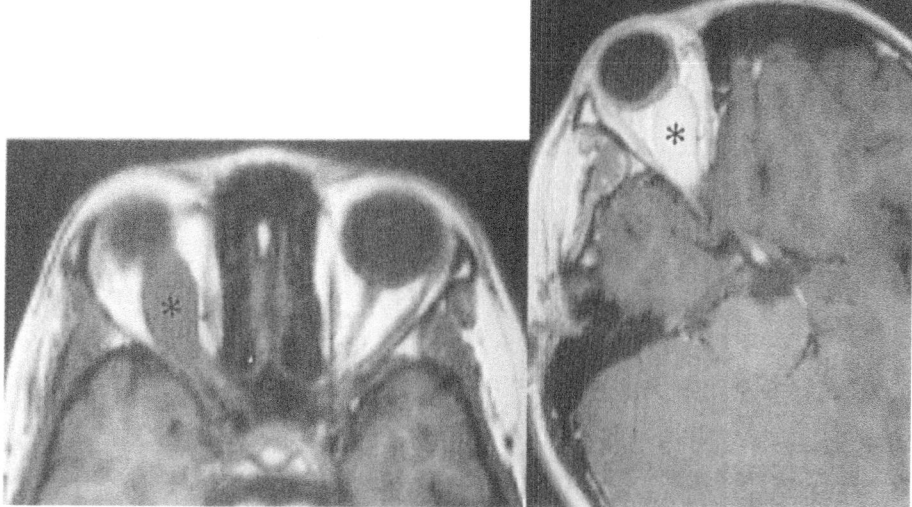

b   c

Figure 5.35 (*legend overleaf*)

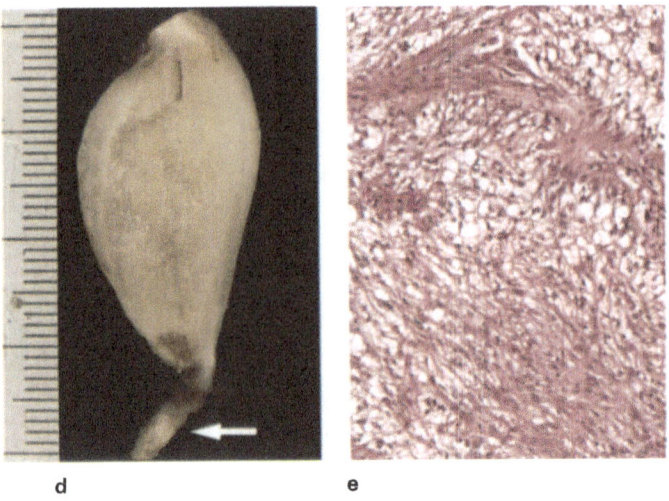

d   e

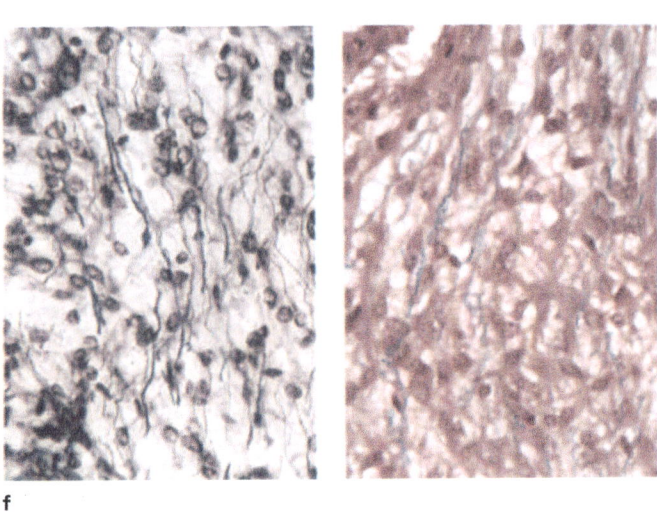

f

Figure 5.35   Optic nerve astrocytoma (glioma): (a) CT + C, **(b)** axial T1WI, **(c)** paraxial T1WI + C, **(d)** surgical specimen, **(e)** HE × 200, **(f)** Holmes LB/HELB × 400; images show homogeneous cortex-isointense expansion of optic nerve (asterisk), diffusely enhancing.

Histology shows characteristic JPA (e) diffusely infiltrating the optic nerve fibres (f). Tumour did not involve intracanalicular portion (d, arrow) of the nerve, which is therefore presumably oedematous

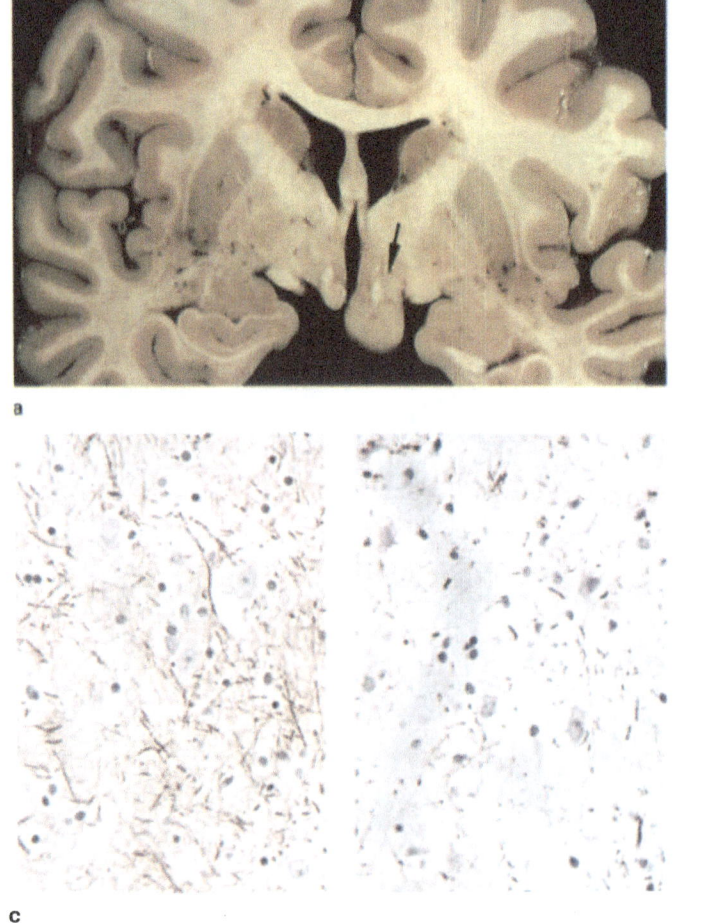

a

c

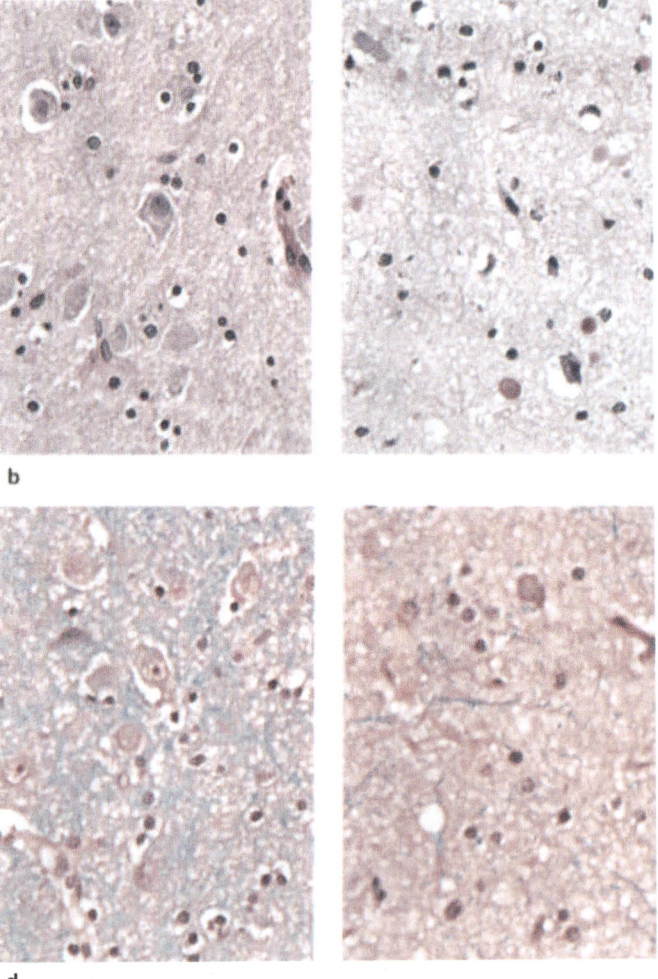

b

d

Figure 5.36   Hamartoma, hypothalamus: **(a)** fixed specimen, **(b)** PAS × 400, **(c)** NF × 400, **(d)** HE/LB × 400; coronal section of brain shows grey-matter mass expanding the mamillary body and

hypothalamus (a, arrow). Sections (b–d) show general paucity of neurones, neuritic processes and myelinated fibres with mild spongiosus (b), which could account for slight signal hyperintensity described at long TR (normal control on left, b–d)

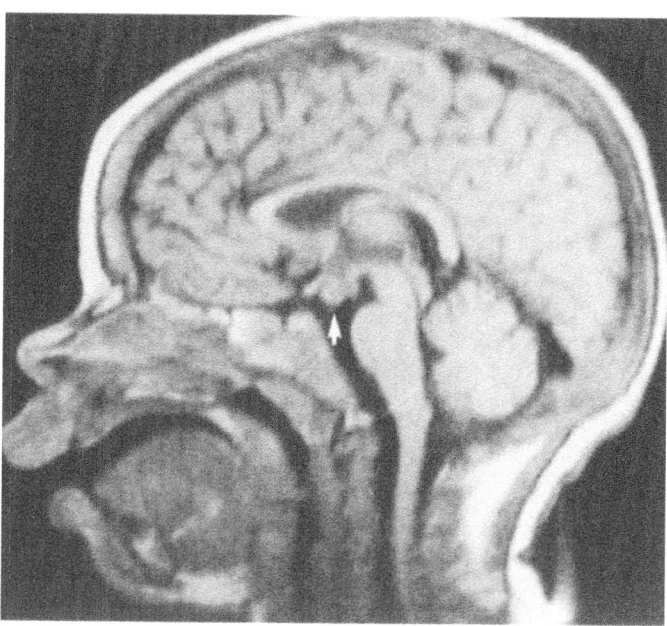

Figure 5.37 Hamartoma, hypothalamus: T1WI shows rounded mass (arrow) projecting downwards between the mamillary bodies and chiasm. Lesion was isointense on all sequences. The correlative pathology of this lesion is illustrated in **Figure 5.36**. (Prof B Cremin, Red Cross Children's Hospital)

Extraparenchymal, meningocerebral, parenchymal and ventricular lesions of the posterior fossa and craniocervical junction

6

6.1. PRIMARY CYSTS

The characterization of *primary or developmental cysts* is discussed in section 3.1. All the main varieties with the exception of colloid cyst have been described in the posterior fossa, and it is worth recalling the histological and immunocytochemical similarities between that entity and the neurenteric cyst. Within the posterior fossa, arachnoid and neurenteric cysts are usually restricted to the subarachnoid space, the former most often within the dorsal cerebellomedullary and quadrigeminal plate cisterns (Figure 6.1), whilst the latter extends with multiple loculations, through the prepontine and cervical subarachnoid space. Intra–extraparenchymal and intraventricular locations are more in favour of neuroepithelial cyst (Figure 6.2). Epidermoidoma (see below), which is also the commonest of the congenital cysts, favours the prepontine–cerebellopontine cistern. Fluid which is T1 hyperintensive relative to CSF suggests protein secretion or keratin. In all these examples, spurious enhancement may be caused by compressed choroid and meninges, and all may be mimicked by cysticercus (Figure 6.8).

6.1a. Neurenteric (enterogenous) cyst

Perimedullary location with caudal extension through the foramen magnum is usual, where loculation may be apparent, particularly with CT myelography (Figure 6.3). Cerebellopontine angle location, and fourth ventricular or intra–extramedullary extension are non-specific variants[1,2]. Consistent with their secretory function, neurenteric cysts display variable density and signal intensity, including T1 hyperintensity/T2 hypointensity[3,4]. The epithelial lining is columnar-cuboidal, mucin and PAS-positive (Figure 6.1), usually heavily ciliated, with interspersed elements having microvilli[5]. Goblet cells are often present, and a collagenous stroma may contain small vascular channels which do not enhance.

6.1b. Epidermoidoma (epidermoid cyst, cholesteatoma) (See also sections 2.4 (skull); 3.1 (supratentorial extraparenchymal); 4.2 (supratentorial parenchymal) and 5.1a (suprasellar).)

The imaging features of the typical cerebellopontine angle and prepontine epidermoidoma are well established in the literature[6,7], being characterized as a lobulated, hypodense, T1 hypointense–T2 hyperintense mass, compressing the brainstem, enveloping the basilar artery, and filling every interstice with tongues of tissue which may appear to penetrate the parenchyma and the internal meatus (Figures 6.4 and 6.5). Lesions entirely confined within the fourth ventricle are also characteristic[8] (Figure 6.6). Desquamated keratin, which in our opinion is sometimes incorrectly quoted as being the source of the cholesterol present in these lesions[7], often exhibits diffuse microscopic mineralization, may be loosely or densely packed, imparts the visually pearly quality to the mass (Figure 6.7). The keratinizing, squamous epithelial wall, invisible on CT and MR and usually non-enhancing, is several cells thick, resting on a collagenous adventitia containing numerous thin-walled vessels (Figure 5.1). Although

mimicking CSF, laminar keratin imparts a certain quality of inhomogeneity to the short TR sequence, but is always CSF-hyperintense at long TR/short TE (proton density) (Figure 6.6).

The reports of epidermoidomas sometimes exhibiting marked T1 and T2 hyperintensity, so-called 'white' or type II epidermoid[9,10], raise biochemical, pathological and taxonomic issues. The view that these lesions are in fact haemorrhagic retention cysts (chocolate cyst/cholesterol granulomas)[11] is supported by surgical evidence[12] that such cysts contain haemorrhagic fluid (methaemoglobin) and not keratin. The question then arises as to whether an epidermoidoma can ever turn into a haemorrhagic retention cyst; apart from the suprasellar region no obvious relics of flaky keratin are to be found in chocolate cysts. Significantly, haemorrhage retention cysts are not described in the usual calvarial sites where epidermoidomas typically occur, the common denominator being the skull base and, specifically, the epithelial-lined air spaces. Even in this location, however, secondary epidermoidomas of the mastoid remain visibly pearly and non-haemorrhagic in the presence of gross infection (see haemorrhagic retention cyst of the petrous apex, section 2.5, and haemorrhagic craniopharyngiomas, section 5.2).

Unfortunately the site and surgical approach to these lesions makes it impossible to obtain all the lining tissue for examination, and therefore to exclude the existence of residual epithelium. In this regard it is a pity that the pathology of epithelial inclusions has been sometimes dismissed as mundane[13].

6.2. PARASITIC CYSTS (see also section 3.3)

Cysticercus cysts affect the brainstem parenchyma very much less commonly than the hemispheres, but intraventricular location is well documented and of great neurosurgical importance[14]. As a rule the protoscolex is visible in intraparenchymal bladders, but not those lying entirely within the ventricle, whilst enhancement is absent until the bladder wall decays (Figure 6.8). Enhancement of a roundly dilated fourth ventricle is typical of ependymitis and choroid plexitis (Figure 6.9). Parenchymal hydatid cyst (Figure 6.10) is usually larger than *Cysticercus*, and the wall may or may not enhance. Compared with *Cysticercus*, location of hydatid cyst within the fourth ventricle is seldom reported.

6.3. INFLAMMATORY MASSES (see also section 4.4)

In the cerebellum, origin (mastoiditis), sulcation and volume combine to ensure that pyogenic abscesses of any size almost invariably involve the meninges and parenchyma together, with obvious morphological and vascular implications, including particularly the tendency for multiloculation (Figure 6.11). The infoldings of choroid plexus and tonsillar cortex have a similar effect on haematogenous masses within the ventricle.

The classification and imaging features of granulomas are discussed in section 3.2. Cerebellar lesions are less

Figure 6.1 Arachnoid cyst, posterior fossa: female, 65 years, episodic dizziness and headache of 3 years duration; resolved following operation; (**a**) sagittal T1WI, (**b**) T2WI; CSF isointense cyst occupies the quadrigeminal plate cistern, with evidence of deformation of the surrounding structures, including the midbrain tectum (a, arrow); at operation, surgeon described cyst wall (b, arrow) as arachnoid

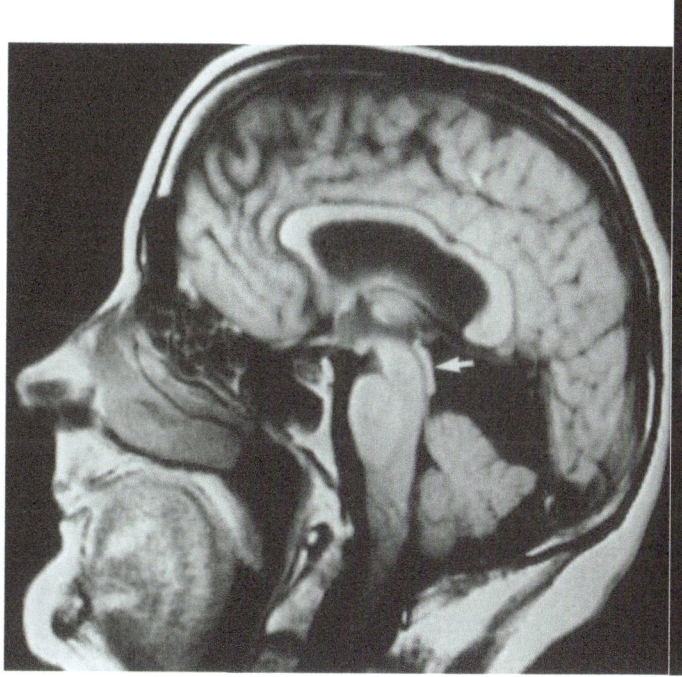

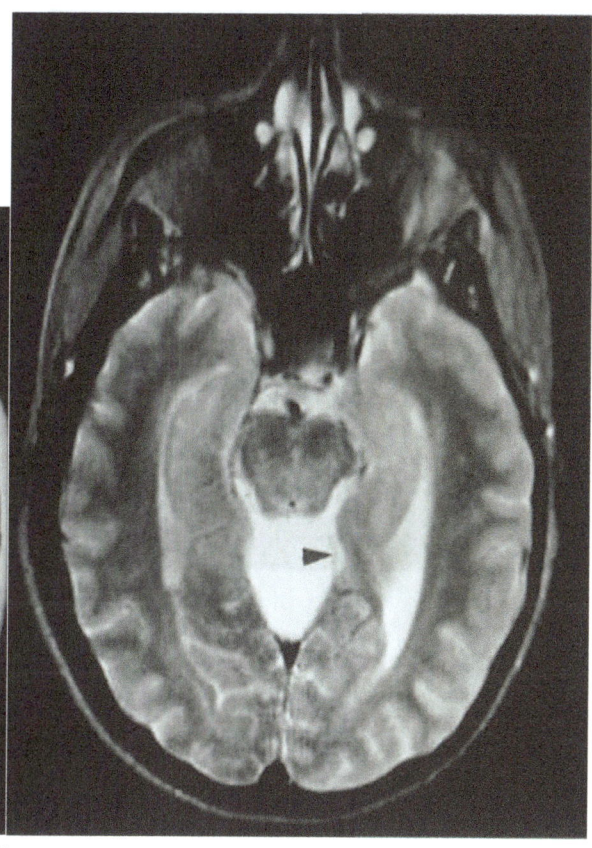

a   b

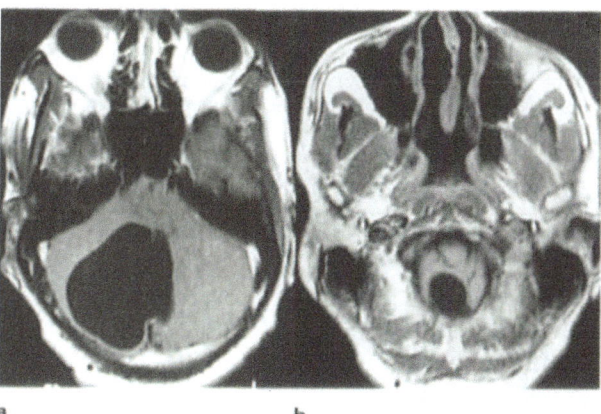

a   b

Figure 6.2 Neuroepithelial (ependymal) cyst, posterior fossa: male, 46 years, acute hydrocephalus; (**a,b**) T1WI; the uncontrasted images show a large, eccentric lobar cyst, with CSF isointense contents. Inferiorly (b), dorsal superficial component of the wall becomes invisible

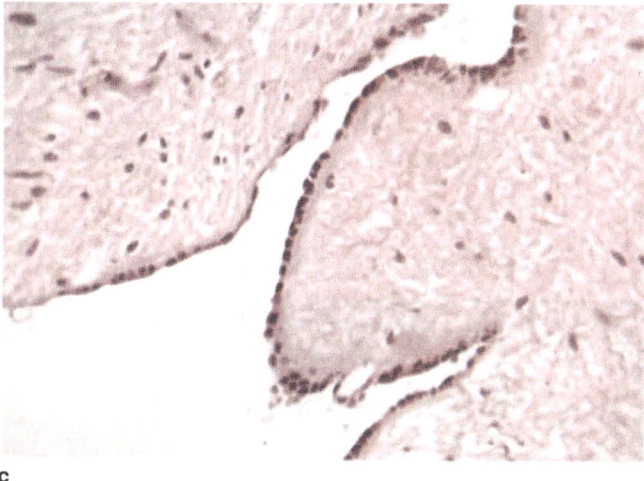

c

(compare with **Figure 7.8**). Cuboidal epithelial lining (c), with basal lamina, was S100-positive/GFAP-negative. No ultrastructure. (Drs M Wright and RM Bowen, Groote Schuur Hospital)

common and, at the same time, usually more complex than supratentorial masses (Figure 6.12), for the anatomical reasons given above. The typical clinical background is that of childhood or adolescent tuberculous meningitis, and depending on the length of history and therapeutic intervention, there may or may not be meningeal enhancement. Adults do not, as a rule, have meningitis, presenting instead with the syndrome of a posterior fossa mass. After tuberculosis, and with less consistent racial bias, parasitic cysts are an important cause of CSF obstruction. These are almost always intraventricular, and may present at any stage of cyst degeneration, including frank granulomatous choroiditis and ependymitis (Figure 6.9).

6.4. EXTRAPARENCHYMAL NEOPLASMS

The cerebellopontine angles constitute the widest part as well as the lateral recesses of the prepontine cistern. Each has as its roof the edge of the anterior cerebellar lobe, with the sloping cerebellar peduncles and the vertical face of the petrous forming the medial and lateral boundaries respectively. The lateral foramen opens into the apex of the recess and its principal contents comprise the flocculus, choroid plexus, VI, VII and VIII nerves, and a number of vessels including the inferior cerebellar and labyrinthine arteries. The approach to masses at this site requires separation of lesions having obvious, gross, associated petrous bony alterations (for which CT is essential), from

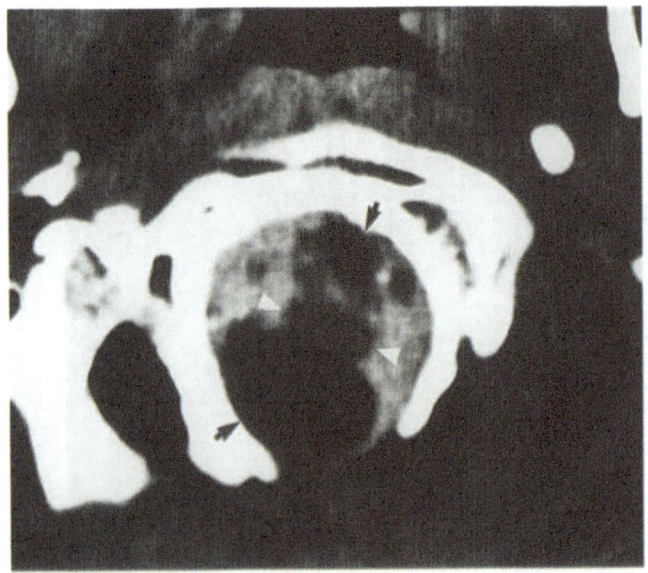

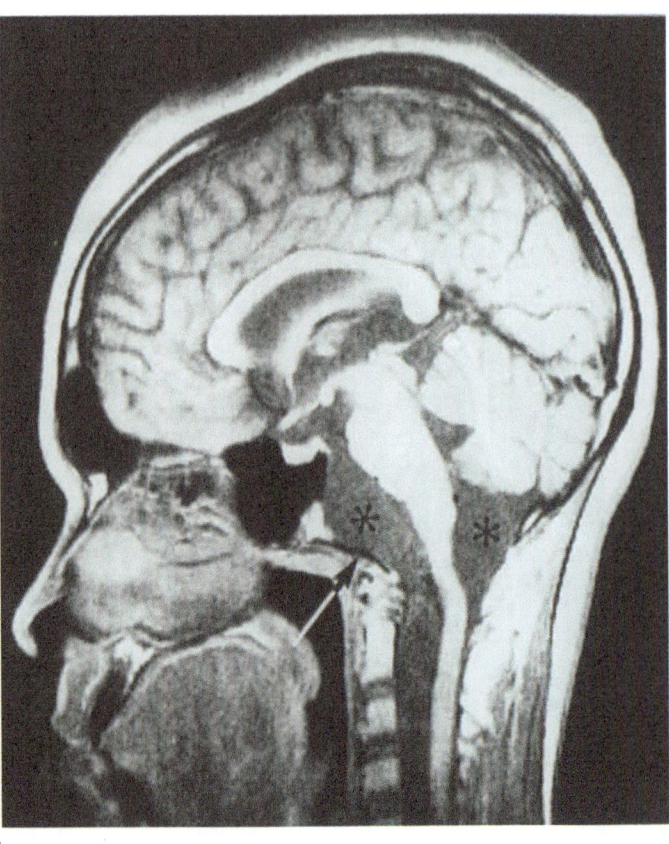

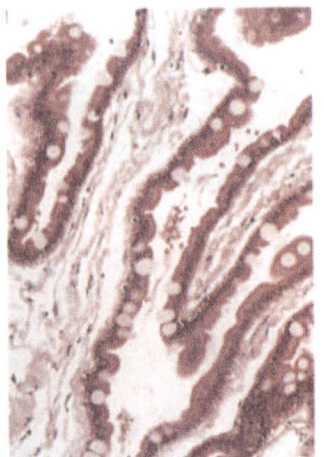
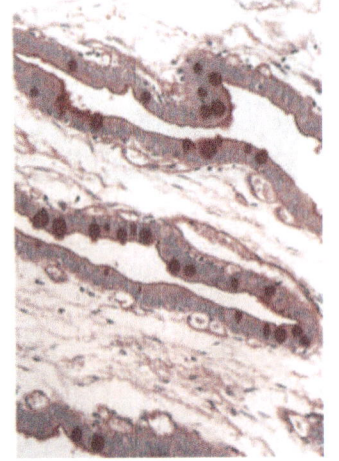

Figure 6.3 Neurenteric cyst, craniocervical junction: (a) CT myelogram, (b) T1WI, (c) HE/APAS ×200; myelogram at level of foramen magnum shows dorsal and ventral cysts (arrows) on either side of a compressed medulla (arrow-heads); sagittal MR demonstrates loss of normal pontomedullary profile with adjacent abnormal CSF isointense encysted spaces (asterisk). Note attenuation and downwards displacement of basi-occiput (arrow). No vertebral abnormalities. Histology shows artefactually folded lining of columnar epithelium, goblet cells and apposed arachnoid

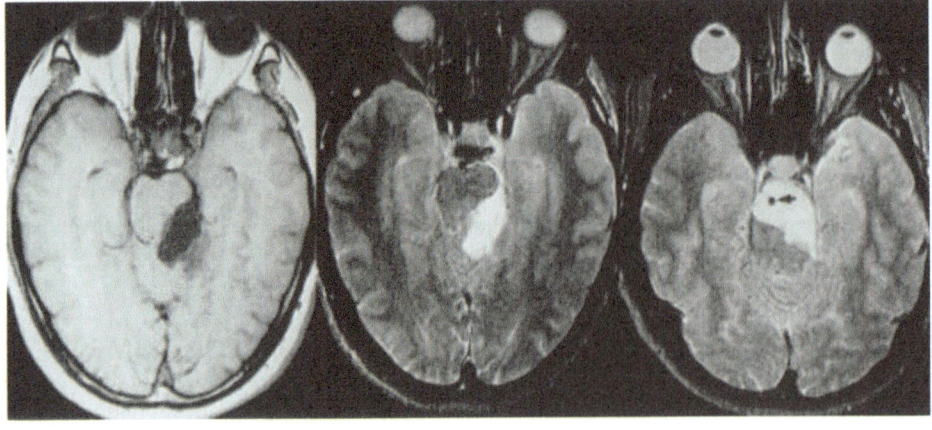

Figure 6.4 Epidermoidoma, ambient cistern: (a) T1WI, (b,c) T2WI; images show T1 hypointense (CSF isointense), T2 hyperintense, faintly inhomogeneous, expansion of ambient cistern with isolation (encasement) of the basilar artery (c, arrow). The border of this lesion is slightly indistinct (blurred) and there is marked deformity of the brainstem. Histology was characteristic

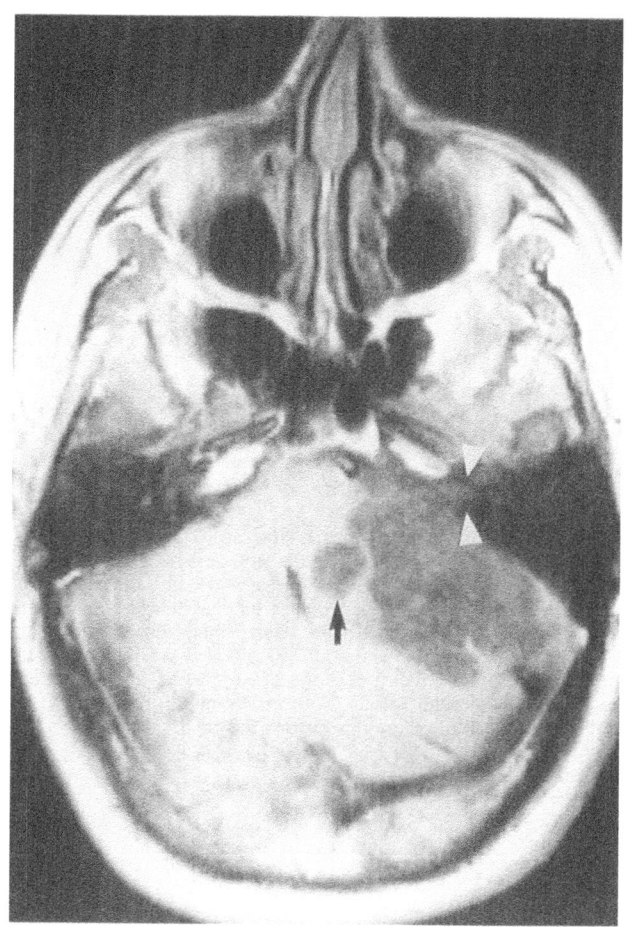

Figure 6.5 Epidermoidoma, CP angle: illustrates extension into the parenchyma of the cerebellum (arrow) and internal auditory meatus (arrow heads)

those without. As far as possible the latter group is then further distinguished according to meningeal, extra- and intraparenchymal origin. Important though uncommon petrous masses impinging upon the cistern include haemorrhagic cyst (Figure 2.13), paraganglioma and rhabdomyosarcoma, whilst acoustic schwannoma, epidermoidoma and meningioma constitute the much commoner, primary occupants[15]. Phacomatoses apart, these latter conditions are restricted to adults, and with the possible exception of tuberculous granuloma there are no common extraparenchymal cerebellopontine angle masses in children.

6.4a. Meningioma

Solitary posterior fossa meningiomas are typically situated on the undersurface of the anterior free margin of the tent (Figure 6.13), the CP angle (Figure 6.14), or the dura anterolateral to the foramen magnum (Figure 6.15). Imaging is required in at least axial and coronal planes to depict topography sufficiently, particularly the flat base with dural tails (Figure 6.16); however, some small, CP angle lesions are indistinguishable from schwannoma, even to the extent of associated widening of the internal meatus. Signal intensities and enhancement are otherwise usual, i.e. brainstem isointense at short TR, and cerebellar cortex isointense at long TR, which is hyperintense relative to white matter (see section 3.4a). Enhancement is diffuse and homogeneous, possibly related to smaller size, on average, than supratentorial masses[16].

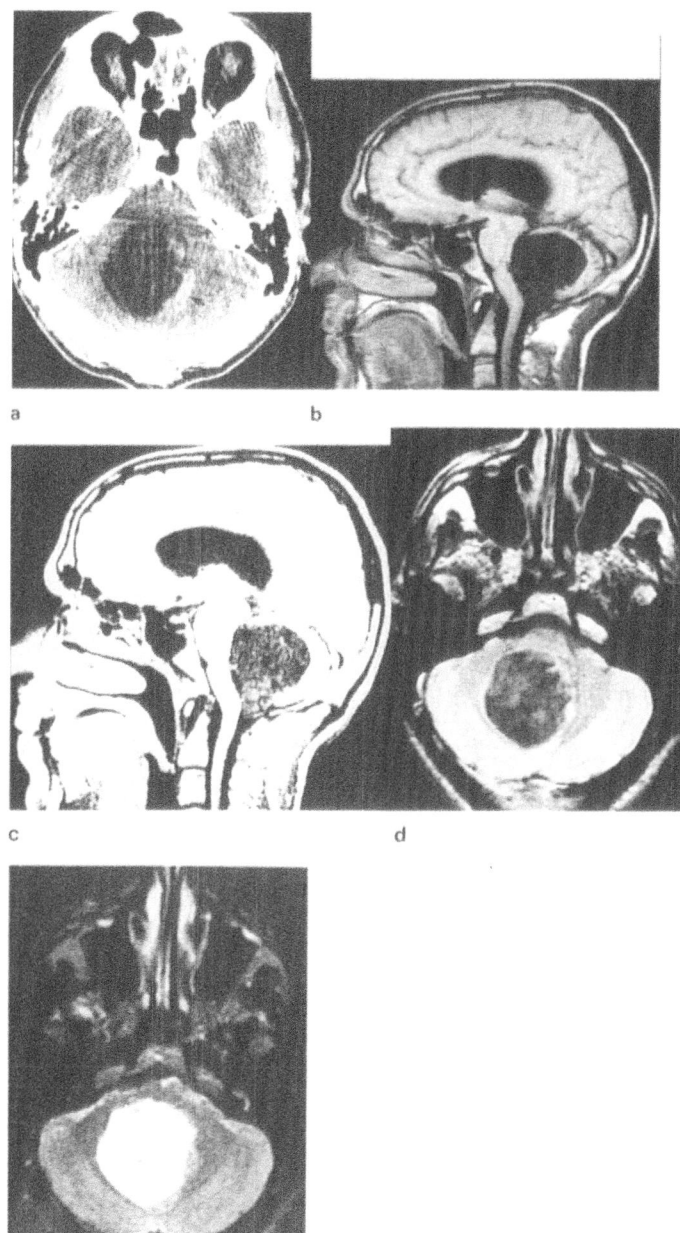

e

Figure 6.6 Epidermoidoma, intraventricular: (**a**) CT + C, (**b,c**) sagittal T1WI, (**d**) PDWI, (**e**) T2WI; CT shows cystic expansion of V4 with feeble incomplete rim enhancement (arrow), probably compressed choroid and meninges. MR images show that the cyst contents resemble CSF at short (b) and long TR (e), but characteristic inhomogeneity of laminar keratin becomes apparent with altered window setting (c) and on PDWI (d). Source of T1 effect in latter is uncertain (see section **6.1b**)

6.4b. Schwannoma

Schwannomas vary greatly in size (Figure 6.17) and shape, and only those lesions filling the cerebellopontine angle from a bell-mouthed internal meatus can really be said to have a typical profile (Figure 6.18). On the other hand, widening of the meatus is reported to be absent in 20% of cases[17], whilst the lobulation so easily seen through the operating microscope is not always apparent on the images. The typical tumour is heterogeneously isointense with the adjacent brainstem, on T1 sequences, becoming homogeneously cortex-isointense at long TR, short TE, and then markedly inhomogeneous at long TE, when it is at its most characteristic (Figure 6.19). This late T2 inhomogeneity results from a composite of brain-

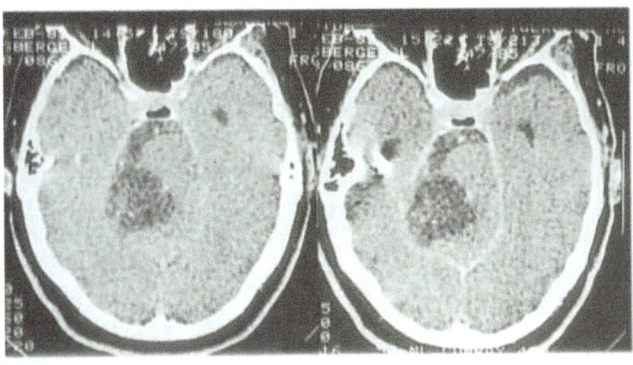

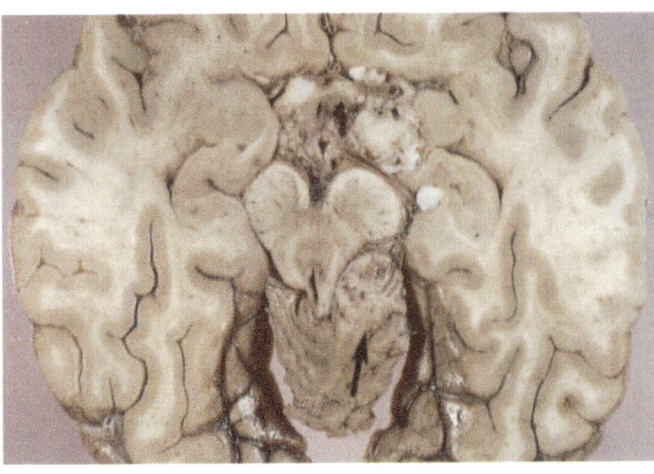

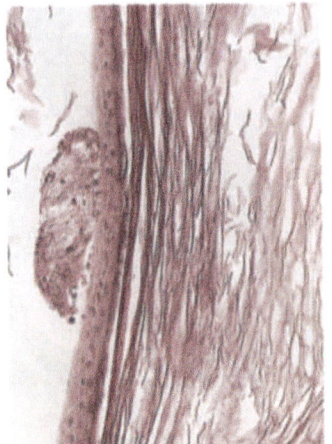
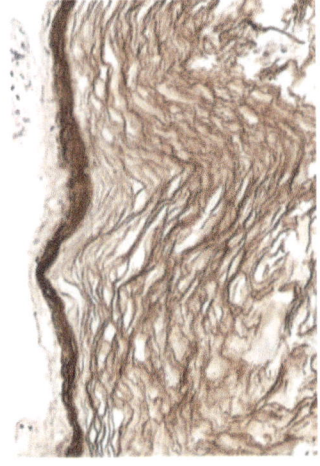

Figure 6.7   Epidermoidoma, suprasellar: (**a**) CT/CT + C, (**b**) fixed brain, (**c**) HE/antikeratin ×200; image shows characteristic non-enhancing, inhomogeneous hypodense tissue indenting the brainstem. Section of fixed brain shows typical pearly material in interpeduncular/suprasellar cistern and choroid fissure; haemorrhage tissue (arrow) is herniated cerebellum overlying tumour. Histology shows characteristic squamous epithelium, devoid of adnexal structures and abundant non-degenerate, laminated keratin, both exhibiting strong labelling by antikeratin antibody (compare with **Figure 5.8**)

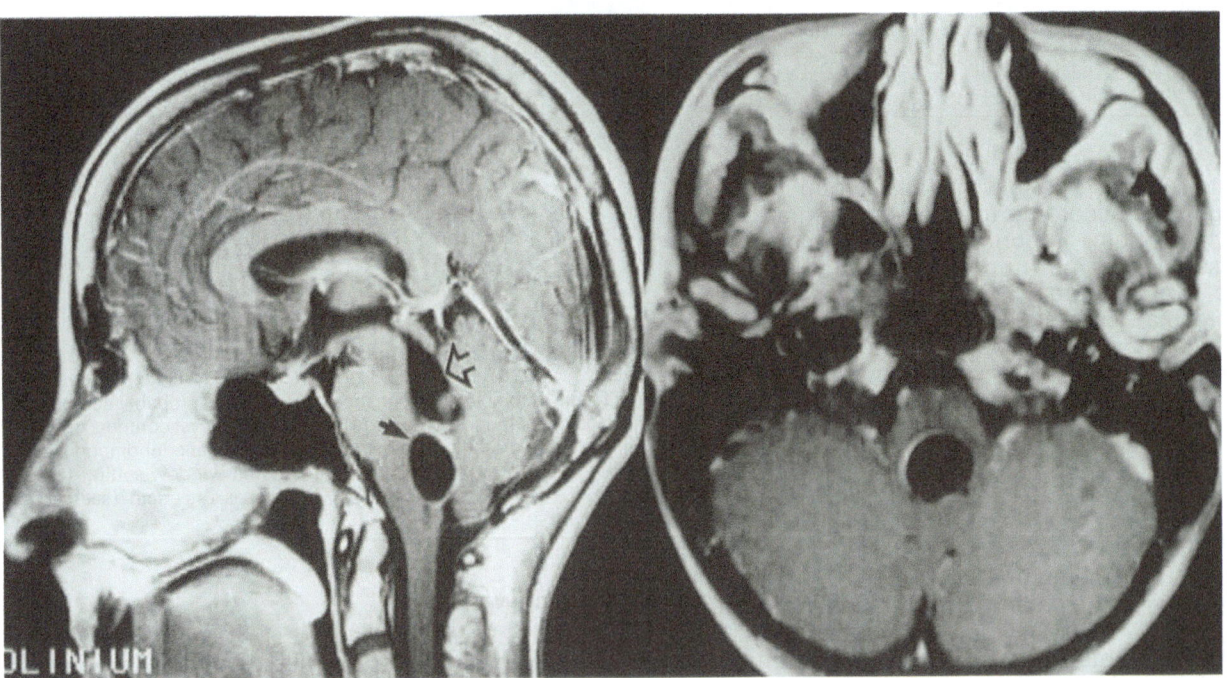

Figure 6.8   Cysticercosis, intraventricular: (**a**) T1WI + C, (**b**) axial T1WI + C; images show circumscribed, incompletely enhancing cyst occupying the inferior 4th ventricle (a, arrow); proximal 4th ventricle is dilated (a, open arrow). The enhancement is probably granulomatous inflammation of the choroid plexus. Histology showed bladder wall germinal tissue only (see **Figure 4.5**)

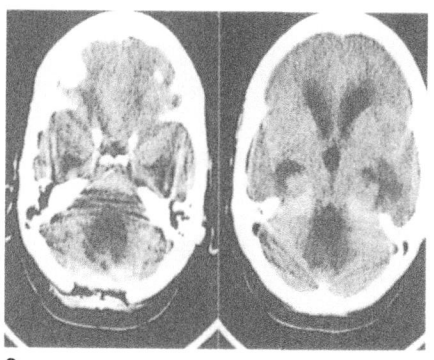

a

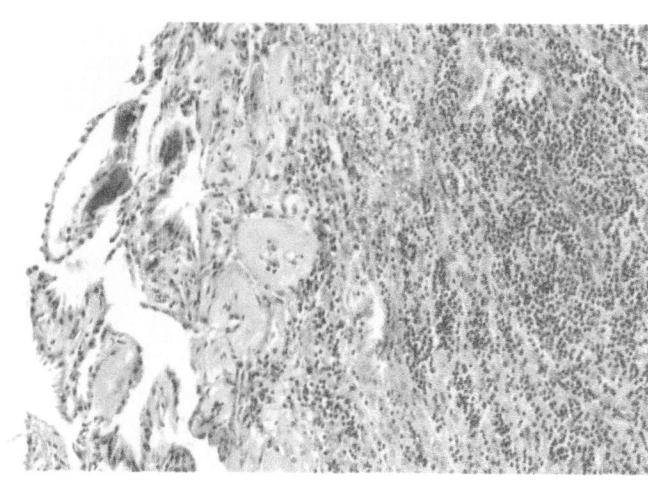

b

Figure 6.9 Cysticercosis, granulomatous choroid plexitis and ependymitis, 4th ventricle: (**a**) CT, (**b**) HE ×200; image shows dilated 4th and lateral ventricles. At operation 4th ventricle contained xanthochromic fluid. Biopsy samples from roof showed fragments of germinal tissue, chronic choroid plexus (b) and ependymitis. Patient has remained permanently obstructed

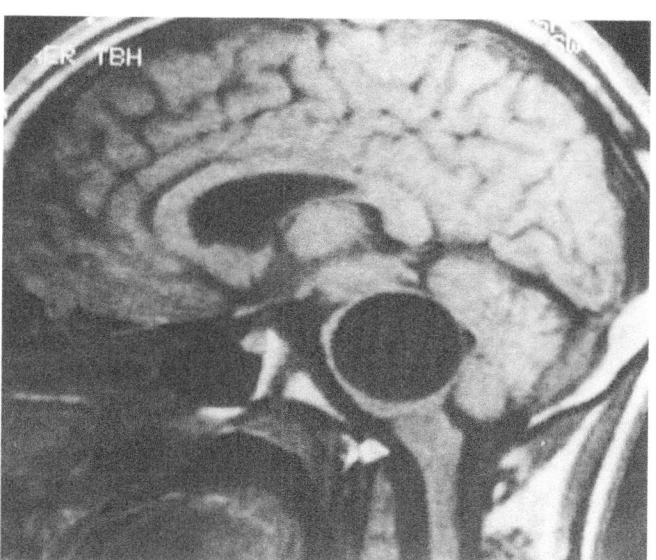

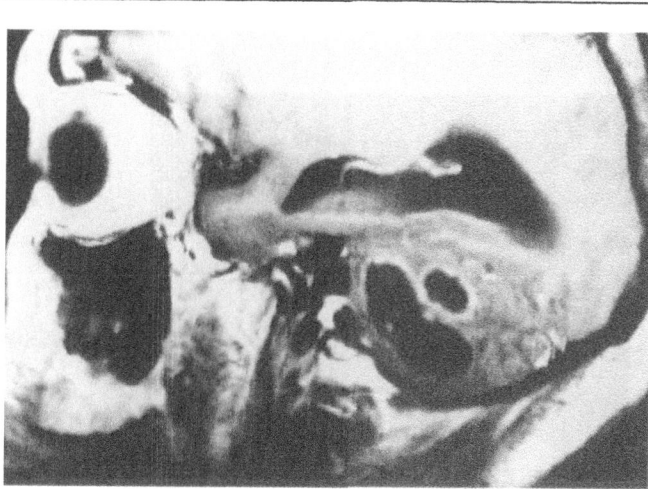

Figure 6.11 Pyogenic abscess, cerebellar: image illustrates mutilocularity of cerebellar abscess, which at this site is characteristic and has no implications of atypicality

Figure 6.10 Hydatitodis, pons: male, 19 years; T1 image shows large, sharply circumscribed pontine cyst with CSF isointense contents. (Histology showed characteristic lamellated cyst wall (see **Figure 7.24**), without evidence of inflammation)

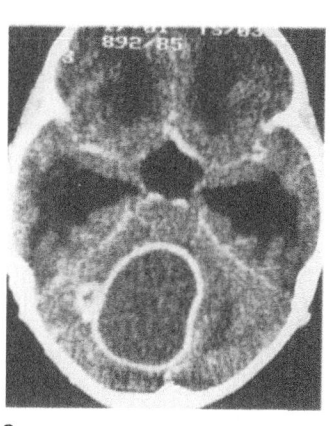

a

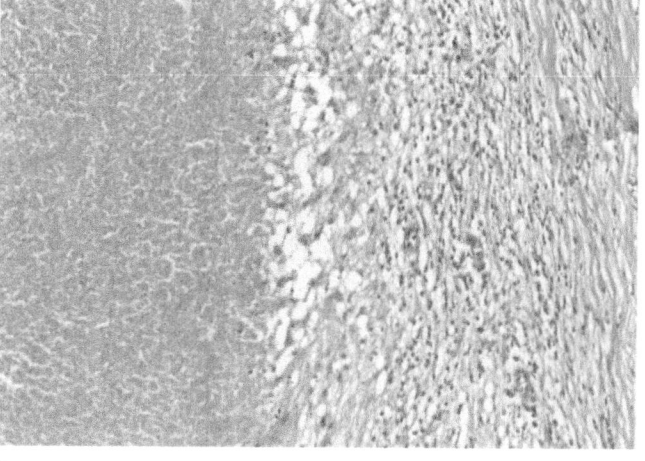

b

Figure 6.12 Granulomatous abscess, cerebellum: (**a**) CT + C, (**b**) HE· ×200; large ring lesion with hypodense contents and exophytic budding of more solid granulomas (a). Histology of abscess wall showed granulation tissue and macrophages, in areas completely devoid of epithelioid and giant cells, giving way abruptly to central caseous necrosis; no organisms demonstrable. (See also discussion of granulomatous inflammation, **section 3.2**)

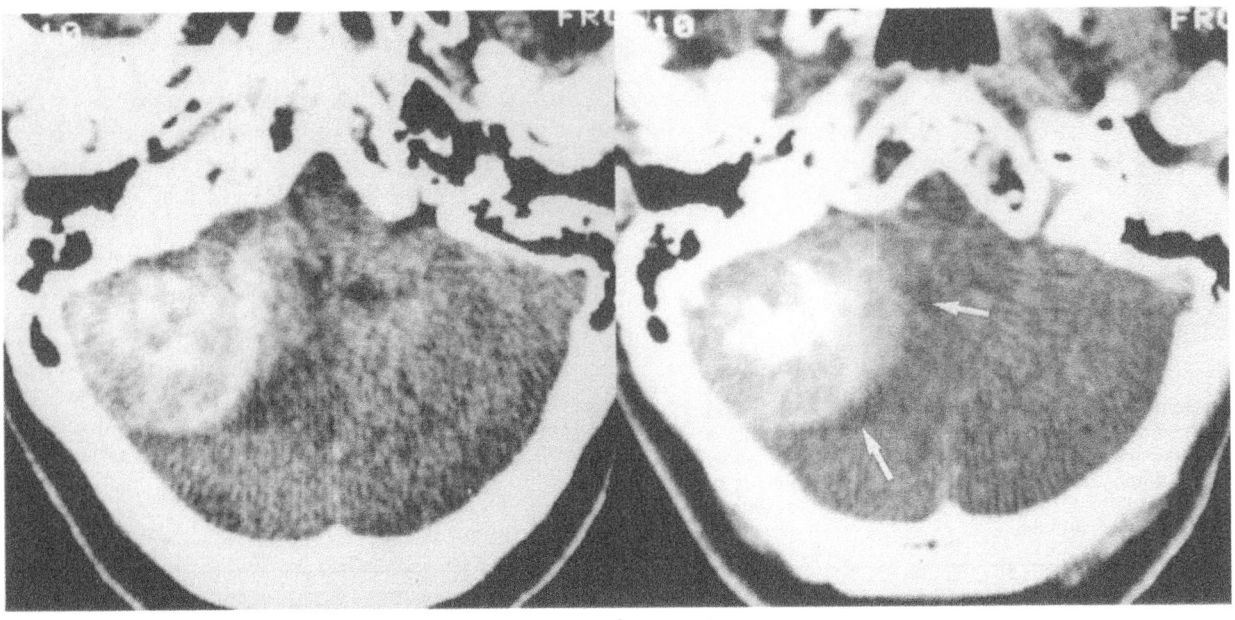

a   b

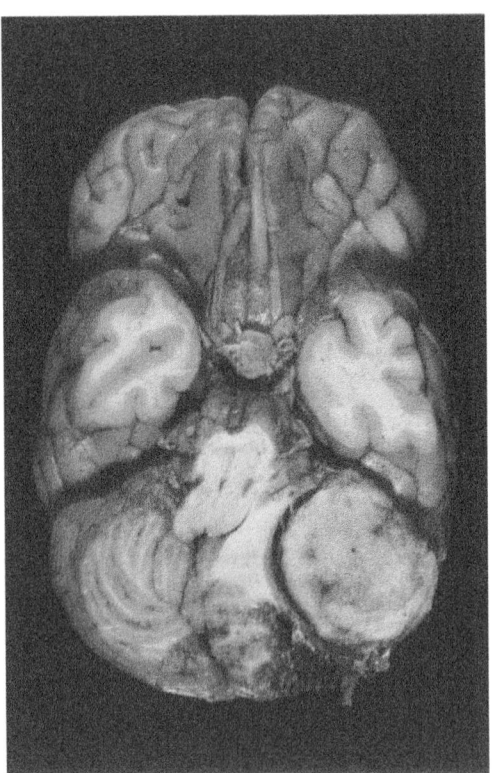

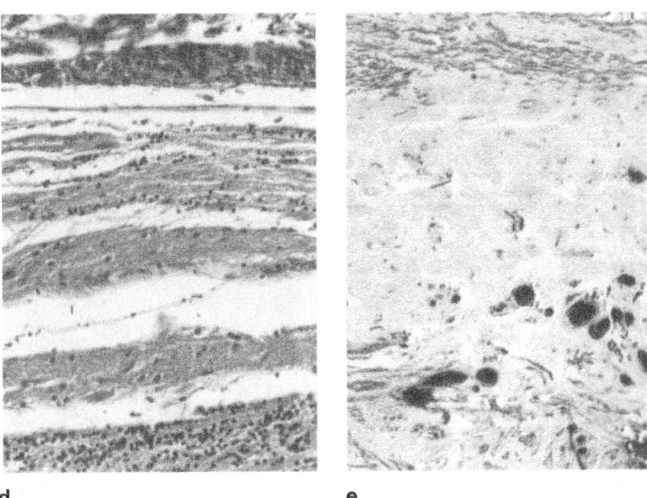

d   e

Figure 6.13 Meningioma, posterior fossa: (a) CT, (b) CT + C, (c) fixed brain, (d) HE × 100, (e) VG × 40; CT shows inhomogeneously hyperdense tumour, with maximal enhancement centrally (b). Fixed brain specimen (c), shows tumour with homogeneous periphery and more granular centre. Tumour–parenchymal cleft is artefactual; section from this site (d), shows compressed atrophic folia, presumed to account for the hypodense rim shown in scan (b, arrows). Section from meningeal surface of tumour (e), shows fibrous capsule with deeper sclerotic and mineralized tissue, latter presumed to be CT hyperdense

c

isointense islands and bands with interspersed hyperintense foci, possibly due to the common occurrence of admixed but sharply delineated tissue types (Figure 6.20). Antoni A tissue, with its many thin, closely packed, interdigitating processes coated with basal lamina, and an intercellular admixture of long-spaced collagen (Luse bodies), together with redundant amorphous/granular 'basement membrane' material, can be reasonably assumed to be (T2) brain isointense (Figure 6.21). The loosely arranged, myxomatous Antoni B tissue, with its greater content of cytoplasmic organelles, paucity of extracellular collagen, and tendency to undergo liquefac-

tive microcystic change[18], must be hyperintense (Figure 6.19). Such expectations are justified until the images are examined after contrast administration, when a different pattern of non-enhancing tissue appears which cannot be satisfactorily equated with the pre-contrast image. For instance, preferential vascularization (or vascular degeneration or mineralization) of either Antoni A or B fields is not apparent from an examination of our material. However, the characteristic smearing pattern (Figure 6.22) of schwannomas supports the difference in reticulin content between the two tissue types.

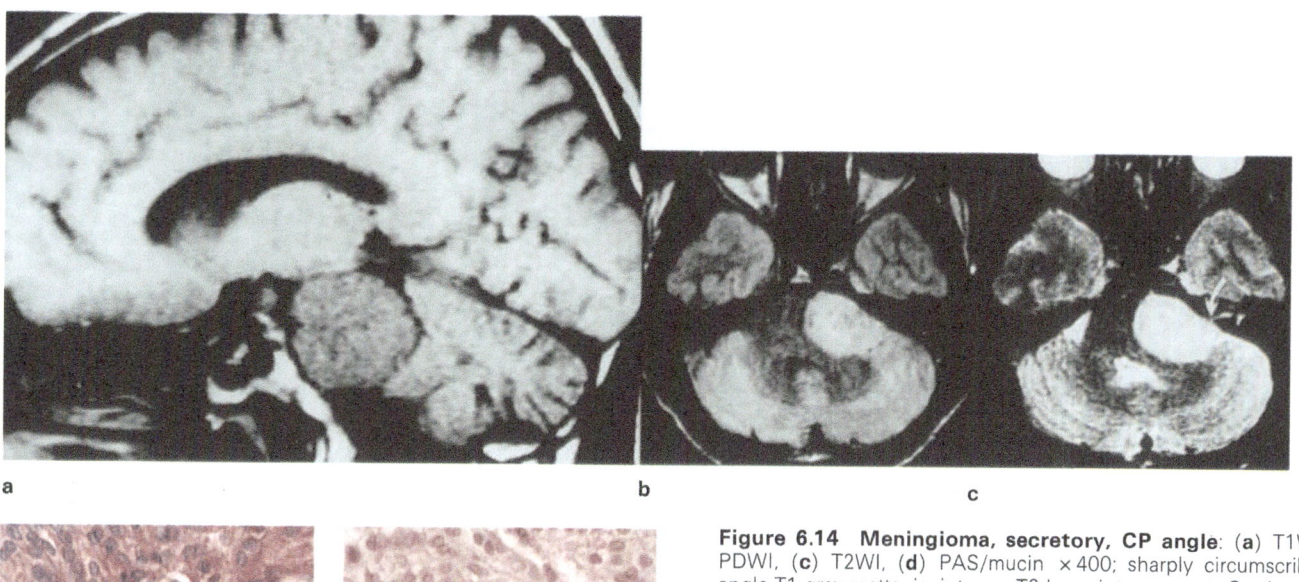

Figure 6.14 Meningioma, secretory, CP angle: (a) T1WI, (b) PDWI, (c) T2WI, (d) PAS/mucin × 400; sharply circumscribed CP angle T1 grey matter isointense, T2 hyperintense mass. On the genuine T1 (a) and PD images (b) the tumour has the same signal intensity as cerebellar cortex, becoming abnormally hyperintense at long TR/TE. Tumour was not microcystic so that T2 hyperintensity is assumed to be due to secretory component (d). Note normal internal meatus (c, curved arrow) (compare with **Figure 6.18**)

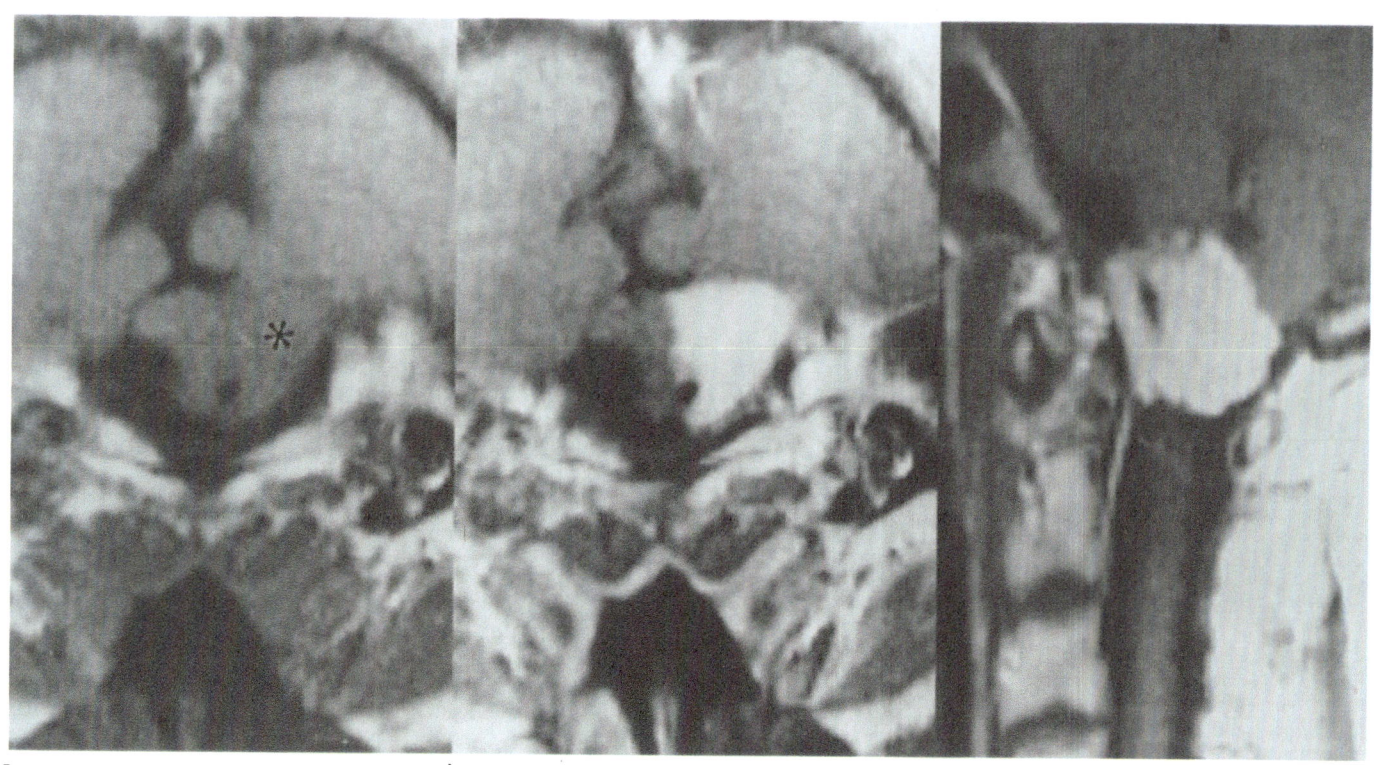

Figure 6.15 Meningioma, foramen magnum: (a) T1WI, (b), T1WI + C, (c) sagittal T1WI + C; lesion (asterisk) is T1 parenchymal isointense with tumour visible only after contrast enhancement. Appearance in axial image (b), is unusual, being indistinguishable from pilocytic astrocytoma; however, sagittal appearance is characteristic

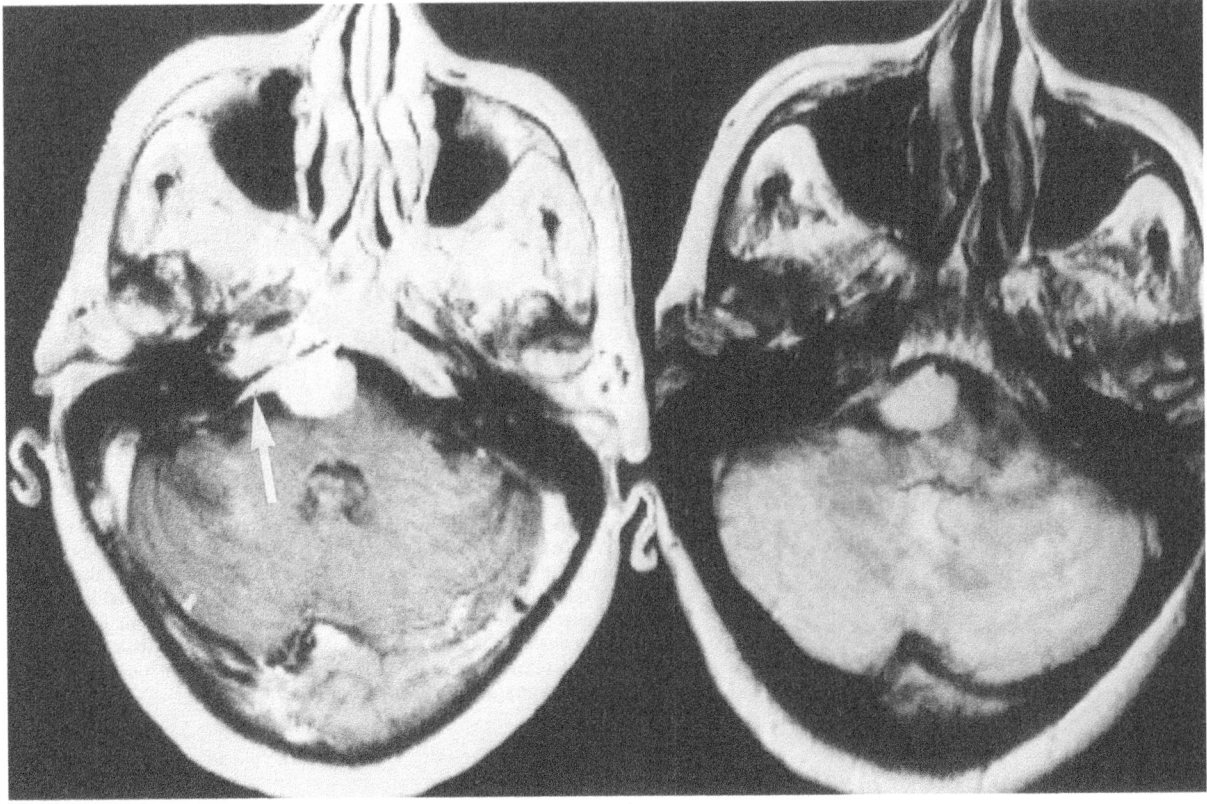

a   b

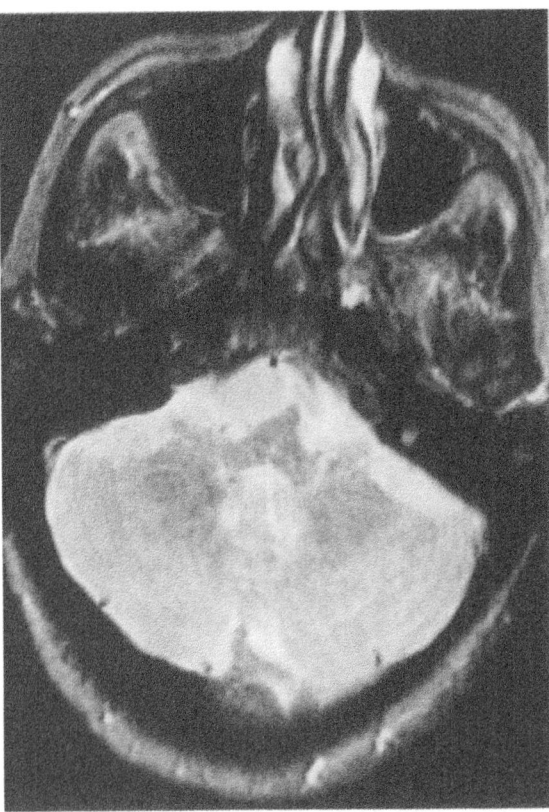

c

Figure 6.16 Meningioma, dural tail, clivus: (**a**) T1WI + C, (**b**) PDWI, (**c**) T2WI; lesion is diffusely enhancing with prominent dural tail (arrow) and thin adjacent cortical bone. Long TR (b,c) shows characteristic grey-matter isointensity

6.5. BRAINSTEM LESIONS

It has been stated unequivocally that investigation of a suspected brainstem lesion begins with MR[19]. This attitude, which summarizes the superiority of MR over CT, is also exemplified in imaging the posterior fossa. In Africa (and presumably many other Third World countries), where CT is the prevailing technique, and where inflammatory disease rivals vascular conditions and neoplasia, the pathologist confronted with a scan and little else will be influenced by patient age and race, and will often require the chest X-ray and CSF findings.

The usefulness of the many groups of statistics quoted with regard to brainstem neoplasms is difficult to assess on account of inconsistent terminology and archiving. For example, MR is said to have reversed the long-held pathological concept of the incidence of infratentorial to supratentorial tumours in childhood[20]. Nowadays, two-thirds occur above the tent; yet the diencephalon is part of the brainstem which is conventionally omitted in favour of the boundaries of the posterior fossa. There also seems little doubt that the term 'brainstem glioma' frustrates imaging, pathological and therapeutic assessment, and ultimately nosology and statistics as well; for the imaging-based figures on brainstem disease to be really meaningful, the features on contrasted, serial MR are needed, together with racial and geographic breakdown.

6.5a. Brainstem astrocytoma (glioma)

The traditional reluctance to biopsy brainstem tumours, despite documented evidence of low morbidity[21], has without doubt been a major factor contributing to the tendency to regard them as a homogeneous group. Attempts to classify these neoplasms on the basis of enhanced imaging alone[22] are likely to be helpful only if made on the assumption of known, biologically distinct variants, including non-astrocytic tumours such as ependymoma which may occasionally appear similar. Aside

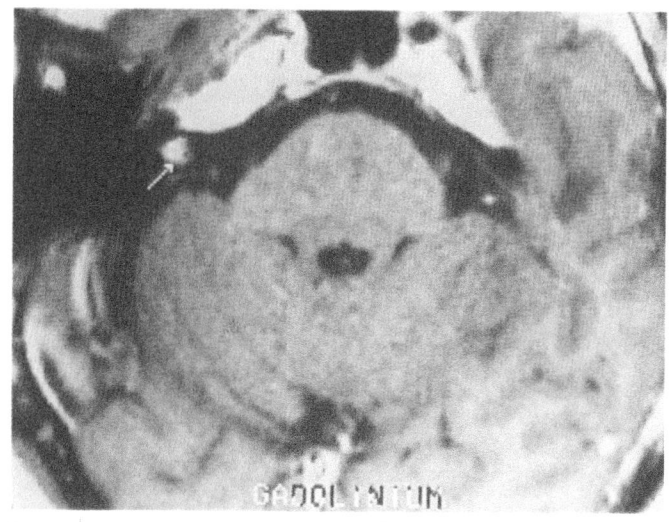

a

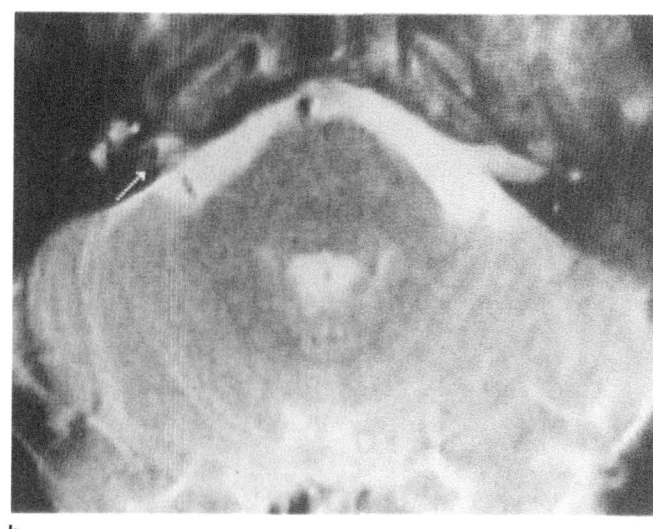

b

Figure 6.17 Schwannoma, intracanalicular: (a) T1WI + C, (b) T2WI; focal, homogeneously enhancing mass in the distal internal meatus (a, arrow), which is T2 brainstem isointense (b, arrow). Tissues from these tiny lesions are seldom available for histological examination

from the obvious differences in MR imaging features of fibrillary and pilocytic astrocytomas, in any case in which tissue diagnosis is contemplated, distinction has to be made between non-enhancing and enhancing components of the same tumour before morphological categorization is possible (Figure 6.23). If this is precluded for technical reasons, diagnosis and prognosis should be based on samples from enhancing tissue. As has been reiterated in this text, the necessity is absolute, for the pathologist not only to be acquainted with the images, but also to view the biopsy site through the operating microscope.

The majority of these lesions are (pontine) fibrillary astrocytomas, appearing on CT as diffuse, hypodense, non-enhancing expansion of the pons, referred to by neurosurgeons as the 'fat pons' (Figure 6.24). MR shows the infiltrated structure to be inhomogeneously T1 hypo-intense, becoming diffusely hyperintense at long TR/TE, when an unexpectedly sharp parenchymal delineation is usually apparent (Figure 6.25). Most characteristic is the bulky, en-plaque growth of tissue over the ventral surface of the pons, enfolding the basilar artery (Figure 6.25). The parenchymal, non-enhancing component of the tumour is composed of fibrillary astrocytes whose nuclear and cytoplasmic morphology is compressed by growth among the fibre tracts blending macroscopically with the colour and texture of normal pons (Figure 6.26). Accretion of tumour cells, still relatively avascular, may lead to degeneration and cyst formation, with concomitant T1 and T2 signal prolongation. Contrary to some[23], in material examined in this laboratory, strong linear or ring enhancement (Figure 6.23), occurring in association with the foregoing features, has as its basis the proliferative vascular changes, anaplastic glial cellularity and focal necrosis comprising the features of malignant glioma (Figure 6.25). Haemorrhage, which may be quite extensive (Figure 6.25) is almost certainly a terminal event induced by the usual mechanism of brainstem displacement.

In a minority of brainstem gliomas the neoplasm conforms entirely or predominantly to that of a well-vascularized (juvenile) *pilocytic astrocytoma* (see also section 6.6a), and presents the images of a circumscribed, diffusely enhancing exophytic mass growing on or in relation to the dorsum of the pons or medulla (Figure 6.27). We have also encountered an exophytic, low-grade, well-

vascularized astrocytic tumour of the brainstem which unaccountably failed to enhance (Figure 6.28).

Gliofibroma is the somewhat presumptive title given to an even rarer subspecies of brainstem tumour consisting of a dense mixture of mature atrocytic and fibroblastic elements whose histogenesis is currently debated[24–26]. CT features include isodensity and strong, homogeneous enhancement (Figures 6.29 and 6.30), consistent with pervasive reticulin content, calcospherite aggregates and capillary angioarchitecture. These features are likely to have the effect of shortening the T2 signal on MR, in common with tumours with an insignificant extracellular space, e.g. medulloblastoma (section 6.6b).

6.6. PRIMARY CEREBELLAR NEOPLASMS
6.6a. Astrocytoma

The great majority of neoplasms of astrocytic type, at this site, are juvenile (dimorphic) pilocytic astrocytomas (JPA), whilst diffuse fibrillary astrocytomas are rare[27]. JPA are found anywhere in the cerebellar grey matter, including intraventricular growth from the vermis (Figure 6.31), and are almost always partially or even wholly cystic. The characteristic dimorphic histology provides significant correlation with the imaging features: areas of compact, vascularized cellularity composed of strongly fibrillated (often bipolar) cells alternate with rarefied, sparsely cellular protoplasmic astrocytic tissue in which microcysts occur (Figure 6.32). At both short and long TR this solid composite has an overall isointensity with cortex, although with a certain quality of T2 hyperintense inhomogeneity which could be the effect of coalescent microcysts (Figure 6.33). Enhancement is strong and diffuse, consistent with the angioarchitecture (Figures 4.51 and 6.34). In some examples examined by us, pronounced and generalized formation of Rosenthal fibres and granular bodies has not appeared to interfere with the signal characteristics described; however, unusually extensive areas of pure protoplasmic tissue (Figure 6.35) might be expected to do so. Despite correlative difficulties, enhancement of the cyst wall is generally assumed to be indicative of tumour (Figure 6.34), and is probably a more reliable means of assessment than microscopy. However, compressed meningeal vessels (Figure 6.36) could give rise to non-neoplastic enhancement. Complete absence

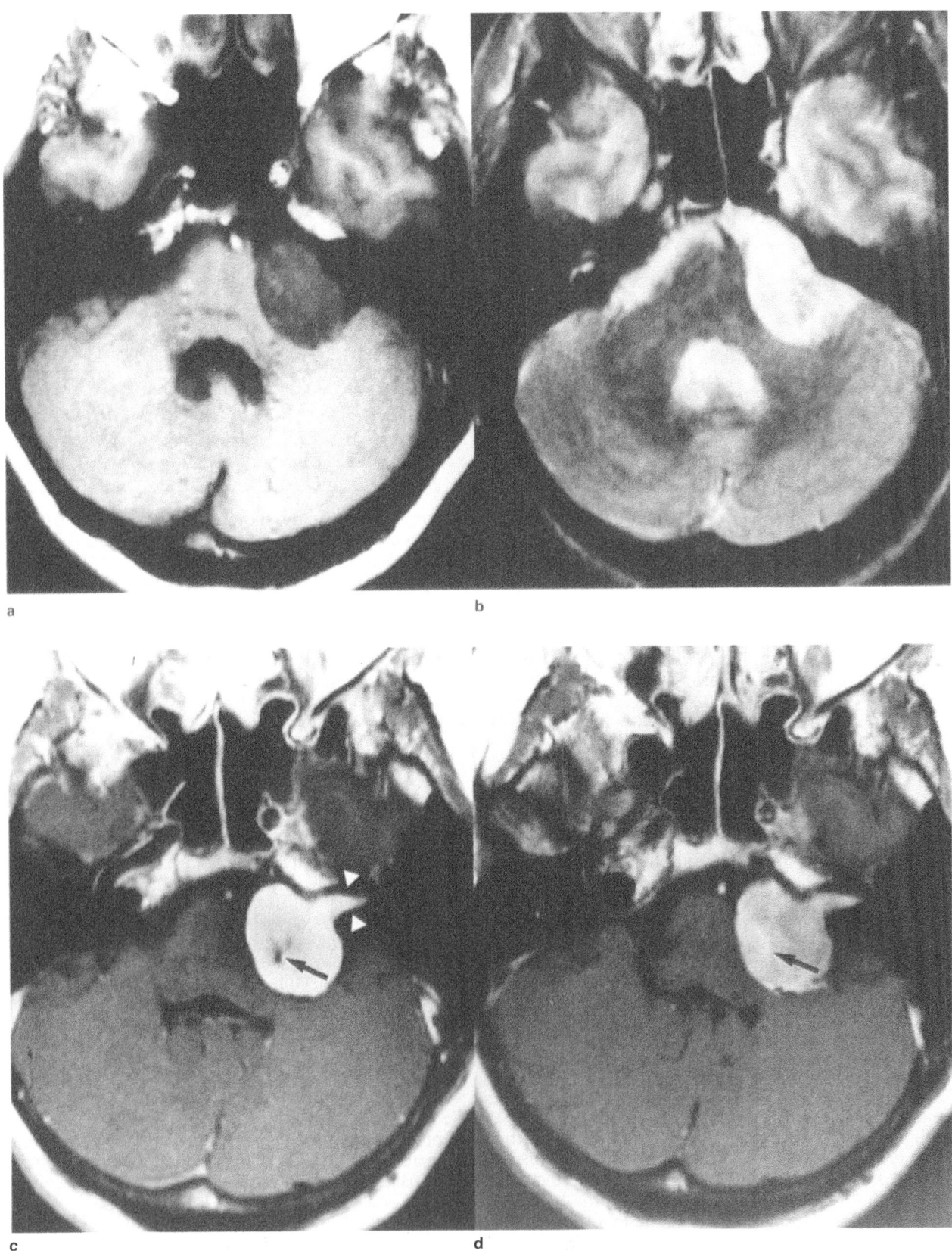

Figure 6.18 Schwannoma, CP angle: (a) T1WI, (b) T2WI, (c) T1WI + C, (d) T1WI + C (delayed); lesion is characteristically T1 hypointense (a), inhomogenously T2 hyperintense (b), with strong diffuse enhancement (c). Non-enhancing focus (c, arrow) accumulates contrast on the delayed study (d, arrow), probably representing accumulation within area of cystic degeneration (see **Figure 6.19d**). Profile of the enhanced lesion, with widened meatus (c, arrow-heads) is pathognomonic. However, signal intensities are otherwise non-specific (compare with **Figure 6.14**)

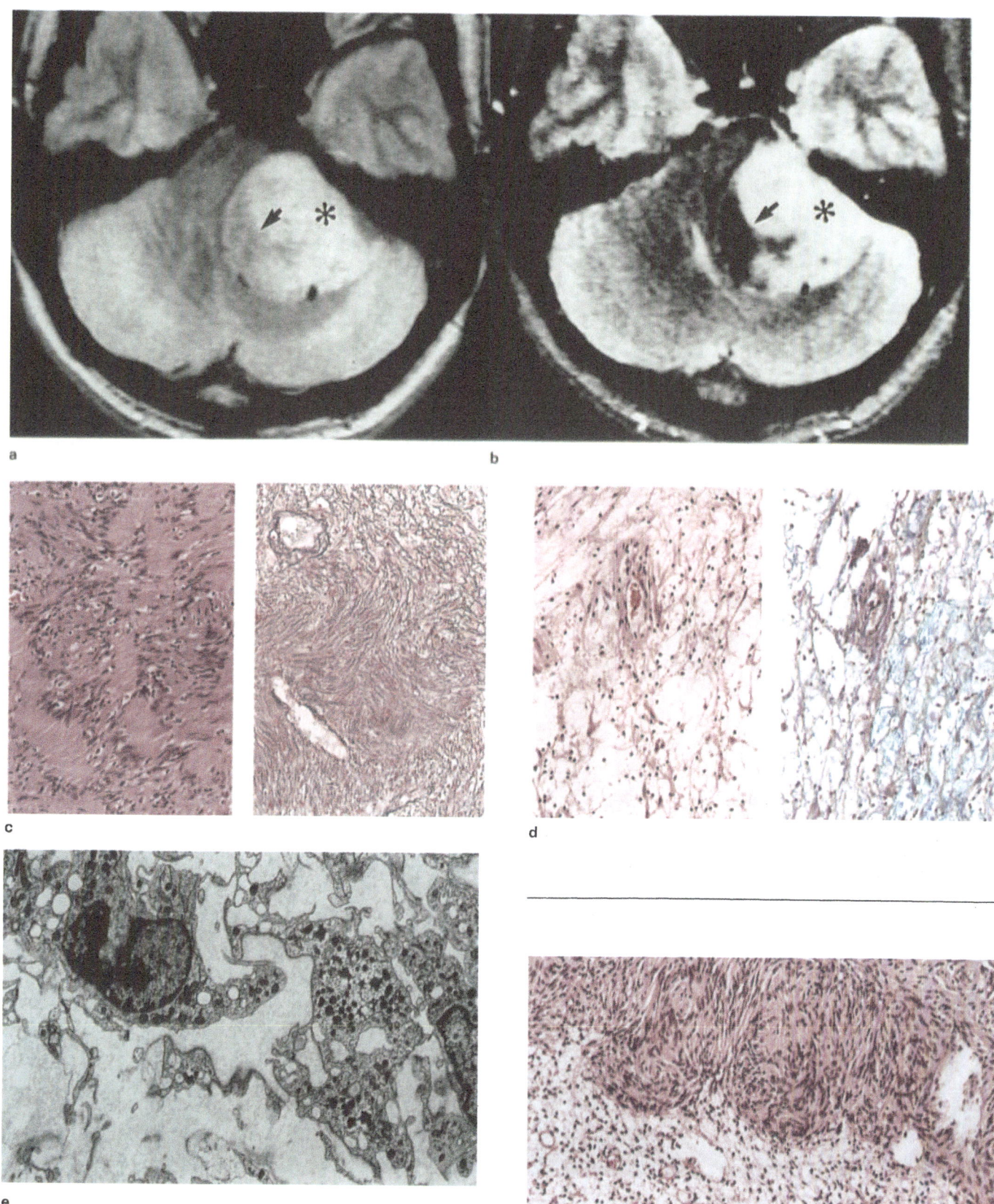

a

b

c

d

e

Figure 6.19 Schwannoma, CP angle: (**a**) PDWI, (**b**) T2WI, (**c**) HE/Retic ×200, (**d**) HE/APAS ×200, (**e**) EM ×4730; tumour has two distinct components, one which is white-matter isointense on proton density and T2 (a,b, arrows), the second being proton density cortex isointense and T2 hyperintense (a,b, asterisks). These are assumed to correspond to Antoni A and B tissues respectively (c,d); note the prominent argyrophilic collagen component in Antoni A tissue (c, right). Ultrastructure of Antoni B tissue (e) emphasizes the abundant interstitial matrix. (See **Figure 6.21** for ultrastructure of Antoni A tissue)

Figure 6.20 Schwannoma: characteristic abrupt transition between Antoni A and B tissue. HE ×200

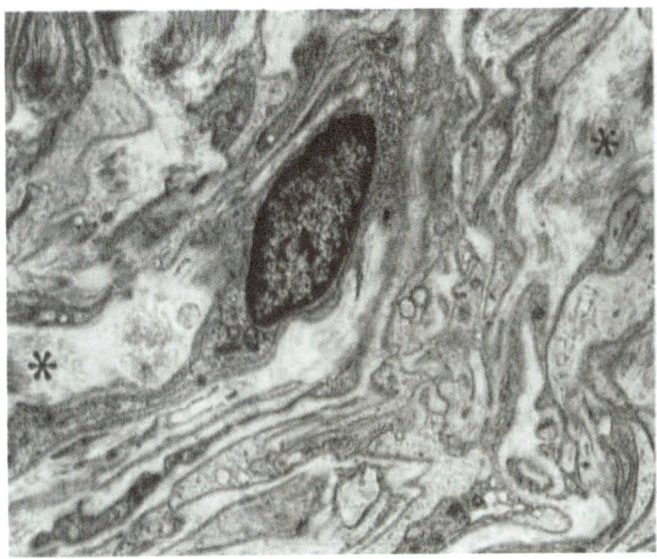

Figure 6.21   Schwannoma: ultrastructure of Antoni A tissue showing compact arrangement of interdigitating processes, with basal laminae and abundant interspersed collagen (asterisk). EM ×5400

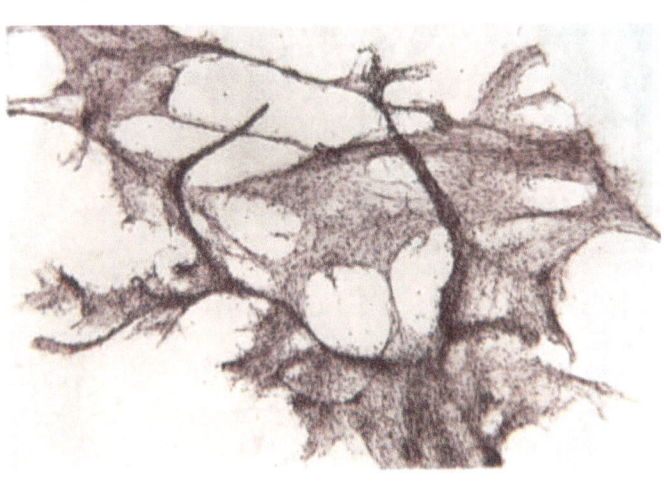

Figure 6.22   Schwannoma: illustrates characteristic smearing pattern of these tumours. HE ×63

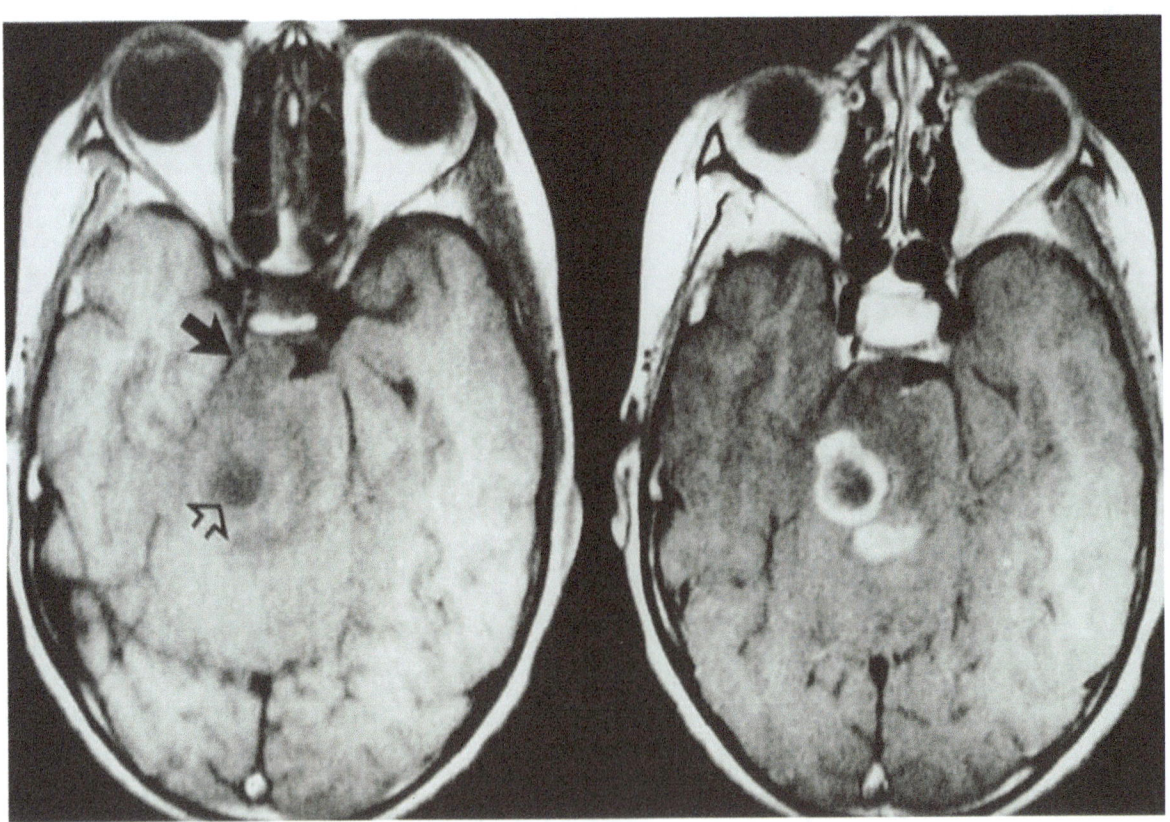

a

b

Figure 6.23   Pontine astrocytoma, focal malignant transformation: (a) T1WI, (b) T1WI + C, (c) T2WI, (d,e) HE ×200; lesion is predominantly right-sided, with typical en-plaque growth (a, arrow) and cystic component (a, open arrow), which also shows strong peripheral enhancement (b). These two components became indis- tinguishable on T2 weighted image (c). Biopsy samples obtained from non-enhancing (d), and enhancing parts (e), showed the latter component to have the features of malignancy. (See also **Figure 6.25** and discussion **section 6.5a**)

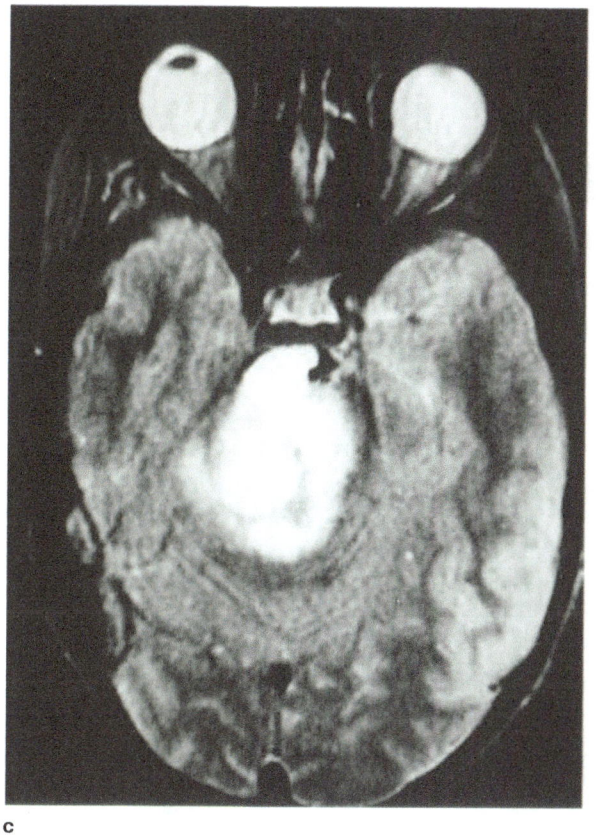

c

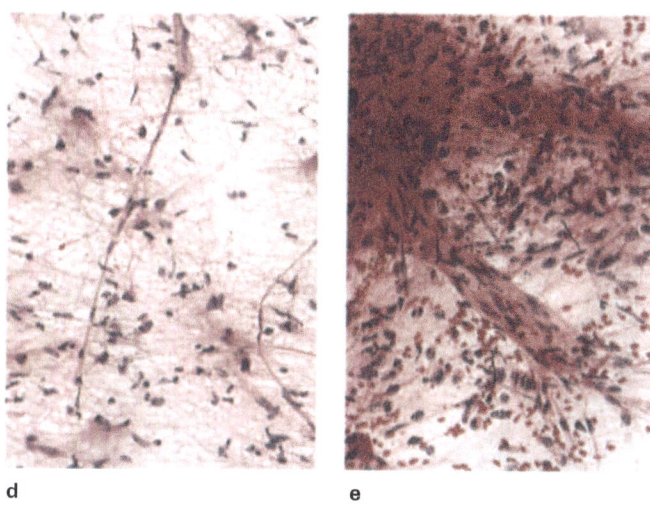

d

e

Figure 6.23 (*continued*)

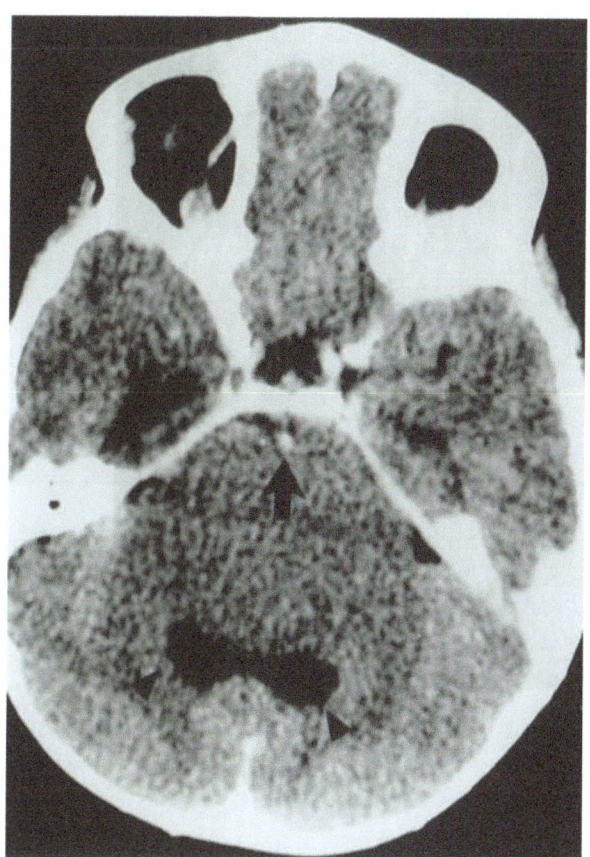

a

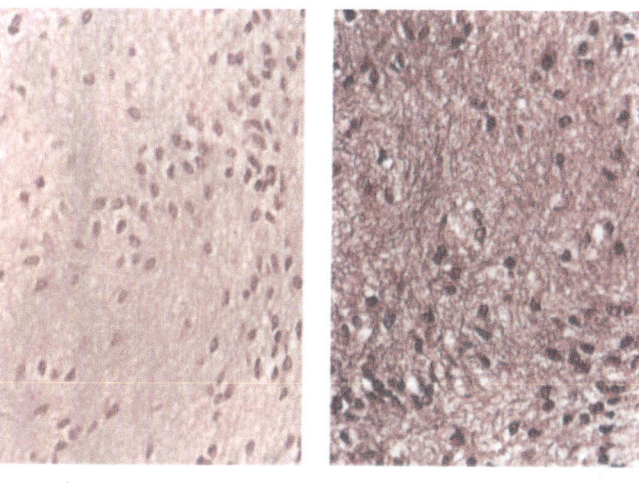

b

Figure 6.24 Pontine astrocytoma: (**a**) CT + C, (**b**) HE/PTAH × 400; enhanced CT shows typical gross non-enhancing, isodense expansion of the pons with cisternal effacement and basilar indentation (arrow); V4 (arrow-heads) is deformed but patent. Histology (rongeur specimen) shows small monomorphic nuclei and a dense fibrillary stroma, shown on PTAH. In the context of the image this sample is considered representative, i.e. necrosis and/or vascular proliferation has not been missed (see **Figure 6.26**)

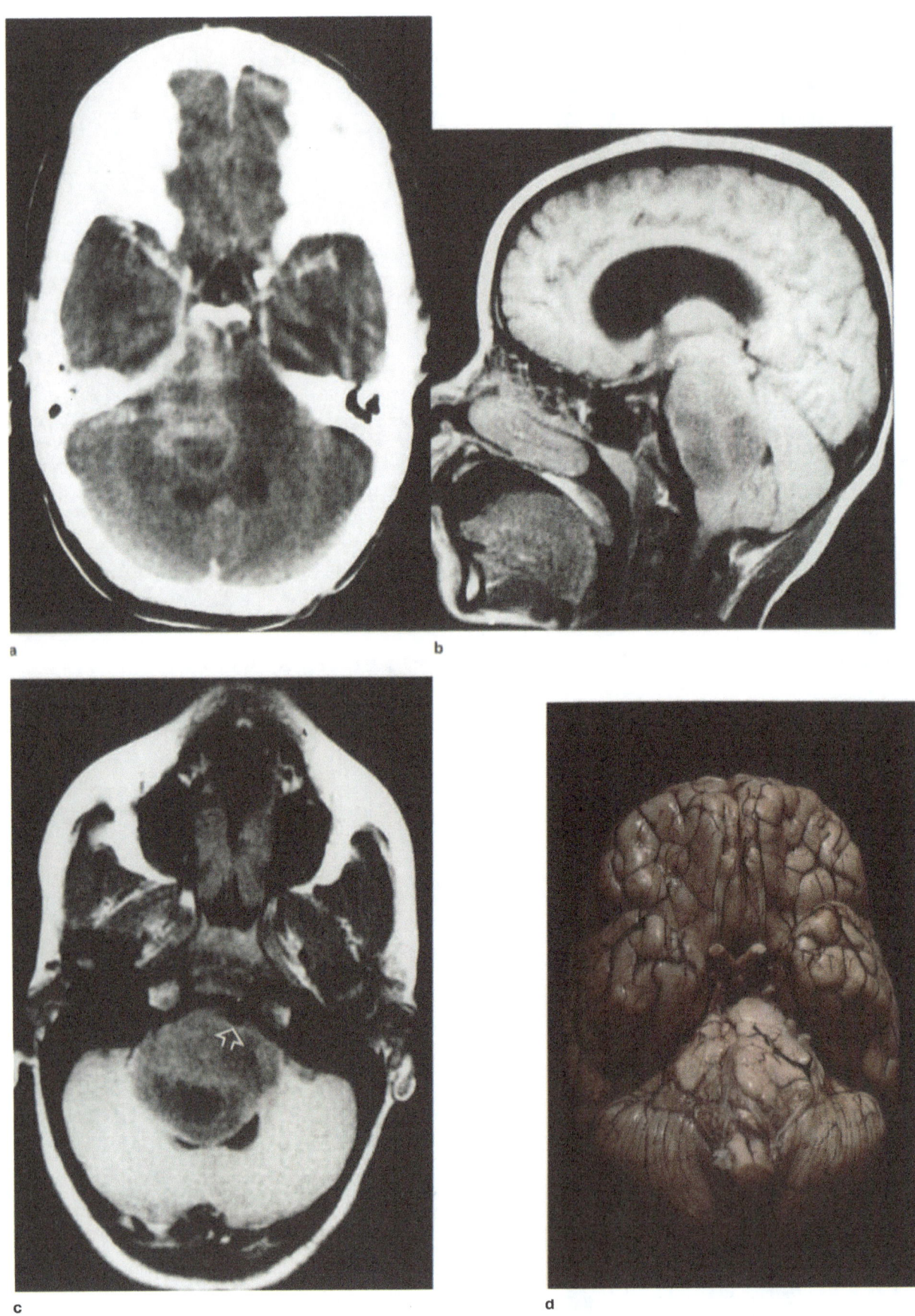

a

b

c

d

Figure 6.25   (*legend opposite*)

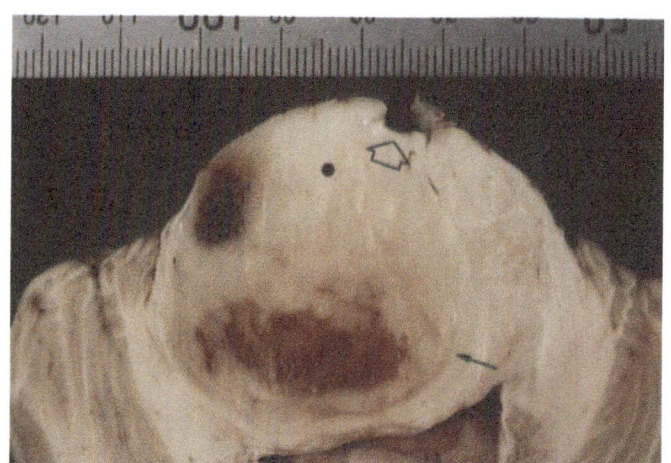

e

Figure 6.25 Pontine astrocytoma, malignant transformation:(**a**) CT + C, (**b**) sagittal T1WI, (**c**) axial T1WI, (**d,e**) fixed autopsy specimens, (**f**) CT, (**g**) CT + C, (**h**) T1WI, (**i**) T2WI, (**j**) fixed autopsy specimen, (**k**) HE ×100, (**l**) HE ×400, (**m**) HE ×100/×400 (all axial images reversed); images show hypodense, hypointense pontine expansion (a–c,f–i), with inhomogeneous, enhancement (a,g); lesion is predominantly unilateral, with en-plaque growth surrounding the basilar artery (c,e, open arrows) and a sharp macroscopic edge (e, closed arrow), shown histologically to be infiltrative (k). Lesion becomes grossly cystic in its rostral extent (h–j, asterisks), with adjacent compressed brainstem (h, arrow-heads). Haemorrhages in fixed specimen (e) are presumably terminal. Histology from pale compact part of tumour (e, dot) shows typical anaplastic astrocytoma (without vascular proliferation or necrosis) (l), while sample from vicinity of haemorrhages . shows tumour to be much more cellular and obviously malignant (m)

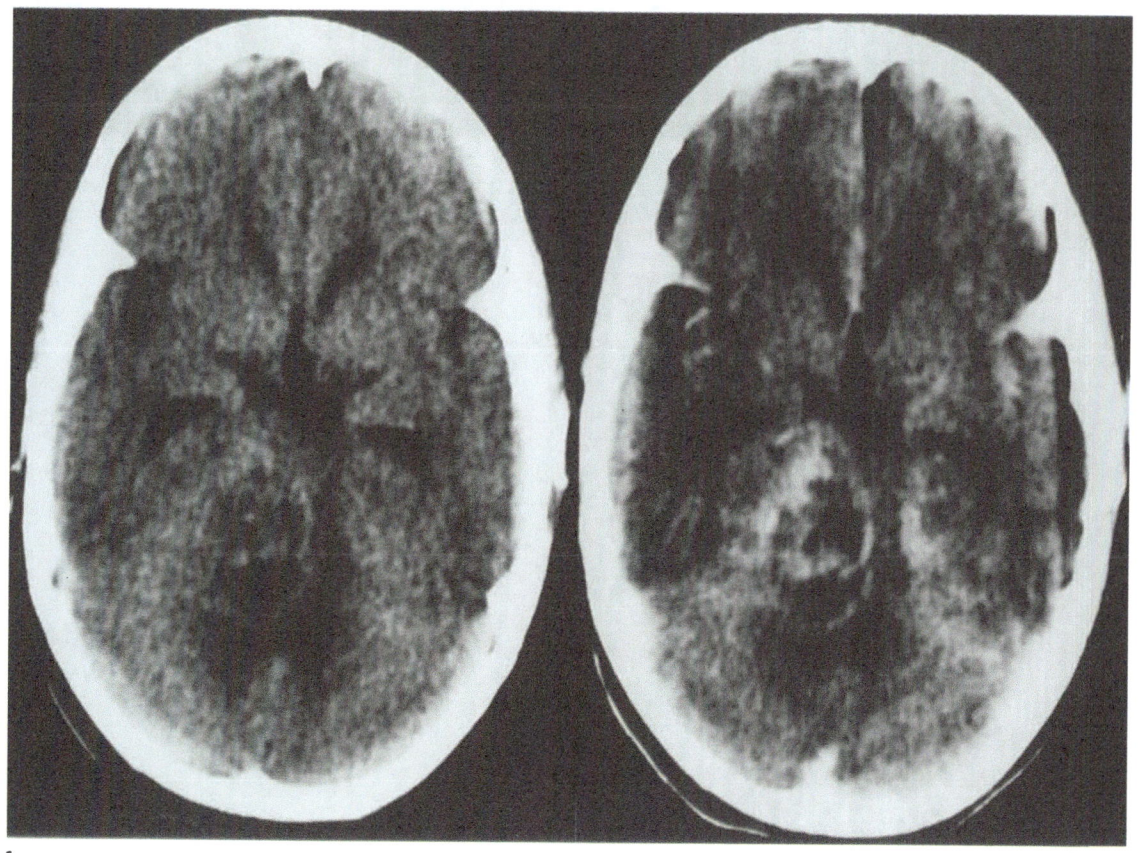

f   g

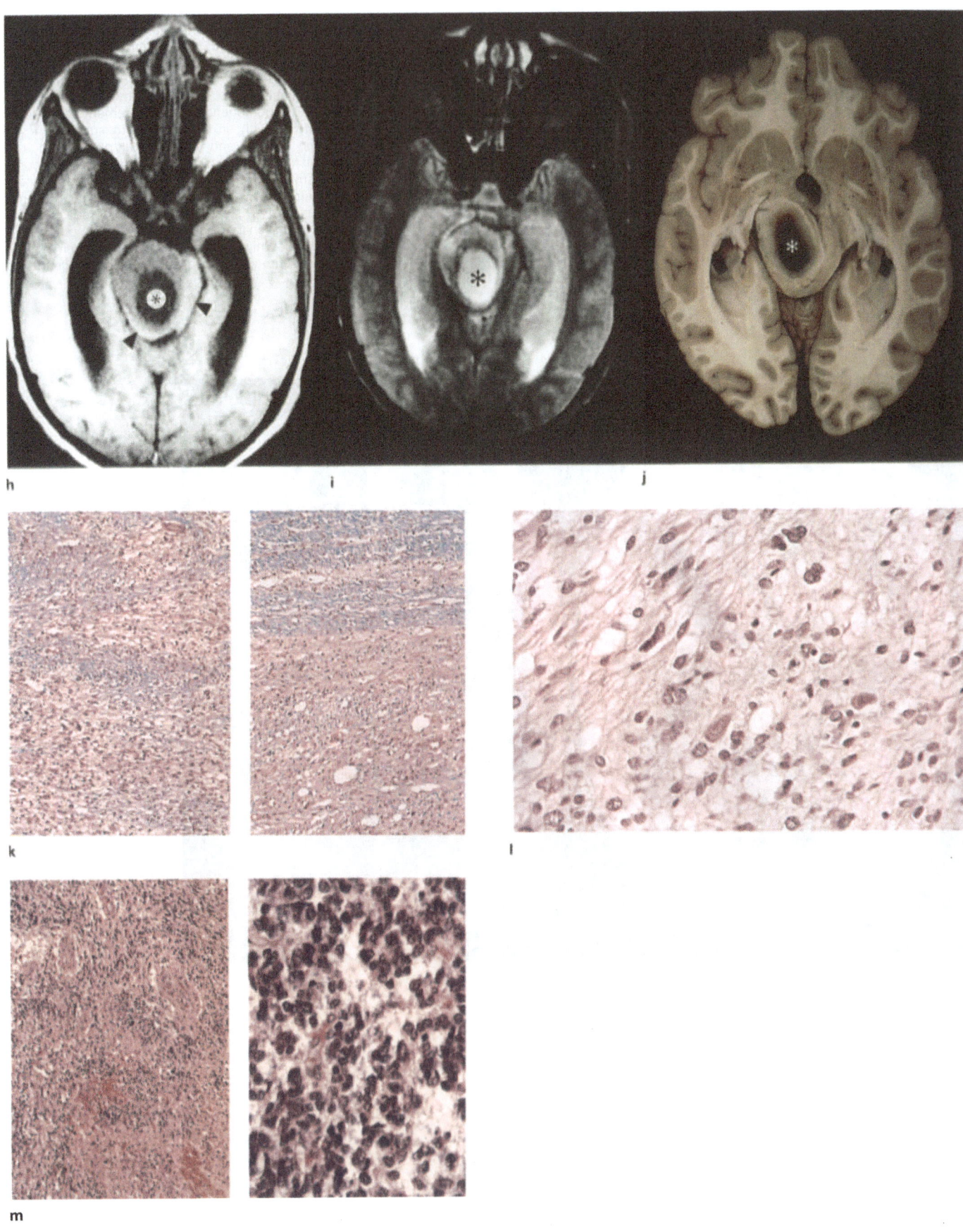

Figure 6.25 (*continued*)

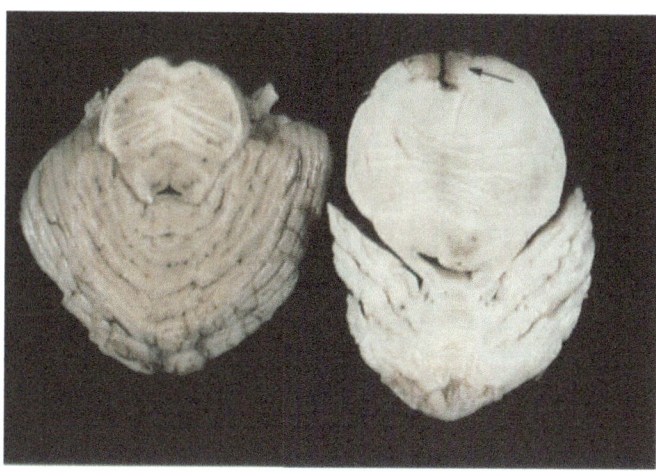

Figure 6.26 Pontine astrocytoma: autopsy specimen showing characteristic homogeneous solid expansion of the pons, with ventral en-plaque growth (arrow); note preservation of pontine fibres and deformed but patent ventricle; compare with normal pons (left). Specimen is a paradigm of images shown in **Figure 6.24**

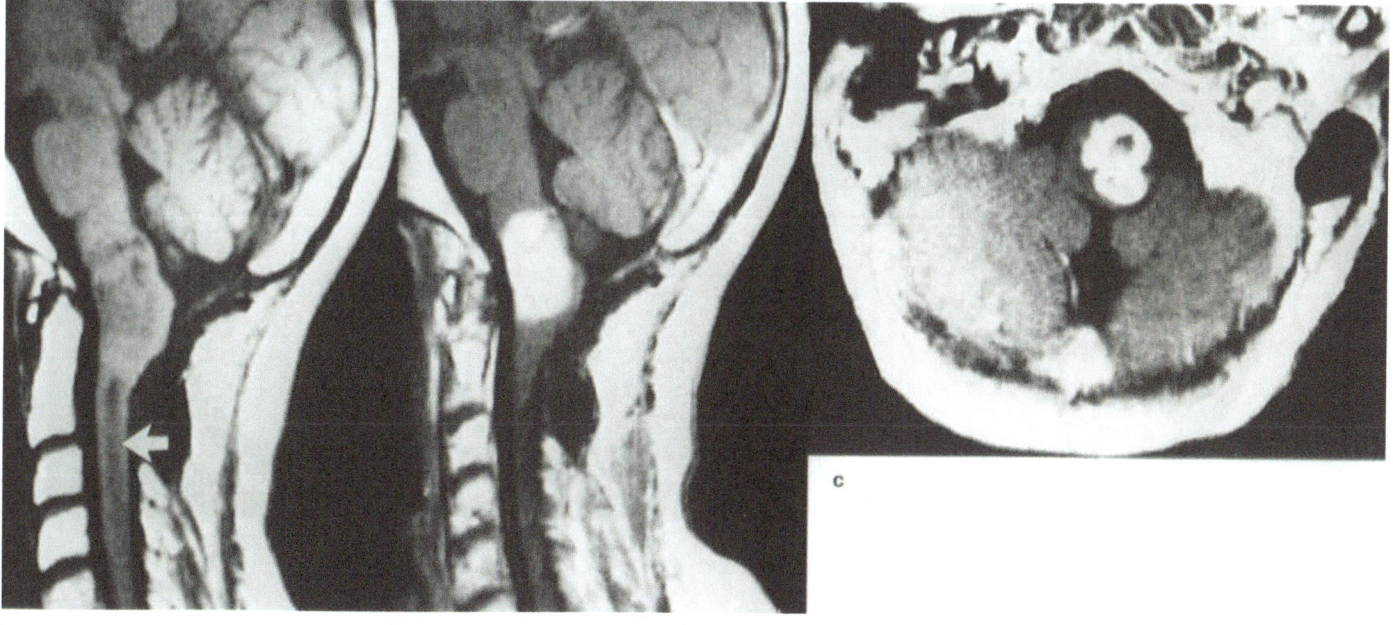

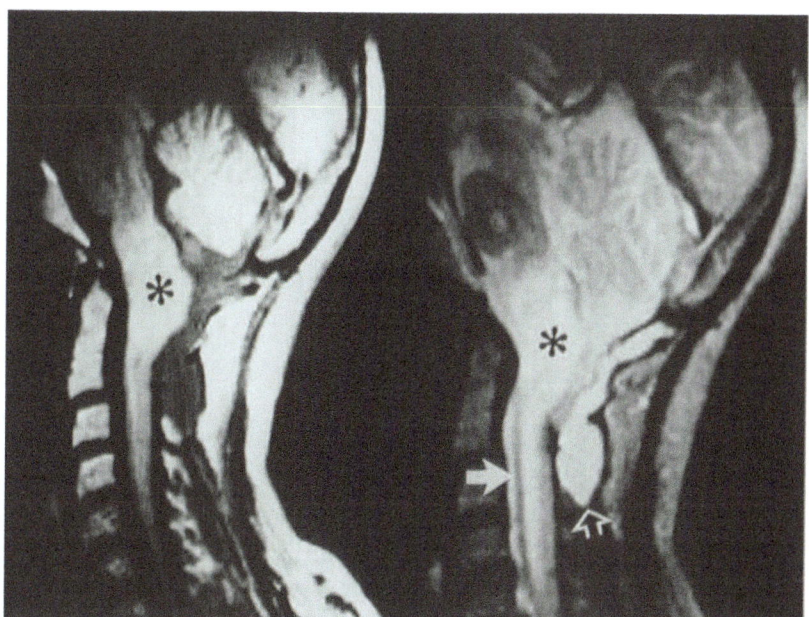

Figure 6.27 Pilocytic astrocytoma, exophytic, medullary: female, 51 years; (a) T1WI, (b) T1WI + C, (c) axial T1WI + C, (d) PDWI, (e) T2WI; images show expansion of the distal caudal medulla by an intra–extraparenchymal, strongly enhancing, lobulated mass with central cyst (a–c). Lesion (asterisk) is hyperintense relative to brainstem and CSF on proton density image (d), becoming CSF isointense on T2WI (e). Rostral cord is cavitated (a,e, arrows). Saccular T2 hyperintense structure (e, open arrow) is a surgical meningocele. Biopsy showed morphologically unremarkable JPA, with slow clinical progression over 4 years. (Dr RM Bowen, Groote Schuur Hospital)

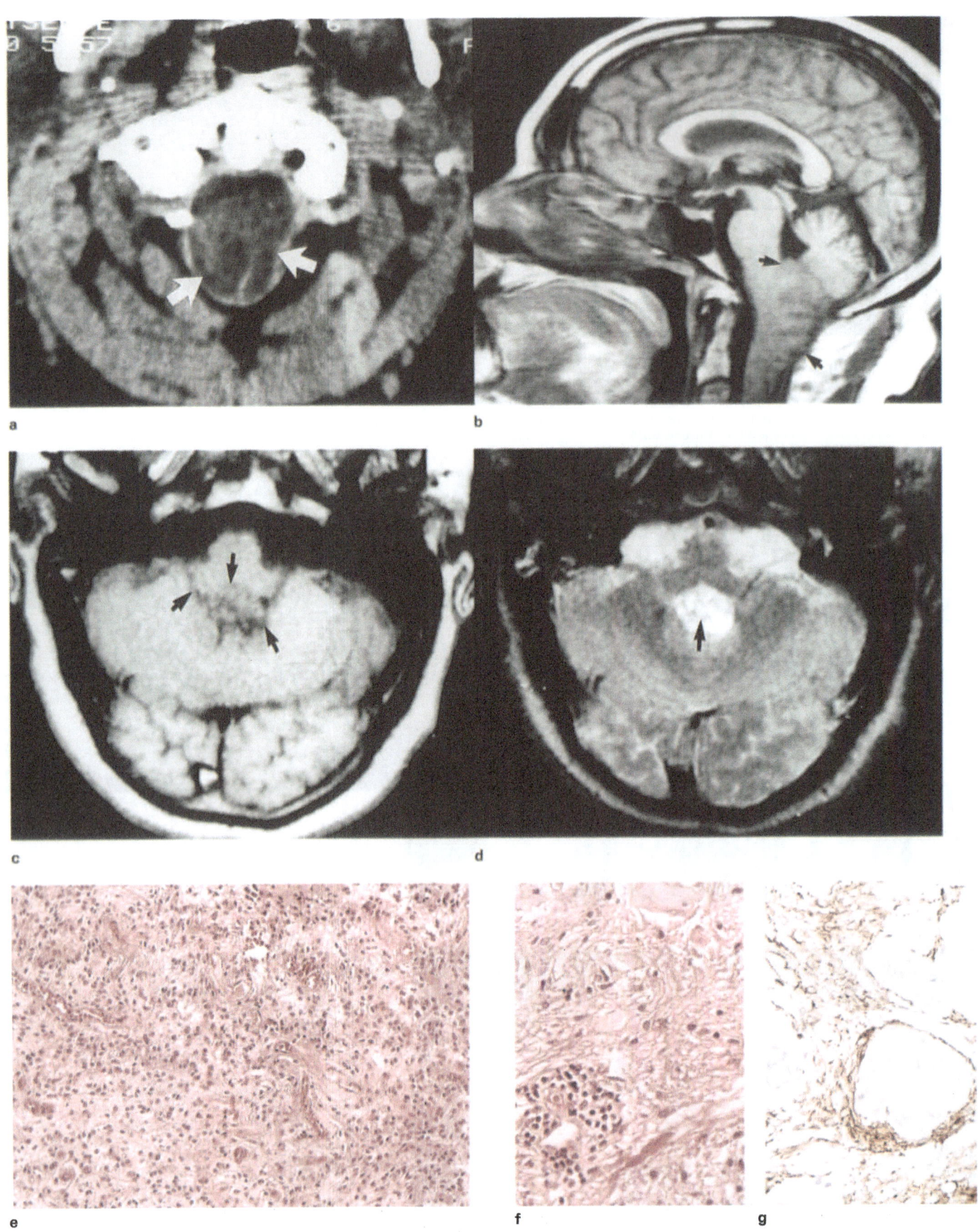

Figure 6.28 'Angioglioma', exophytic, medullary: male, 33 years; (**a**) CT + C, (**b**) sagittal T1WI, (**c**) T1WI, (**d**) T2WI, (**e**) HE ×200, (**f**) HE ×400, (**g**) GFAP ×400, (**h**) VG ×200; postoperative scan shows non-enhancing, hypodense tumour (a, arrows) on dorsum of medulla, extending superiorly into the 4th ventricle, inferiorly to the level of C2 and through the lateral foramen into the subarachnoid space (b,c, arrows). Tumour is inhomogeneous intermediate signal intensity on all sequences, but at long TR (d) is obscured by a mixture of surrounding

CSF hyperintensity and degeneration. Histology shows a fibrillated astrocytoma with typical pilocytic morphology (f,g) and areas which are more cellular where perikarya are prominent (e). The marked proliferative vasculature (h) suggests that non-enhancement on CT is spurious. Collagenous tissue would contribute to T2 hypointensity. There were no features of malignancy and patient has shown prolonged survival (6 years since initial biopsy), consistent with benign exophytic nature of the tumour

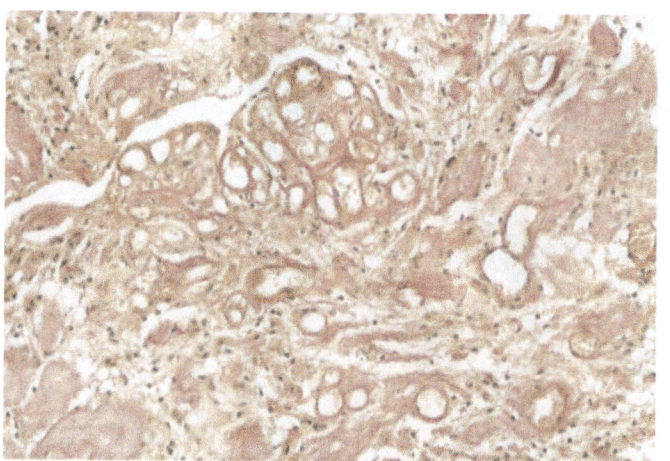

Figure 6.28(h)

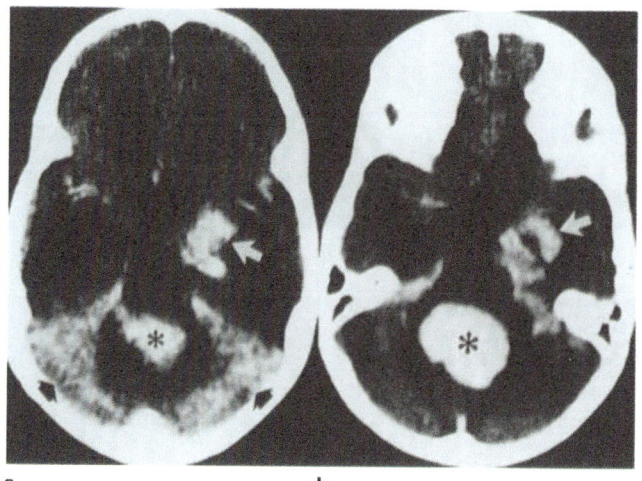

a   b

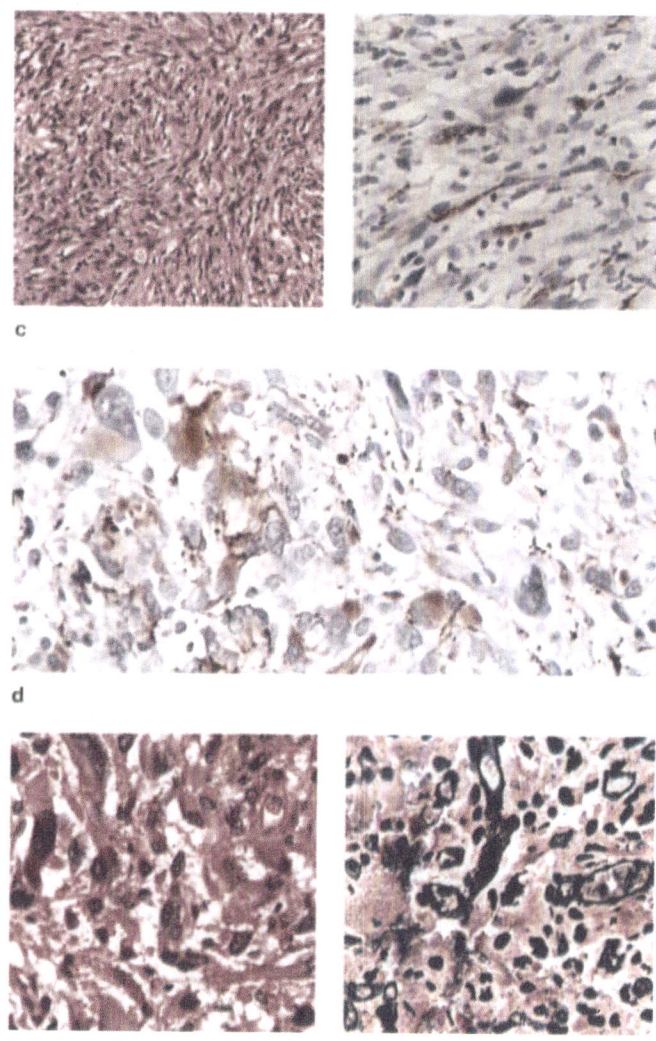

c

d

e

Figure 6.29 Gliofibroma, 4th ventricle, posterior fossa and basal meninges: female, 4 years; (**a,b**) CT + C, (**c**) HE ×100/GFAP ×200, (**d**) GFAP ×400, (**e**) HE ×400/Retic ×200; images show diffusely enhancing tumour occupying 4th ventricle (a,b, asterisks), and growing over the cerebellar surface (a, black arrows) and into the basal cisterns (a,b, white arrows). Histology shows compact, cellular tumour with elongated nuclei (c) (containing abundant reticulin – not shown, but see **Figure 6.30**), and areas of loosely arranged cells with anaplastic nuclei (d,e). GFAP staining is variable (c,d). Angioarchitecture is profuse and capillary in type (e, right). (Sections reviewed by Prof JJ Kepes, University of Kansas)

of enhancement is consistent with a non-neoplastic cyst, whose pathogenesis is uncertain; in these cases the cyst wall is gliotic (Figure 6.35). At short TR, protein concentration often induces loss of differentiation between solid and cystic components (Figure 6.34).

JPA in patients below age 15 has been subdivided into types A and B, having respectively better and worse prognoses[28,29]. However, the only imaging feature incorporated in this classification was topography, so that this important concept awaits many crucial refinements related to enhanced MR.

Fibrillary astrocytoma of the cerebellum appears identical to its hemispheric counterpart (section 4.6a). CT-hypodense, T1 hypointense–T2 hyperintense, non-enhancing parenchymal expansion is centred on white matter, with occasional cyst formation and poorly defined borders (Figure 6.37). In operative specimens from the case illustrated, the cortex was uninvolved.

6.6b. Medulloblastoma (cerebellar PNET)

The concept and morphological implications of the label PNET[30–33] are generally well known, and from the vantage of historical perspective can now be summarized. It is accepted by many, including the WHO[34], that malignant tumours consisting of undifferentiated and thus 'primitive' neuroepithelial round cells should be included, together with the potential for differentiation along glial, neural and even mesenchymal lines, regardless of whether the neoplasm is located in peripheral soft tissues[35], or the CNS. The term is rejected by some neuropathologists[36,37] including the present writers, for a variety of reasons, not least being that in most instances these neoplasms are clear-cut clinicopathological entities which pose no real diagnostic problems when technically adequate material is available. By designating them appropriately, the 'dumping ground' tendency for diagnostically difficult

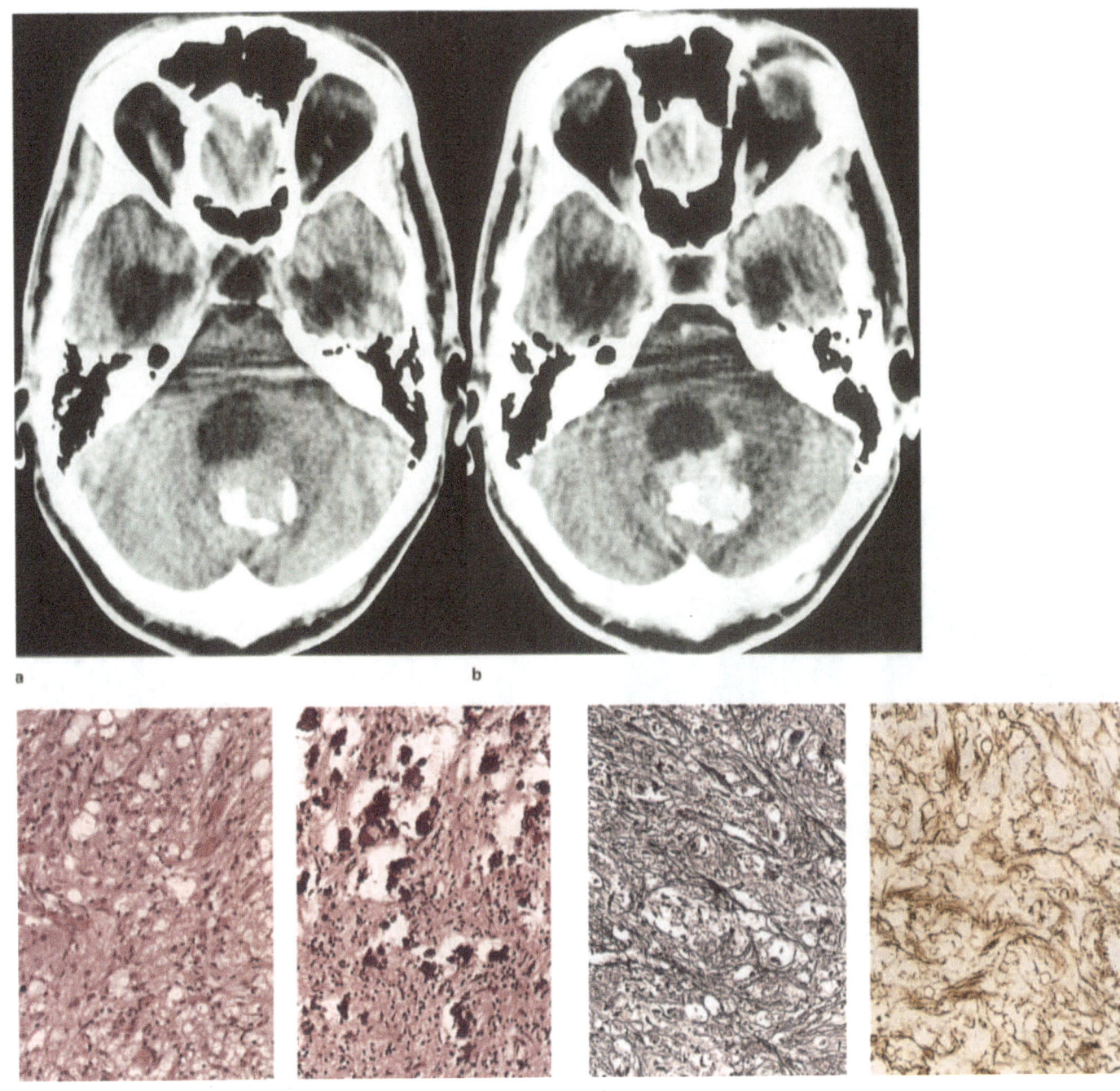

a b

c d

Figure 6.30 Gliofibroma, cerebellar vermis: male, 19 years; (**a**) CT, (**b**) CT + C, (**c**) HE × 200, (**d**) Retic/GFAP × 200; images show an isodense, coarsely mineralized, diffusely enhancing tumour in the cerebellar vermis. Histology shows a mineralized astrocytic tumour. Serial sections (d) show synchronous production of reticulin and GFA protein

tumours is avoided. Radiologists, whilst conceding the difficulties, appear to have accepted the term in a restricted form, to include medulloblastoma, and what they suppose to be its supratentorial equivalent, the cerebral neuroblastoma[20,38,39]. Examination of the relevant cumulative indexes indicates that medulloblastoma is still entrenched in neurosurgical terminology.

The unenhanced imaging characteristic of tumour stroma which is isodense and isointense with cerebellar cortex (Figure 6.38, 6.39 and 6.40), accords well with both the light microscopy and ultrastructure of conventional medulloblastoma: small round perikarya, high nuclear–cytoplasmic ratio and a negligible interstitial space are shared by the cerebellar microneurone population (Figure 6.41). Signal prolongation at both short and long TR is best explained by cyst formation, a process occurring apparently in relation to blood vessels and not associated with tumour necrosis or degeneration (Figures 6.39 and 6.42). In other important respects, however, correlation unaccountably fails. Despite a rather sparse vasculature, most medulloblastomas enhance moderately; some, however, are practically unchanged after contrast, a recognized imaging aberration[40] which is not explained by light microscopy (compare Figures 6.38 and 6.40). Nor does the presence of reticulin appear to confer any significant alteration to the imaging features of desmoplastic medulloblastoma, in spite of the unusual morphology (Figure 6.43).

Most tumours are situated in the midline (vermis), with lateral, meningocerebral location being characteristic of lesions in older subjects (Figure 6.39), but neither CT nor MR has so far provided any additional, site-specific attributes. Indeed, images show the occasional medulloblastoma to resemble a cerebellopontine angle mass.

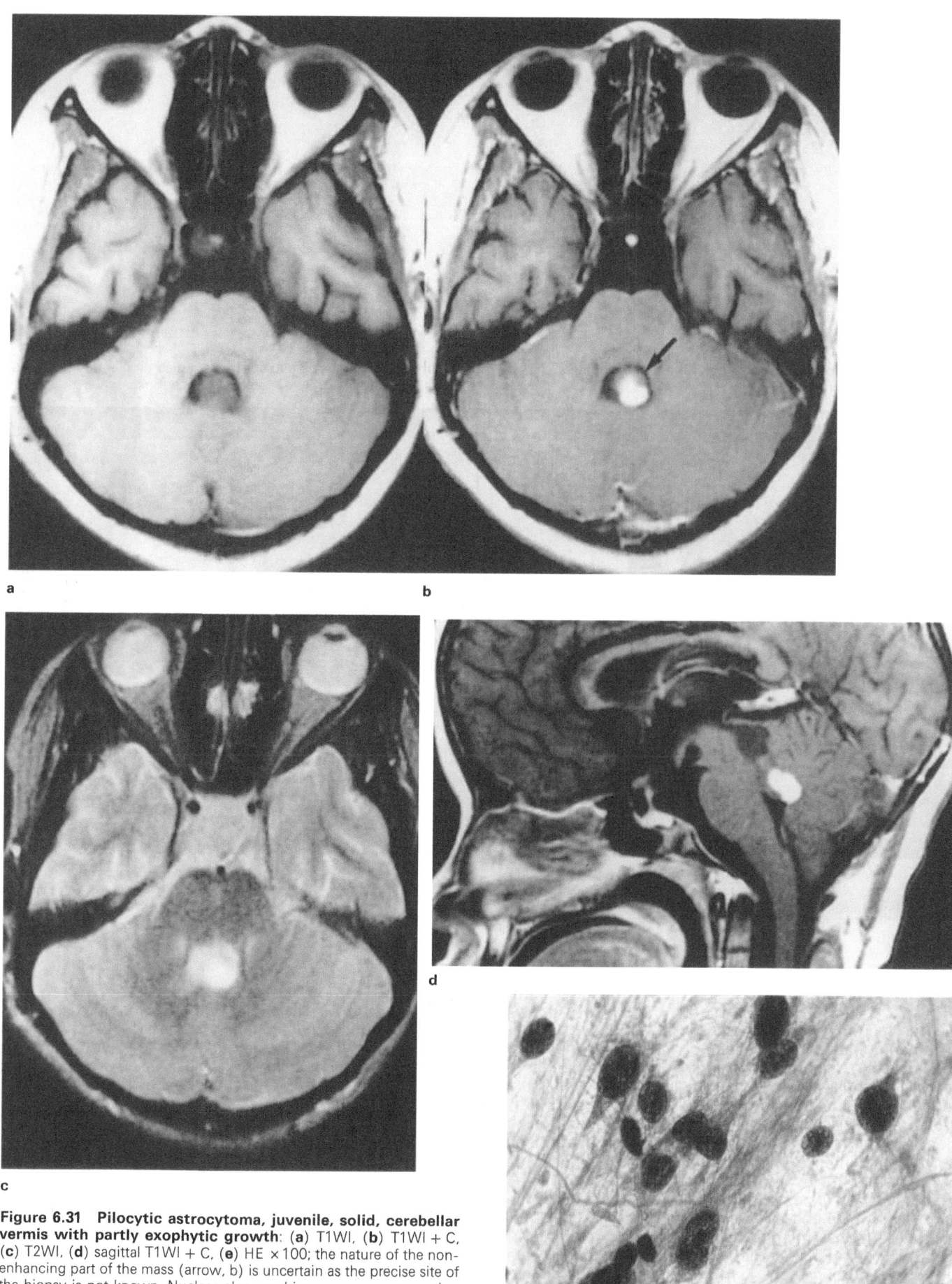

Figure 6.31 Pilocytic astrocytoma, juvenile, solid, cerebellar vermis with partly exophytic growth: (a) T1WI, (b) T1WI + C, (c) T2WI, (d) sagittal T1WI + C, (e) HE ×100; the nature of the non-enhancing part of the mass (arrow, b) is uncertain as the precise site of the biopsy is not known. Nuclear pleomorphism on smear preparation is not unusual

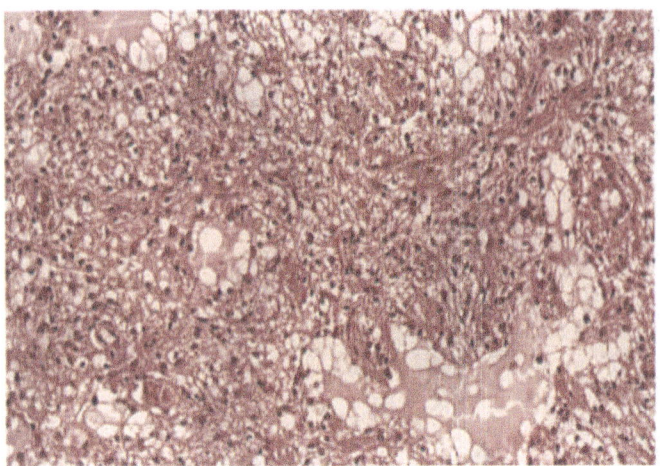

Figure 6.32 Pilocytic astrocytoma, juvenile, cerebellar: characteristic dimorphic growth pattern, with microcysts. HE × 200

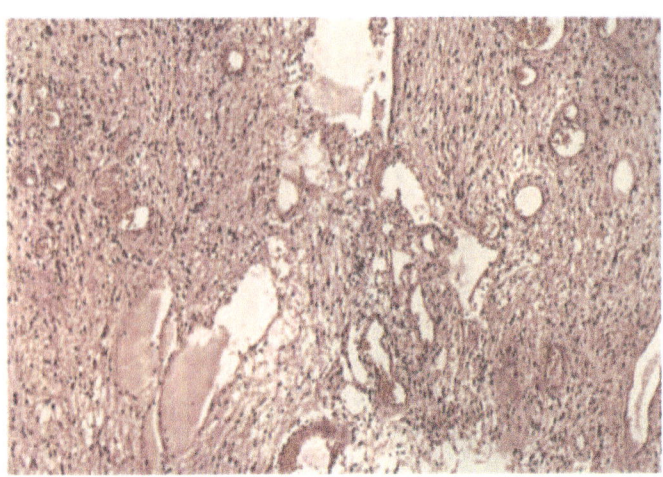

Figure 6.33 Pilocytic astrocytoma: typical proliferative vasculature and solid tumour with interspersed coalescent microcysts

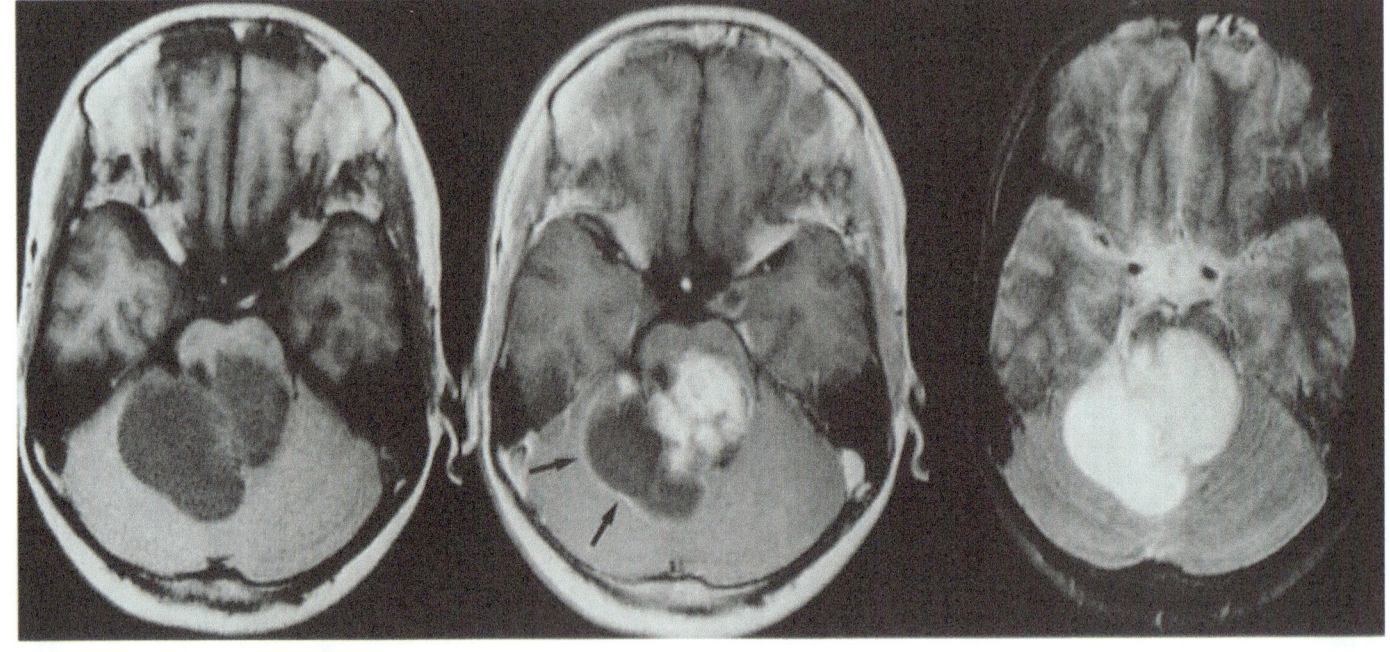

a   b   c

Figure 6.34 (*legend opposite*)

6.6c. Haemangioblastoma

Of the factors which combine to characterize cerebellar haemangioblastoma, presentation in the fourth to fifth decades and meningocerebellar location are probably the most influential. Under these circumstances a cyst with an enhancing nodule can be regarded as pathognomonic[41,42] (Figure 6.44). However, the solid component of the tumour has little imaging specificity, being CT isodense and T1 isointense with cerebellar cortex, moderately T2 hyperintense and strongly enhancing (Figure 6.44), features to be expected from tissue which is composed of cellular, filament-laden vasoformative (mesenchymal) cells with dense intervening reticulin (Figures 6.45 and 6.46). Hyperintensity at long TR, seen best in very small lesions (approximately 1 cm) must reflect a significant extracellular space[43]. The presence of a predominant lipidized stromal cell component (Figures 6.46 and 6.47) might be expected to exert both T1 and T2 signal-shortening, as would the rare event of intratumoural

haemorrhage. The cyst wall is lined by compressed meninges and gliotic cerebellar cortex and does not enhance. Less commonly, the tumour is solid, with contained smaller cysts (Figure 6.48). Whilst vascular signal voids (Figure 6.49) correlate well with the distended vessels which are commonly associated with this tumour (Figure 6.50), spin-echo images do not give any indication of the inconsistent tumour vasculature as revealed by angiography[44], and large vascular channels within the tumour might also explain the T1-mottling effect seen on some images.

6.7. PREDOMINANTLY INTRAVENTRICULAR PRIMARY NEOPLASMS

6.7a. Ependymoma and subependymoma (see also sections 4.10a and 7.5d)

Fourth ventricular ependymomas, by the time they present, occlude the entire space, and their purported origin

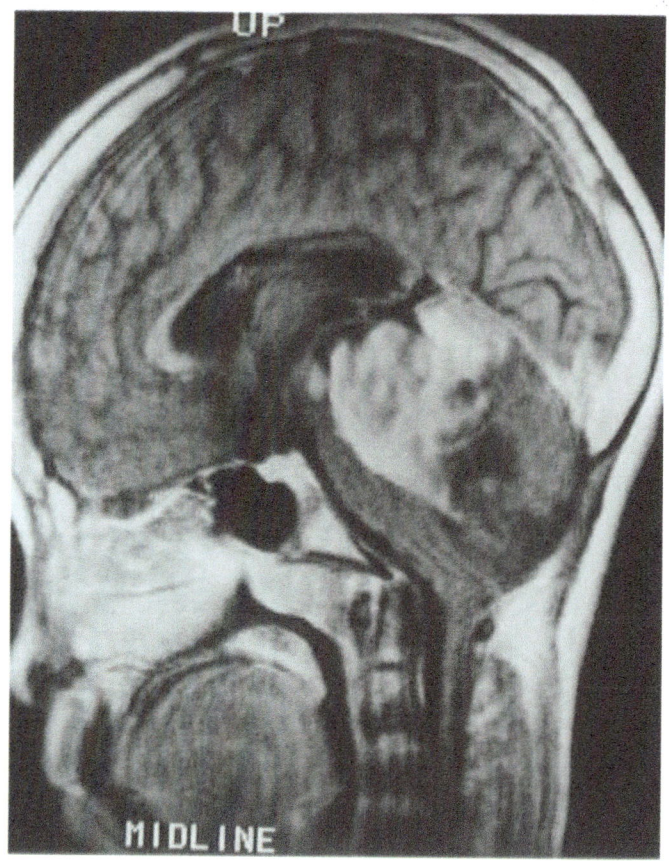

d

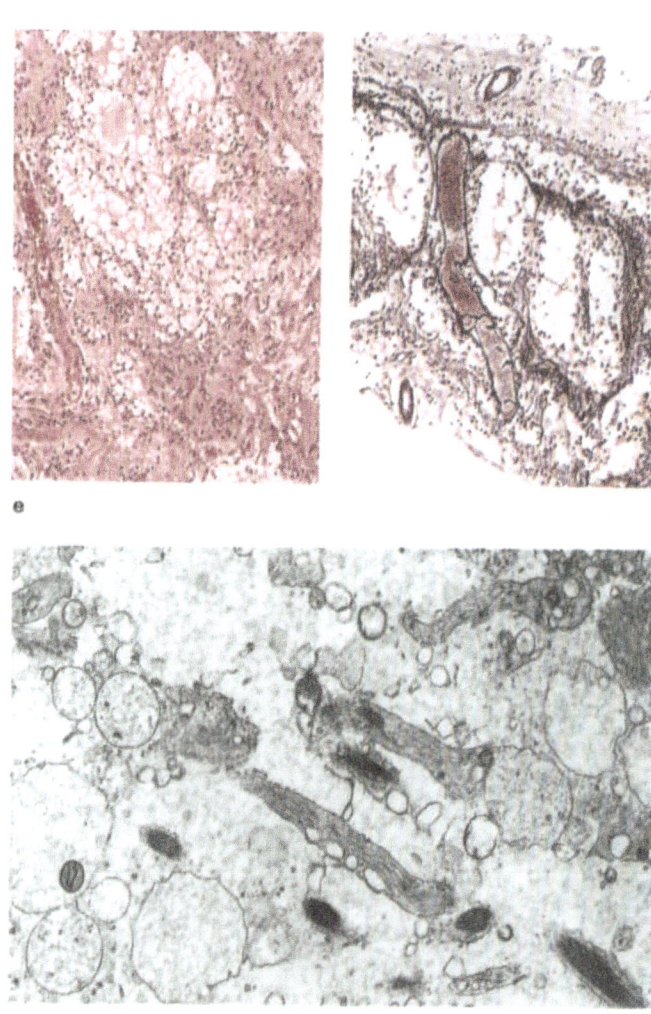

e

f

Figure 6.34 Pilocytic astrocytoma, juvenile, cystic, cerebellar:
(**a**) T1WI, (**b**) T1WI + C, (**c**) T2WI, (**d**) sagittal T1WI + C, (**e**) HE/reticulin ×100, (**f**) EM ×10 800; lobulated tumour occupying 4th ventricle with adjacent parenchymal cyst; both solid and cystic components are similarly T1 hypointense (a), becoming differentiated on T2 image (c); enhancement is diffuse, but reveals tumour lobulation. Cyst wall exhibits rim enhancement (b, arrows), confirmed at operation to be characteristic tumour tissue (e). EM shows abundant intercellular matrix (some membrane-bound), assumed to be responsible for signal prolongation

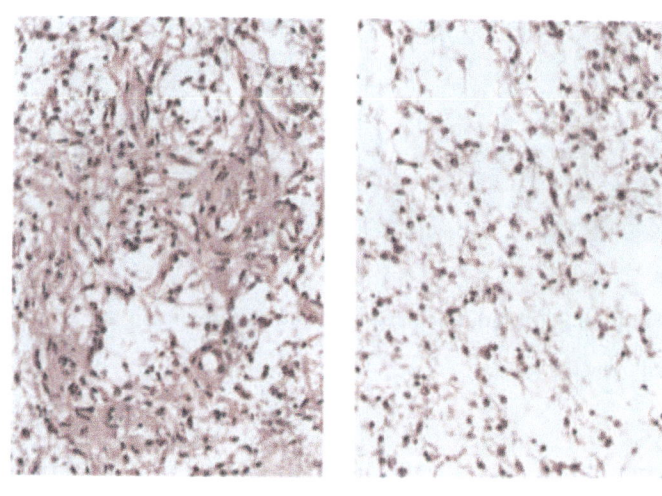

a

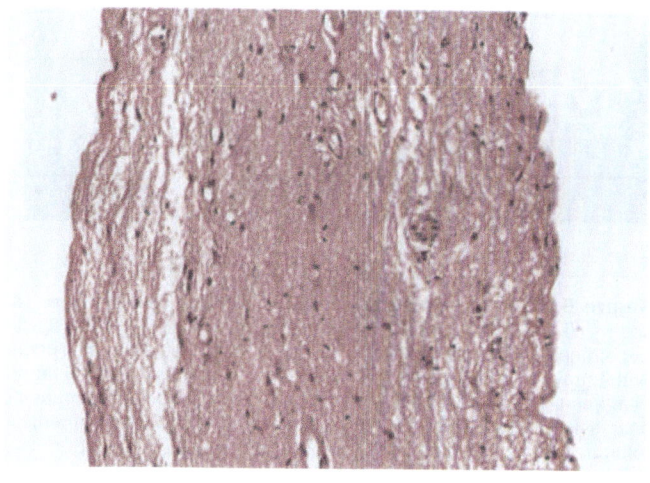

b

Figure 6.35 Pilocytic astrocytoma, juvenile, cystic, cerebellar:
(**a,b**) HE ×200; biopsy showing prominent protoplasmic component (a, right) which probably explains the moderate and inhomogeneous enhancement encountered in some cases. Cyst wall (b) shows gliosis only, consistent with total lack of enhancement

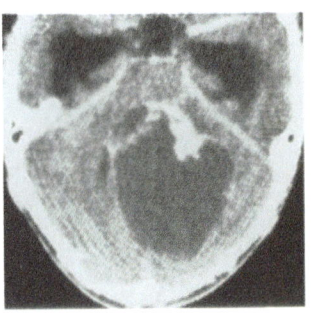

a

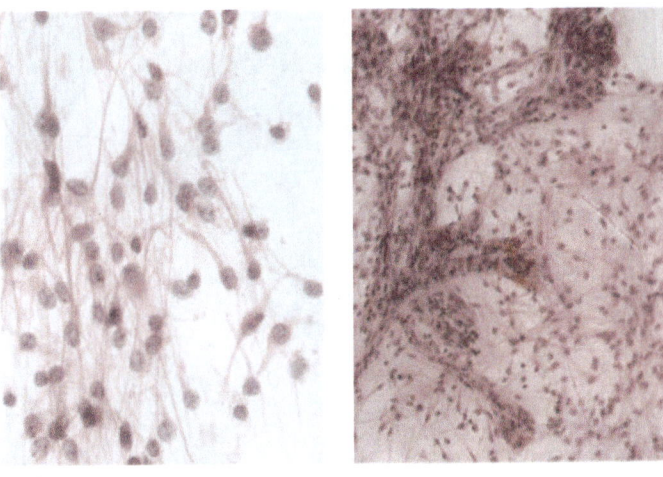

b

c

Figure 6.36 Pilocytic astrocytoma, juvenile, cerebellar, cystic with mural nodule: (**a**) CT + C, (**b**) HE × 400, (**c**) HE × 200 (**d**) HE ×400, (**e**) VG ×100; CT shows strongly enhancing nodule and incomplete cyst wall enhancement. Smears illustrate characteristic cytology and vascular leashes (a,b). Paraffin section (c) shows dimorphic nature of tumour, while sample from cyst wall (e) shows abundant abnormal vasculature, presumably derived from compressed meninges, but no tumour

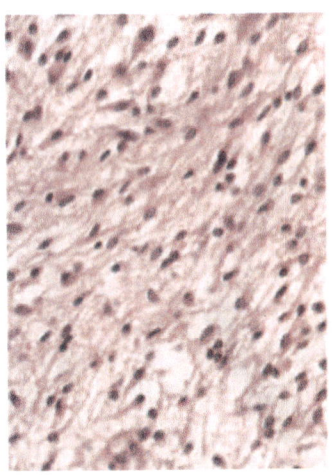

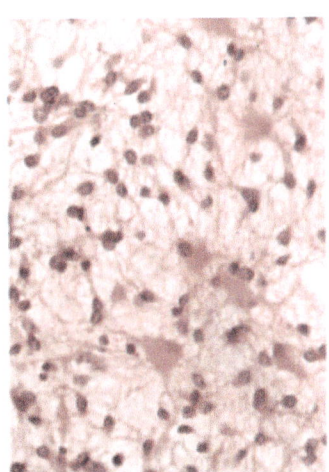

d

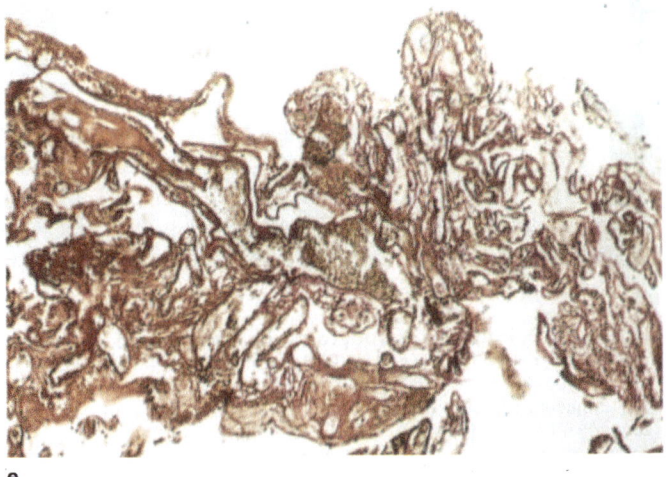

e

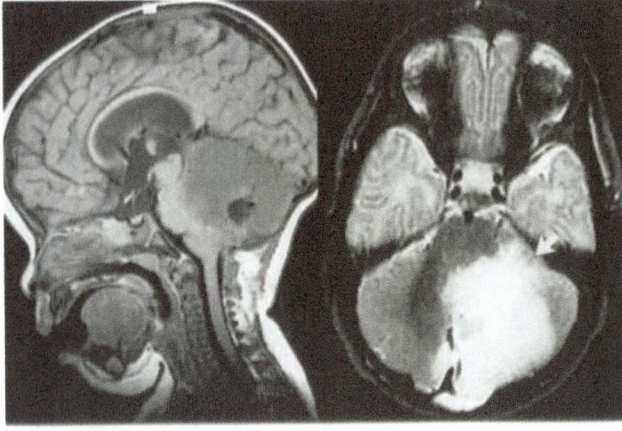

a   b

Figure 6.37 Astrocytoma, fibrillary, diffuse, cerebellum: (**a**) sagittal T1WI, (**b**) axial T2WI; infant with diffuse hypodense, T1 hypointense, T2 hyperintense expansion of L cerebellar hemisphere, with intraventricular and en-plaque growth (arrow) and cyst formation. Features are typical of diffusely infiltrating fibrillary or non-enhancing anaplastic astrocytoma. Biopsy, presumably taken from superficial inferior part of cerebellum, which is not involved by tumour, was inconclusive

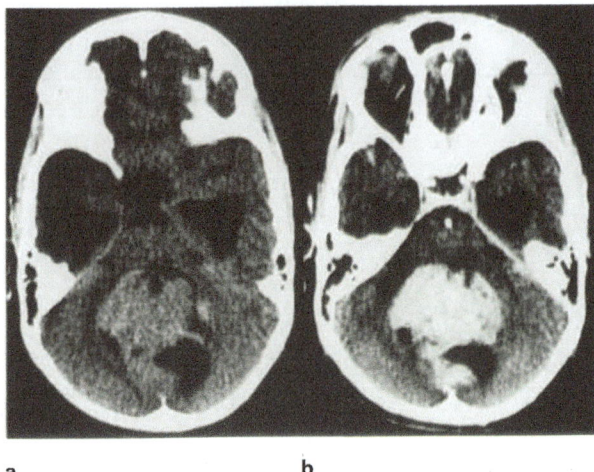

a   b

Figure 6.38 Medulloblastoma, central, enhancing: (**a**) CT, (**b**) CT + C; large, circumscribed mass with cyst formation, strongly and diffusely enhancing

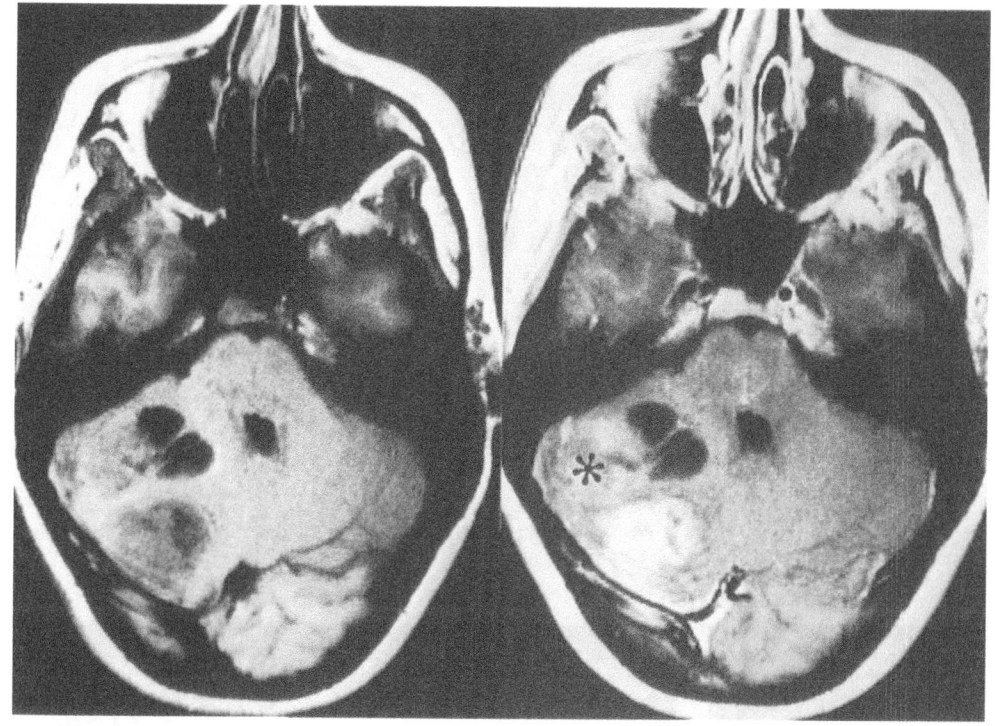

a   b

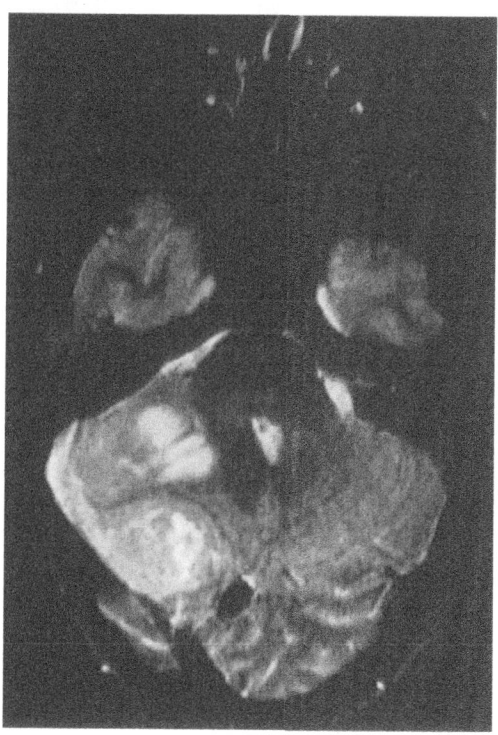

c

Figure 6.39 Medulloblastoma, desmoplastic: (a) T1WI; (b) T1WI + C, (c) T2WI. Lesion is characteristically cortex isointense on all sequences, with cyst formation. Note anterior component (asterisk) barely enhances, unexplained by biopsy morphology, which was unremarkable

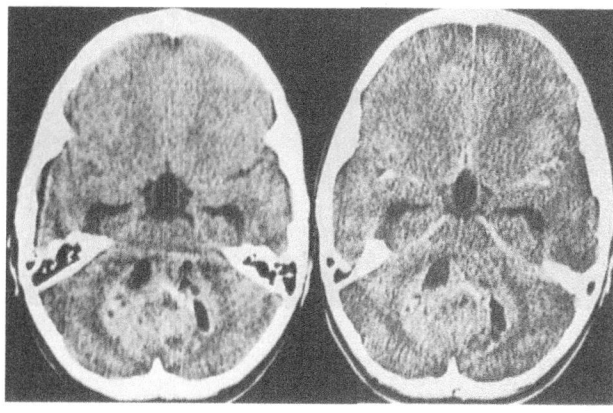

a   b

Figure 6.40 Medulloblastoma, non-enhancing: (a) CT, (b) CT + C; solid cystic midline tumour with focal mineralization (arrow), unchanged following contrast administration. Histology unremarkable. (Dr RM Bowen, Groote Schuur Hospital)

from the ventricular floor[45] is not demonstrable even with MR. This exophytic form of growth, which is emphasized by extrusion through a lateral foramen (Figure 6.51) helps to distinguish ependymoma from JPA and medulloblastoma, both of which may efface the ventricle from without. The rather consistent cytological monomorphism and vasculature tend to brain isodensity and T1 isointensity, with inhomogeneity being principally attributable to the lobulated growth pattern (Figure 6.51). Although the quality of (T1) inhomogeneity is bound to be augmented by the effects of necrosis (Figure 6.53), small cysts and haemorrhage, the conventional morphology of ependymoma does not support the imaging-literature impression that (mineralization excepted) these are either common or characteristic features[46]. The basis of the usual moderate T2 hyperintensity compared with JPA can only be surmised. The extracellular space is somewhat restrained by ubiquitous desmosomes and interdigitating processes (Figure 7.46), but this may be offset by ependymal lumina and/or tubules (Figure 7.46) and interlobular clefts.

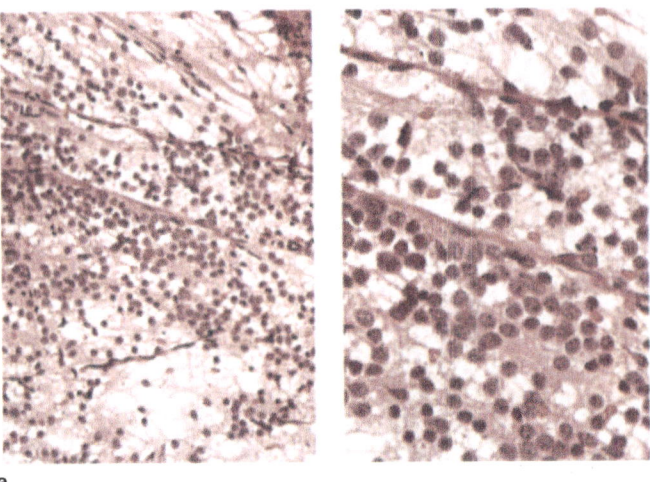

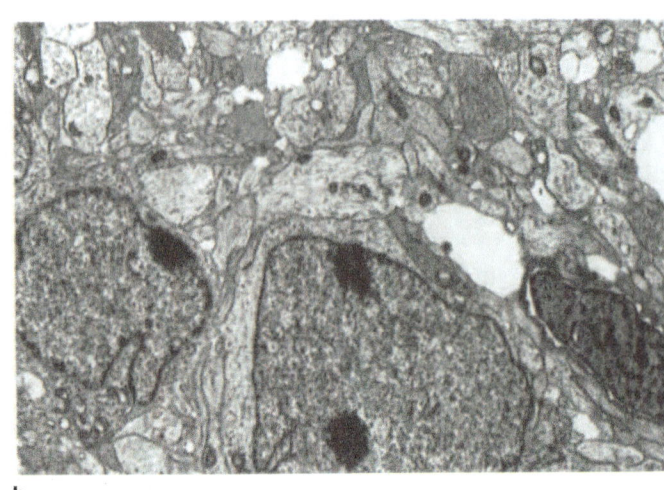

a

b

Figure 6.41 Medulloblastoma: (**a**) HE ×100/×200, (**b**) EM ×6750; characteristic smear showing tendency to cell disruption and inconspicuous capillary vasculature (a). Ultrastructure (b) shows tumour cells with high nuclear/cytoplasmic ratio and closely packed processes with sparse junctions (spaces are artefactual)

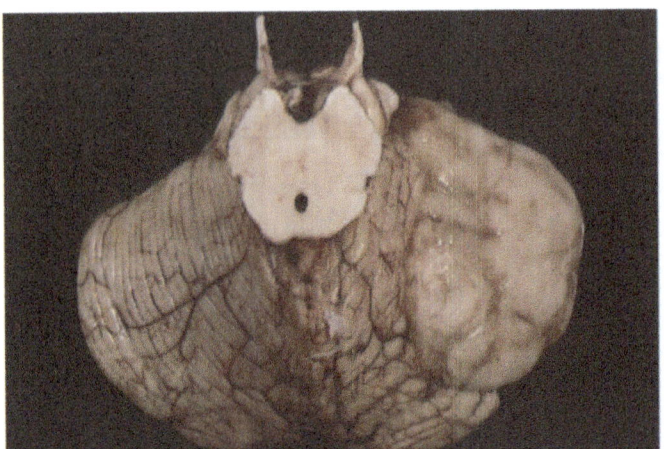

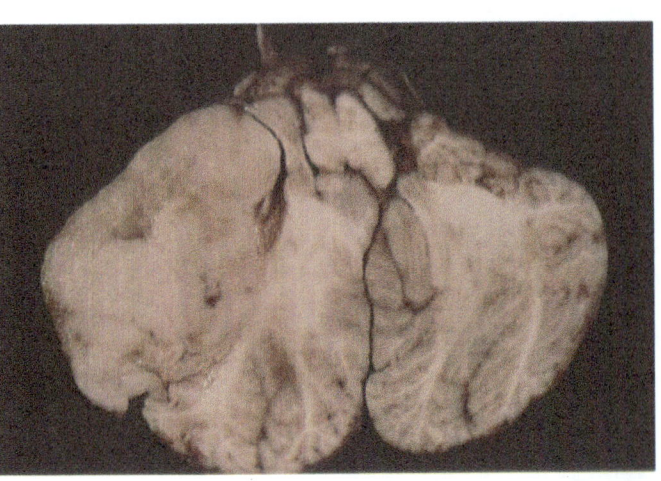

a

b

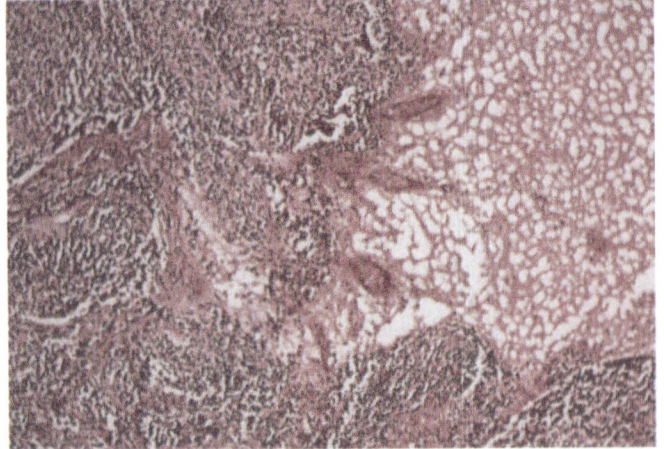

c

Figure 6.42 Medulloblastoma, desmoplastic: (**a**) macroscopic specimen shows characteristic en-plaque meningoparenchymal lobar lesion; (**b**) cut surface showing cystic degeneration and infiltrating edge; (**c**) histology shows cystic degeneration commencing around blood vessels. HE ×100

As with medulloblastoma, enhancement is variable[47,48], sometimes remarkably so, with some components of the solid tumour seemingly refractory (Figures 6.51 and 6.52); in the cases illustrated, biopsy morphology was unremarkable, and this feature remains an enigma (see also section 4.6).

Since the majority of ependymomas appear to be histologically mature, the factors operating to give childhood lesions a typically poor prognosis are not cytologically obvious, although it has been suggested that very high cell density (Figure 6.54) and mitotic activity are indicative of malignancy[49]. In this context the imaging exhibition of variations in enhancement and occasional haemorrhage may *not* have the same predictive significance of other enhancing astrocytic gliomas.

Subependymoma
Opinion is still divided concerning the microscopic criteria for proper identification of this uncommon tumour, being considered a distinct entity by some[50], but classed as a type of mixed ependymal–astrocytic glioma by the WHO[34]. Apart from its occurrence in older individuals, imaging features are reported as being indistinguishable from ependymoma on MR[46]. Morphologically, however, it is much less cellular than ependymoma, and its vasculature may be much more abundant (Figure 4.69) contribu-

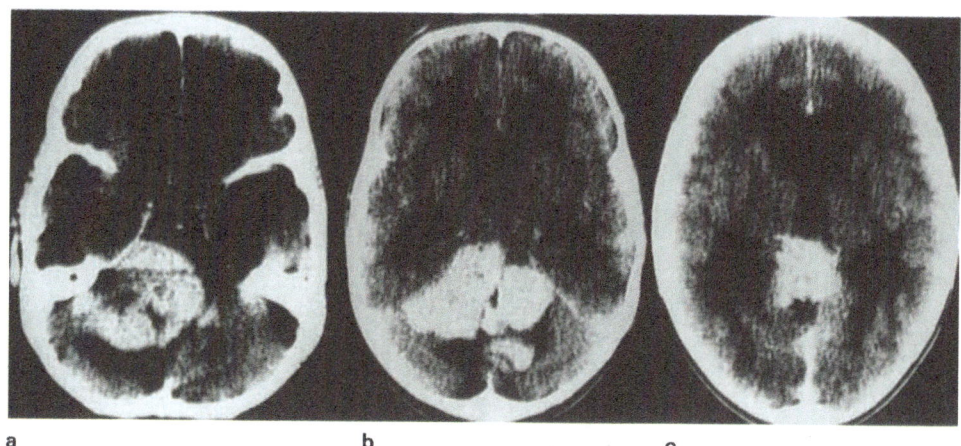

a   b   c

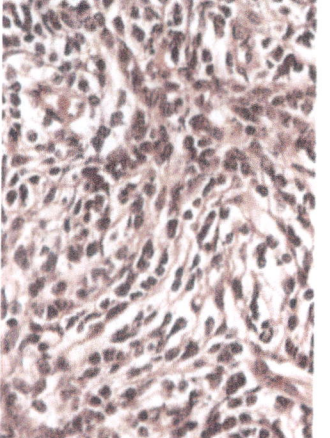
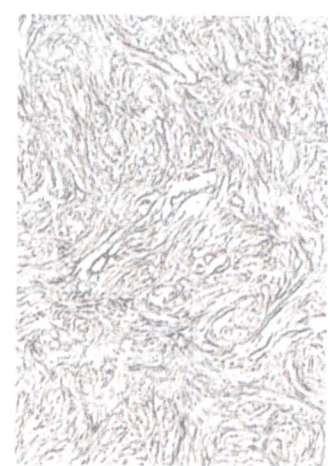

d

Figure 6.43 Medulloblastoma, desmoplastic: (**a–c**) CT + C, (**d**) HE ×400/reticulin ×200; contrasted CT scan shows lateral, solid, lobulated, diffusely enhancing cerebellomeningeal tumour, effacing 4th ventricle (a,b) and extending upwards to the pineal region (c). Histology (d) shows characteristic cellular morphology with prolific reticulin stroma

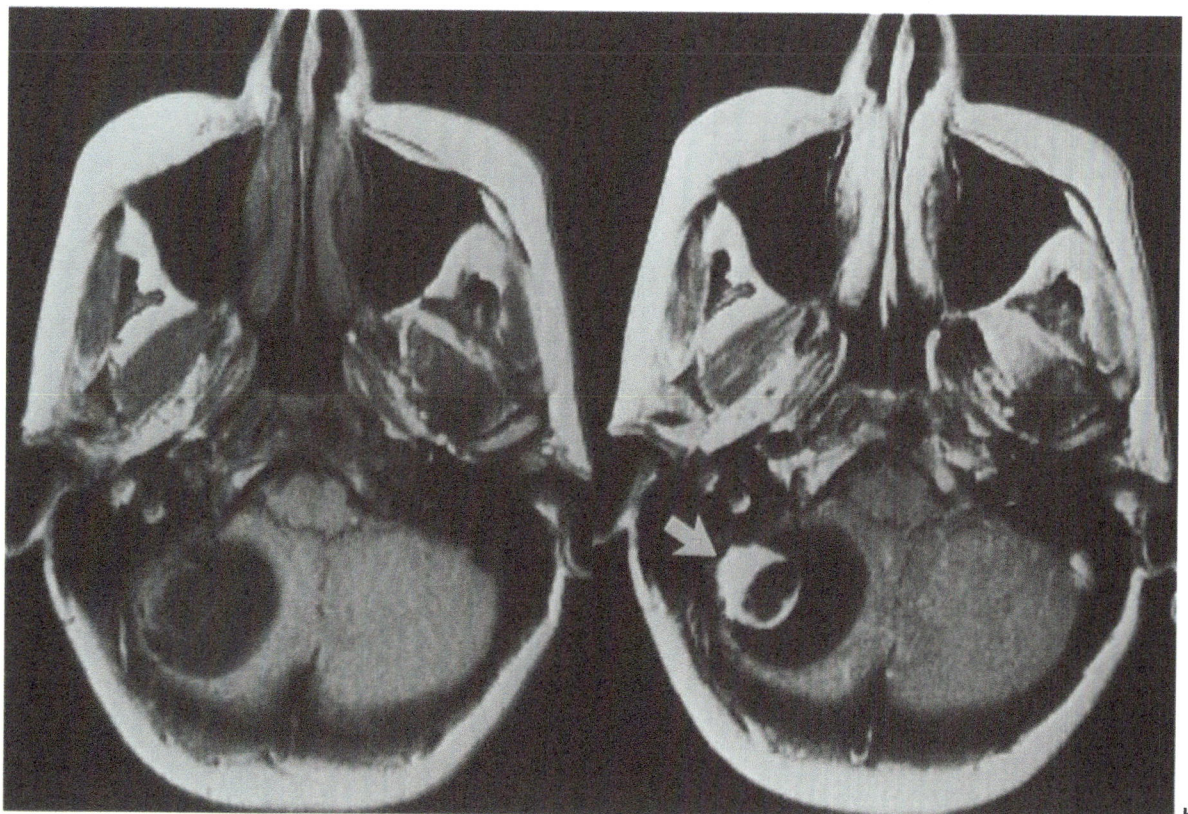

a   b

Figure 6.44 Haemangioblastoma, cystic: (**a**) T1WI, (**b**) T1WI + C; lobar cyst with cystic mural nodule; enhancing tissue is partly meningoparenchymal (b, arrow); wall of cerebellar cyst does not enhance; cyst fluid (a) is hyperintense relative to CSF (lesion shares imaging features with cystic pilocytic astrocytoma – compare with **Figure 4.49**). (Dr JW Lotz, City Park Hospital)

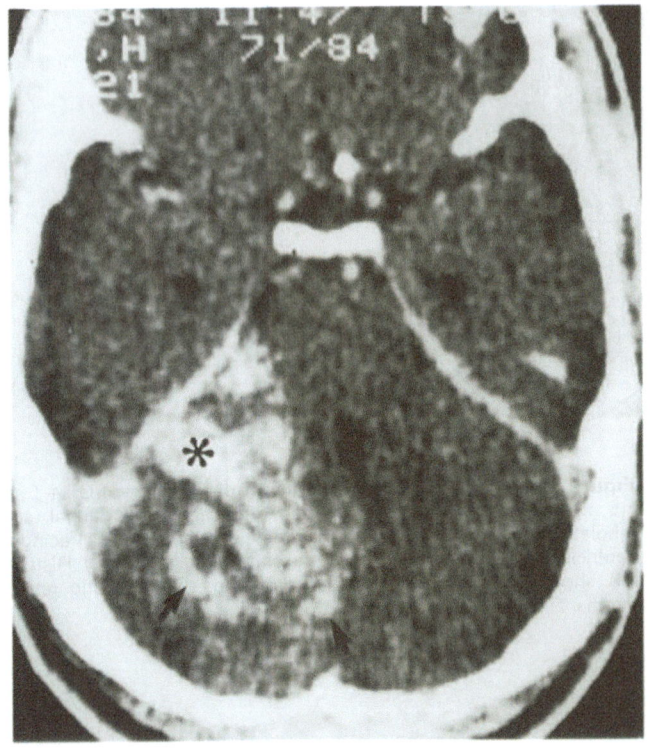

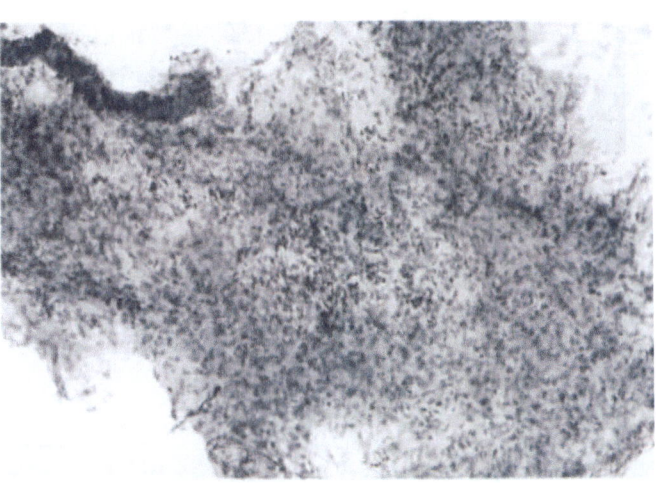

a

b

Figure 6.45 Hemangioblastoma, solid: (**a**) CT + C, (**b**) Tol blue ×200; image shows strong but patchy/inhomogeneous enhancement, presumably partly due to large ectatic vessels (arrows); more circumscribed part of the lesion (asterisk) is characteristically intra–extra-

cerebellar. Smear preparation shows characteristically dense and untidy tissue caused by adhesion of cells and vessels, due to abundant reticulin (see **Figure 6.46**)

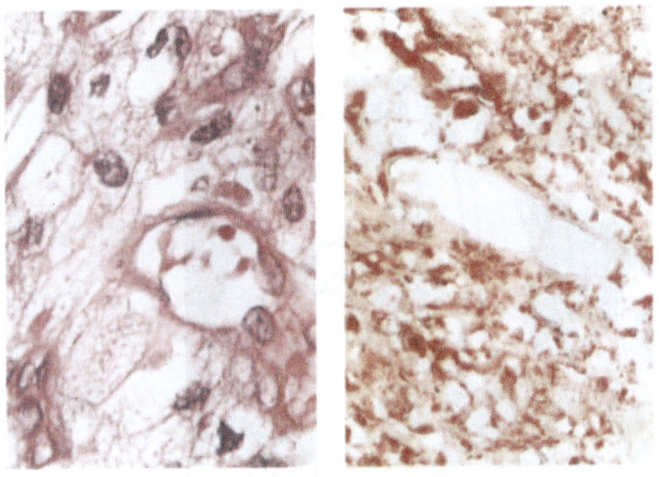

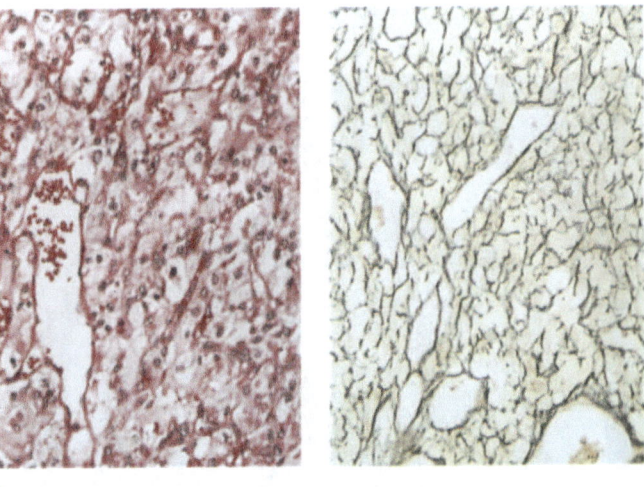

a

b

Figure 6.46 Haemangioblastoma (**a**) HE ×400/FF ×200, (**b**) HE/Retic ×200; illustrates lipidized stromal cells, theoretically respon-

sible for T1 signal shortening; high reticulin content usually makes intraoperative smear preparation difficult (see **Figures 6.45** and **6/47**)

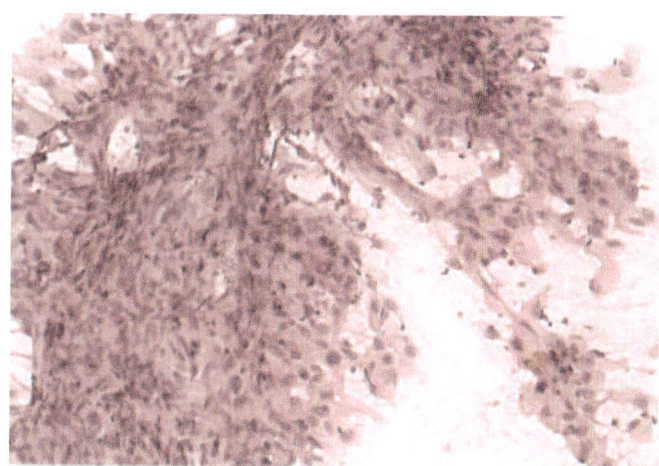

Figure 6.47 Haemangioblastoma: intraoperative smear showing unusual preponderance of plump, finely vacuolated, stromal cells. HE ×200

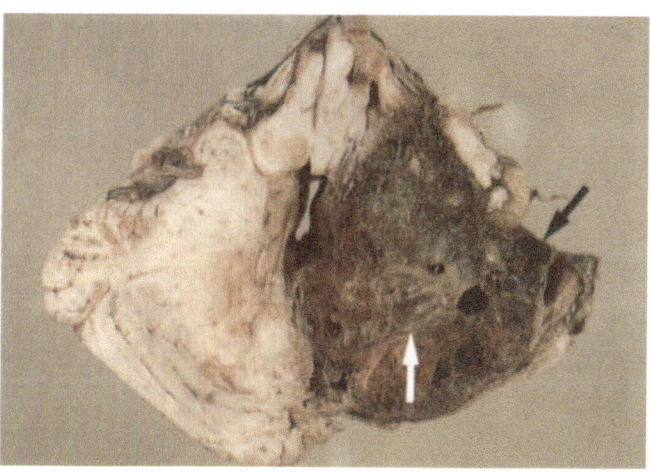

Figure 6.48 Haemangioblastoma: large solid superficial tumour containing admixed cystic and vascular spaces (arrows); note gelatinous quality of central cystic degeneration, consistent with its transudative nature*. (Dr DB Brownell, Frenchay Hospital)
*Cumings JN. The chemistry of cerebral cysts. Brain. 1950;73:244–50.

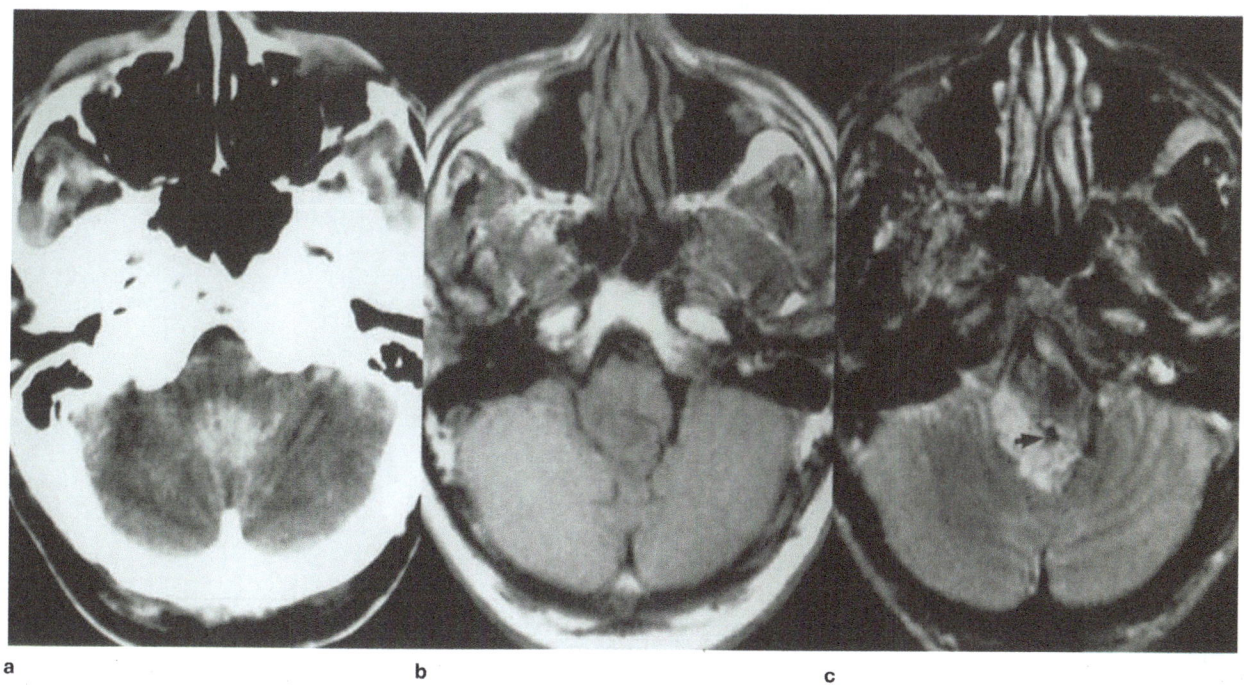

a   b   c

Figure 6.49 (*legend overleaf*)

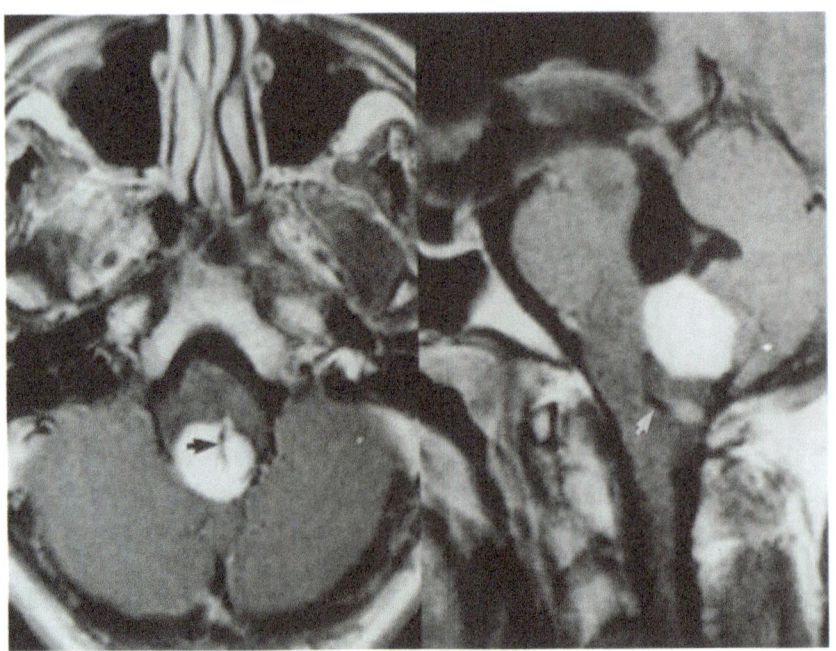

d   e

Figure 6.49 Haemangioblastoma, dorsal medulla: (**a**) CT + C, (**b**) T1WI, (**c**) T2WI, (**d**) axial T1WI + C, (**e**) sagittal T1WI + C, (**f**) EM x9000; poorly demonstrated, enhancing lesion on CT (a) is shown on MR to be a circumscribed, lobulated T1 isointense (b), T2 hyperintense mass (c), with strong homogeneous enhancement (d,e); vascular flow voids are visible in c–e (arrows). Electron microscopy (f) shows abnormal vessel, probably fenestrated, with prominent, perivascular, replicated basal laminar material (asterisk) and adjacent lipid vacuoles (arrow)

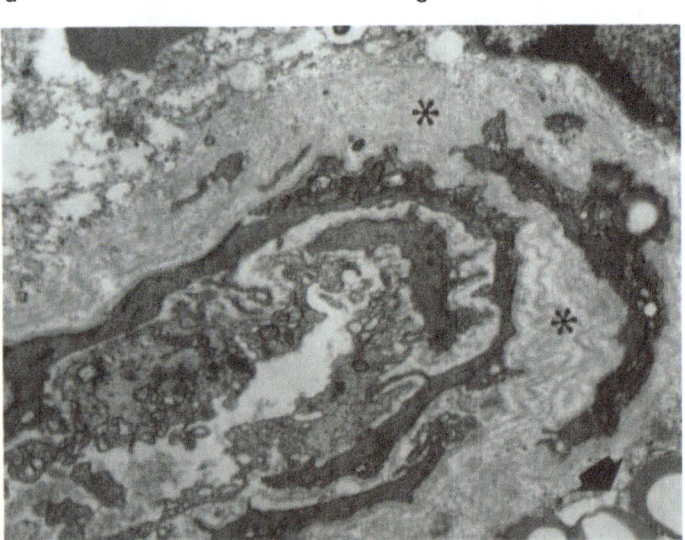

f

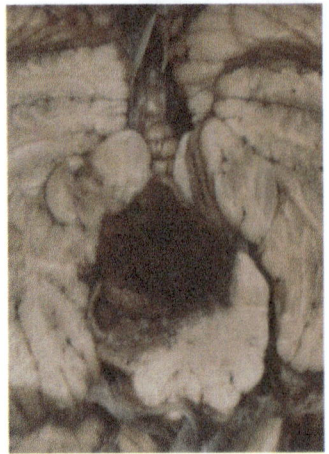

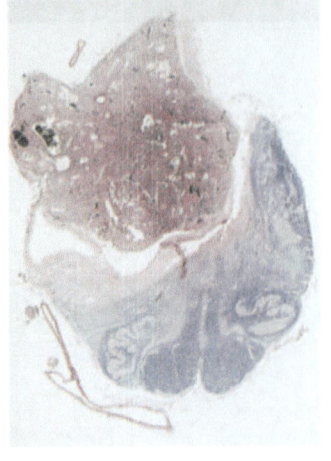

a   b

Figure 6.50 Haemangioblastoma: (**a**) fixed autopsy specimen, (**b**) whole mount; discrete yellow/haemorrhagic tumour, probably originating from · medullary floor of the 4th ventricle; parenchyma shows commencing cystic degeneration. Whole mount (b) reveals vascular honeycombing of tumour

ting, at least in some instances, to the focal nature of T2 inhomogeneity and enhancement.

6.8. METASTASIS

The morphology and signal characteristics of metastatic epithelial neoplasms are discussed in section 4.12. The reputation of metastatic carcinoma to be the commonest neoplasm of the adult posterior fossa[51], applies principally to the cerebellum and its coverings; intraparenchymal brainstem lesions are rare by comparison. The principal source of T2 signal prolongation (hyperintensity) in otherwise cortex isointense tissue (Figure 6.55), is cystic necrosis, also a singular feature of bronchial carcinoma. Conversely, acute haemorrhage or mucin induce T2 hypointensity (Figure 6.56).

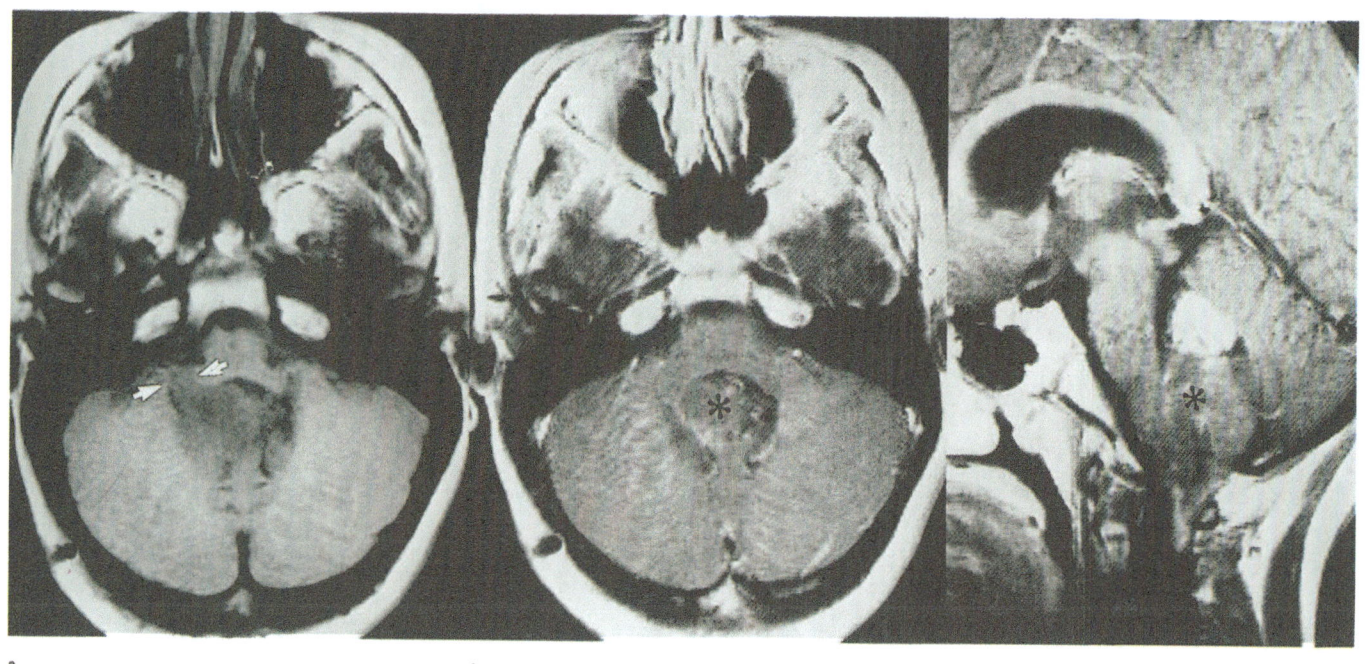

a   b   c

Figure 6.51 Ependymoma, intraventricular: (**a**) T1WI, (**b**) T1WI + C, (**c**) sagittal T1WI + C; lobulated, T1 hypointense, intraventricular tumour growing through lateral foramen (a, arrows); tumour shows focal diffuse enhancement (c), with areas which are non-enhancing (b,c, asterisks). Histology showed ependymoma with no unusual features and pattern of enhancement is unexplained

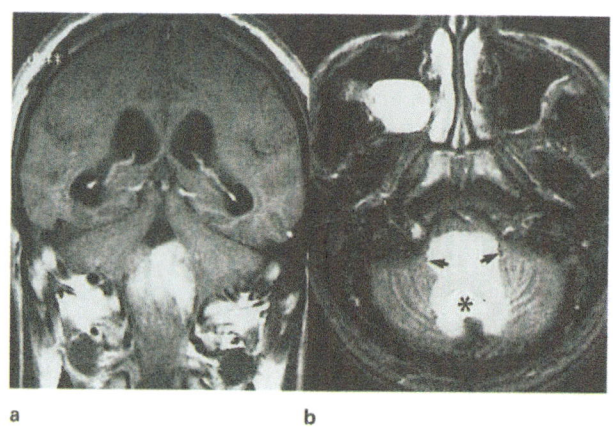

a   b

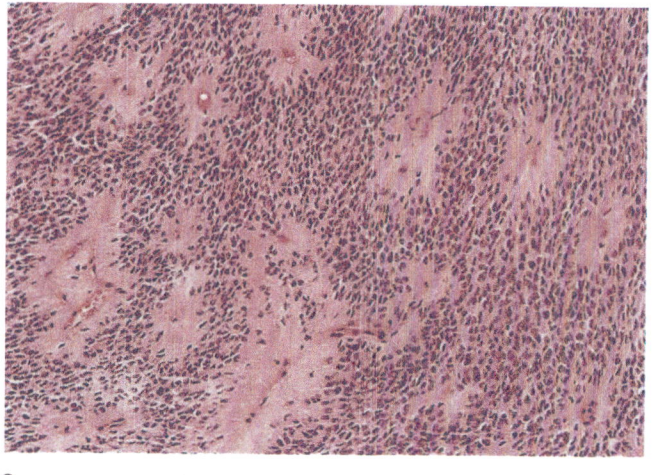

c

Figure 6.52 Ependymoma, intraventricular: (**a**) T1WI + C, (**b**) T2WI, (**c**) HE × 200; mass obliterates inferior 4th ventricle and is partially enhancing (a); T2 weighted image shows untidy infiltrative edge of neoplasm (arrows), with focal homogeneous component (asterisk) shown at operation to be haematoma (likely to be pressure-related). Tumour is histologically unremarkable (c), despite imaging and surgical evidence of infiltration

6.9. RARE LESIONS

6.9a. Choroid plexus papilloma[52]

While lateral ventricular papillomas (section 4.10c) are found most frequently in children, infratentorial examples usually present in the late teenage and early adult years. The imaging features are non-specific, being iso- to hypointense at short TR and iso- to hyperintense on T2 weighted sequences. Enhancement is moderate to intense, consistent with the vasculature of these tumours. Calcification may result in a degree of inhomogeneity. Like ependymomas, papillomas may extend through the exit foramina of the 4th ventricle.

6.9b. Vascular lesions

The recognized natural history of capillary–cavernous or 'angiographically occult' angioma has led to an aggressive neurosurgical approach to these lesions occurring in the brainstem[53], where they present as acute, spontaneous intraparenchymal haematomas (Figure 6.57). Hypertensive haemorrhages, although infrequently a neurosurgical problem, also occur at this site (Figure 6.58). The imaging features of parenchymal haemorrhages are discussed in section 4.1b.

6.9c. Chordoma (see also section 2.6f)

Cranial lesions are usually related to the clivus, from where they may grow upwards into the suprasellar cistern, or posteriorly into the prepontine cistern and cerebellar pontine angle, with painless destruction of bone. Chordoma forming a CP angle mass will have originated from the adjacent bone, usually the clivus, which will show evidence of destruction as seen on the CT (Figure 2.27).

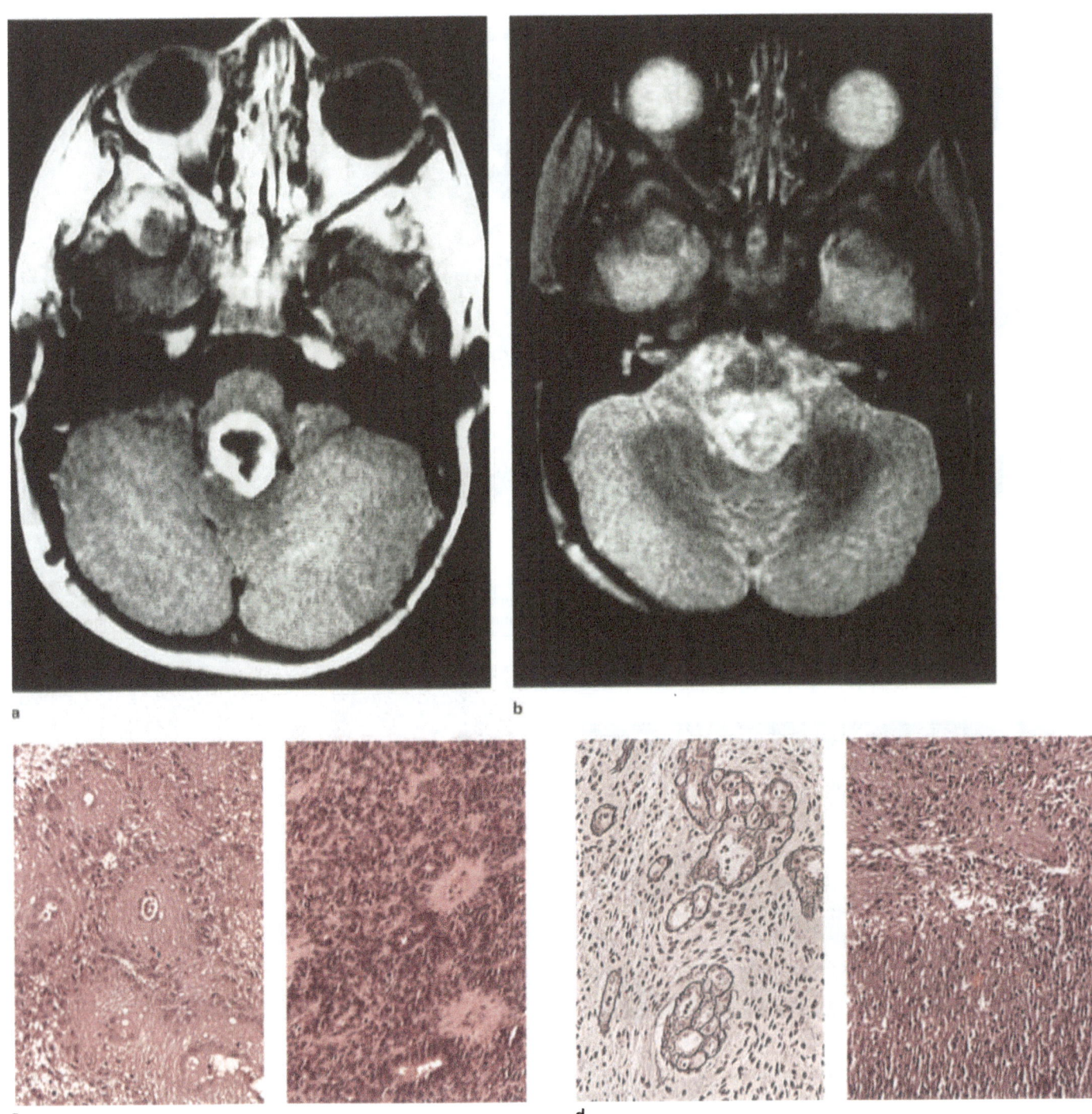

Figure 6.53   Ependymoma, ring-enhancing, 4th ventricle: (a) T1WI + C, (**b**) T2WI, (**c**) HE × 200, (**d**) Retic/HE × 200; circumscribed enhancement with central hypointensity (a), becomes inhomogeneous on T2 weighted image (b); peripheral signal hyperintensity is oedema and CSF. Histology shows typical nuclear-free perivascular rosettes with variation in cellularity (c), and florid proliferative vasculature (d, left), with adjacent necrosis (d, right). Although biopsy was not stereotactic, necrosis was thought to explain the central non-enhancement. The significance of proliferative vessels in these tumours is uncertain

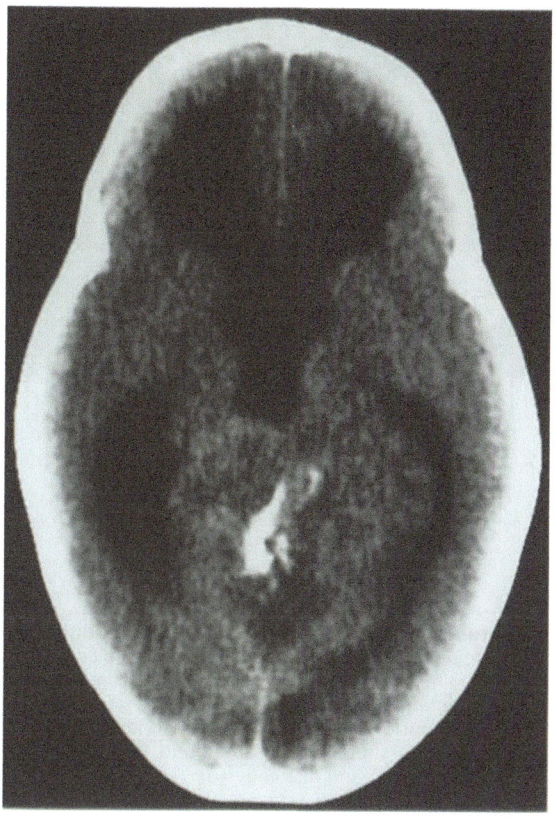

a

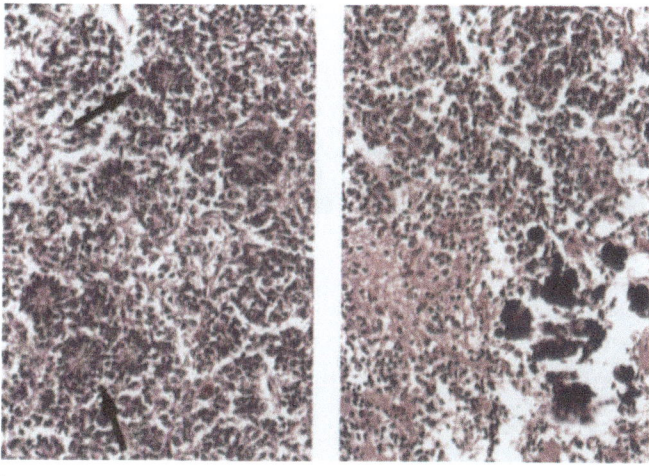

b

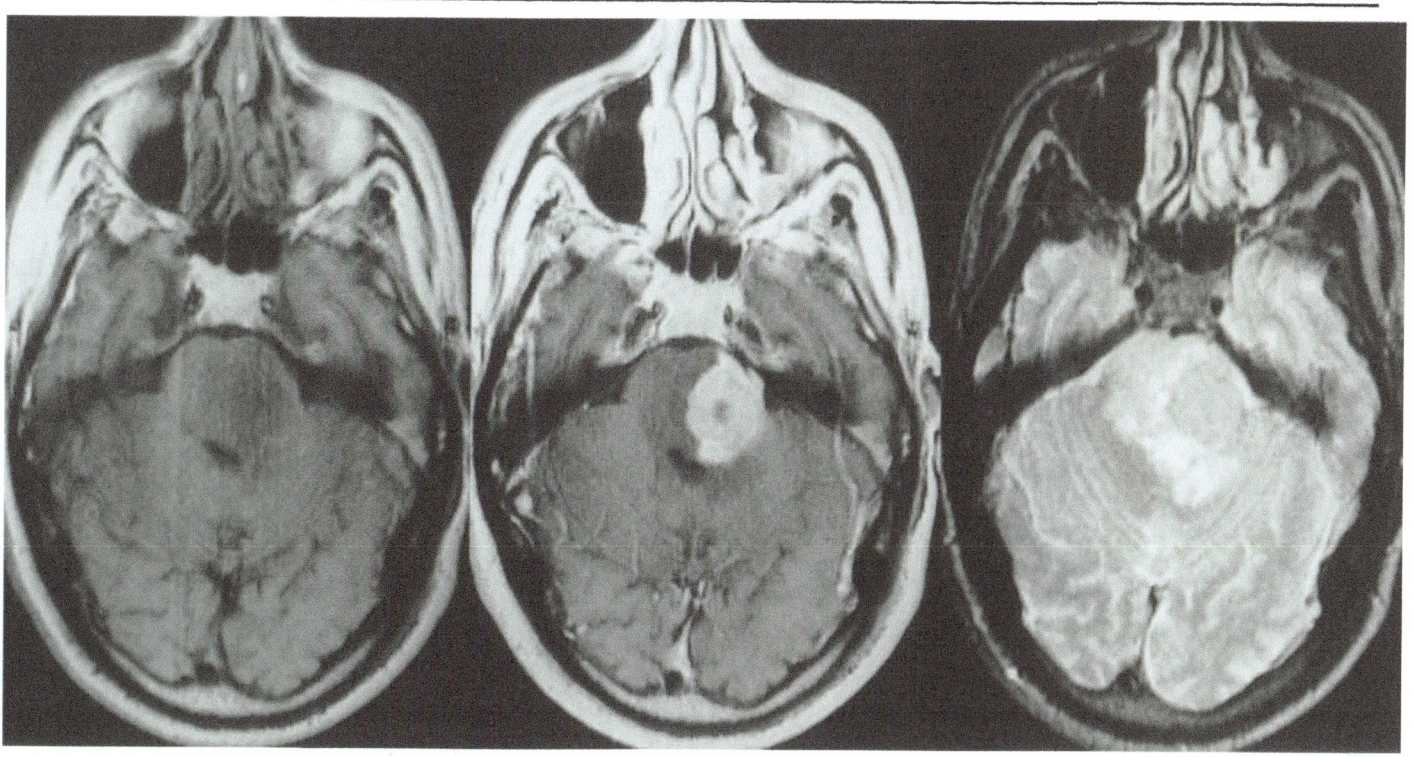

a

b

c

Figure 6.55 Metastatic disease, pons: (**a**) T1WI, (**b**) T1WI + C, (**c**) T2WI; circumscribed T1/T2 brain isointense mass, with diffuse enhancement, except for centre (unexplained, but possibly coagulative necrosis); peripheral parenchymal enhancement, presumably due to rapid extravasation from the tumour. T2 isointensity favours a solid, non-secreting epithelial metastasis (compare with Figure 6.56)

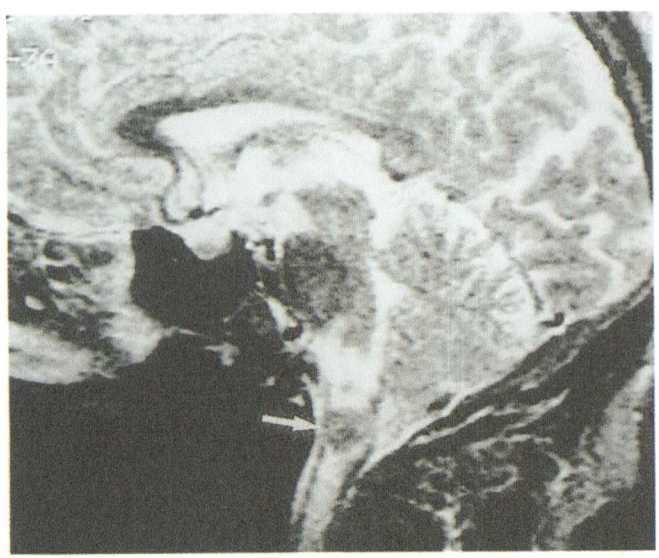

a

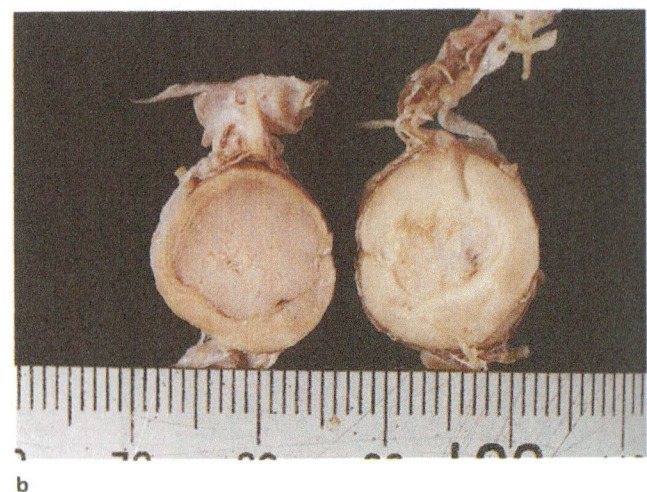

b

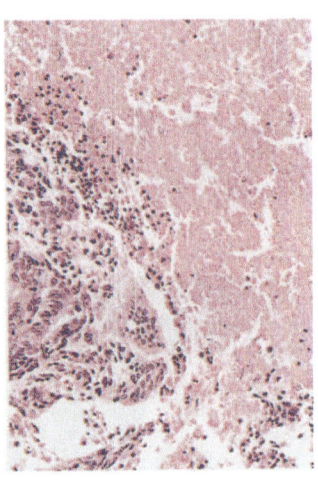

c   d

Figure 6.56   Metastatic disease, adenocarcinoma, medulla: (**a**) T2WI, (**b**) fixed specimen, (**c,d**) HE × 200; caudal medulla contains a slightly brain T2 hypointense mass (a), demarcated by adjacent CSF and/or oedema hyperintensity (arrow). Relative T2 signal shortening (hypointensity) is in favour of a mucin-secreting secondary neoplasm (c). Slight T2 hyperintense stippling corresponds to foci of necrosis apparent in fixed specimen (b) and histology (d)

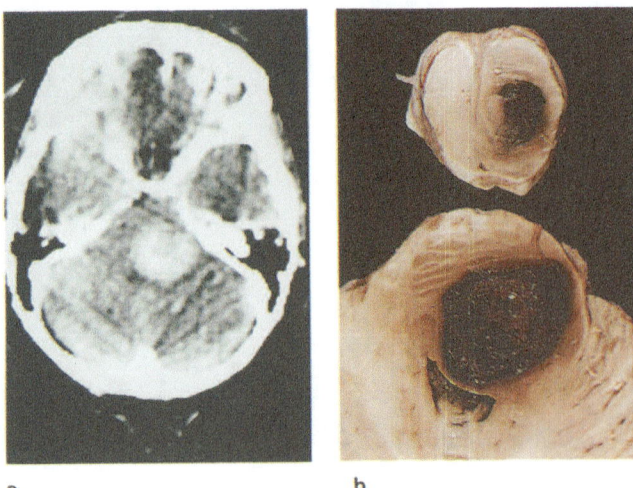
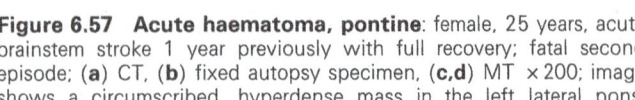
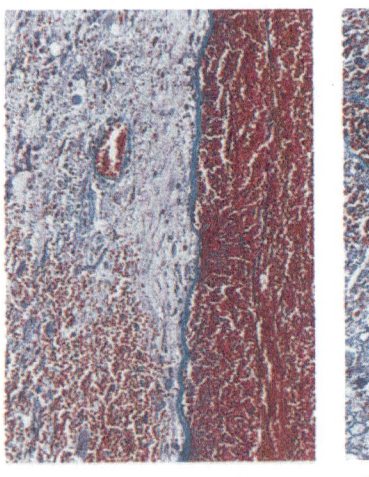
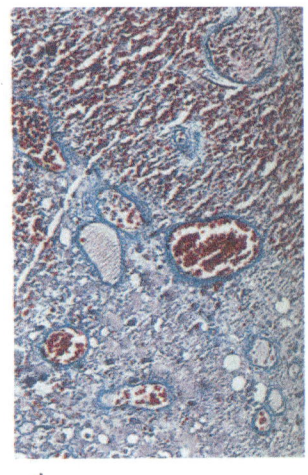

a   b   c   d

Figure 6.57   Acute haematoma, pontine: female, 25 years, acute brainstem stroke 1 year previously with full recovery; fatal second episode; (**a**) CT, (**b**) fixed autopsy specimen, (**c,d**) MT × 200; image shows a circumscribed, hyperdense mass in the left lateral pons, corresponding to acute haematoma shown in fixed specimen (b). Histology shows haematoma to be partly circumscribed by a thin collagenous wall (c), contiguous at other sites with numerous abnormal capillary vessels (d)

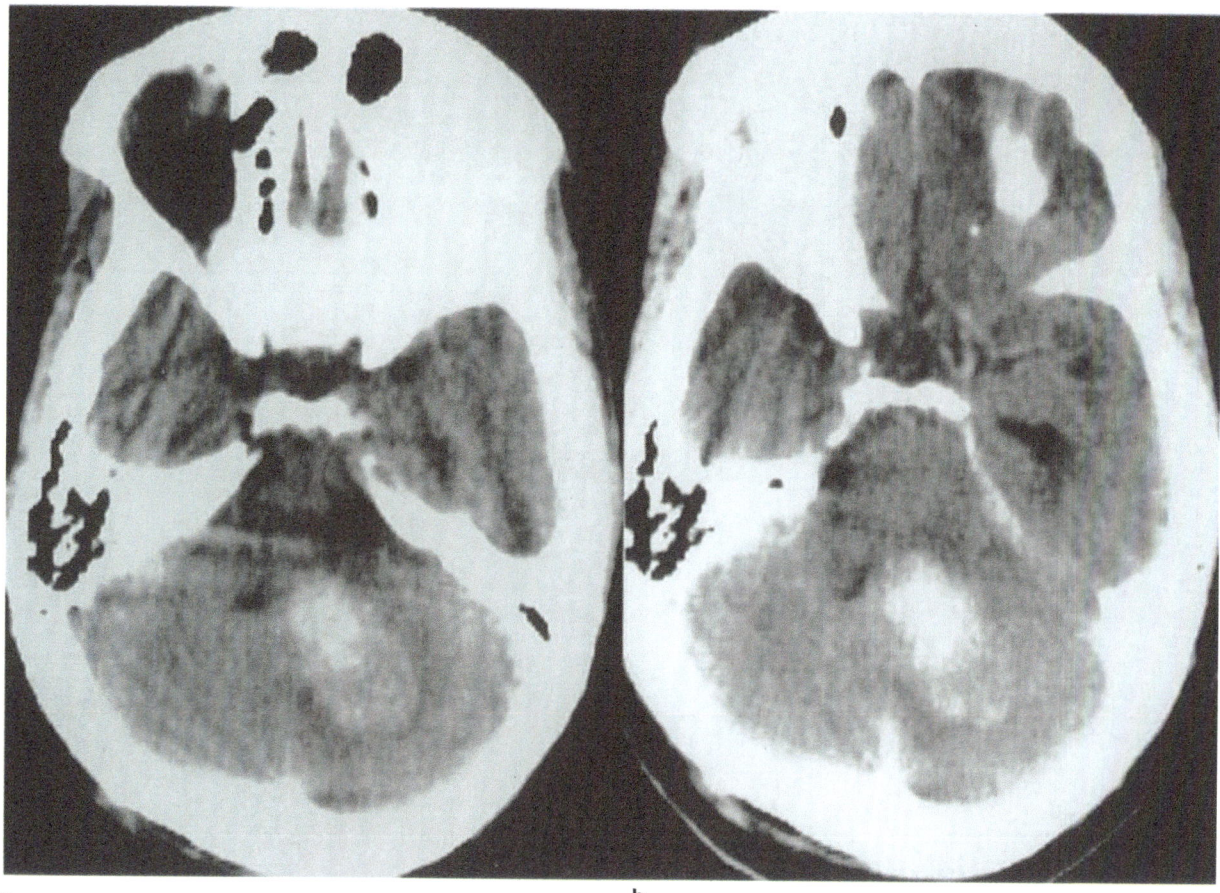

a   b

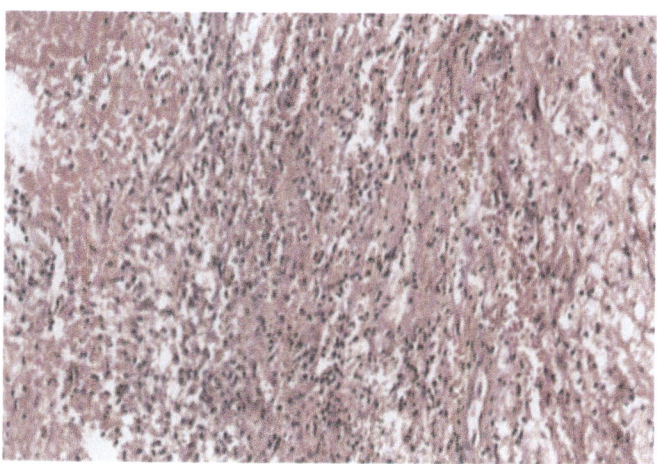

c

Figure 6.58 Acute haematoma, cerebellar: male, 50 years, hypertensive; (**a**) CT, (**b**) CT + C, (**c**) HE ×200; image shows inhomogeneous mass, with marked central hyperdensity, and slight diffuse brightening after contrast (b). Solitary haemorrhagic metastasis was suspected. Biopsy shows haematoma with commencing organization, without prominent vascular reaction, and contrast enhancement is therefore presumed to be due to vessel disruption

REFERENCES

1. Kak VK, Gupta RK, Sharma BS. Craniocervical enterogenous cyst: MR findings. JCAT. 1990;14:470–2.
2. Afshar F, Scholtz CI. Enterogenous cyst of the 4th ventricle. J Neurosurg. 1981;54:836–8.
3. Romero FJ, Ortega A, Ibarra B et al. Craniocervical neuroepithelial cysts. AJNR. 1987;8:1001–2.
4. Malcolm GP, Symon L, Kendall B et al. Intracranial neurenteric cysts. J Neurosurg. 1991;75:115–20.
5. Morita Y, Kinoshita K, Wakisaka S et al. Fine surface structure of an intraspinal neurenteric cyst: a scanning and transmission electron microscopy study. Neurosurgery. 1990;27:829–33.
6. Latack JT, Kartush JM, Kemink JL et al. Epidermoidomas of the cerebellopontine angle and temporal bone: CT and MR aspects. Radiology. 1985;187:361–6.
7. Tampieri D, Melanson D, Ethier R. MR imaging of epidermoid cysts. AJNR. 1989;10:351–6.

8. Yuh WTC, Barloon TJ, Jacoby CG et al. MR of fourth ventricular epidermoid tumors. AJNR. 1988;9:794–6.
9. Horowitz BL, Chari MV, James R et al. MR of intracranial epidermoid tumors: correlation of in vivo imaging with an in vitro 13C spectroscopy. AJNR. 1990;11:299–302.
10. Vion-Dury J, Vincentelli F, Jiddane M et al. MR imaging of epidermoid cysts. Neuroradiology. 1987;29:333–8.
11. Gentry LR, Jacoby CG, Turski PA et al. Cerebellopontine angle-petromastoid lesions: comparative study of diagnosis with MR imaging and CT. Radiology. 1987;162:513–20.
12. Alschuler EM, Jungreis CA, Sekhar LN et al. Operative treatment of intracranial epidermoid cysts and cholesterol granulomas. Neurosurgery. 1990;26:606–14.
13. Burger PC, Scheithauer BW, Vogel FS. Surgical pathology of the nervous system and its coverings, 3rd edn. New York: Churchill Livingstone; 1991:106.
14. Chang KH, Cho SY, Hesselink JR et al. Parasitic diseases of the central nervous system. Neuroimag Clin N Am. 1991;1:159–78.
15. Bilaniuk LT. Adult infratentorial tumors. Semin Roentgenol. 1990;25:155–73.
16. Press GA, Hesselink JR. MR imaging of cerebellopontine angle and internal auditory canal lesions. AJNR. 1988;9:241–51.
17. Sterkers JM, Perre J, Vial P et al. The origin of acoustic neuromas. Acta Otolaryngol (Stockh). 1987;103:427–31.
18. Murray MR, Stout AP. Characteristics of human Schwann cells in vitro. Anat Rec. 1942;84:275 (quoted in Russel and Rubinstein, [ref. 27] p. 543).
19. Smith RR. Brainstem tumors. Semin Roentgenol. 1990;25:249–62.
20. Zimmerman RA. Pediatric supratentorial tumors. Semin Roentgenol. 1990;25:225–48.

In the following sections, the material presented has been restricted to the sort commonly encountered in purely neurosurgical practice. The effect of such arbitrary selection is immediately apparent with regard to vertebral lesions, where primary neoplasms are omitted; apart from discogenic disease the neuropathologist will only receive extradural tissues when parenchymal or radicular impingement occurs and, even then, primary osseous conditions are excluded, being normally handled by the orthopaedic surgeons. Conversely, the routine management of discogenic and other mechanical disturbances of root and cord function in most neurosurgical units, constitutes a unique area of extrameningeal pathology, which MR has made very much more relevant than formerly.

The ascendency of MR over myelography and CT-myelography is documented[1], as well as generally acknowledged, but creates a curious anomaly in respect of the venerated neuroradiological approach of defining pathological processes in relation to the dura; for this densely collagenous structure is normally invisible, and its profile is assessed by technical means, particularly gradient echo, which is inimical to pathology. Although we endeavour to satisfy the neurosurgeon on the point, the usefulness of defining the dura in the anatomical diagnosis nowadays strikes us as only marginal, mainly because the MR scanner defines osseous–intraspinal masses so consistently.

7.1. DISCOGENIC AND JOINT-RELATED DISEASE

Emanating from the specialized MR units in North America, a systematized approach to discogenic disease has now cleared up the confusion which resulted from the lack of specificity in the terms 'herniation' and 'prolapse'. Displacement of the disc annular fibrocartilage and nucleus is now defined as protrusion, extrusion and sequestration[2], and pathologists should not attempt to provide a specific anatomical diagnosis without this information. Although histopathological assessment of disc material aims to confirm the clinical and imaging diagnosis of displacement of the nucleus pulposus, morphological criteria that allow this are complicated by age-related degenerative changes such as fibrillation, 'chrondrocyte cloning', and granular change[3] (Figure 7.1). These alterations are probably causally related to disc displacement, but their presence is inferential, a more reliable feature being that of 'edge neovascularization'[4], to be found in about 50% of cases (Figure 7.1). However, it must be emphasized that the biochemical and mechanical factors which are also associated with disc disease make it unlikely that histology will have much diagnostic specificity[5]. In cases of re-operation (failed-back syndrome), the pathologist needs to take particular note of the fact that fibrous tissue, on account of its early and preferential enhancement, can frequently be clearly distinguished from recurrent or residual disc material[6,7] (Figure 7.2), a matter of great clinical importance[8]. The pathogenesis of the extensive spontaneous fibrous stenosis illustrated in Figure 7.3 is unknown; fragmented elastic fibres implicate ligamentum flavum degeneration. Degenerative joint-related cysts, usually presenting as a disc syndrome, are discussed below.

7.2. CYSTS

The precise identification of spinal cysts is dependent on a combination of CT myelography, MR imaging, surgical inspection and histological examination. In the vertebral canal the presence of an epidural space, adjacent joint structures and a long history of myelographic investigation, probably account for differences in terminology compared with equivalent intracranial lesions[9,10].

Our approach to the characterization of *primary, development cysts* is discussed in section 3.1. Meningeal (or arachnoid) cysts[11] comprise the majority, being situated outside (Figure 7.4) or inside the dura (Figure 7.5), and filled with CSF-physiologically identical fluid, whether or not subarachnoid space communication is demonstrable (as may be shown with myelographic contrast media); below the conus, origin is from a nerve root or its sheath, which may be adherent to, or lie within the cyst[12] (Figure 7.6). As with their intracranial counterparts, there is no enhancement with intravenous contrast. Non-arachnoid, intradural cysts include dermal inclusion (epidermoidoma, dermoid (Figure 7.7), neuroepithelial (i.e. ependyma)[13], and enterogenous types. Lesions lined by neuroepithelium may be completely intraparenchymal, but with such a degree of superficial attenuation that this feature can be recognized only microscopically (Figure 7.8).

The *apophyseal joints* are associated with synovial[14] and periarticular ganglion cysts[15]. However, the taxonomy of the latter is confusing, as the term 'ganglion' has also been applied to perineurial[16] and synovial cysts[17]. The genuine ganglion cyst should have no synovial lining membrane and no communication with the joint cavity[18], features which differentiate it from a true synovial cyst, while perineurial cysts, now classified as type 2 meningeal cysts[19], contain spinal nerve root fibres within the cyst wall or cavity (see above).

A distinctive form of non-synovial cyst, usually presenting as a disc syndrome[20], appears both topographically and on account of its elastic tissue content, to originate from the *ligamentum flavum*. In the series collected by us, a macroscopically characteristic feature is its resemblance, at surgery, to a blood-engorged tick (Figure 7.9). Although the enhancing wall of the lesion correlates with its vasoformative nature (Figure 7.10), the haemorrhagic contents may not induce T1 signal shortening (Figure 7.9). In the case illustrated in Figure 7.11 a clinically acute, spontaneous extradural haematoma contained fragments of proliferative vascular tissue typical of this type of cyst, implying its pathogenesis in some intraspinal bleeds.

7.3. INFLAMMATION

7.3a. Epidural inflammation and pachymeningitis

The submission of epidural inflammatory tissue for histological examination appears to be a function of the clinical picture and neurosurgical interest. The acute, liquid purulent collection typical of a haematogenous lesion in younger patients, although strikingly hyperintense on T2 weighted images (Figure 7.12), is a microbiological problem; in more protracted disease the mass includes granulation and/or granulomatous tissue (Figure 7.13),

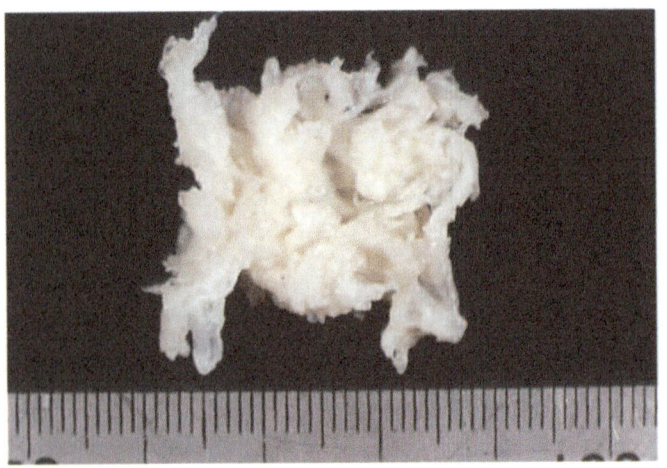

a

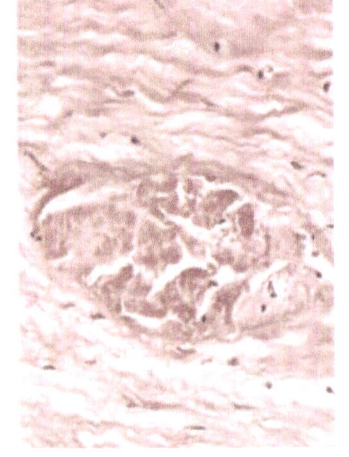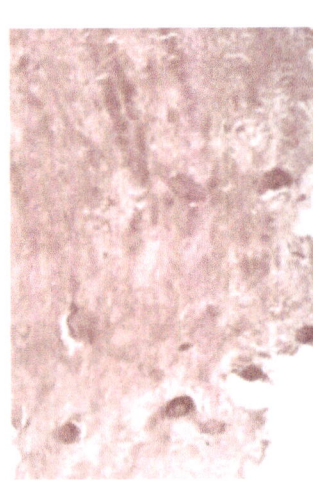

b

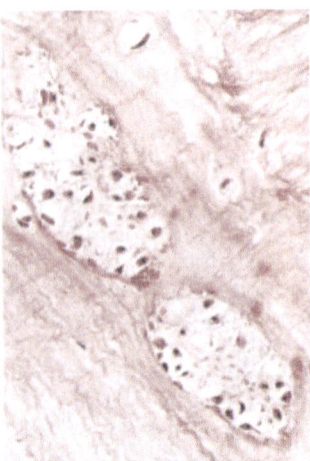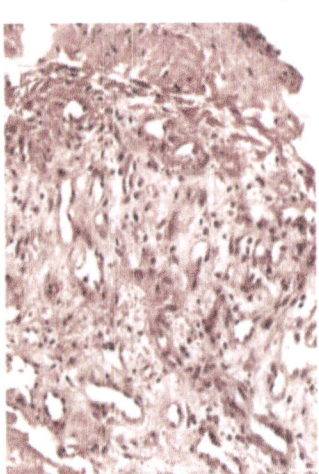

c

Figure 7.1 Disc extrusion: (a) fixed specimen, (b,c) HE × 200; typical disorganized, extruded fibrocartilaginous disc material, lifted from the epidural space (a); histology shows granular change, necrosis with dead chrondrocytes (b, left and right), and chrondrocyte cloning (c, left); edge neovascularization (c, right) is presumably the source of contrast enhancement and subsequent fibrous organization (see **Figure 7.2**)

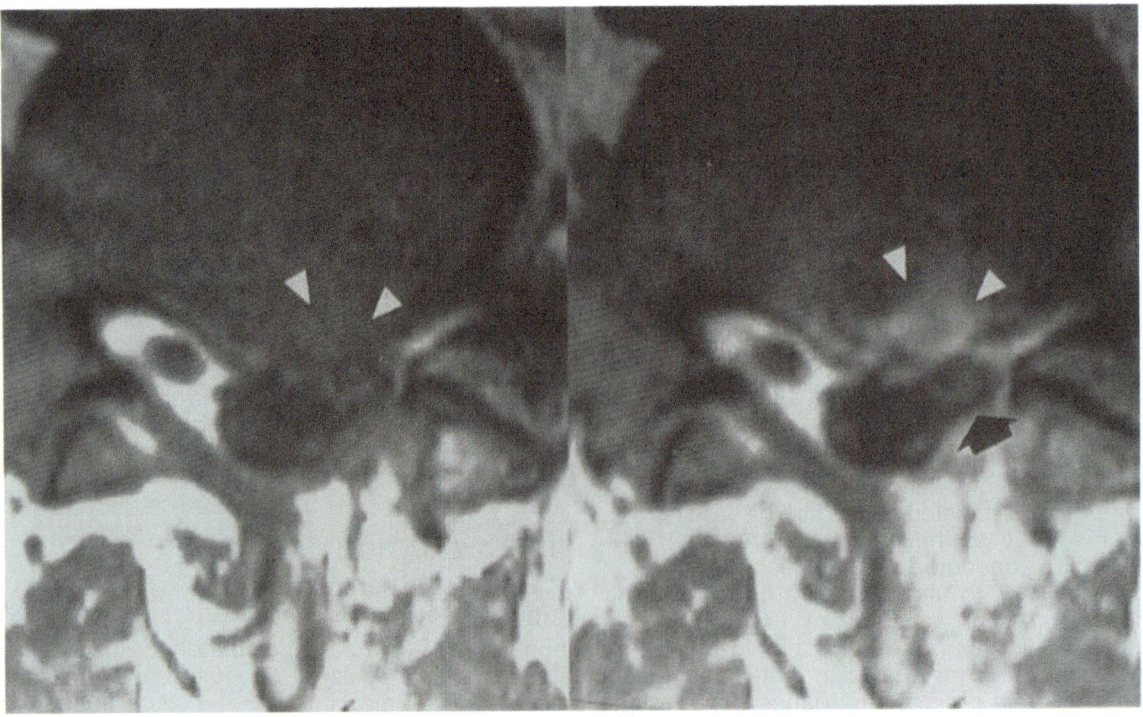

a   b

Figure 7.2 Lumbar intervertebral disc, protrusion and postoperative fibrosis: (a) T1WI, (b) T1WI + C; contrasted image (b) shows enhancement of formerly indistinguishable tissues (arrow-heads) occupying the lateral recess, with swollen nerve root in relief (b, arrow)

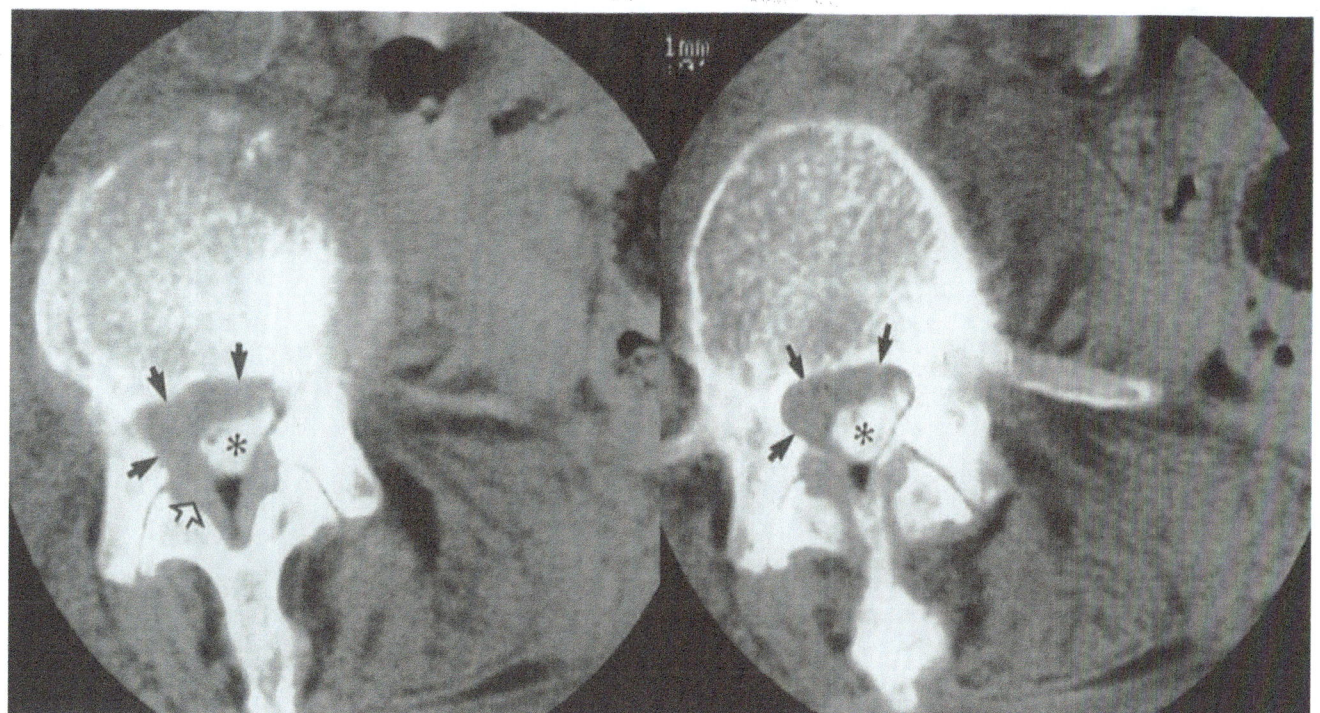

a

b

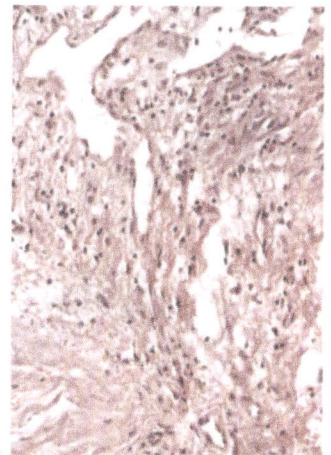

c

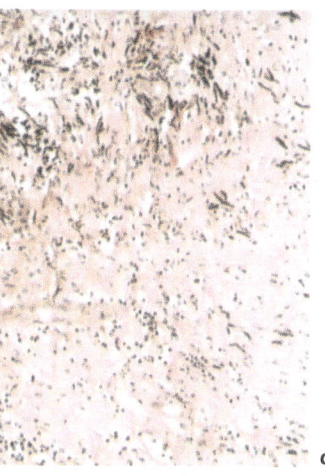

d

Figure 7.3 Spinal stenosis, extradural fibrosis, aetiology unknown: female, 60 years, transient subacute myelopathy and residual paraparesis; (**a,b**) CT myelogram, (**c**) HE × 200, (**d**) EVG × 100; images show soft tissue extradural mass (arrows), resembling disc material in density, with compression and displacement of the dural sac (asterisk). Note apparent continuity with ligamentum flavum (a, open arrow). Histology shows reactive fibrovascular tissue containing degenerate elastic fibres (d), presumed to be of ligamentum flavum origin

associated with bony changes, either pyogenic discitis (Figure 7.14) or tuberculous spondylitis[21], and may or may not contain pus (Figure 7.15). However, extraparenchymal granulation tissue has no specific imaging features, being T1-isointense with cord and soft tissues, and strongly enhancing. The thecal profile is deformed and obliteration of the dural margin by contrast is consistent with focal pachymeningitis (Figures 7.14 and 7.15), which is usually focally necrotizing (Figure 7.16). Unfortunately, in the Cape Town teaching hospitals, improved imaging of spinal tuberculosis has served merely to decrease interest in histological correlation.

Granulomatous disease of the epidural space, presenting as an enhancing epidural mass with or without central liquefaction (T1 hypointense/T2 hyperintense), can also occur without concurrent bony changes, and should always be considered in the appropriate geographic and clinical setting. While usually tuberculous (Figure 7.17) (section 3.2), fungal and parasitic aetiologies are possible, schistosomiasis being of importance in endemic areas (Figure 3.18). Although manifestly extradural, granulomatous disease at this site is probably always pachymeningitic to a degree.

Occasionally, the insidious onset of root or cord compression is the result of obliteration of the epidural space by a form of hypertrophic pachymeningitis morphologically identical to the conditions affecting the cavernous sinus and tentorium[22,23] (section 3.2b). MR reveals the process of inflammatory fibrosis to be T1 soft-tissue hypointense and enhancing, and may involve the length of the cord[24] (Figure 7.18).

7.3b. Focal (lepto)meningeal and meningoparenchymal inflammation

Granulomatous disease of the spinal cord, although very much rarer, follows similar diverse aetiologies as occur intracranially[25]. Tuberculosis may present on MR as multifocal, enhancing nodules whose profiles indicate parenchymal, nerve root or dural (subdural) apposition, referred to as a form of radiculomyelitis[26]. In the case illustrated in Figure 7.19 the lesions included homogeneous and inhomogeneous enhancement consistent with the biopsy demonstration of proliferative and necrotizing granulomas, presumed tuberculous; however, there was no response to anti-tuberculosis therapy, and luetic serology was positive, with resolution on appropriate treatment. Sarcoidosis may be morphologically indistinguishable[27].

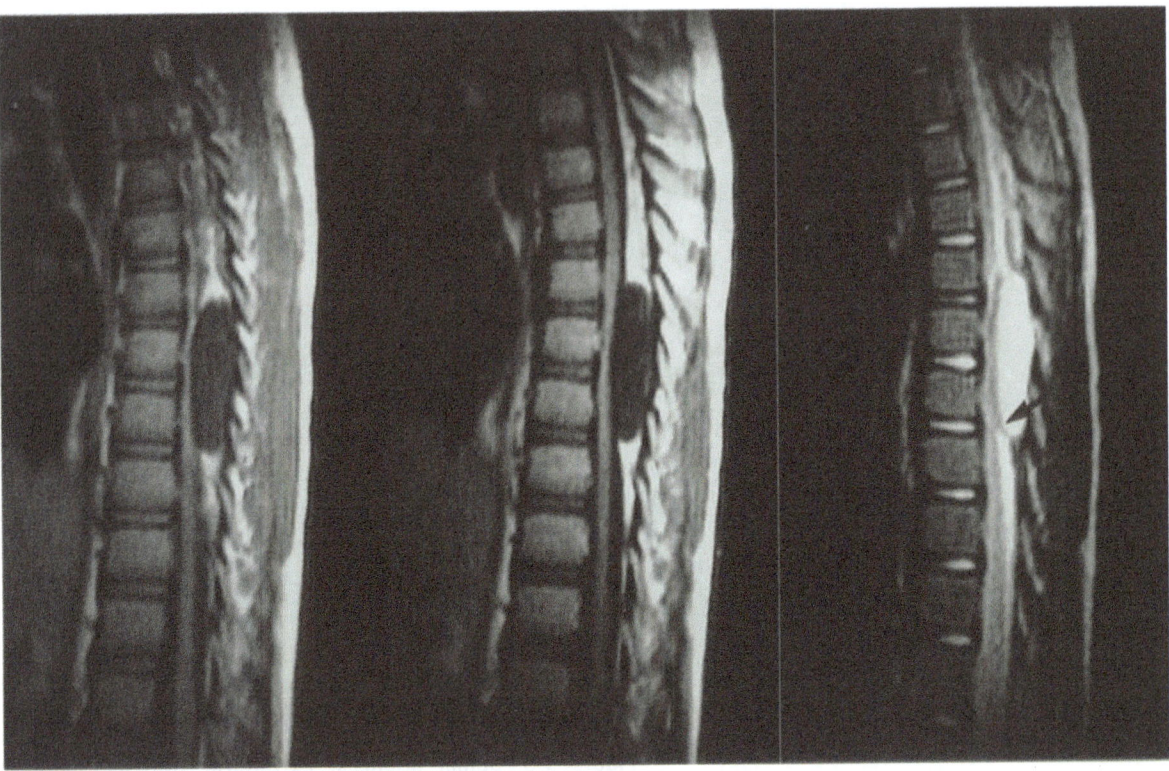

a   b   c

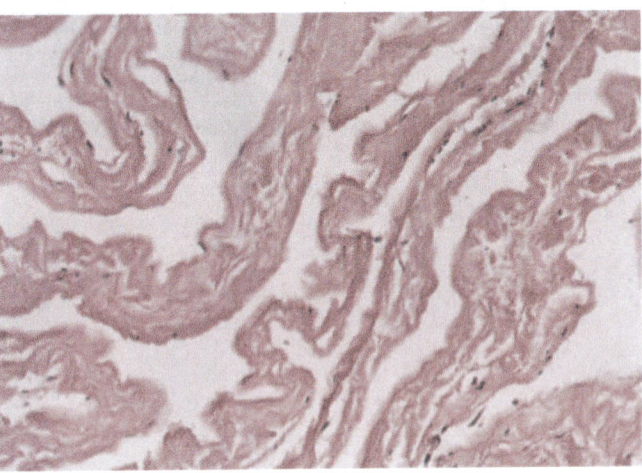

d

Figure 7.4 Cyst, arachnoid, spinal extradural, communicating (meningeal type I): male, 17 years, 5-month history of progressive paraparesis; **(a)** T1WI, **(b)** T1WI + C, **(c)** T2WI, **(d)** HE × 200; images show sharply circumscribed extradural CSF intensity cyst, with associated epidural fat above and below (a), further delineated by epidural contrast enhancement (b). Dura is apparent on T2WI (c, arrow). At surgery controlled aspiration yielded ∼20 ml clear fluid, with subsequent slow reaccumulation; cyst pedicle found to be attached to left T7 nerve root sheath. Histology (d) shows cyst wall consists of a thin fibrocollagenous membrane, devoid of lining cells (compare with **Figure 7.5**)

7.3c. Parenchymal inflammation

In 20 years of clinical neuropathology we have not experienced a request to examine inflammatory tissue biopsied from within the cord parenchyma, and have encountered only one case of intramedullary abscess[28]. In the cases of focal, inflammatory demyelinating disease illustrated in Figures 7.20 and 7.21 no specific primary imaging diagnosis was made, although an unusual tumour was suspected. However, the cases also illustrate how the refinements of imaging and neurosurgery have combined to make biopsy of small intraparenchymal lesions perfectly feasible.

7.4. PARASITES

Vertebral cysts with extradural cord compression from *Echinococcus*, are of great clinical and pathological importance, not least being their resistance to both surgical and medical management[29]. The usual plain film and CT picture of bizarre, scalloped expansion of bone is augmented by the MR demonstration of cyst multiplicity,

with characteristic paraspinal extension (Figure 7.22). The hydatids which erupt into the spinal canal do not seem to exceed 20 mm in diameter (Figure 7.23), and are not clearly visualized as individual structures on the images. In spite of the presence of intraosseous granulomata (Figure 7.24), the epidural cysts do not exhibit the surrounding inflammatory changes seen in the orbit soft tissues and, less commonly, the brain. Encysted metacestodes of any genus are rarely found within the spinal canal, and most intradural examples are cysticerci.

7.5. NEOPLASTIC DISEASE

7.5a. Tumours with intraosseous–extradural growth

Primary, expansile neoplasms of a single vertebra comprise a considerable list whose popularity with radiologists has at least something to do with the art of plain film examination. As has been already pointed out, these lesions are seldom seen by neurosurgeons, whilst metastatic disease and the reticuloses are subject to surgical intervention when a number of factors combine to convince the clinician that this forms an essential aspect of management, foremost among which are decompression for acute myelopathy, and precise histological diagnosis. On MR, non-sclerotic infiltration of vertebral bone causes a striking loss of the marrow signal at short TR, with relative hyperintensity at long TR, explained simply by

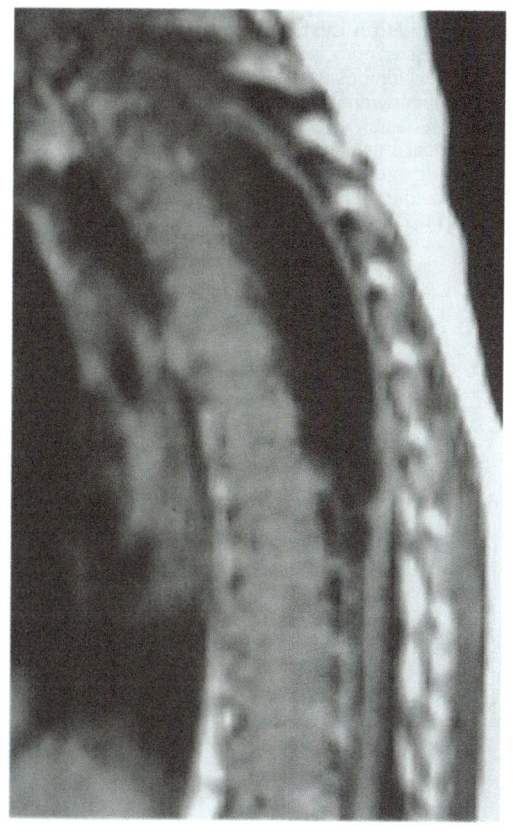

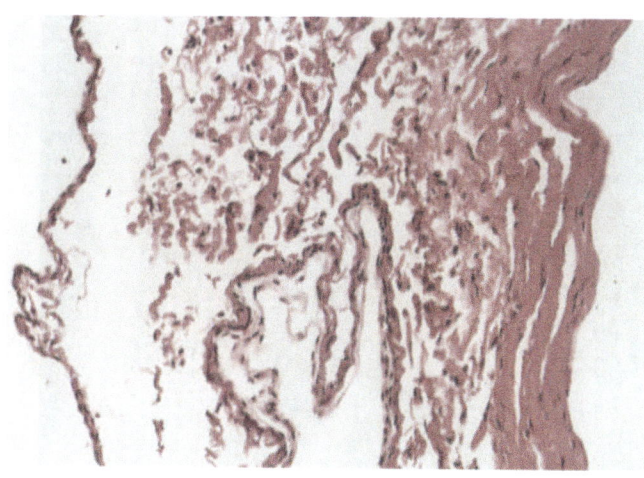

b

Figure 7.5 Cyst, arachnoid, spinal intradural (meningeal type III): (**a**) T1WI, (**b**) HE × 200; image shows lesion extending over several segments, posterior displacement of the cord and widening of the spinal canal. Intradural location confirmed at surgery; biopsy of cyst wall (b) shows internal lining of folded arachnoid (left), blending with connective tissue of ventral dura (right) (compare with cyst wall shown in **Figure 7.4**)

a

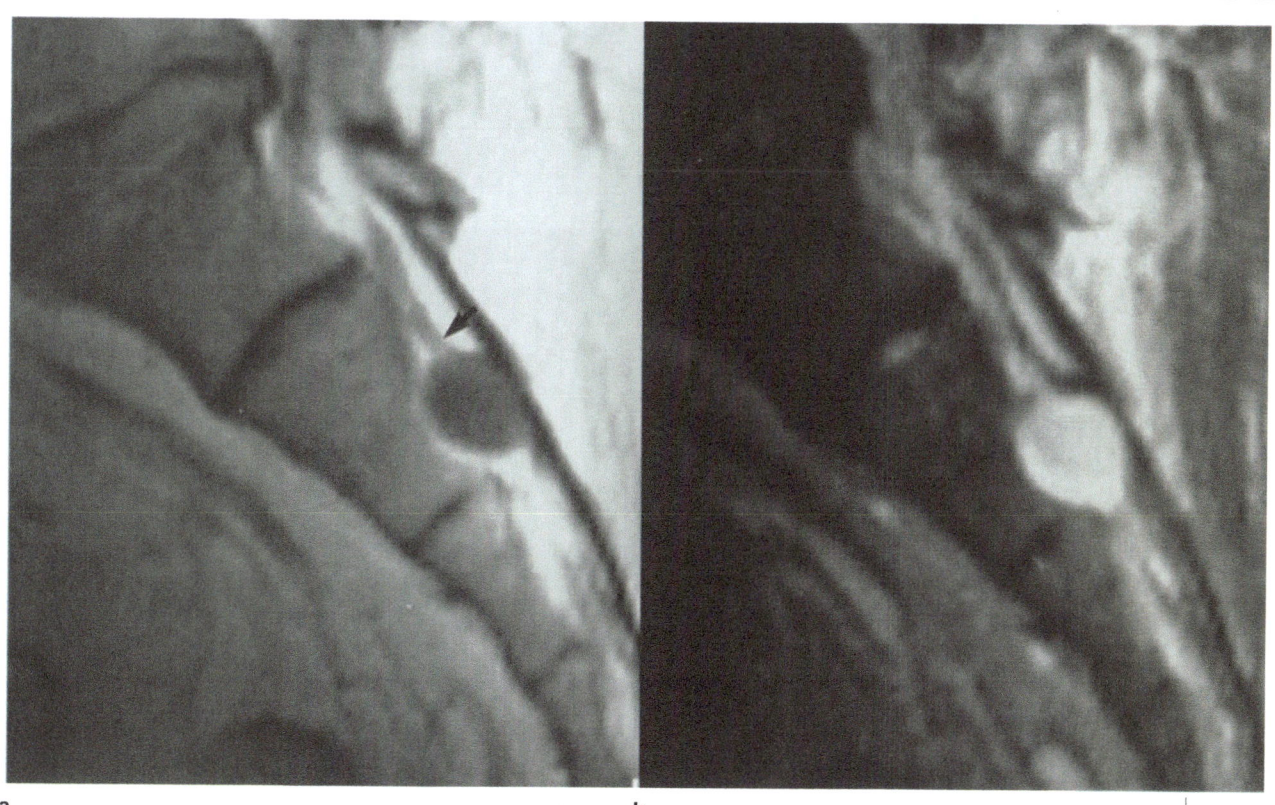

a   b

Figure 7.6 Cyst, sacral nerve root (meningeal type II): (**a**) T1WI, (**b**) T2WI; images show association of cyst and nerve root (a, arrow), with CSF T2 isointense contents (b). No tissue available for histology

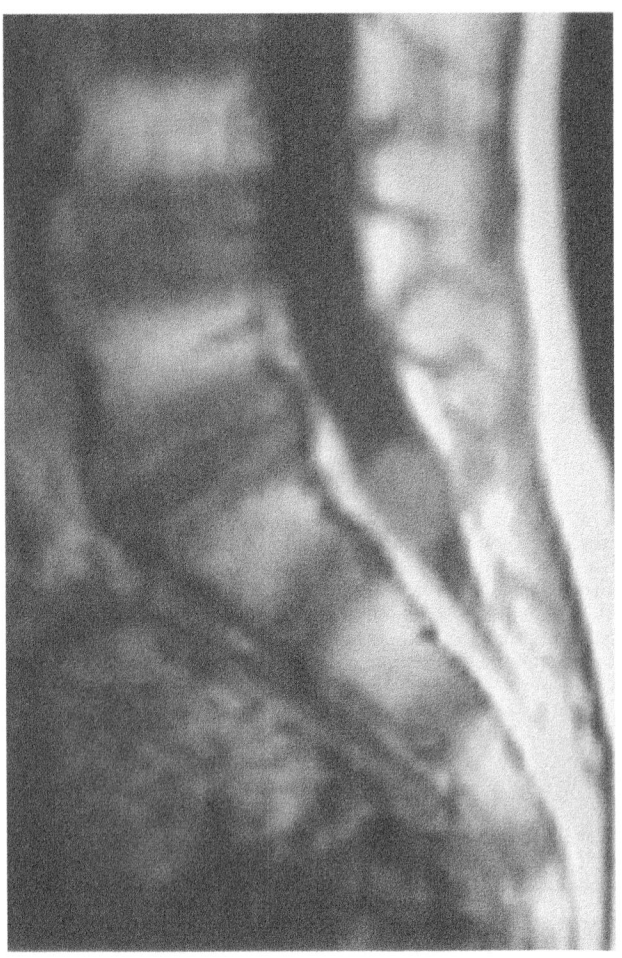

Figure 7.7 Dermal inclusion cyst, cauda equina: male, 4 years; PDWI shows oval, soft tissue/cord isointense (T2 hyperintense) mass in the inferior part of the lumbosacral subarachnoid space. Imaging diagnosis was that of ependymoma, and although histology showed sparse adnexal structures, lesion was filled with flaky keratin, without any adipose tissue. Signal intensity is therefore appropriate for epidermoidoma, despite disc protocol sequences (TR1500/TE15), with adjacent epidural fat providing reference hyperintensity (compare with **Figures 7.39** and **7.41**). (Prof ROC Kaschula, Red Cross Children's Hospital)

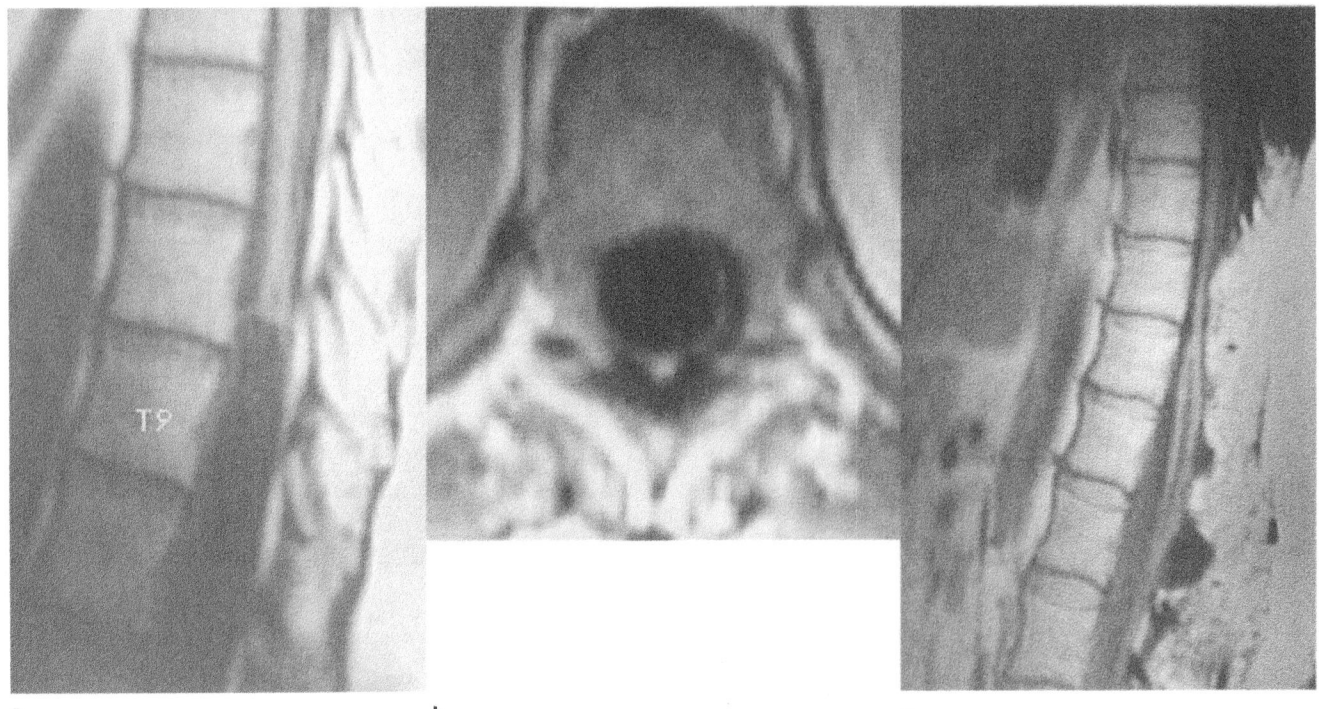

a　　　　　　b　　　　　　c

Figure 7.8 (*legend opposite*)

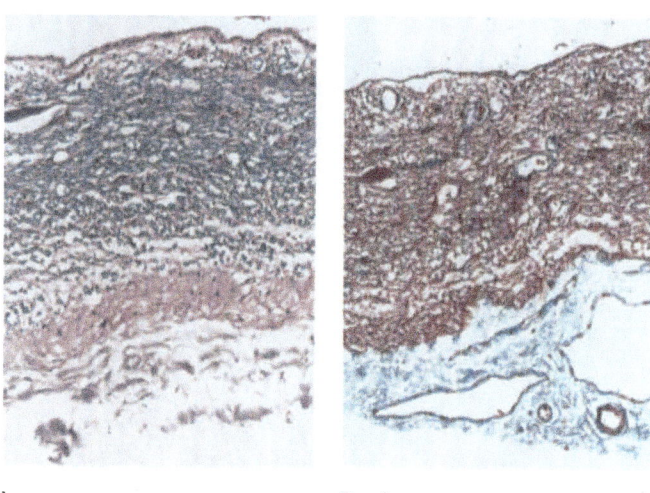
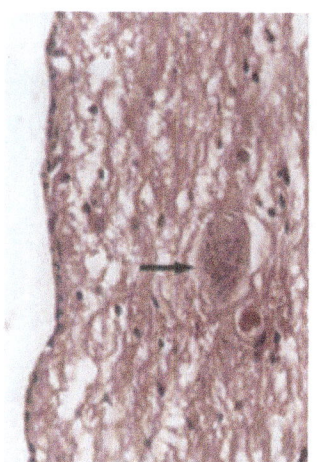
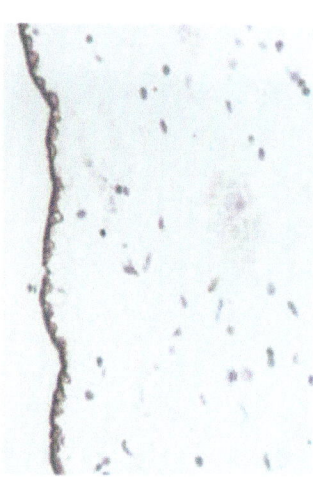

d   e   f

Figure 7.8 Ependymal cyst: female, 51 years; (**a**) sagittal T1WI, (**b**) axial T1WI + C, (**c**) postoperative sagittal T1WI, (**d**) LBHE × 200, (**e**) MT × 200, (**f**) HE/keratin × 400, (**g**) EM × 16 200; images show non-enhancing, lumbar intra–extramedullary cyst with CSF isointense contents (a,b). (At operation cyst was thought to be extramedullary.) However, sample obtained from superficial aspect of cyst shows lining to consist of flattened cuboidal epithelium (keratin-positive (f), GFAP-negative), resting on a thin layer of neural parenchyma with adjacent fibrotic arachnoid (note neuronal perikarya – f, arrow). EM shows microvilli, interdigitating processes, complex junctions (arrow-heads), pinocytotic vesicles (open arrows) and intermediate filaments. Basal membrane and collagen (asterisk) separates abluminal surface from underlying neuropil. Postoperative image (c) shows residual cyst with considerable parenchymal restitution

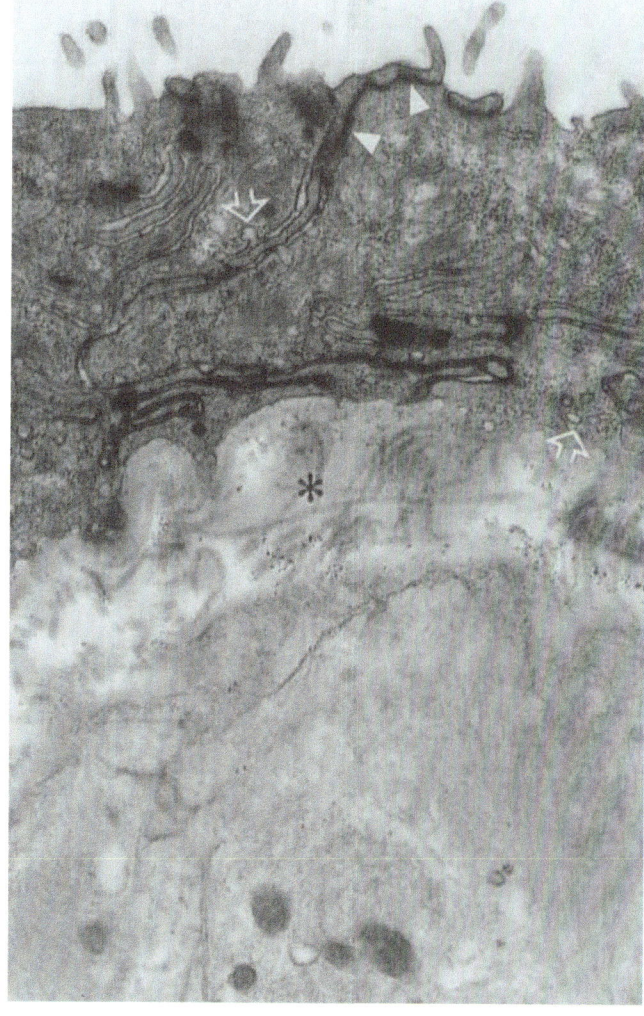

g

the replacement of marrow fat by tumour tissue (Figures 7.25 and 7.26), which may at the same time permit more interstitial water. These signal alterations are usually combined with obvious disturbance of the normal profile (Figure 7.27). Extradural tumour tissue is expectedly cord isointense and enhancing (see also section 2.6d). The pathologist should also be prepared to be confronted with gradient echo sequences which highlight the bony component of the lesion, whilst obscuring the intraspinal tissue (Figure 7.27). Although these features are rather characteristic of metastatic disease in general, they are not specific and there are currently no useful correlative aspects, either with regard to distinguishing epithelial and reticular neoplasms from one another, or identifying features of epidural fat infiltration and tumour necrosis (Figure 7.28).

7.5b. Diffuse intraspinal–extraparenchymal tumours

Although enhanced MR is the only effective imaging technique for demonstrating diffuse tumour growth in the peridural spaces, signal characteristics are variable and non-specific[1], as is to be expected. Lymphoma is the single most important malignancy having a propensity for epi- or subarachnoid spread, although without any tendency to penetrate the dura in either direction. Extra-dural lymphoma is always secondary, and subarachnoid spread almost always; occasional cases exhibiting only the latter location being assumed, by default, to be primary. As in the brain, meningeal and nerve root involvement exhibits strong enhancement[30], presumed to result from relatively leaky vessels. Myeloma may be sometimes most easily biopsied in the epidural space, where growth

is focal and associated with a florid tumour vasculature without necrosis (Figure 7.29). Subarachnoid spread from primary CNS tumours such as medulloblastoma is usually multifocal (seeding), whereas growth from extra-CNS malignancies, whether epithelial or reticular, tends to be diffuse or en plaque.

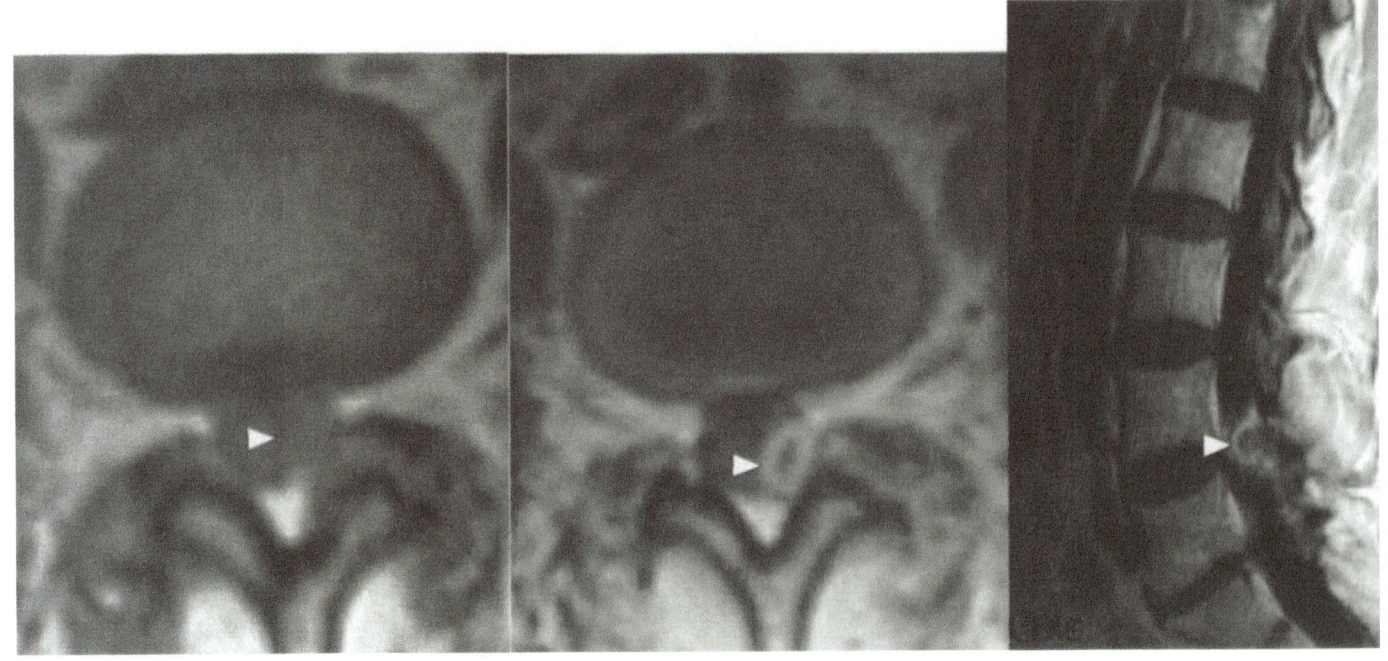

a   b   c

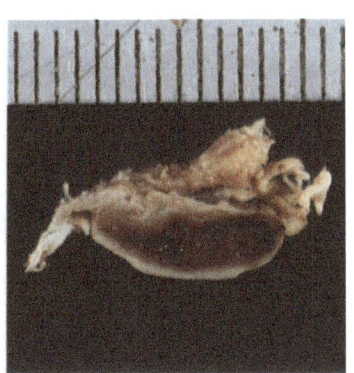

d

Figure 7.9 Cyst, haemorrhagic, intraspinal, extradural: adult presenting with localized back pain; (**a**) T1WI, (**b**) T1WI + C, (**c**) sagittal T1WI + C, (**d**) fixed specimen, (**e**) HE × 200, (**f**) EVG × 200; cyst is invisible on T1 sequence (a), but shows peripheral enhancement with contrast (b,c). Note that contents are tissue isointense, in spite of the fact that cyst contains fresh and organizing haemorrhage (d). Histology shows wall to contain abundant vasoformative tissue, with recent and organizing haemorrhage (e). At operation surgeon did not demonstrate any connection with facet joint, but black-staining elastic fibre remnants (f), indicates association with ligamentum flavum

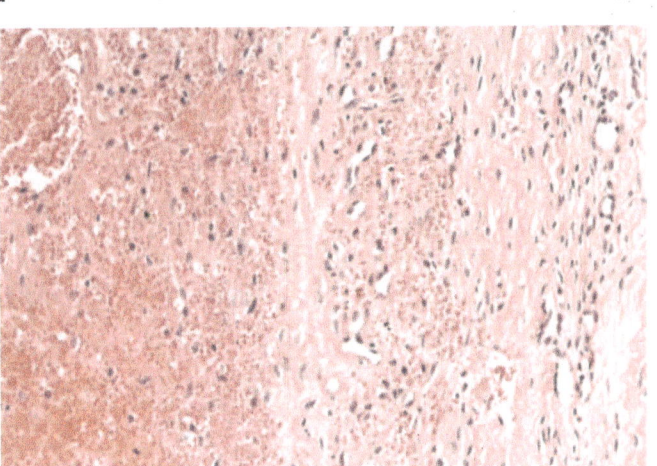

e

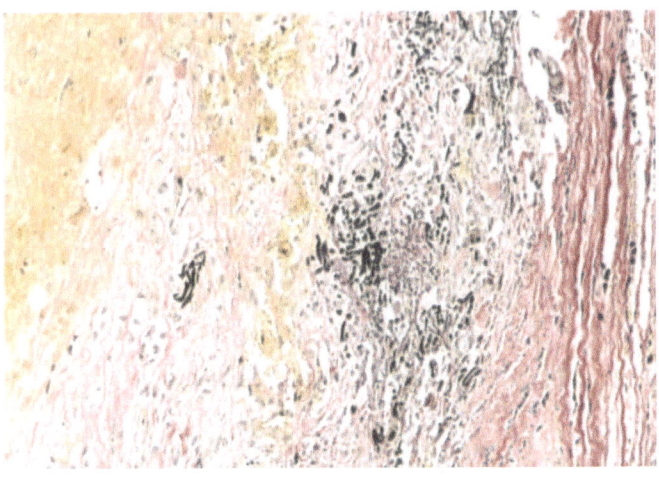

f

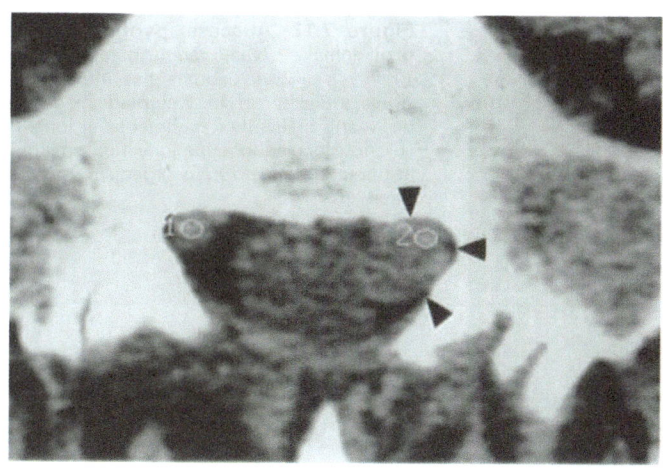

a

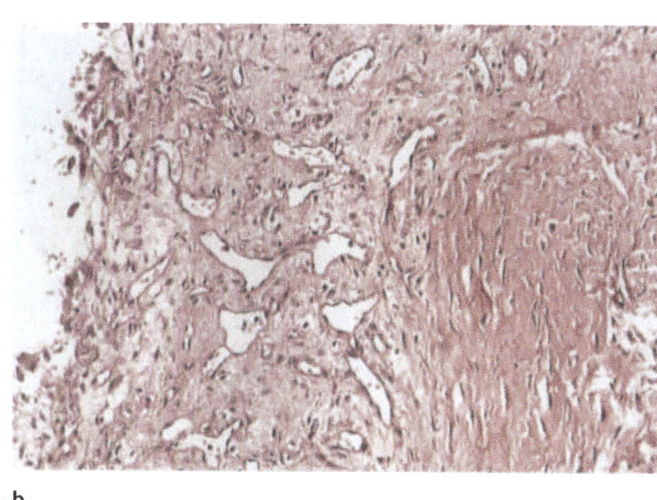

b

Figure 7.10 Cyst, haemorrhagic, intraspinal, extradural: (a) CT, (b) HE ×200; image shows extradural mass (a, arrow-heads) having a density consistent with disc material. At operation a blue-tinged cyst was dissected from the apophyseal joint/ligamentum flavum;

lesion did not communicate with the joint space. Histology (b) shows the wall to be composed of collagen lined by 'vasoformative' tissue, with a central space containing red cells. Degenerate elastic fibres as illustrated in **Figure 7.9** were also present

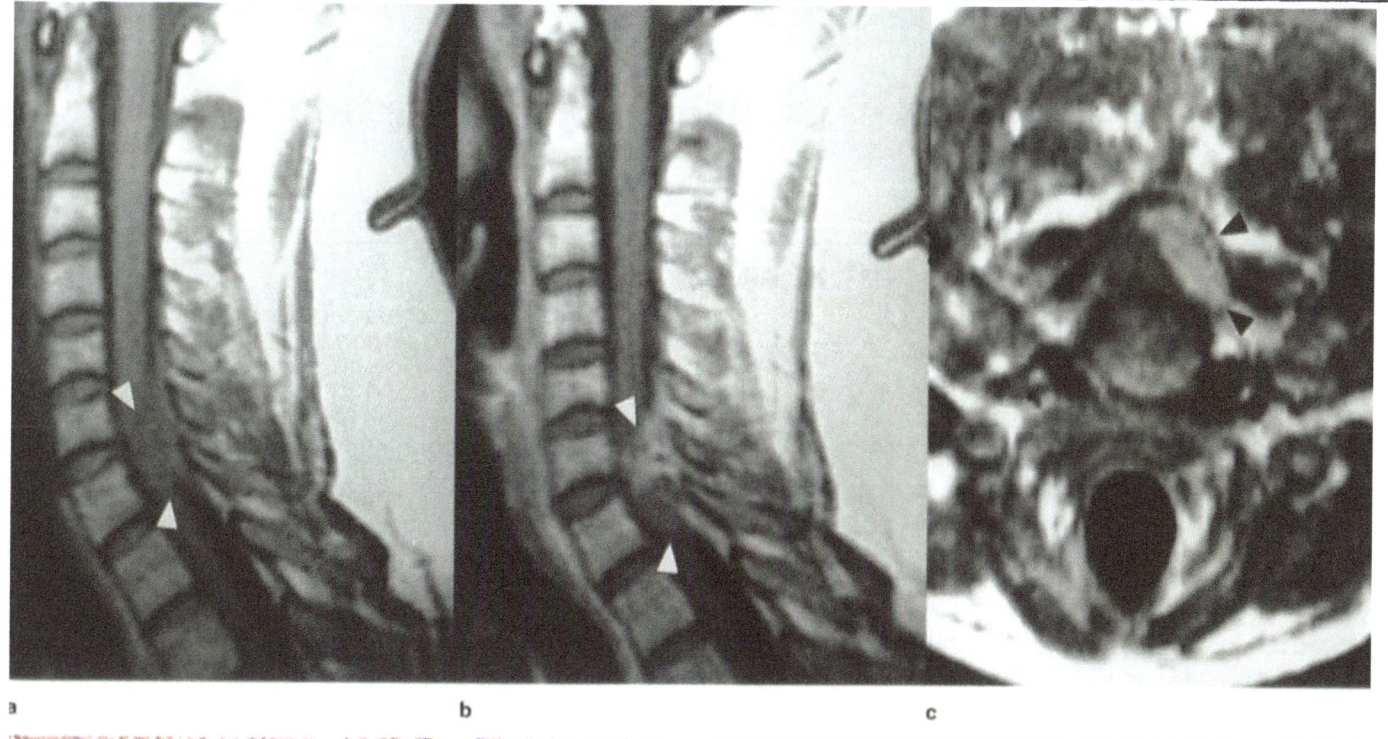

a   b   c

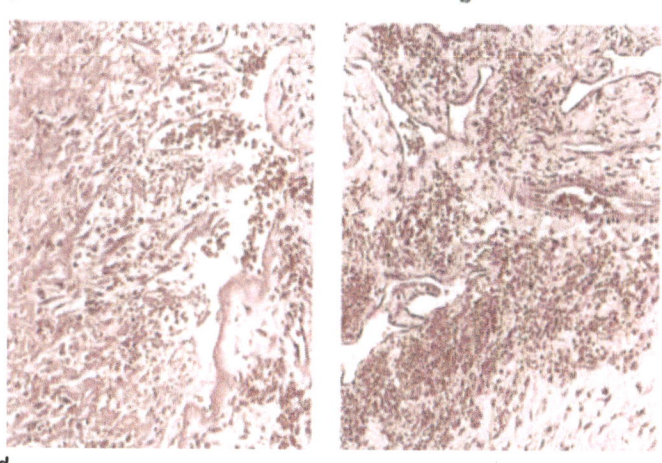

d

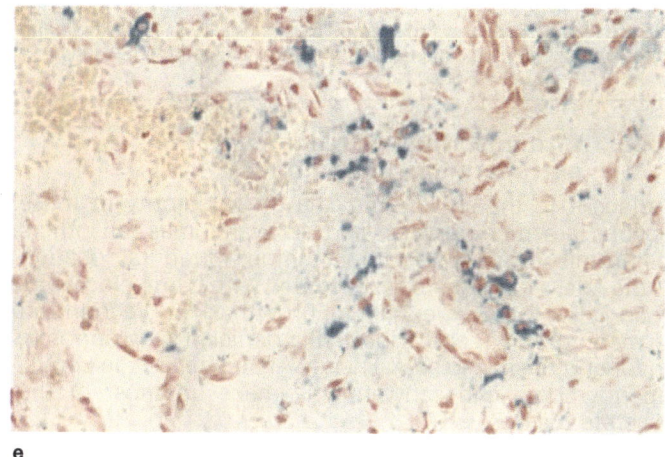

e

Figure 7.11 Acute spontaneous epidural haematoma: (a) T1WI, (b) T1WI + C, (c) axial T1WI + C, (d) HE ×200, (e) Perl's ×400; images show a poorly defined cord isointense, extradural mass (a,

arrows), which enhances inhomogeneously (b,c, arrows). Histology shows florid vasoformative tissue (d), recent and old haemorrhage with iron deposition (e)

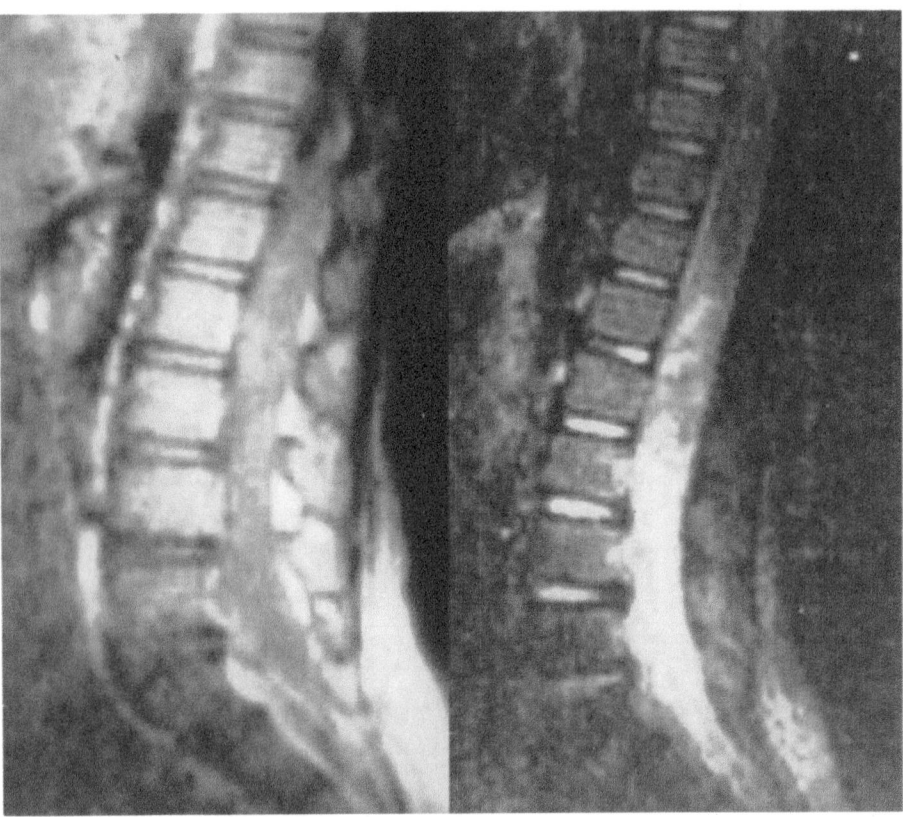

a   b

Figure 7.12 Abscess, pyogenic, epidural: female, 6 years, acute paraplegia: (**a**) T1WI, (**b**) T2WI; exudate has intermediate signal intensity on T1 weighted image (a), becoming brilliantly hyperintense at long TR (b); note loculations superiorly. Pus was liquid at operation and *Proteus* organism was cultured

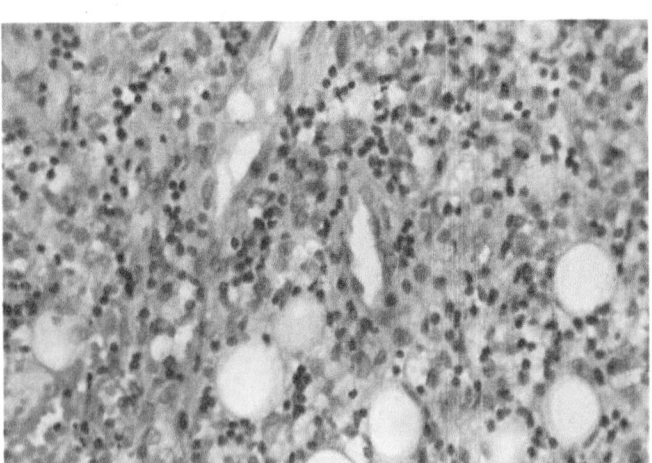

Figure 7.13 Epidural infection: paraparesis 5 days post-trauma with myelographic block; operative specimen showing panniculitis and granulation tissue. HE × 400

7.5c. Circumscribed intraspinal–extraparenchymal tumours

Adjacent to the spinal cord, the great majority of these lesions are meningiomas and schwannomas, all others being miscellaneous and uncommon. Intradural location is the rule, a point more easily settled with CT myelography than MR. However, extradural growth is well recognized in meningioma[31], and is inevitably partial in schwannoma, involving the mixed spinal nerve. At and below the conus, ependymoma and schwannoma make up most of the discrete masses.

Meningioma

The MR imaging characteristics of meningioma are described in detail in section 3,4, and spinal examples are typical, being isointense with cord at short TR, and slightly hyperintense at long TR (Figure 7.30), although this feature is usually obscured by the surrounding CSF signal. Enhancement is strong and homogeneous (Figure 7.31) without revealing a dural tail, and in most cases the general profile is not different to schwannoma. Mineralized, psammomatous-type morphology is said to be commoner in the spine[25], but even the rare en plaque and subdural growths[32,33] are not histologically unusual.

Schwannoma

The correlative features of discrete, intradural spinal schwannoma conform to those of the acoustic nerve described in section 6.4b. Signal characteristics include T1 cord-isointensity, with inhomogeneous hyperintensity at long TR (Figure 7.32). Cystic change is common (Figure 7.33), apparently due to progressive degeneration of Antoni B tissue and is occasionally subtotal (Figure 7.34). Mineralization of dystrophic type may be extensive (Figure 7.35). These alterations, including hyalinization, are the principal source of signal inhomogeneity, whilst Verocay body architecture and melanin production[34] (Figures 7.36 and 7.37) might be expected to contribute to T2 and T1 shortening respectively. When the schwannoma involves the combined nerve roots, it assumes an elongated, dumbell shape (Figure 7.36), and the tendency to cyst formation seems to be lost. This form is often diagnosed as neurofibroma clinically, but is usually unexceptionally schwannian. Extensive destruction of bone illustrated in Figure 7.38 was associated with histological malignancy, including invasion of connective tissue and muscle, but MR was not done. Rarely, an extraparenchymal schwannoma may grow into the cord parenchyma, suggesting a meningoparenchymal tumour[35] (Figure 7.37 – see also section 7.5).

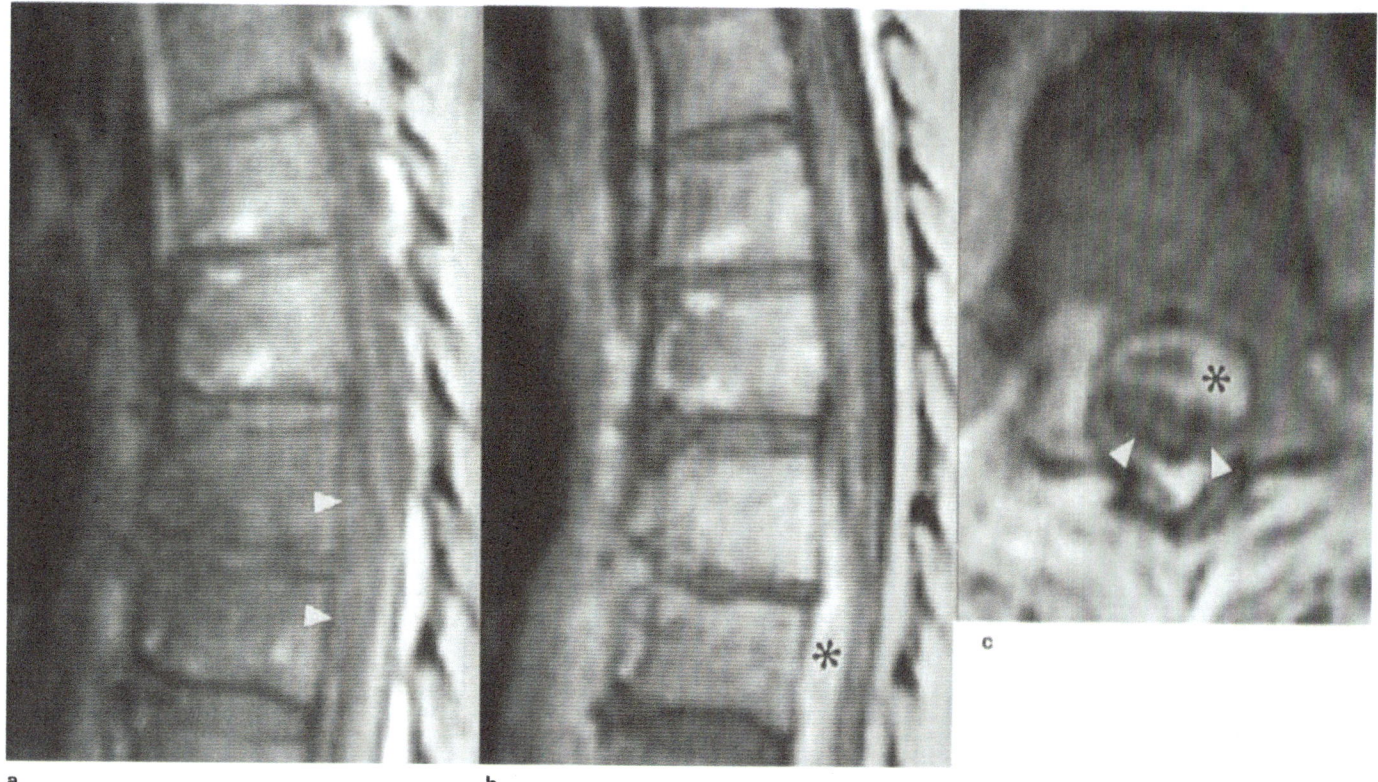

a   b

c

Figure 7.14   Epidural abscess and discitis, thoracic spine: (a) T1WI, (b) T1WI + C, (c) axial T1WI + C; sagittal T1 image (a) shows hypointensity of disc and adjacent bone, with soft tissue isointense extradural mass (arrow-heads) compressing cord. entire mass enhances following contrast (b, asterisk). Axial view (c) shows enhancing mass (asterisk) with hypointense centre (pus), loss of thecal outline (pachymeningitis) and cord compression (arrow-heads)

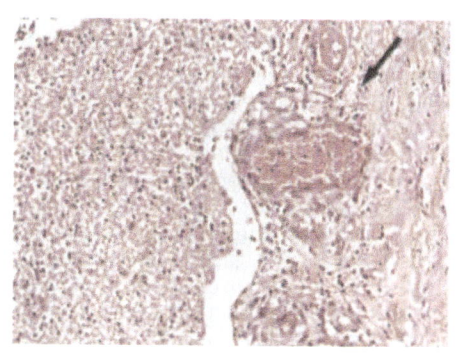

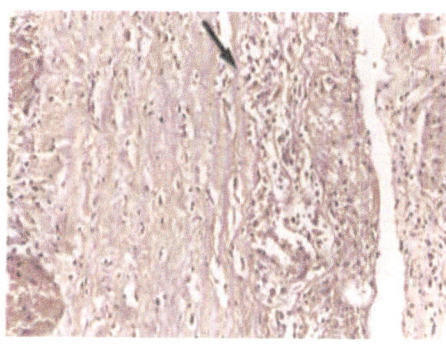

a   b

Figure 7.15   Epidural abscess: (a) epidural space, with dura (right), granulation tissue (arrow) and inflammatory exudate (left); (b) subdural space, with dura (left), reactive vessels and exudate (arrow) and leptomeninges (right). These morphological features explain why dura can not be distinguished on enhanced images (see **Figure 7.14**). HE × 200

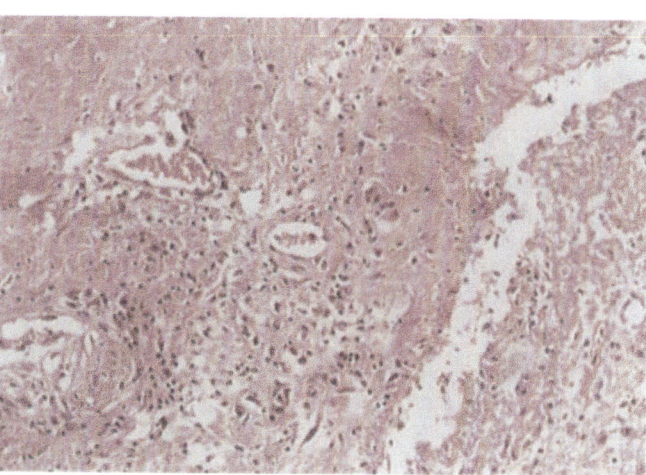

Figure 7.16   Epidural abscess: illustrates pachymeningitis with focal necrosis of dura. HE × 200

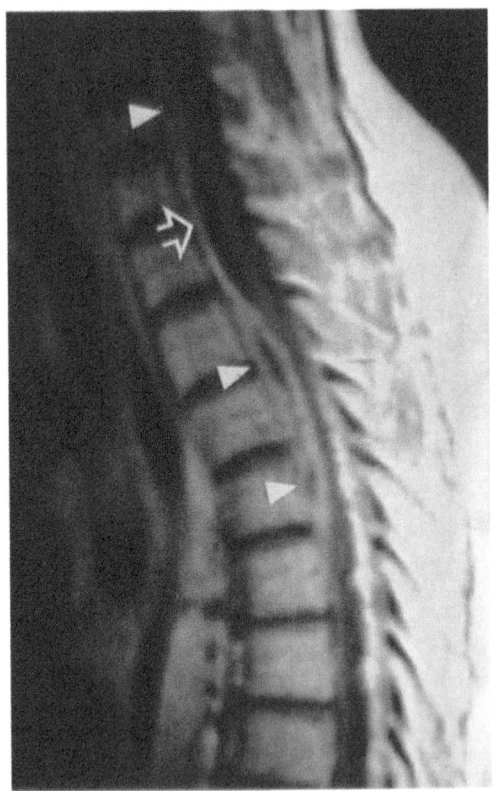

a

Figure 7.17 Granulomatous abscess, epidural: (**a**) T1WI + C, (**b**) HE × 200; enhanced T1 image shows two smooth extradural masses (arrow-heads), lower lesion with central hypointensity, confirmed at operation to be purulent. Histology shows granulomatous pachymeningitis, with prominent vessels responsible for abscess wall and intervening dural enhancement (a, open arrow); no demonstrable organisms, but patient responded to antituberculous treatment

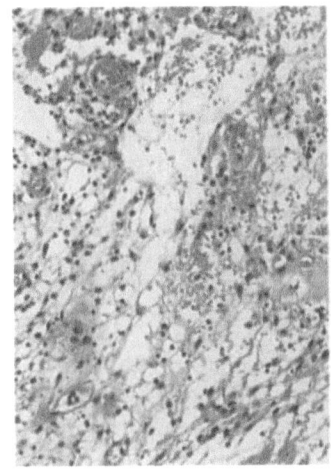 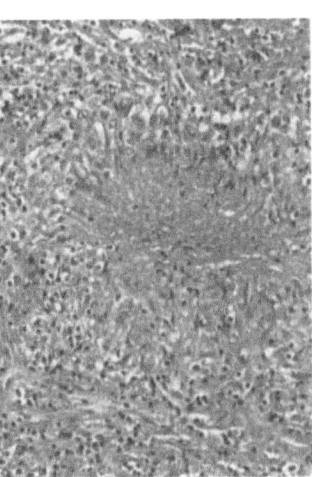

b

Ependymoma of the filum
These lesions, the majority of which are myxopapillary type[36], occur anywhere along the filum, where they present as circumscribed masses with the signal characteristics of glial tumours, being T1 isointense/T2 hyperintense, with moderate, diffuse enhancement (Figure 7.39). Occasional tumours having compact, clear-cell morphology do not appear to exhibit any imaging features different to the conventional myxopapillary type (Figure 7.40). As with schwannoma, the discrete mass may be cystic[25], but with growth the characteristic profile is lost and the lumbosacral CSF space is obliterated, with expansion of the bony canal (Figure 7.41). Neither this form[37], nor the tumour seeding illustrated in Figure 7.42 was associated with histological evidence of malignancy.

Rare lesions
Paraganglioma and epidermoidoma are uncommon tumours, usually of the cauda equina region, which mimic the common residents on account of macroscopic profile and signal intensity. The histology of paraganglioma (Figure 2.28) is consistent with reported T1 cord isointensity, T2 hyperintensity[38] (section 2.6g). Epidermoidoma (Figure 7.7) may resemble cystic schwannoma or ependymoma, with peripheral enhancement. Haemangioblastoma may occur within the cord or as a superficial mass; in the latter site it is invariably associated with angiomatous ectasia of the superficial vessels, presenting as punctate signal voids which demarcate the tumour, accounting for the spotty tissue inhomogeneity at both short and long TR[39] (Figure 7.43); as with intracranial lesions, enhancement is strong. Teratoma is the primary diagnosis when the images display prominent fat-consistent density or signal intensity (T1 hyperintense/T2 hypointense), with lobulation and septation (Figure 7.44).

7.5d. Circumscribed intraparenchymal tumours

Prior to MR, the presence or absence of circumscription of an intrinsic cord lesion was a purely neuropathological parameter. As with intracranial glial neoplasms, enhanced MR not only provides the basis for macroscopic definition, but is also essential to some aspects of histological definition. The principal examples of primary intramedullary neoplasms having an edge clearly demarcated by either contrast enhancement or cord-signal difference (T2 hyper- or hypointense) are ependymoma and juvenile pilocytic astrocytoma. Haemangioblastoma and schwannoma are also circumscript, but rare, as are metastases within the cord.

Extrapolating from the correlative appearances of intracranial astrocytomas (see the discussion in section 4.6), it is reasonable to expect that a purely protoplasmic astrocytic cord lesion could have a sharp margin on the long TR/TE sequence, but that a fibrillary tumour would not, and neither type would exhibit any genuine enhancement. Inhomogeneous enhancement (not arising spuriously from the meninges of the spinal fissures) ought to imply malignant transformation, whilst only (juvenile) pilocytic astrocytoma and ependymoma should enhance diffusely. The radiological literature, however, does not properly support these precepts, suggesting instead, that low-grade astrocytic tumours of the cord are peculiar in that enhancement is a characteristic[1], whilst examination of illustrative cases shows most to be circumscribed. Since the respective histologies of fibrillary (Figure 7.51) and juvenile pilocytic astrocytoma (Figure 7.48) are identical whether in the hemisphere or cord, the imaging conclusion that cord gliomas differ basically from their supratentorial counterparts, could be explained in a number of ways, the most important being inaccurate histological diagnosis arising from the inherent difficulty in

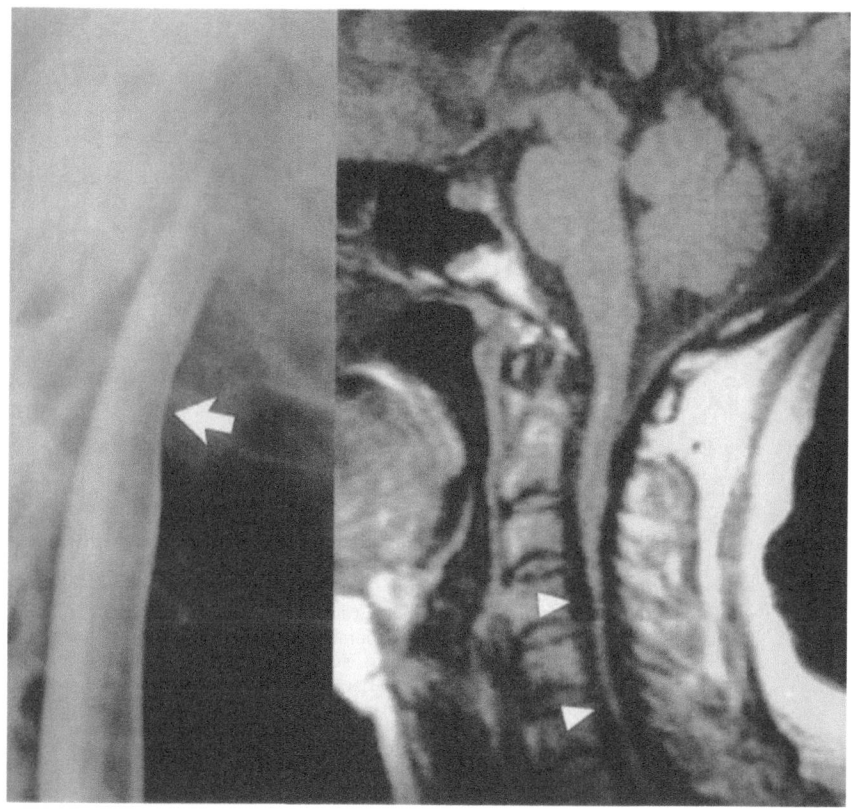

a

b

Figure 7.18 Hypertrophic pachymeningitis, spinal: female, 46 years; long history of spinal cord dysfunction; (**a**) myelogram, (**b**) T1WI, (**c**) CT + C, (**d**) HE ×100; myelogram shows arachnoid space constriction (a, arrow), which is T1 hypointense (b, arrow-heads). Biopsy of dura (d) shows dense fibrosis with non-specific chronic inflammation. Abnormal enhancement of orbit and cavernous sinus (c, arrow), not biopsied, suggests similar pathology (see discussion in section **3.2b** and **Figure 3.12**)

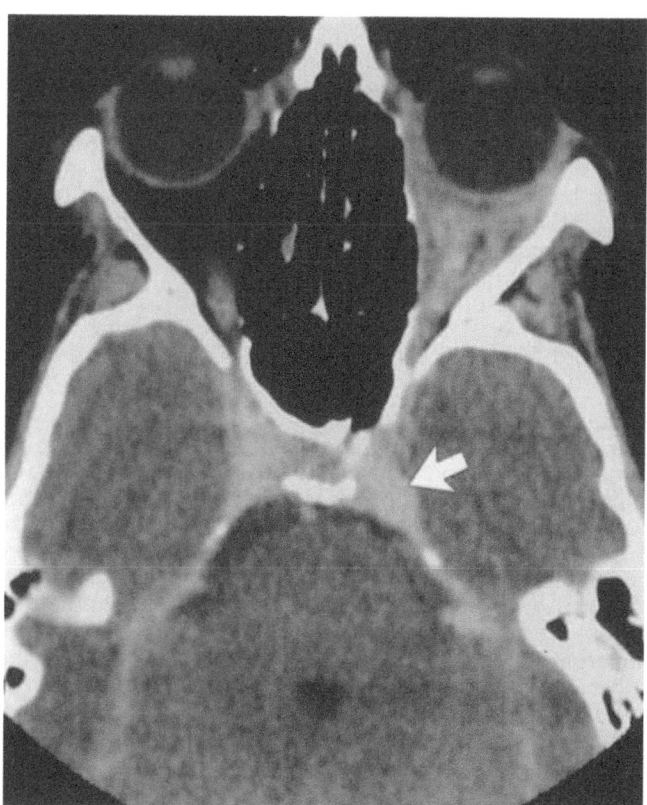

c

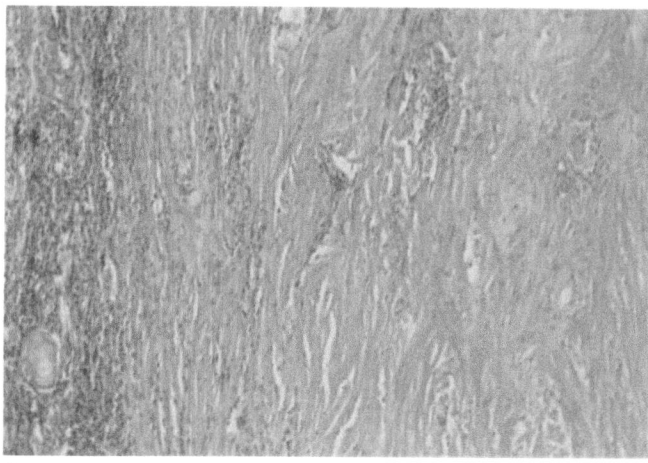

d

Table 7.1 Spinal cord 'gliomas' at TBH, 1980–1992

Ependymoma NOS	4
Classic ependymoma	4
Myxoid ependymoma	1
Myxopapillary ependymoma	4
Astrocytoma NOS	2
Fibrillary astrocytoma	1
Pilocytic astrocytoma	4
Glioma NOS	1
Mixed glioma	1
Ganglioglioma	1
Malignant glioma	1
Sarcoglioma	1

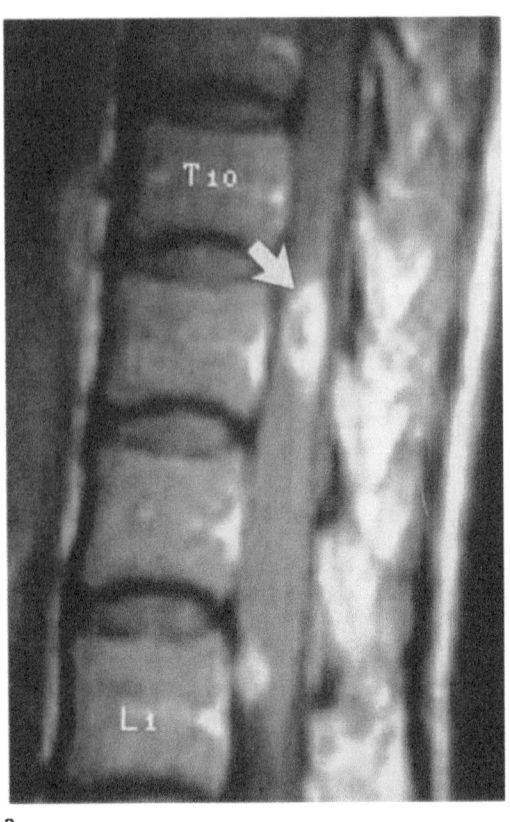

a

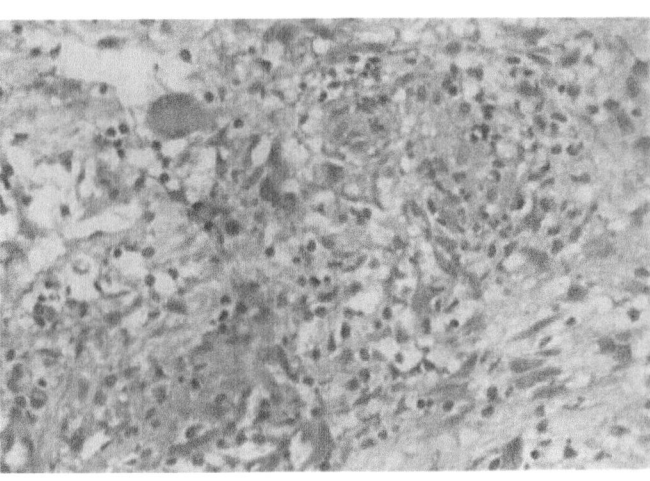

b

Figure 7.19 Granulomatous radiculomyelitis, syphilitic: (a) T1WI + C, (b) HE ×400; image shows multiple elongated, enhancing lesions appearing to be either adherent to or infiltrating the cord; central inhomogeneity of larger lesion (arrow) is probably volume averaging, and not tissue breakdown. At operation pale, granular nodules embedded on the pial surface of the cord, some involving the nerve roots, were found. Histology shows non-necrotizing epithelioid granulomas with no demonstrable organisms. Initially assumed to be tuberculous, but failed to respond to treatment; positive lues serology which responded to antisyphilitic therapy

obtaining tissue samples adequate for paraffin processing. That this has happened is immediately evident from the general lack of histomorphological detail with consequent 'lumping'[40–42], or such stated incongruities as the possibility of a (low-grade) astrocytoma exhibiting central necrosis[43]. However, it is apparent from a review of the pathological material in this teaching hospital (Table 7.1, p.221), that apart from the clear-cut examples of fibrillary and juvenile pilocytic neoplasms, the majority of astrocytic tumours conform to the adult type of compact pilocytic astrocytoma (Figure 7.49) in which there is additionally a prominent vasculature. The source of these vessels is speculative; they may be part of the intrinsic fascicular angioarchitecture. It may also be predicted that some cases of cord glioma, exhibiting inhomogeneous or patchy enhancement, will represent either focal malignant transformation or else mixed cell populations (or even both of these). Bearing in mind the volume of tissue removed by a micro-rongeur, only multiple biopsies could identify such lesions. Inadequate material is also implied in the designation NOS with regard to our own material (Table 7.1).

Intramedullary ependymoma
Although ependymoma is quoted as being the commonest primary cord neoplasm[1], it is difficult to find out the incidence of those lesions which are properly within the parenchyma as opposed to the relatively common extrinsic conus region tumour (section 7.5c). In the material from this hospital, 4/13 cord ependymomas diagnosed between 1980 and 1992, were classic myxopapillary tumours (Table 7.1).

The histomorphology of intramedullary ependymoma is regarded as being identical to the intracranial counterpart[25], which is discussed in section 6.7a. Lesions may be extended over one or several segments and are delineated by adjacent cord cavitation (Figure 7.45) or contrast

(Figure 7.46) or both. Cord T1 isointensity, with moderate, inhomogeneous T2 hyperintensity is consistent with densely cellular tissue organized into lobules with intervening clefts (Figure 7.46). However, lesions of identical morphology lying wholly outside the parenchyma have been reported to be uniformly T2 hyperintense[37], as might be expected from a purely glial neoplasm. Tumour vasculature is plentiful and diffuse, and necrosis is not a feature. Surgery demonstrates continuity of the surrounding parenchyma, although this may be so attenuated as to be invisible on the images (Figure 7.46). The presence of multiple ependymomas or subependymomas within the cord is characteristic of type 2 neurofibromatosis (Figure 7.47).

Pilocytic astrocytoma
The morphology and imaging features of pilocytic astrocytoma are described under section 6.6a. Its incidence in relation to other gliomas is said to be unknown[25], but combined MR and histology will foreseeably establish this. In our series 4/7 non-malignant astrocytomas were pilocytic (Table 7.1). Strong homogeneous enhancement (Figures 7.48 and 7.49) distinguishes the tumour from diffuse fibrillary astrocytoma and malignant glioma, but not from ependymoma. T1 cord isointensity favours the compact variety of morphology (Figure 7.49), whilst T1 hypointensity would favour the dimorphic variety of pilocytic astrocytoma (JPA).

Rare circumscribed, intramedullary tumours
Intramedullary schwannoma[44,45], haemangioblastoma[46] and metastasis[47] comprise the less common discrete neoplasms, all of which are known to enhance strongly. The schwannoma illustrated in Figure 7.50 was identified by means of a small rongeur biopsy only, and the reason for its relative T2 hypointensity (i.e. cord isointense) is unknown. Non-necrotic metastatic carcinoma is expected to be cord isointense and to exhibit surrounding oedema.

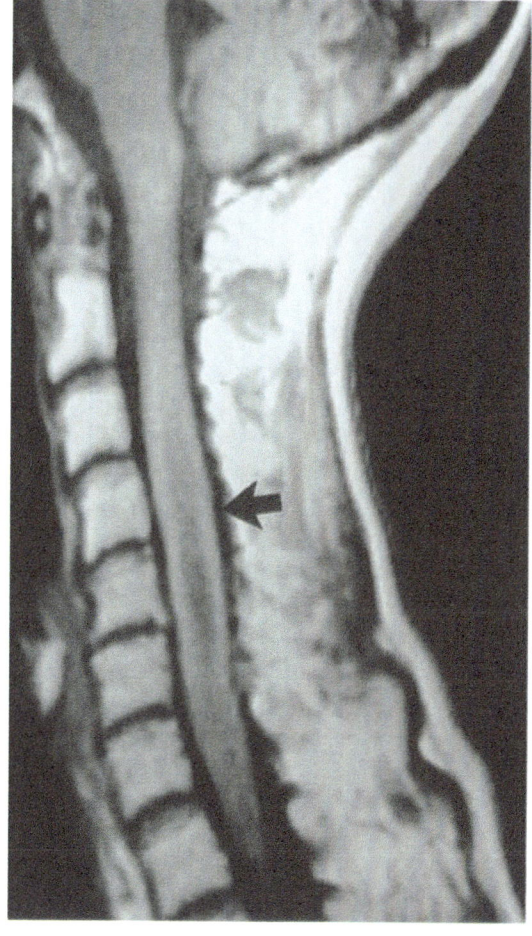

.a

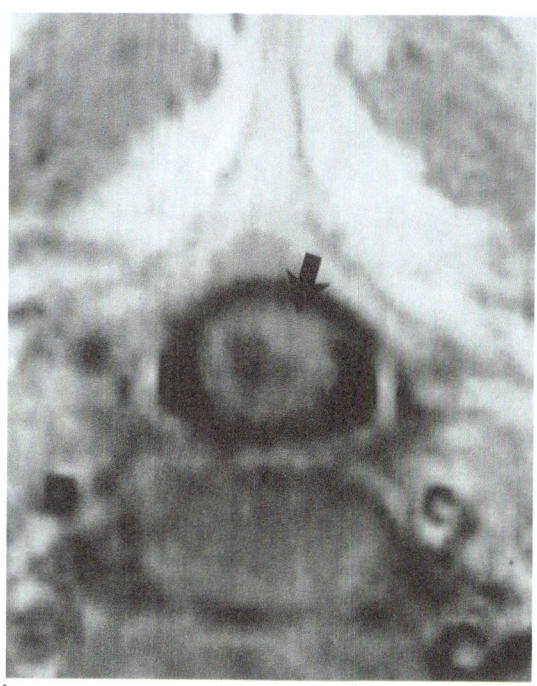

b

Figure 7.20   Necrotic myelopathy with cord cavitation: female, 50 years; recent onset of hemiparesis; no history of trauma; (**a**) T1WI + C, (**b**) axial T1WI + C, (**c**) HE × 100, (**d**) HE × 400; images show swelling and central hypointense abnormality with weak peripheral enhancement (a,b, arrows), thought to be a tumour syrinx. Specimen obtained through myelotomy shows abnormal proliferating vessels (c), macrophages and gliosis (d); features were considered consistent with liquefactive necrosis or myelinolysis. Follow-up scan 6 months later showed a syrinx and multiple enhancing lesions, considered to be demyelinative

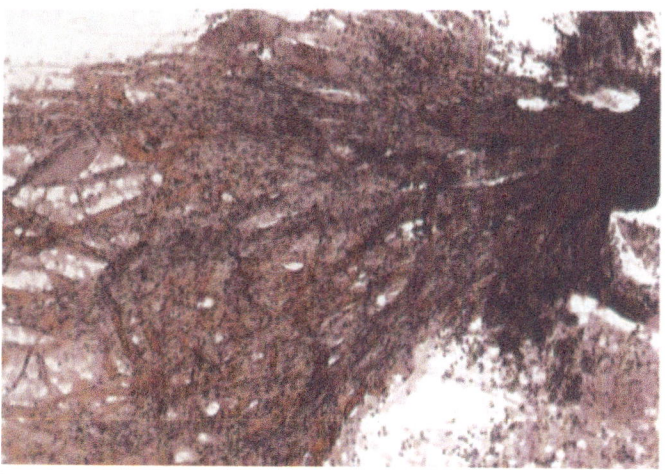

c

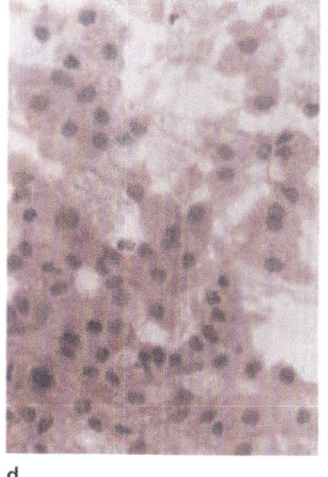
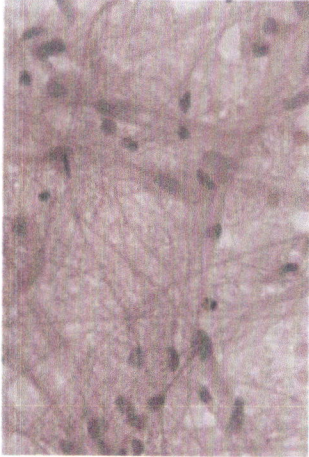

d

7.5e.   Diffuse neoplastic expansion of the cord (astrocytoma–malignant glioma, oligodendroglioma, mixed glioma) (see also the discussion in section 7.5d above)

Fibrillary astrocytoma, in our experience, rare (Table 7.1), is typically associated with a diffuse, T1 hypointense, T2 hyperintense expansion of the cord, with little or no enhancement (Figure 7.51), signal characteristics identical to those of its intracranial counterpart (see section 4.6). The morphological basis of occasional foci of enhancement is unknown, but malignant transformation has to be considered (Figure 7.52).

7.5f.   Rare primary intramedullary tumours

The number of rare primary neoplasms of mixed (Figure 7.53) or indeterminate cell type (Figure 7.54) will probably be found to obey the same rule of proportion that the commoner lesions follow, but will constitute unique cases in individual departments. Ganglioglioma[48–50] is probably the most important unusual neoplasm of the spinal cord (Figure 7.55), whose imaging features are nevertheless non-specific. The intramedullary sarco-glioma[51] illustrated in Figure 7.56 exhibits a smooth, moderately T2 hyperintense expansion of the conus; contrast was not given but the tumour cord interface is abrupt, and vessels are prominent, so that enhancement could be expected.

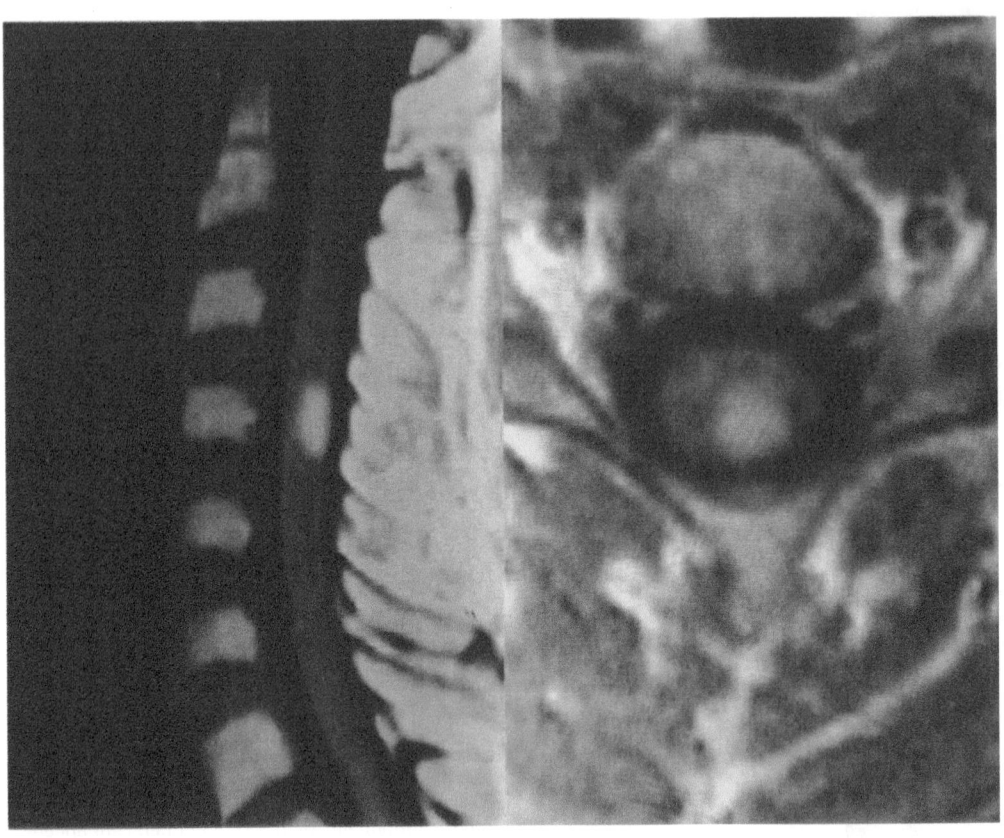

a   b

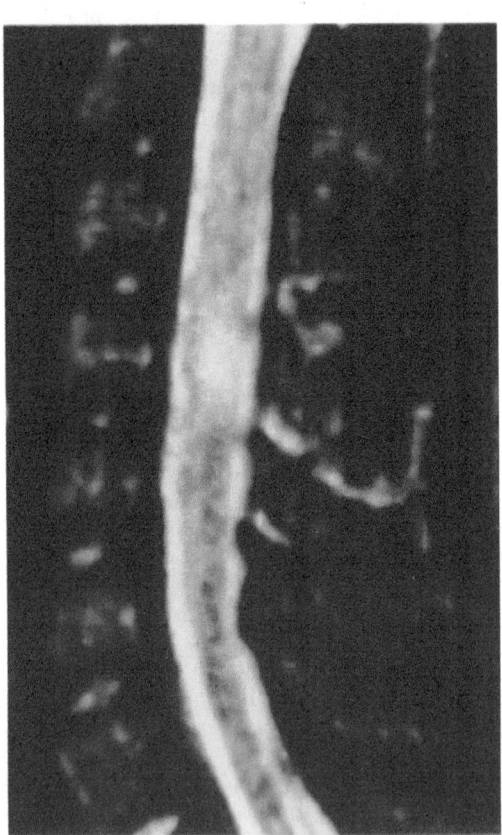

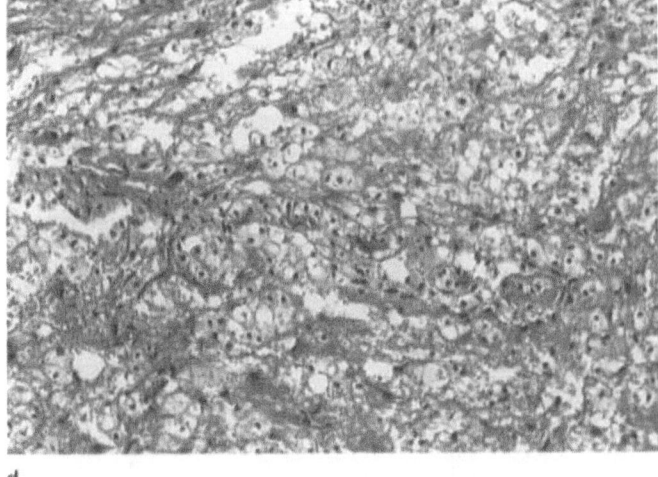

d

c

Figure 7.21   Focal demyelination, spinal cord: female, 26 years;
subacute history of progressive hemisensory disturbance and paresis;
(**a**) T1WI + C, (**b**) axial T1WI + C, (**c**) T2WI, (**d**) LBHE ×200, (**e**)
Holmes LB/Retic ×200; images show a circumscribed enhancing focal
lesion (a,b), which is T2 hyperintense (c). Volumetric expansion is
scarcely apparent. Histology shows active demyelination (note preservation of axons (e, left), with remarkable small-vessel proliferative
alteration (e, right) and sparse chronic inflammatory cell infiltrate

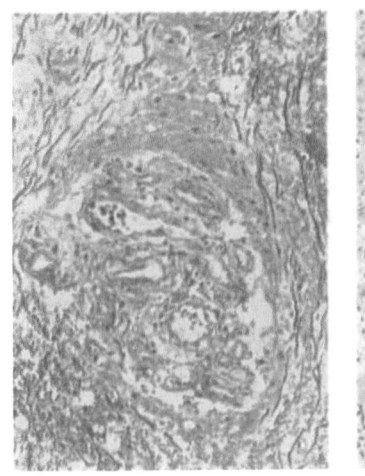
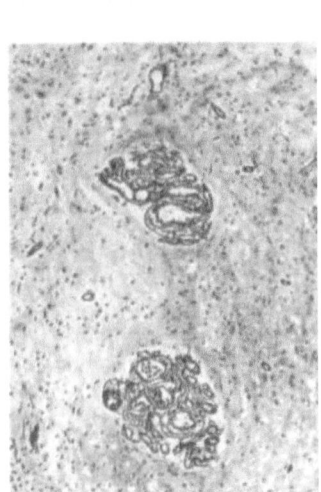

e

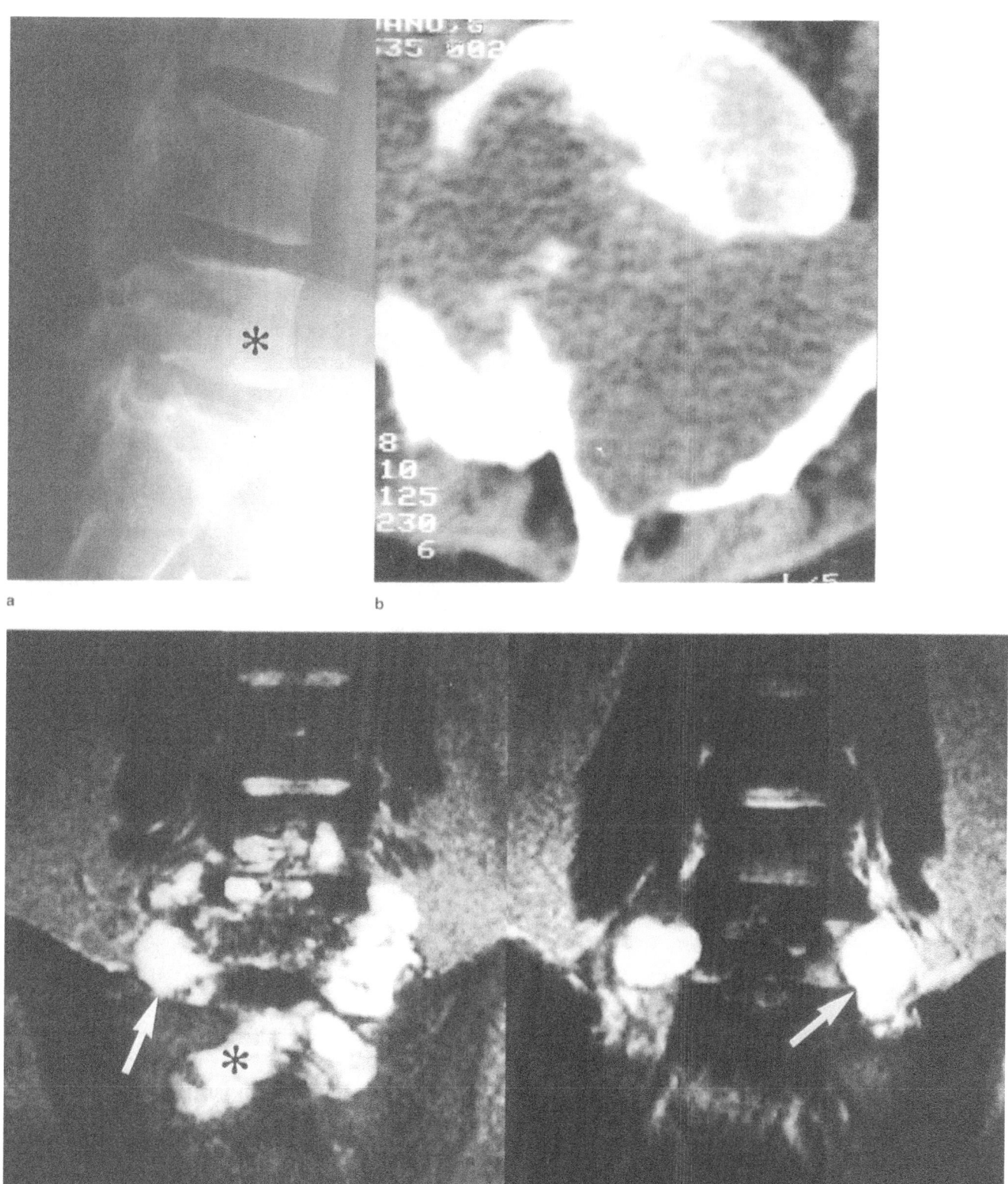

Figure 7.22 Hydatidosis, spinal: (**a**) X-ray spine, (**b**) CT, (**c,d**):
T2WI; plain film shows bubbly expansion of pedicles and spinous
process of L5 (a, asterisk), also seen on the axial CT, with obliteration
of the spinal canal. MR shows multiple variably sized hyperintense cysts,
including within the disc (c), paravertebral tissues (c,d, arrows) and
sacrum (c, asterisk)

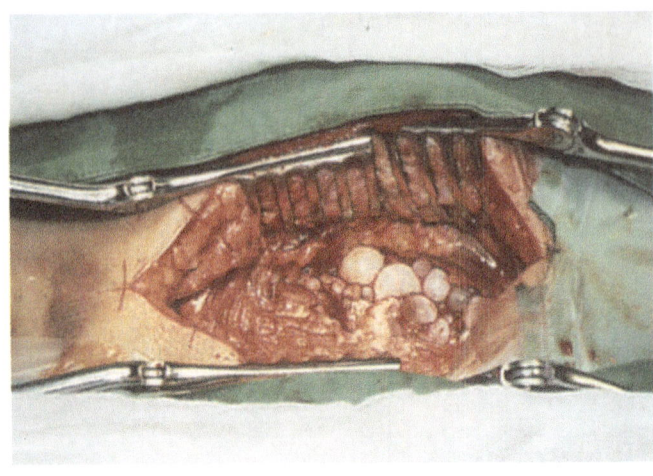

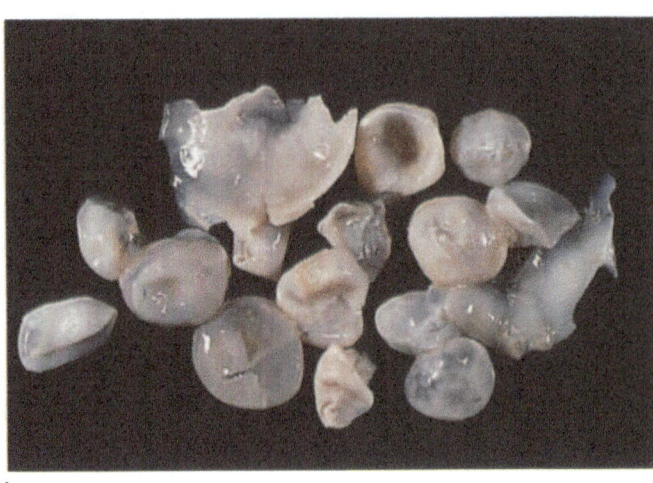

Figure 7.23 Hydatidosis, spinal, extradural: (**a**) operative view, (**b**) fixed specimen; operative view shows innumerable cysts of different sizes prolapsing spontaneously into the field. Fixed cysts, illustrating variable thickness of cyst wall lamellation. No viable protoscolisces seen on histology

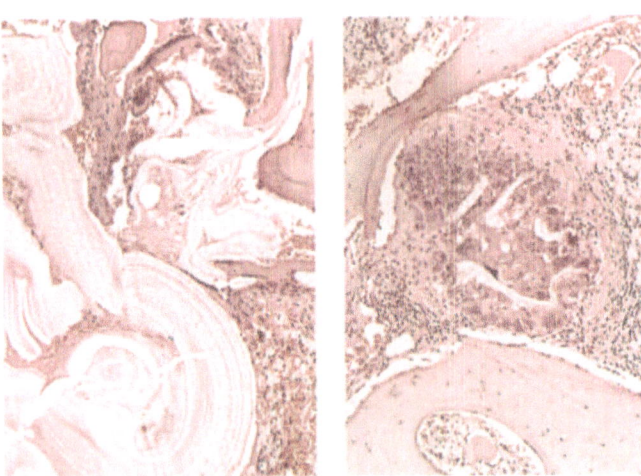

Figure 7.24 Hydatidosis, intraosseous: histology of necrotic cysts, granulomata and replacement of marrow by macrophages and myxomatous granulation tissue. HE ×100 (Dr RM Bowen, Groote Schuur Hospital)

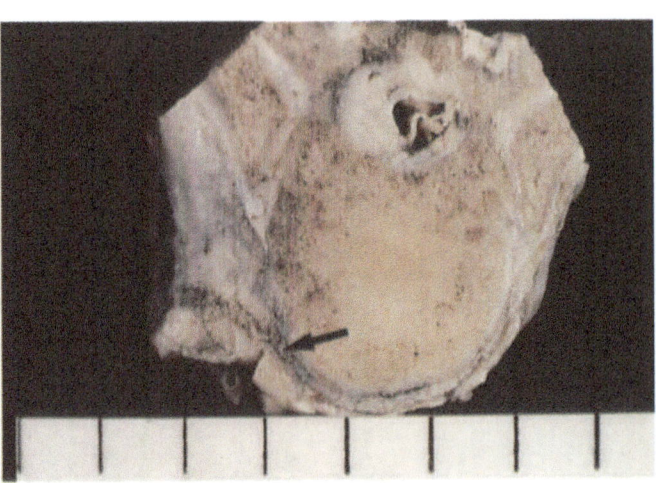

Figure 7.25 Metastatic disease, local, epidural: pulmonary tumour is adherent to vertebral body (arrow) and partially fills the epidural space (necrotic cord is artefactually cavitated)

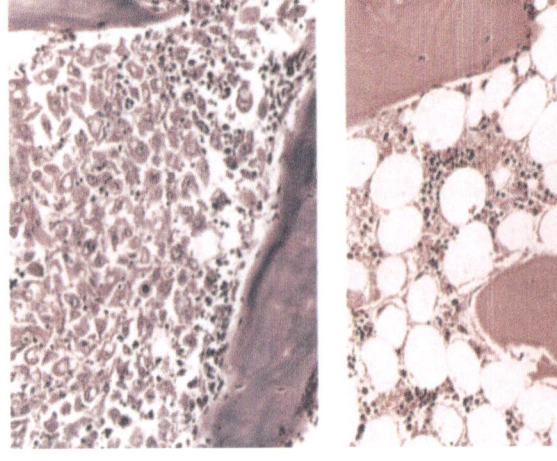

Figure 7.26 Metastatic disease, vertebral: shows replacement of vertebral marrow by metastatic tumour, responsible for loss of normal marrow signal at short TR (compare with normal marrow, right). PAS/HE 200

7.6. MISCELLANEOUS SPINAL AND INTRASPINAL LESIONS NOT ILLUSTRATED

Aneurysmal bone cyst, giant-cell tumour, osteochondroma, lipomatosis[52].

References

1. Sze G, Twohig M. Neoplastic disease of the spine and spinal cord. In: Atlas SW, ed. Magnetic resonance imaging of the brain and spine. New York: Raven Press; 1991:921–65.
2. Modic MT. Degenerative diseases of the spine. In: Modic MT, Masaryk TJ, Ross JS, eds. Magnetic resonance imaging of the spine. Chicago: Yearbook Medical Publishers; 1989:75–119.
3. Yasuma T, Koh S, Okamura T, Yamauchi Y. Histological changes in aging lumbar intervertebral discs. Their role in protrusions and prolapses. J Bone J Surg. 1990;72(2):220–9.

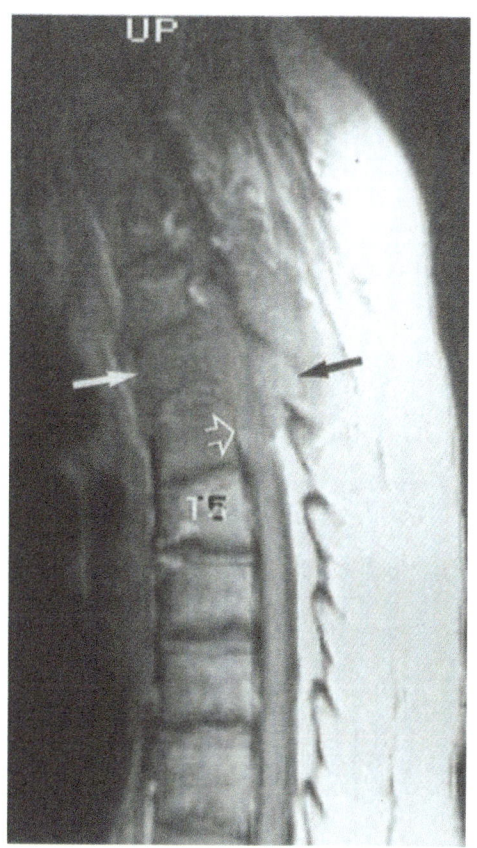

Figure 7.27 Metastatic disease, vertebral (breast): T1 weighted image of thoracic spine showing loss of normal marrow signal of vertebral bodies (white arrow), cord–theca delineation (open arrow) and epidural fat (dark arrow). (Tumour tissue is also T2 intermediate signal intensity.) These images are now so characteristic that, in the presence of known primary malignancy, they are no longer biopsied

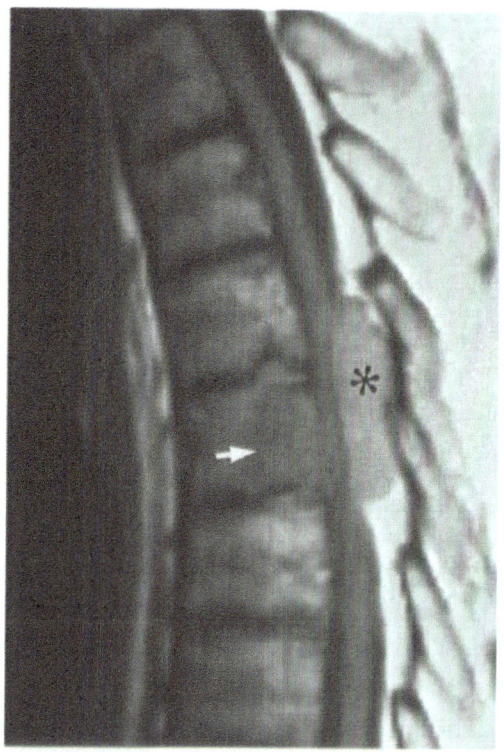

a

b

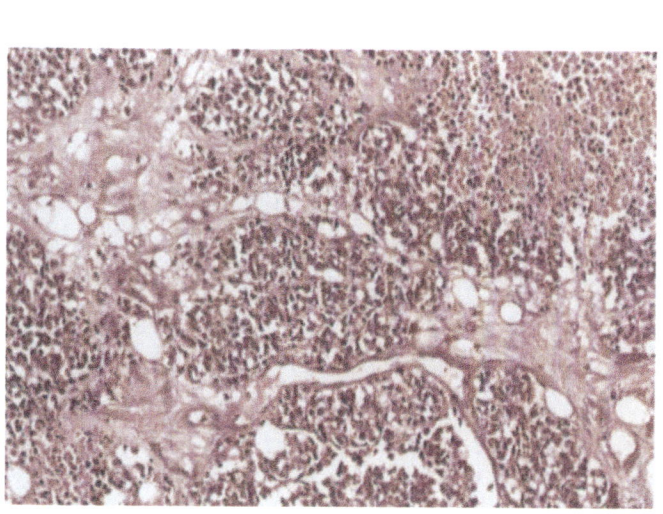

c

Figure 7.28 Metastatic disease, epidural (bronchial carcinoma): (**a**) T1WI, (**b**) T1WI + C, (**c**) HE ×200; sharply circumscribed homogeneous T1 cord isointense mass (a, asterisk), is diffusely enhancing (b, asterisk); note adjacent vertebra (a, arrow) is abnormal, but does not enhance. Despite image homogeneity tumour shows focal necrosis and admixed epidural fat; vasculature is probably also epidural

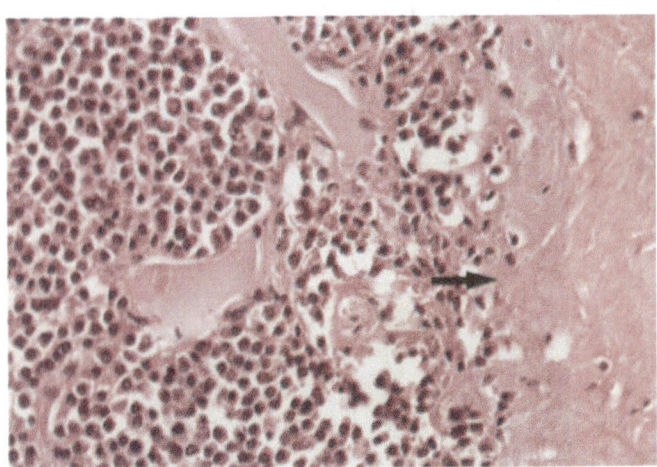

Figure 7.29 Myeloma, epidural, spine: illustrates tumour adherent to dura (arrow), and prominent blood vessels. HE × 200

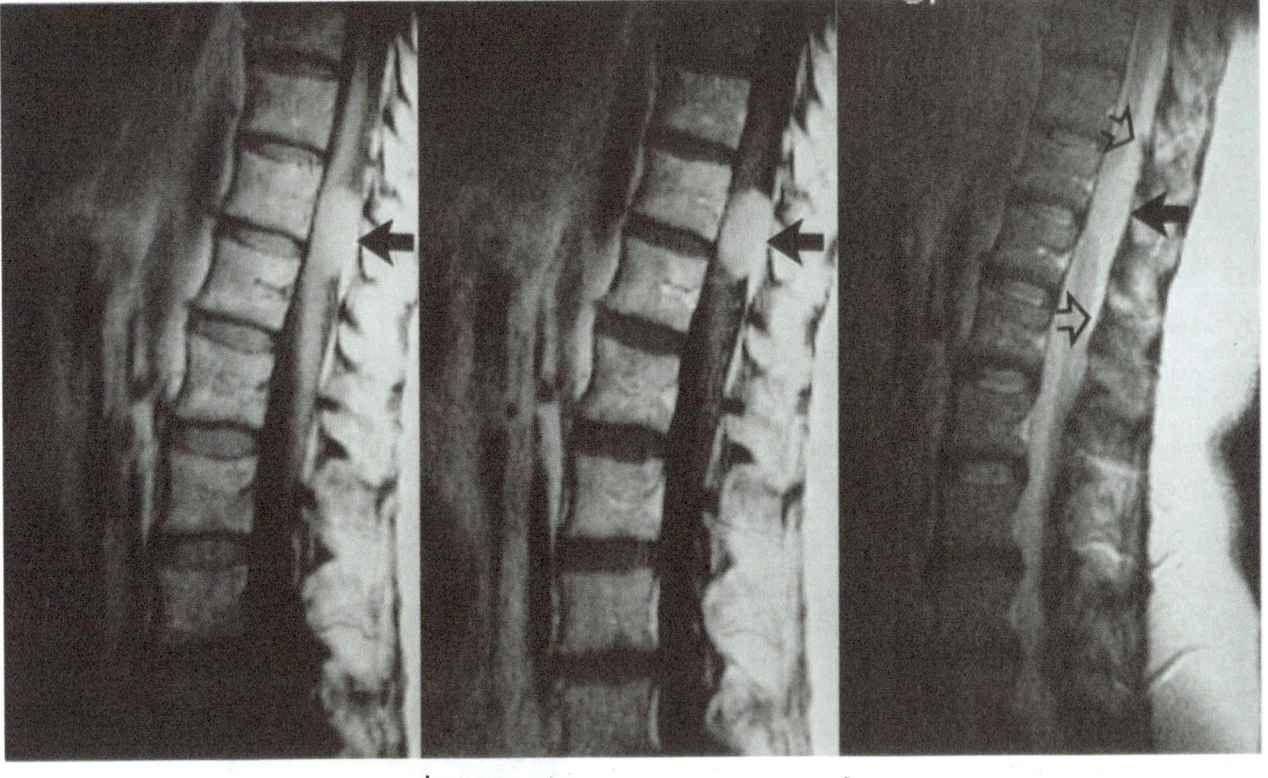

a   b   c

Figure 7.30 Meningioma, psammomatous, thoracic, intradural: (a) T1WI, (b) T1WI + C, (c) T2WI; circumscribed, extramedullary mass exhibits expected cord/parenchymal isointensity at short and long TR, with diffuse enhancement (arrows, a–c). Bright tapering signal adjacent to the lesion (c, open arrows) is CSF. Spurious, mild T2 hyperintensity is considered to be partial volume effect. Histology was uniformly that of a psammomatous meningioma

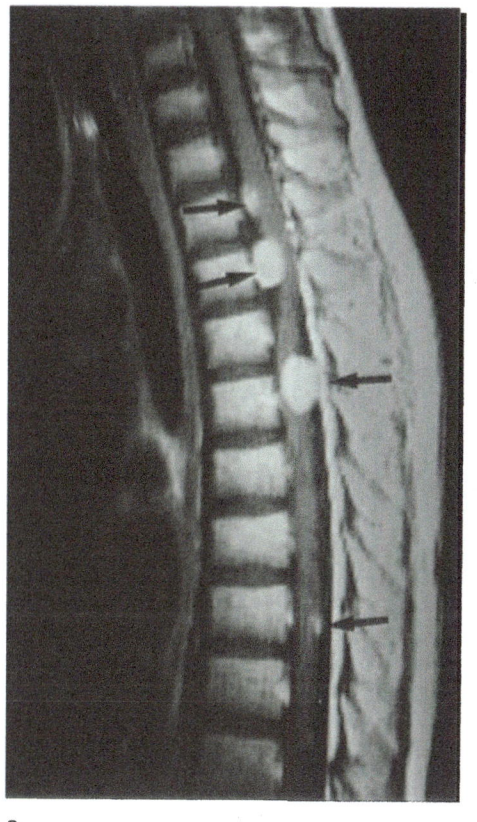

a

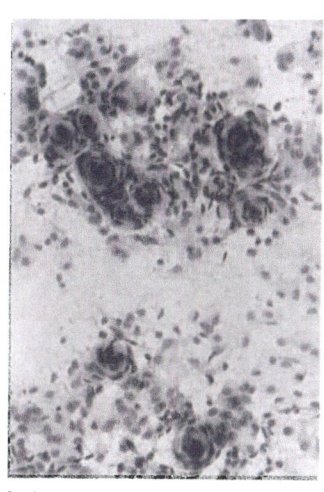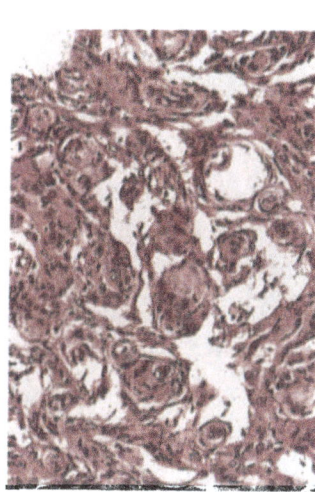

Figure 7.31 Meningiomas, multiple, presumed metastatic: previously resected intracranial meningioma (see **Figure 3.21**); (a) T1WI + C, (b) Tol blue/HE × 200; multiple circumscribed, extraparenchymal lesions are apparent on account of diffuse enhancement (arrows). Despite the inferred metastatic nature of the tumour the morphology is unremarkable, including classical meningiomatous whorls (b). (Follow-up CT scan did not show evidence of intracranial recurrence.)

b

4. Weidner N, Rice DT. Intervertebral disc material: criteria for determining probable prolapse. Hum Pathol. 1988;19:406–10.
5. Modic MT, Herfkens RJ. Intervertebral disc: normal age-related changes in MR signal intensity. Radiology. 1990;177:332–4.
6. Bundschuh CV, Stein L, Slusser JH et al. Distinguishing between scar and recurrent herniated disc in postoperative patients: value of contrast-enhanced CT and MR imaging. AJNR. 1990;11:949–58.
7. Heuftle MG, Modic MT, Ross JS et al. Lumbar spine: postoperative imaging with Gd-DTPA. Radiology. 1988;167:817–24.
8. Cervellini P, Curri D, Volpin L et al. Computed tomography of epidural fibrosis after discectomy; a comparison between symptomatic and asymptomatic patients. Neurosurgery. 1988;23:710–13.
9. Wilkins RH, Odom GL. Spinal intradural cysts. In: Vinken PJ, Bruyn GW, eds. Handbook of clinical neurology. Tumors of the spine and spinal cord, Part II. Amsterdam: North-Holland; 1976:20:55–102.
10. Breeze RE, Nichols P, Segal H et al. Intradural epithelial cyst at the craniovertebral junction. J Neurosurg. 1990;73:788–91.
11. Nabors M, Pait TG, Byrd EB et al. Updated assessment and current classification of spinal meningeal cysts. J Neurosurg. 1988;68: 366–77.
12. Hemmati M, Thomas C, Patel DV. Symptomatic intraspinal ganglion cyst of the nerve root sheath. AJNR. 1989;10(S):100.
13. Robertson DP, Kirkpatrick JB, Harper RL, Mawad ME. Spinal intramedullary ependymal cyst. Report of three cases. J Neurosurg. 1991;75:312–16.
14. Mercader J, Gomez J, Cardenal C. Intraspinal synovial cyst: diagnosis by CT. Neuroradiology. 1985;27:346–8.
15. Chung CK, Uihlein A, Bickel WH, Soule EH. Lumbar intraspinal extradural ganglion cyst. J Neurosurg. 1968;29:168–72.
16. Hemmati M, Thomas C, Patel DV. Symptomatic intraspinal ganglion cyst of the nerve root sheath. AJNR. 1989;10:S100.
17. Bhushan C, Hodges FJ, Wityk JJ. Synovial cyst (ganglion) of the lumbar spine simulating extradural mass. Neuroradiology. 1979;18:263–8.
18. Carp L, Stout AP. A study of ganglion. With special reference to treatment. Surg Gynecol Obstet. 1928;47:460–8.
19. Nabors MW, Pait TG, Byrd EB et al. Updated assessment and current classification of spinal meningeal cysts. J Neurosurg. 1988;68:366–77.
20. Vernet O, Frankhauser H, Schnyder P et al. Cyst of the ligamentum flavum: report of 6 cases. Neurosurgery. 1991;29:277–83.
21. Bates DJ. Inflammatory diseases of the spine. Neuroimag Clin N Am. 1991;1:231–50.
22. Rosenfeld JV, Kaye AH, Davis S et al. Pachymeningitis cervicalis hypertrophica. J Neurosurg. 1987;66:137–9.
23. Adler JR, Sheridan W, Kosek J et al. Pachymeningitis associated with a pulmonary nodule. Neurosurgery. 1991;29:283–7.
24. Digman KE, Partington CR, Graves VB. MR imaging of spinal pachymeningitis. JCAT. 1990;14:988–90.
25. Burger PC, Scheithauer BW, Vogel FS. Surgical pathology of the nervous system and its coverings, 3rd edn. New York: Churchill Livingstone; 1991:605–60.
26. Chang KH, Han MH, Choi YW et al. Tuberculous arachnoiditis of the spine. AJNR. 1989;10:1255–62.
27. Ulmer JL, Elster AD. Sarcoidosis of the central nervous system. Neuroimag Clin N Am. 1991;1:141–58.
28. Blacklock JB, Hood TW, Maxwell RF. Intramedullary cervical cord abscess. J Neurosurg. 1982;56:270–4.
29. Eckert J. Prospects for the treatment of the metacestode stage of echinococcosis. In: Thompson RCA, ed. The biology of echinococcus and hydatid disease. London: George Allen & Unwin; 1988:251–84.
30. Burns DH, Blaser S, Ross JS et al. MR imaging with GdDTPA of leptomeningeal spread of lymphoma. JCAT. 1988;12:499–500.
31. Levy WJ, Bay J, Dohn D. Spinal cord meningioma. J Neurosurg. 1982;57:804–12.
32. Stechison MT, Tasker RR, Wortzman GW. Spinal meningioma en plaque. J Neurosurg. 1987;67:452–5.
33. Carter DA, Rowed DW, Lewis AJ. Subdural meningioma of spinal cord. J Neurosurg. 1985;63:800–3.
34. Lowman RM, Livolsi VA. Pigmented (melanotic) schwannomas of the spinal canal. Cancer. 1980;46:391–7.
35. Tabatatabai A, Jungreis CA, Jonas H. Cervical schwannoma masquerading as a glioma: MR findings. JCAT. 1990;14:489–90.
36. Sonneland PR, Scheithauer BW, Onofrio BM. Myxopapillary ependymoma: a clinicopathological and immunocytochemical study of 77 cases. Cancer. 1985;883–93.
37. Wagle W, Jaufman B, Mincy JE. Intradural extramedullary ependymoma: MR-pathologic correlation. JCAT. 1988;12:704–7.
38. Hayes E, Lippa C, Davidson R. Paragangliomas of the cauda equina. AJNR. 1989;10:S45–7.
39. Kaffenberger DA, Chunilal P, Shah F et al. MR imaging of spinal cord hemangioblastoma associated with syringomyelia. JCAT. 1988;12:495–8.

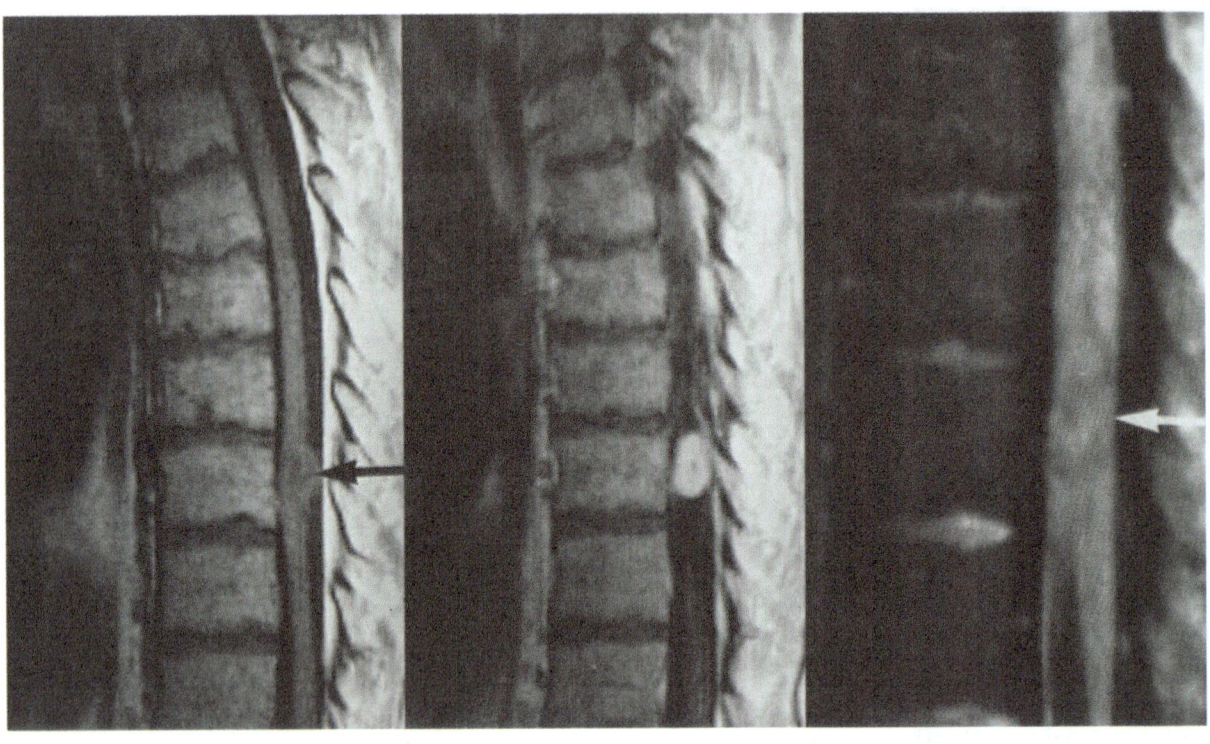

a   b   c

Figure 7.32 Schwannoma, intradural: (**a**) T1WI, (**b**) T1WI + C,
(**c**) T2WI, (**d**) HE × 200; lesion is inhomogeneous at both short (a)
and long TR (c), but enhancement is almost diffuse (b). Thin capsule
(probably meningeal in origin), with vascularized Antoni A tissue (d).
(Dr J Lotz, City Park Hospital)

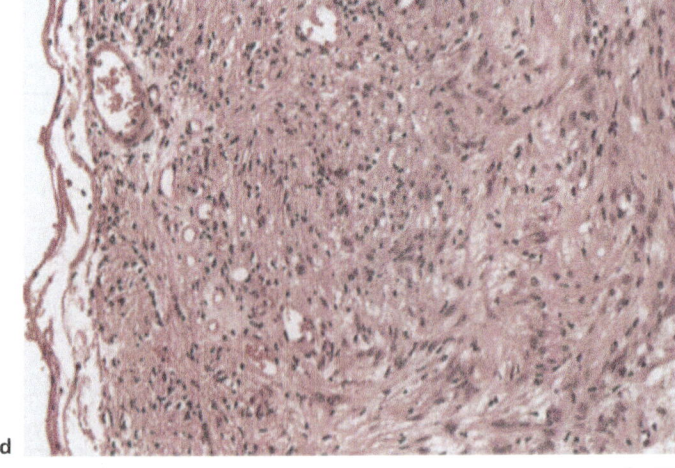

d

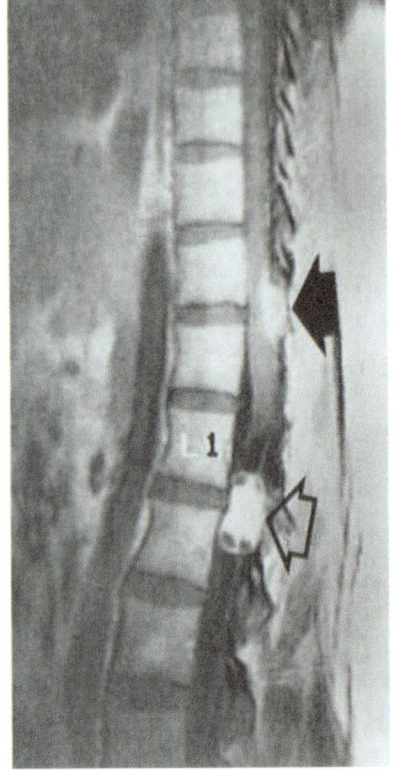

a

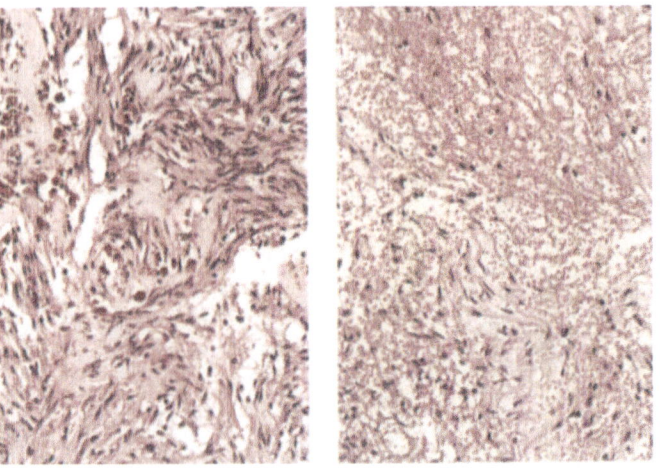

b

Figure 7.33 Schwannoma, multiple intradural: (**a**) T1WI + C,
(**b**) HE × 200; circumscribed cauda equina region mass (open arrow),
with cyst formation commencing beneath the capsule of the tumour.
Enhancing 'tails' (solid arrow) of upper lesion are thought to be part
of the attached nerve; histology shows Antoni A tissue with haemosiderophages (b, left) and recent non-surgical haemorrhage (b, right).
(Dr J Lotz, City Park Hospital)

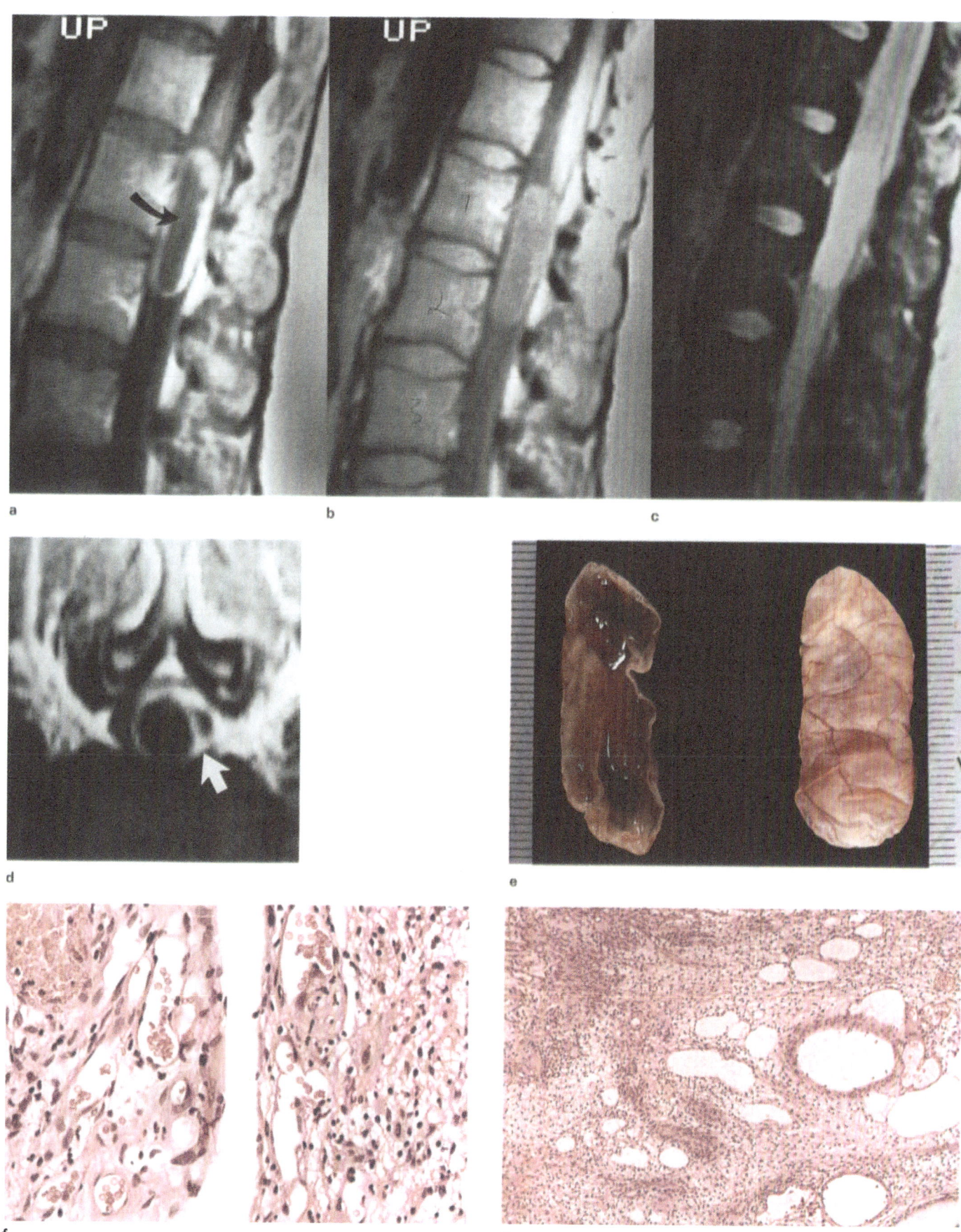

Figure 7.34 Schwannoma, cystic, cauda equina: (a) T1WI + C, (b) PDWI, (c) T2WI, (d) axial T1WI + C, (e) fixed specimen, (f) HE × 400, (g) HE × 100; enhanced T1 scan (a) shows central, cystic hypointensity (curved arrow), with an enhancing rim; homogeneity on proton density (b) and T2 weighted images (c) reflects protein content and water, respectively. Cyst loculation apparent on axial views (d, arrow) is seen in fixed specimen. The enhancing rim histologically consists of vascularized Antoni A and B tissue (f). Gelatinous cyst contents which have the brick-red colour of old haemorrhage (e) have not induced T1 signal shortening (a and d). Origin of cyst formation is suggested by presence of confluent microcysts (g)

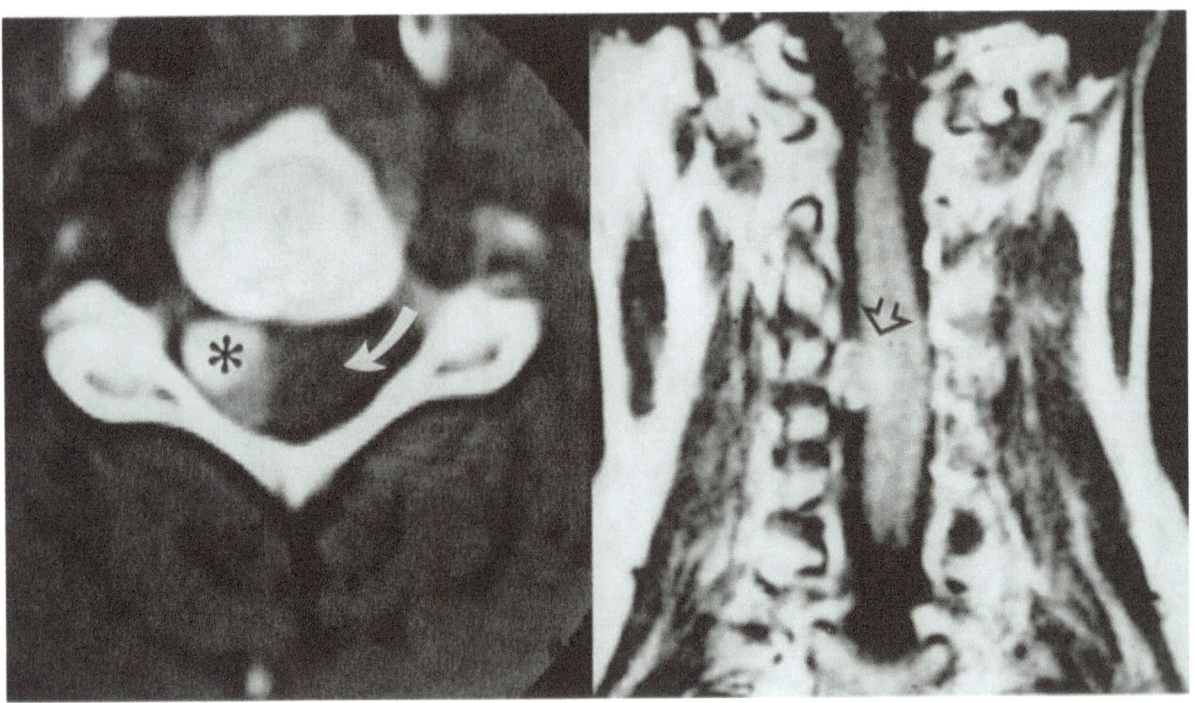

a   b

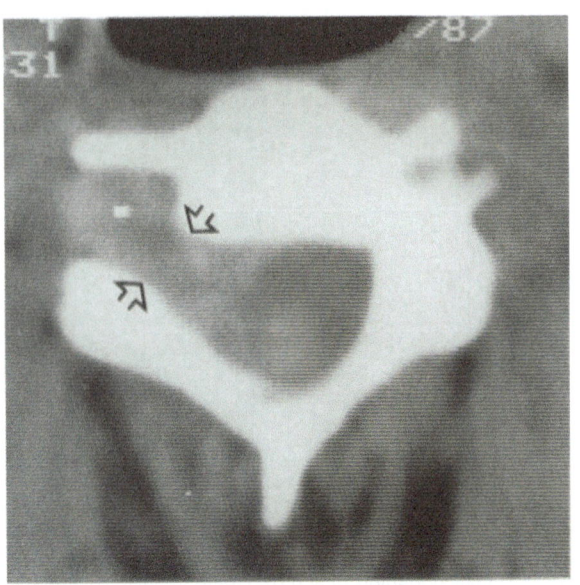

c

Figure 7.35 Schwannoma, mineralized: (**a**) CT myelogram, (**b**) T1WI + C, (**c**) HE ×400/LBHE ×200; CT hyperdense mass (asterisk), displacing the cord (a, curved arrow), also displays irregular peripheral enhancement (b, open arrow). Dystrophic mineralization (c, right) (responsible for CT hyperdensity), is not readily evident on routine HE (c, left)

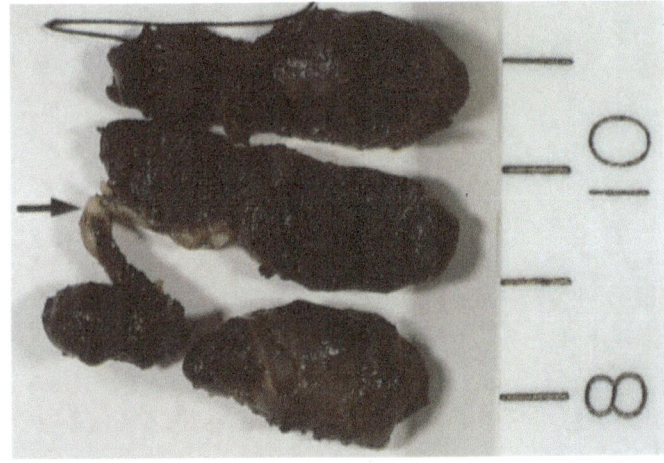

a   b

Figure 7.36 (*legend opposite*)

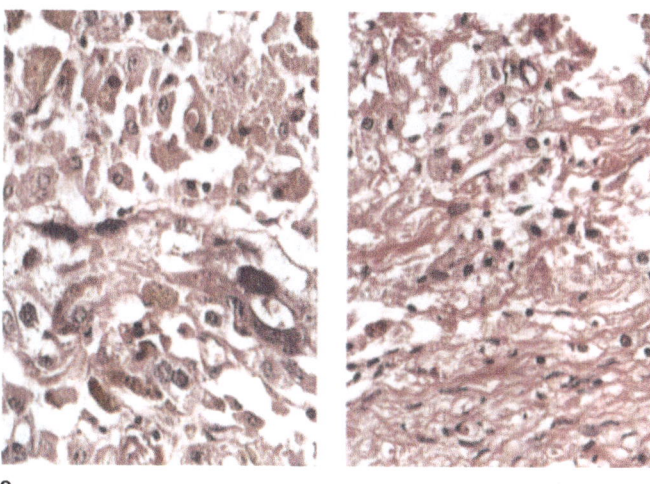

c

Figure 7.36 **Nerve sheath tumour, melanotic, radicular, intra–extradural**: (**a**) CT + C, (**b**) fixed specimen, (**c**) HE ×100/×200; axial CT scan shows a lobulated, diffusely enhancing mass, extending from within the spinal canal, through a dilated neural foramen (arrows). Operative specimen illustrates intensely melanotic tumour, with a dumbell profile and attached nerve root (b, arrow). Lesion is histologically pleomorphic (c, left), but retains a well defined capsule (c, right) (compare with **Figure 7.37**)

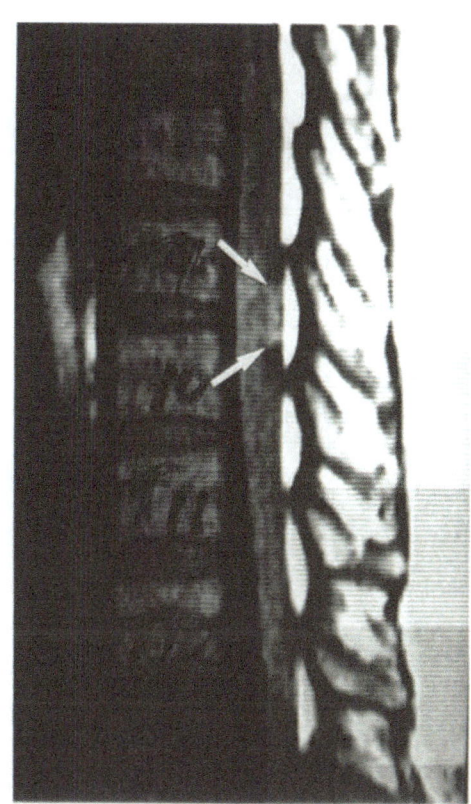

a

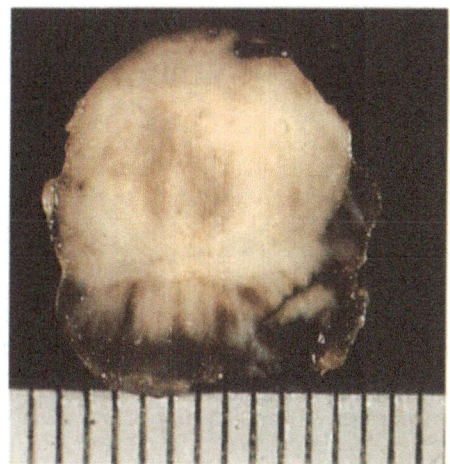

c

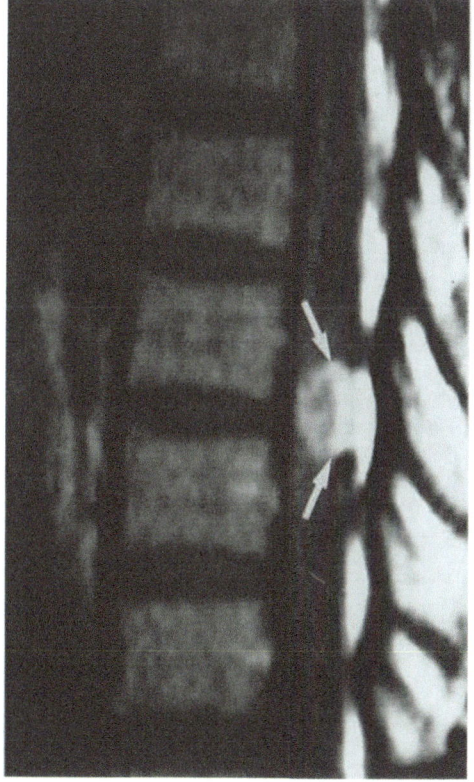

b

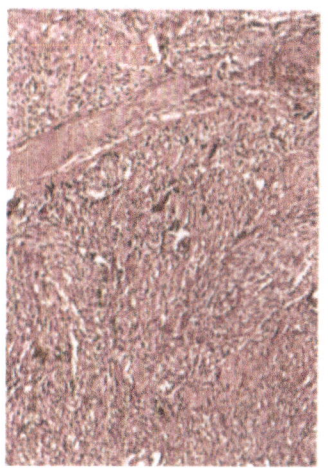 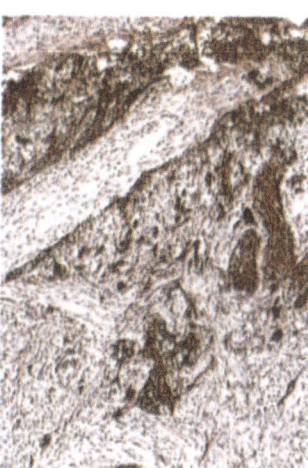

d

Figure 7.37 **Schwannoma, melanotic, intra–extramedullary**: (**a**) T1WI, (**b**) T1WI + C, (**c**) fixed specimen, (**d**) HE/GFAP ×100; exophytic component of lesion is initially faintly hyperintense (a, arrows), enhances strongly (b, arrows) with more inhomogeneous parenchymal component. Mass (c) was obviously pigmented at operation and histology (d) shows melanotic schwannoma cells (left) and GFAP-positive glial component (right) marking tumour–cord interface without cleavage plane. (Dr A Bok, Panorama Hospital)

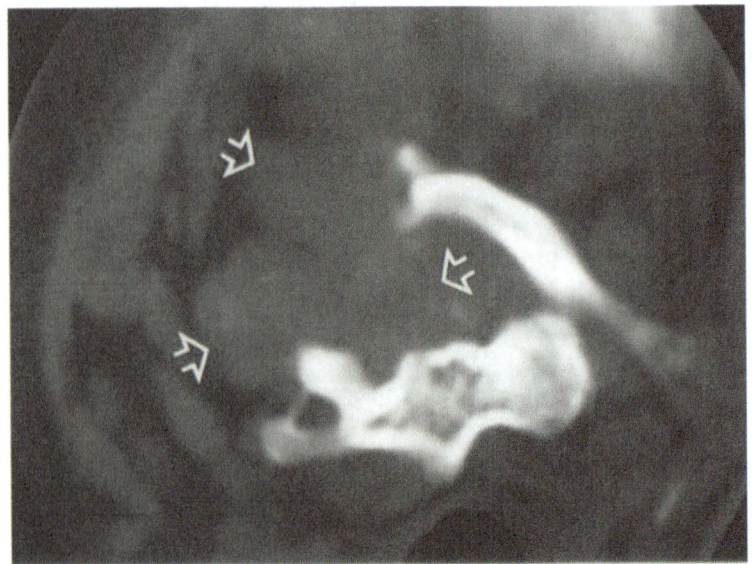

a

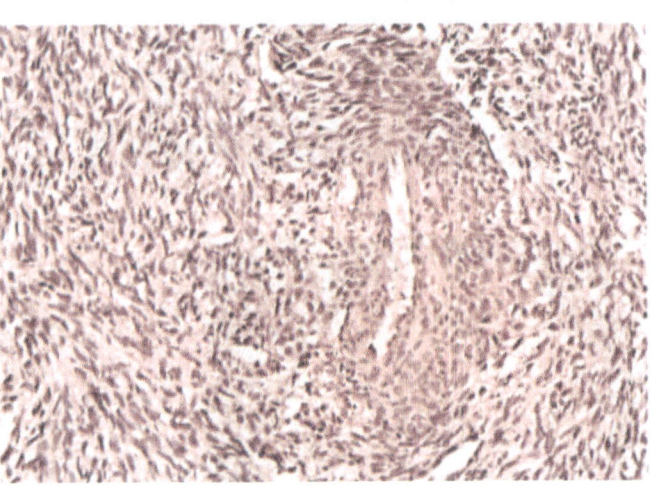

b

Figure 7.38 Schwannoma, malignant: (**a**) CT, (**b**) HE × 200; lobulated mass (arrows) arising within the spinal canal, is eroding vertebral lamina and extending into cervical soft tissues. Histology illustrates characteristic cellularity and perivascular congregation of malignant schwannoma, consistent with the invasive appearance on the images

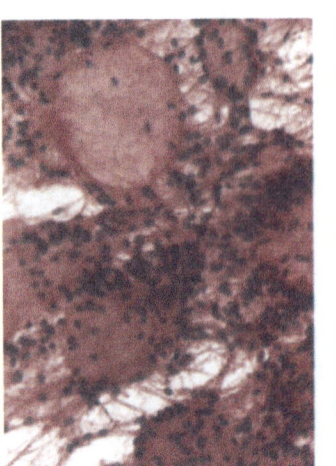

c

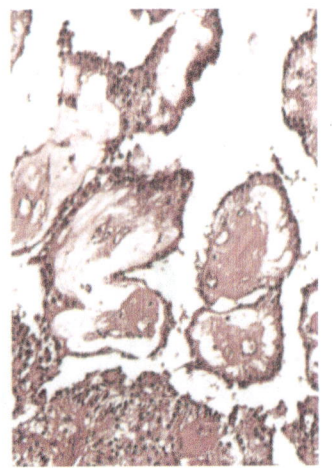

d

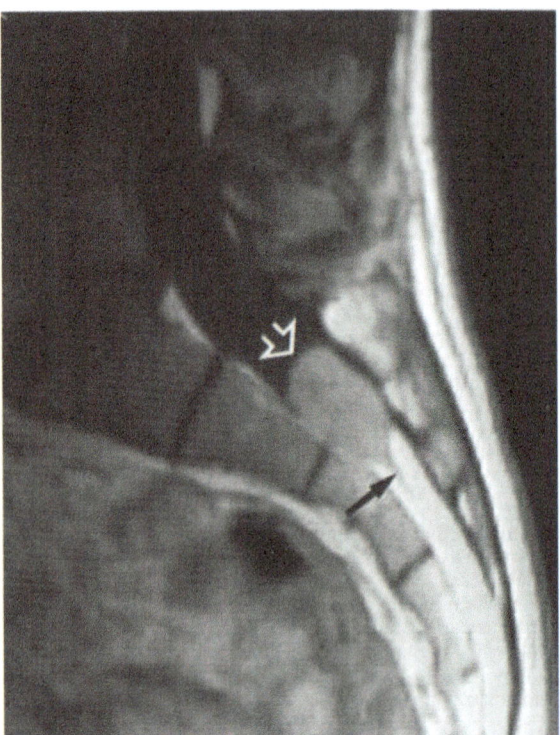

a

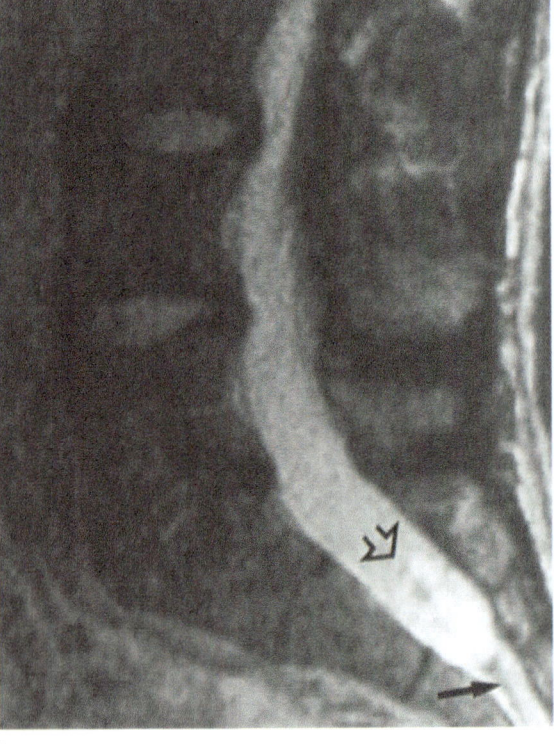

b

Figure 7.39 Ependymoma, myxopapillary, sacral: (**a**) T1WI, (**b**) T2WI, (**c,d**) HE × 200; circumscribed, homogeneous cord T1 isointense, lobulated T2 hyperintense mass (open arrows, a,b), occupies the distal sacral canal; linear structure is the filum (closed arrows, a,b) (compare with images of **Figure 7.7**). Smear (c) and paraffin section (d) shows a characteristic myxopapillary tumour; signal intensities at both short and long TR can be attributable only to protein content of myxoid material

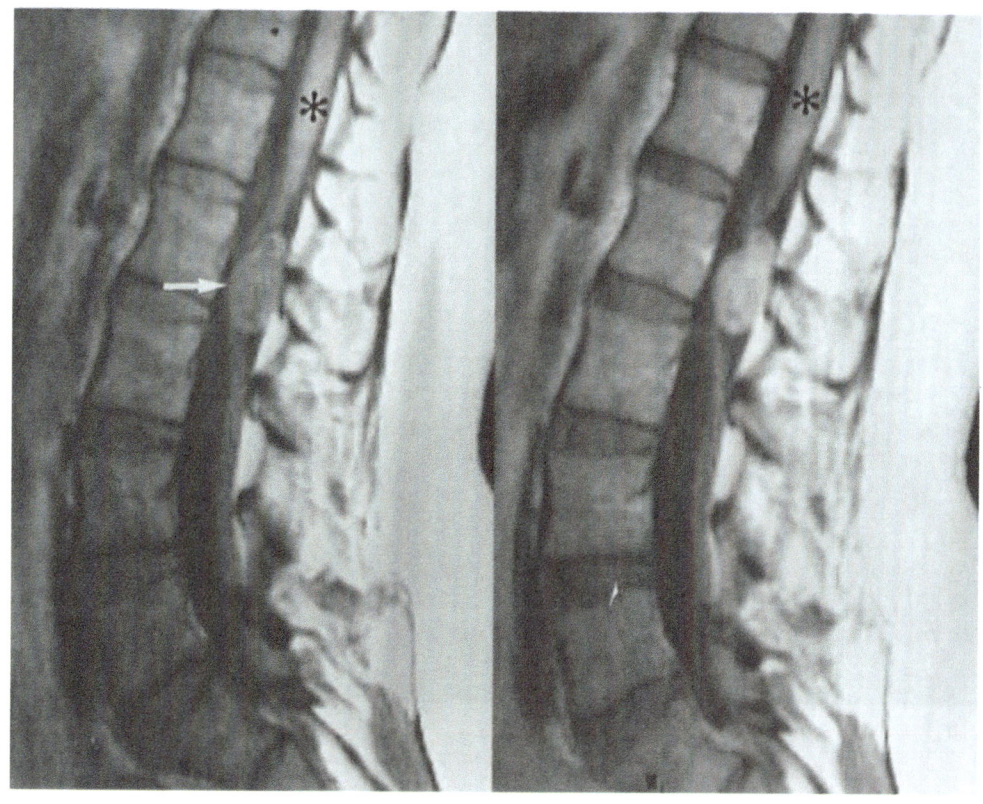

a
b

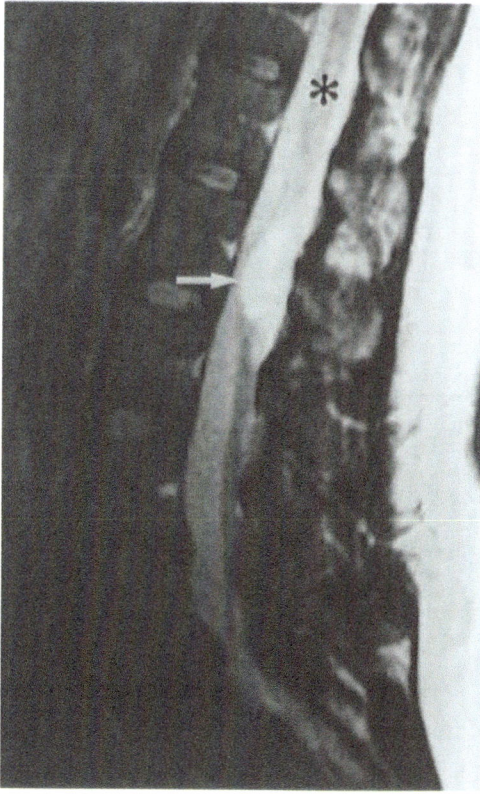

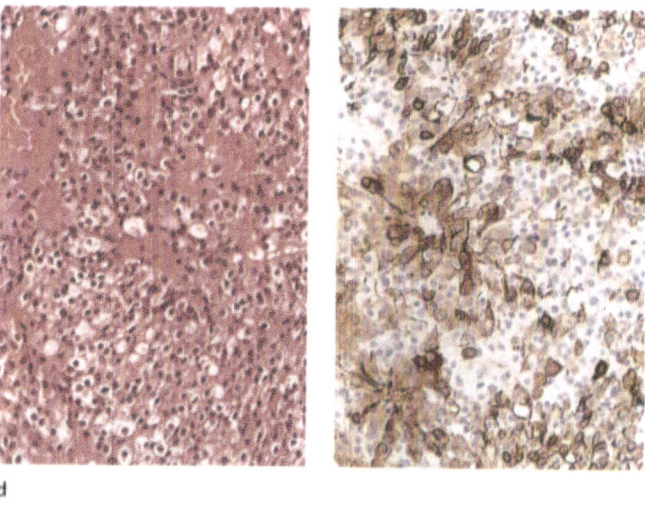

d

c

Figure 7.40 Ependymoma, clear cell, conus: female, 27 years; (**a**) T1WI, (**b**) T1WI + C, (**c**) T2WI, (**d**) HE/GFAP ×200, (**e**) Retic ×200; circumscribed conus lesion (a, arrow), is cord isointense, moderately enhancing (b) and hyperintense relative to CSF (c, arrow). (Asterisks identify cord parenchyma.) Histologically the tumour conformed to the rare clear-cell type of ependymoma, with strong overall GFAP positivity (d); numerous simple vessels and clefts are apparent with the silver stain (e)

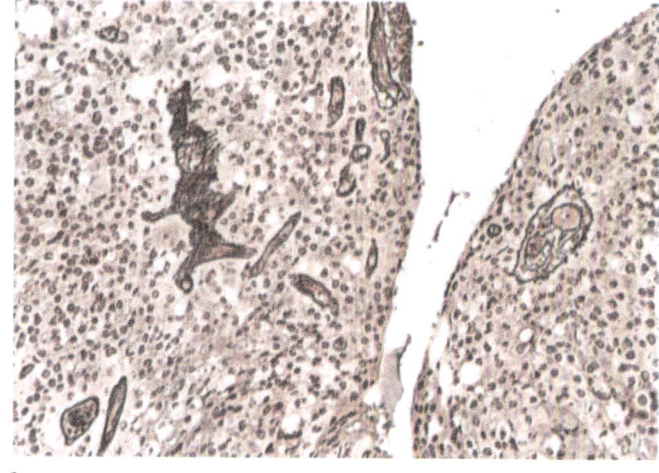

e

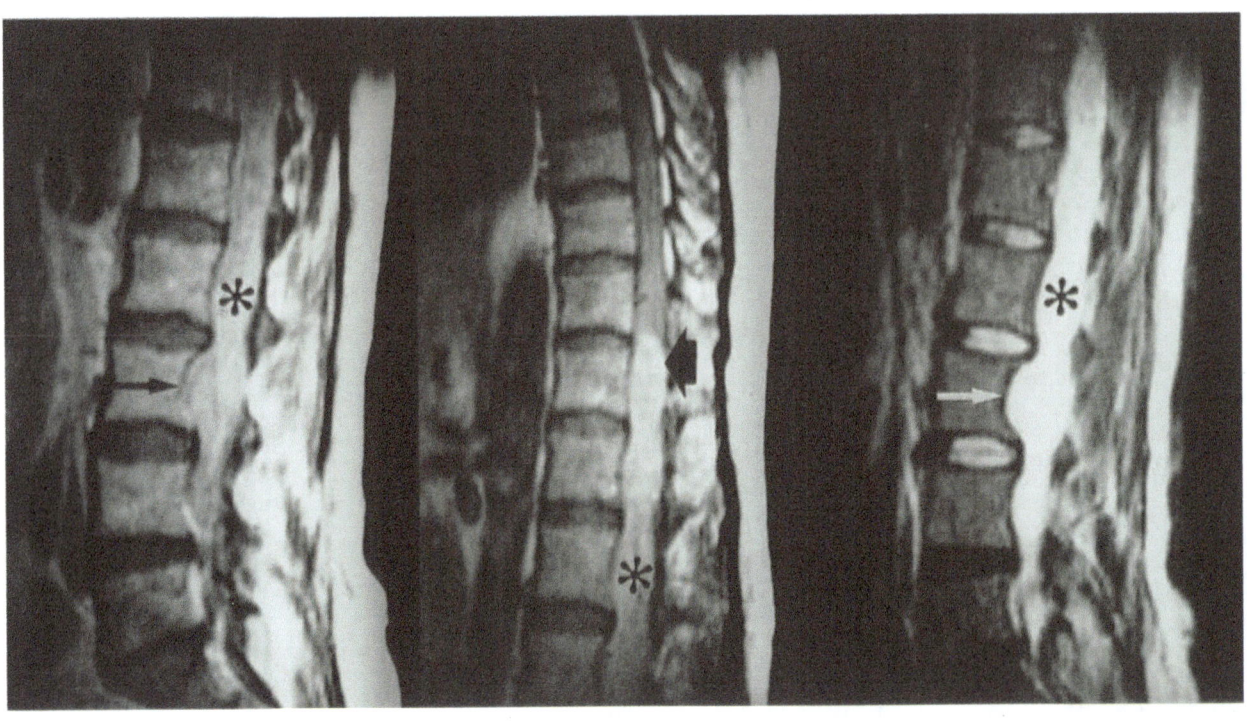

a   b   c

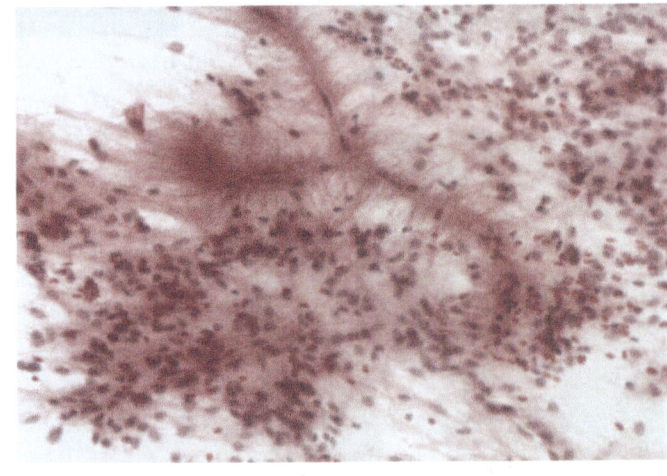

Figure 7.41 Ependymoma, myxopapillary, sacral with sub-arachnoid space effacement: female, 30 years; (**a,b**) T1WI + C, (**c**) T2WI, (**d**) HE ×200; the tumour (asterisk), which is moderately enhancing (a,b), and strongly T2 hyperintense (c), fills the lumbosacral canal, with vertebral scalloping (arrows, a,c). Note sharply circumscribed rostral border (b, arrow), only apparent after contrast administration. Smear preparation illustrates perivascular, nuclear-free organization of cells typical of ependymoma (d)

d

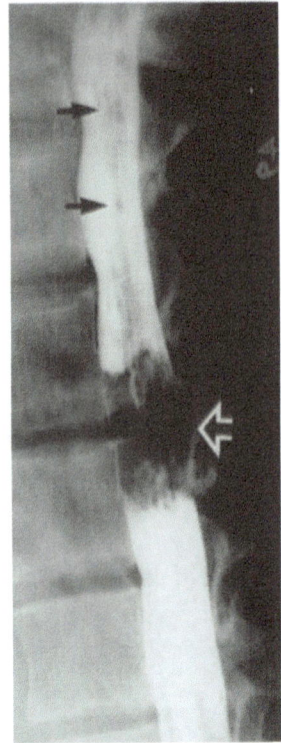

a

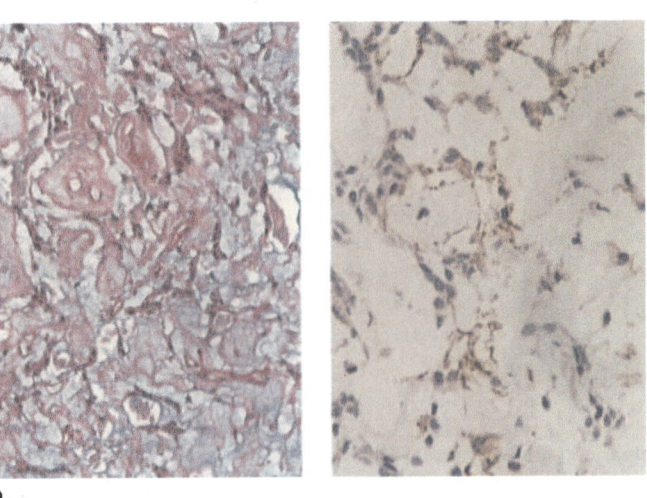

b

Figure 7.42 Ependymoma, myxopapillary, recurrence with seeding: (**a**) myelogram, (**b**) APAS ×200/GFAP ×400; postoperative myelogram shows extensive, but non-obstructive, tumour growth with seeding (arrows), above and below the main lesion (open arrow). Biopsy shows characteristic papillary morphology, with vascular myxoid degeneration (b, left), but without overt evidence of malignancy; note scattered GFAP-positive processes (b, right)

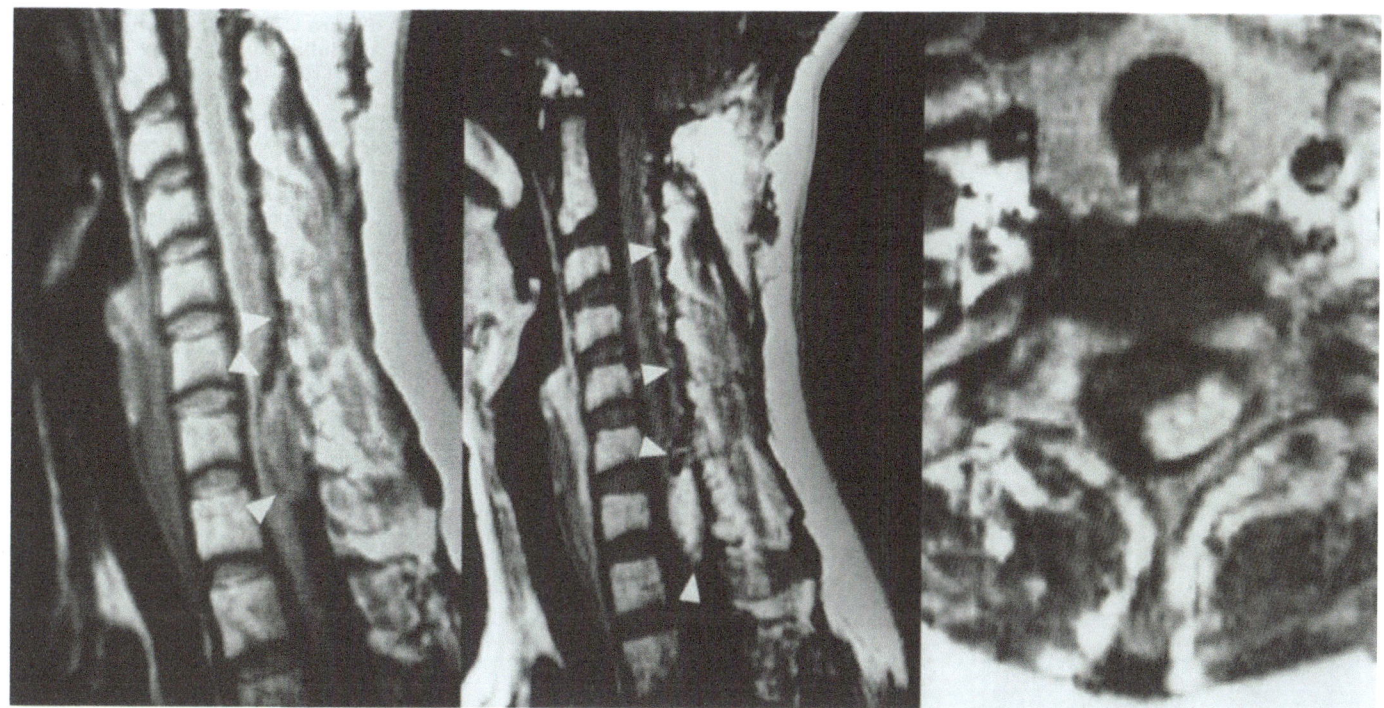

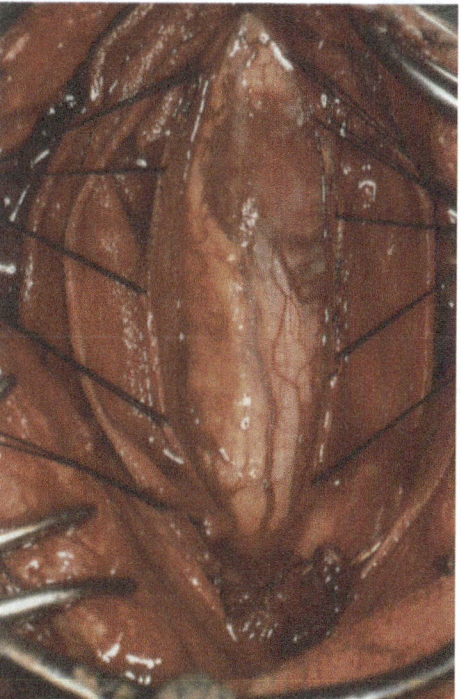

Figure 7.43 Haemangioblastoma, spinal cord: (**a**) T1WI, (**b**) T1WI + C, (**c**) axial T1WI + C, (**d**) operative view; en-plaque, isointense, diffusely enhancing lesion is demarcated from the cord by irregular, punctate signal voids, which continue upwards on the dorsum of the cord (arrow-heads), corresponding to grossly ectatic vessels observed at operation (d). Exophytic nature of tumour is shown in axial enhanced image (c) and operative view (d). (Dr JW Lotz, City Park Hospital)

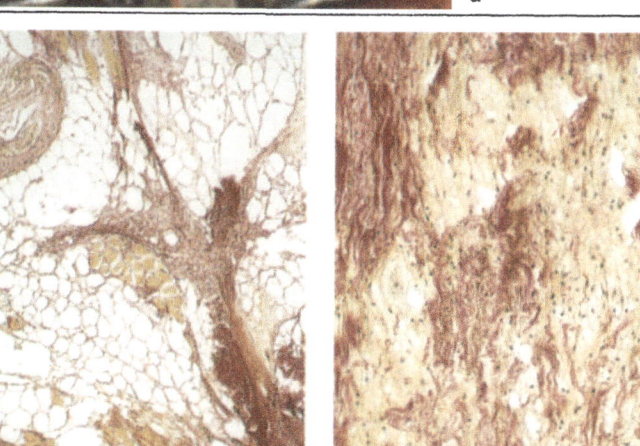

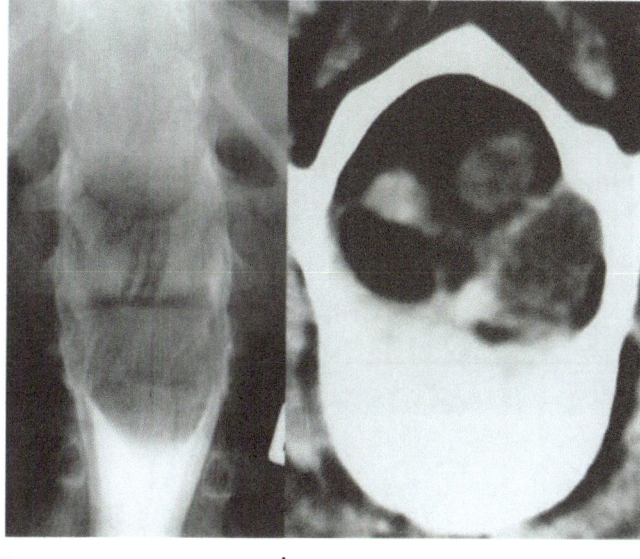

Figure 7.44 Teratoma, conus: (**a**) myelogram, (**b**) CT myelogram, (**c**) VG ×100, (**d**) VG ×200; conventional myelogram (a) shows gross expansion of the lumbar canal; mass on axial CT scan (b) has striking negative Hounsfield unit components, together with lobulated soft tissue isodensity. There is no evidence of a posterior arch defect. Histology confirms the benign teratomatous nature of the lesion, with adipose and other connective tissues (c). Nature of isodense tissue is not known, but could represent disorganized neural tissue (d)

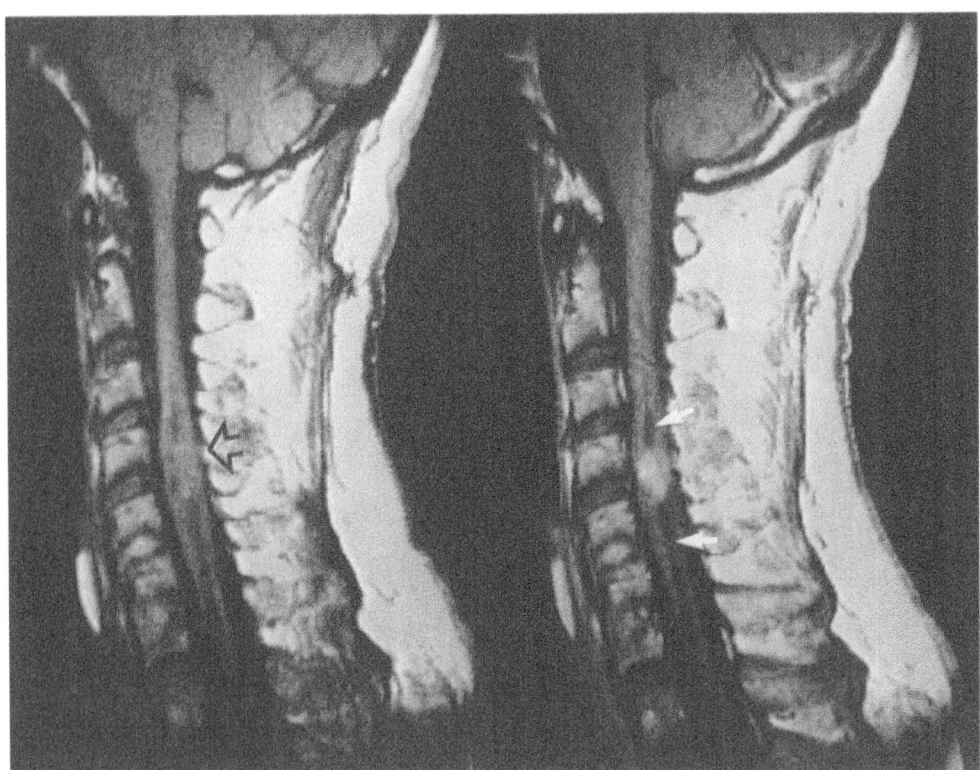

a   b

Figure 7.45 Ependymoma, intramedullary, with syrinx: male, 72 years; (a) T1WI, (b) T1WI + C; circumscribed T1 isointense (a, open arrow), moderately, diffusely enhancing, cervical, intramedullary mass with associated cavitation (b, closed arrows). (Imaging diagnosis includes pilocytic astrocytoma, haemangioblastoma and metastatic disease.)

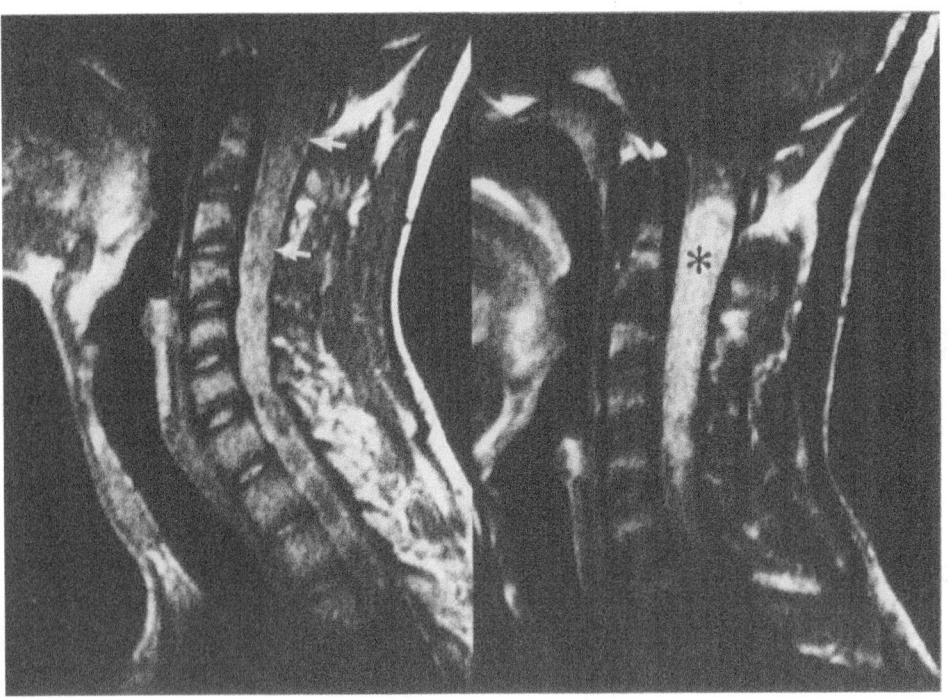

a   b

Figure 7.46 Ependymoma, intramedullary: (a) T1WI (b) T1WI + C, (c) axial T1WI + C, (d) HE ×200, (e) HE ×100, (f) VG ×100; (g) EM ×10000; tumour which is cord T1 isointense (inhomogeneously T2 hyperintense), effaces the normal anatomical profile (a, arrows), becomes delineated after contrast administration (b, asterisk). Axial view (c) shows central location of tumour with surrounding cord parenchyma (open arrows). At operation an easily defined cleavage plane was confirmed. Although the cellular morphology is characteristic of ependymoma (d), the tumour contains dilated clefts, into which fibrin-like exudation is occurring (e), with apparent organization (f, arrow). Absence of intercellular space on EM (g), suggests that clefts are responsible for grainy inhomogeneity at short and long TR

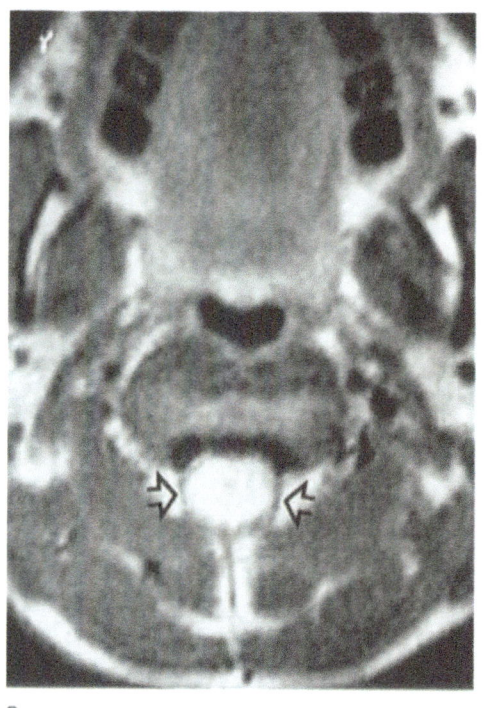

c

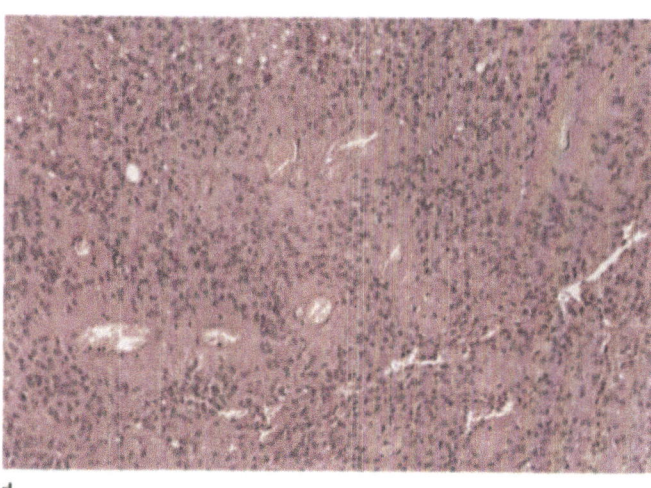

morphic fibrillated cells with abrupt tumour/parenchymal interface.
HE × 200

d

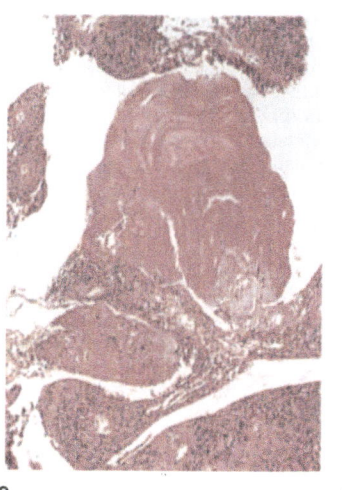

e

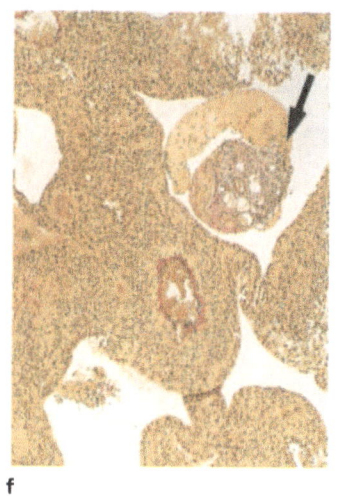

f

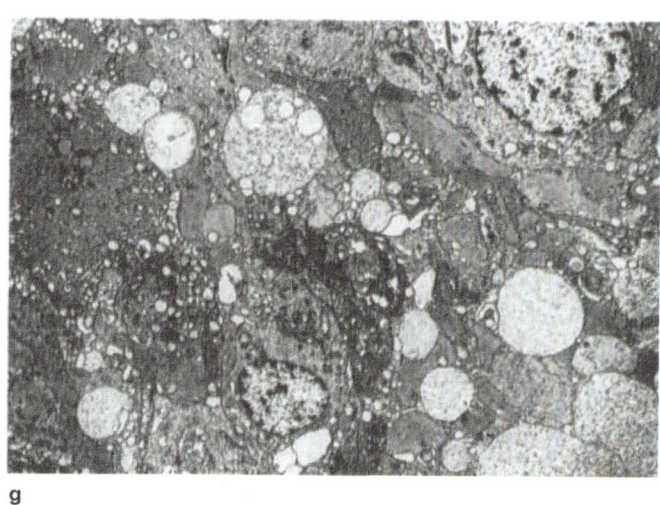

g

Figure 7.46 (*continued*)

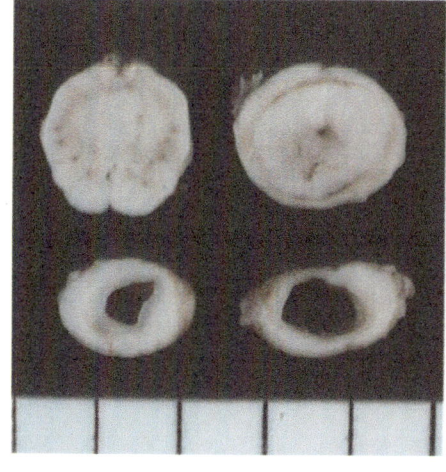

a

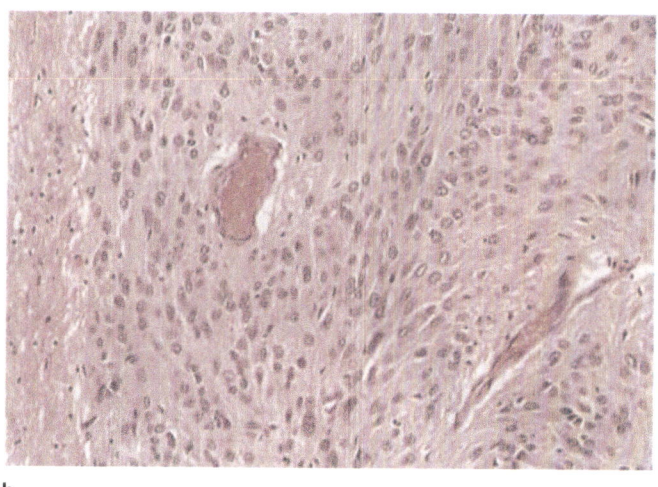

b

**Figure 7.47 Ependymomas/subependymomas, multiple, type
2 neurofibromatosis**: (**a**) sharply circumscribed pearly white, intramedullary tumour with adjacent syrinx; (**b**) histology shows monomorphic fibrillated cells with abrupt tumour/parenchymal interface.
HE × 200

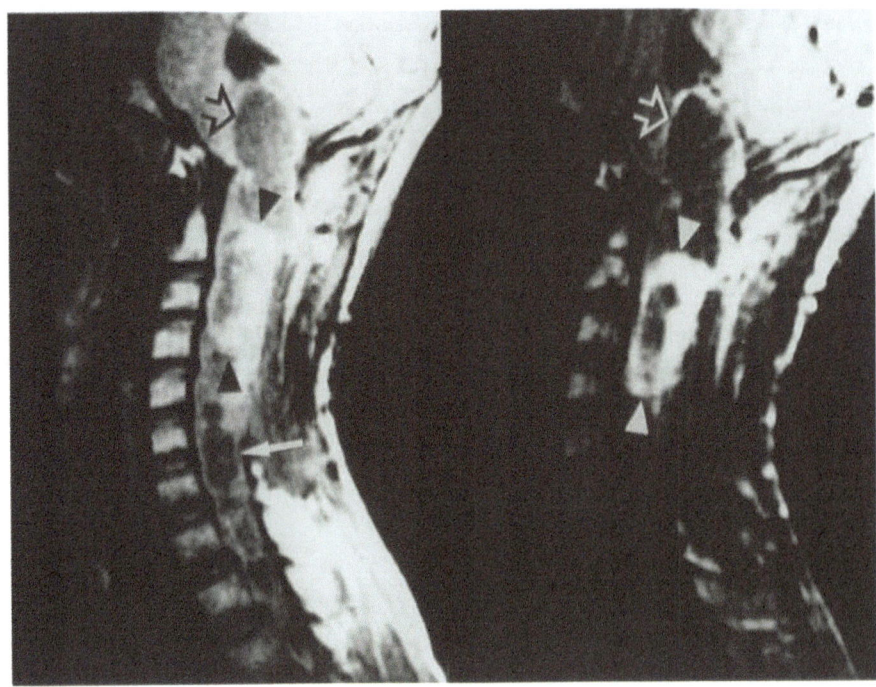

a   b

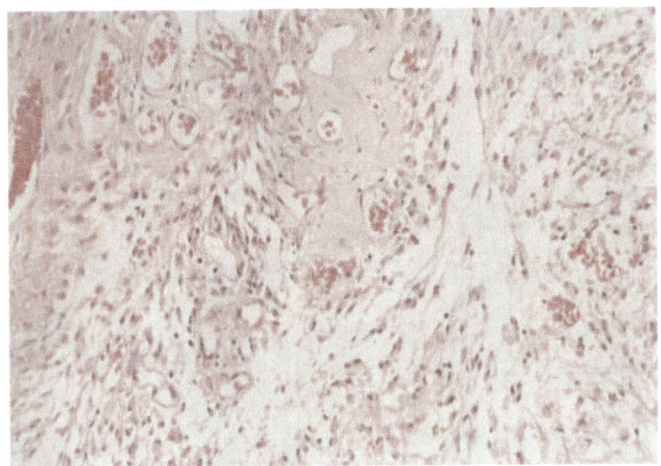

c

Figure 7.48 Pilocytic astrocytoma, juvenile, cystic, cervico-medullary: male, 12 years; (**a**) PDWI, (**b**) T1WI + C, (**c**) HE ×200; brainstem, hyperintense, circumscribed mass, with central cyst (arrow-heads, a,b) and strong enhancement (b). Nature of brainstem cavitation (open arrows, a,b) is uncertain; morphology and rim enhancement suggest this is neoplastic. Cord cavitation (a, arrow), is secondary. Histology is typical, including bipolar cells and prominent benign vasculature (c)

40. Bydder GM, Brown J, Niendorf HP. Enhancement of cervical intraspinal tumors in MR imaging with intravenous gadolinium-DTPA. JCAT. 1985;9:847–51.

41. Parizel PM, Baleriaux D, Rodesch G. GdDTPA-enhanced imaging of spinal tumors. AJNR. 1989;10:249–58.

42. Brunberg JA, DiPietro MA, Venes JL et al. Intramedullary lesions of the pediatric spinal cord: correlation of findings from MR imaging, intraoperative sonography, surgery and histologic study. Radiology. 1991;181:573–9.

43. Dillon WP, Norman D, Newton TH et al. Intradural spinal cord lesions: GdDTPA-enhanced MR imaging. Radiology. 1989; 170:229–37.

44. Giampiolo C, Ciapetta P, Delfini R et al. Intramedullary spinal neurinomas. J Neurosurg. 1982;57:143–7.

45. Rout D, Pillay SM, Radhakrishnan VV. Cervical intramedullary schwannoma. J Neurosurg. 1983;58:962–4.

46. Silbergeld J, Cohen WA, Maravilla KR et al. Supratentorial and spinal cord hemangioblastomas: gadolinium-enhanced MR appearance and pathologic correlation. JCAT. 1989;13:1048–51.

47. Costigan DA, Winkelman MD. Intramedullary spinal cord metastasis. J Neurosurg. 1985;62:227–33.

48. Kalyanaraman UP, Henderson JP. Intramedullary ganglioneuroma of spinal cord: a clinicopathological study. Hum Pathol. 1982;13:952–5.

49. Wald U, Levy PJ, Rappaport ZH. Conus ganglioglioma in a 2 and a half year old boy: case report. J Neurosurg. 1985;62:142–4.

50. Cheung Y-K, Fung C-F, Chan F-L. MRI features of spinal ganglioglioma. Clin Imag. 1991;15:109.

51. Lalitha VS, Rubinstein LJ. Reactive glioma in intracranial sarcoma: a form of mixed sarcoma and glioma ('sarcoglioma'). Report of eight cases. Cancer. 1979;43:246–57.

52. Quint DJ, Boulos RS, Sanders WP et al. Epidural lipomatosis. Radiology. 1988;169:485–90.

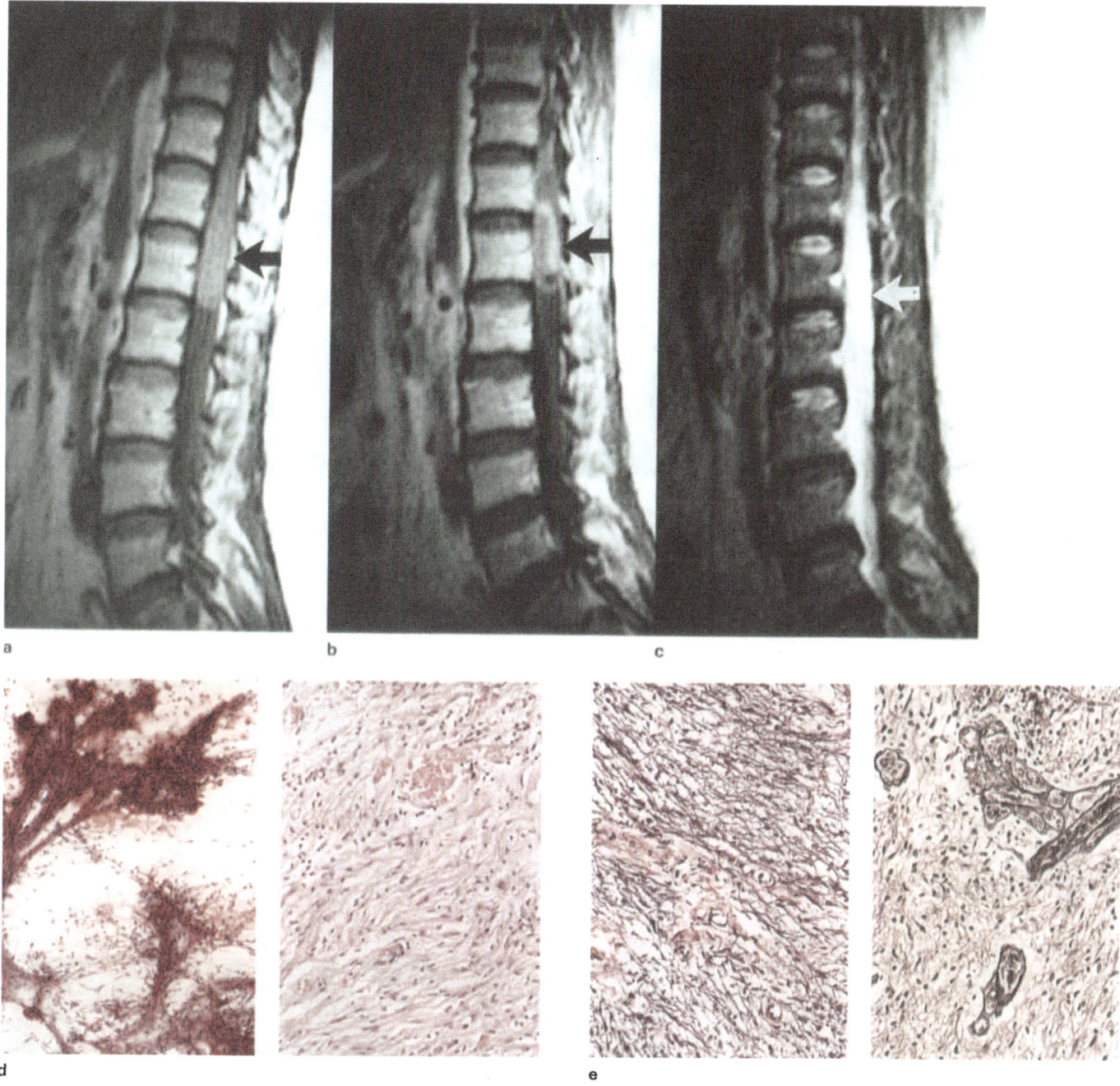

Figure 7.49   Pilocytic astrocytoma, compact, conus: female, 48 years; (**a**) T1WI, (**b**) T1WI + C, (**c**) T2WI, (**d**) HE ×100/×200, (**e**) PTAH/Retic ×200; conus is expanded by a T1 cord isointense (a), inhomogeneously enhancing mass (b), uniformly T2 hyperintense.

Cytological preparation shows perivascular arrangement of fibrillated cells (d, left), and a compact arrangement of pilocytic astrocytes in the paraffin section (d, right and e, left). Silver stain confirms prominent vasculature (e, right)

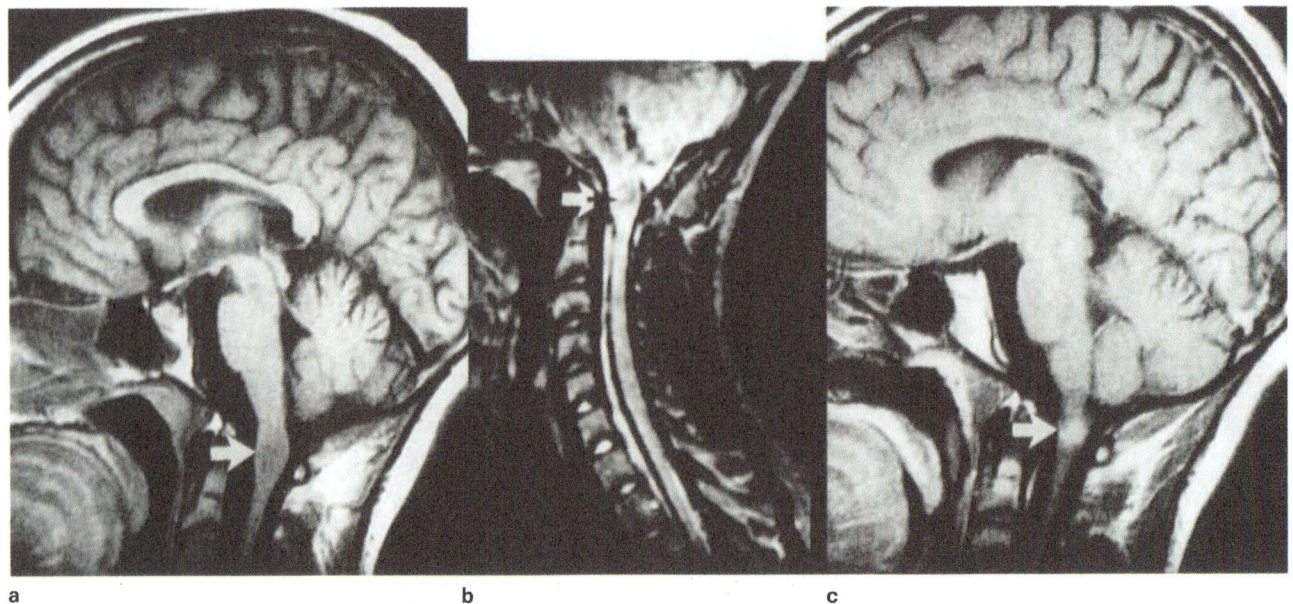

a   b   c

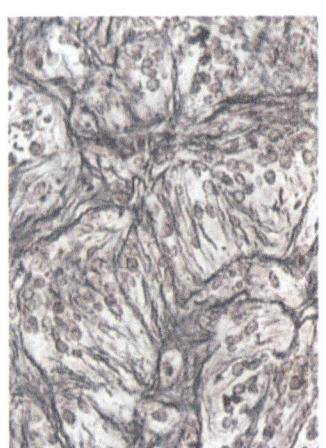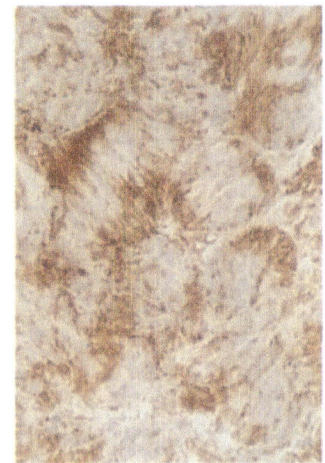

d

Figure 7.50   Schwannoma, intramedullary: (**a**) T1WI, (**b**) T2WI, (**c**) T1WI + C, (**d**) Retic/S100 ×400; lesion, which appears to expand the cord, is T1 cord isointense, predominantly T2 isointense, but with focal hyperintensity, and diffusely enhancing (arrows, a–c); surrounding hyperintensity (b) is probably parenchymal oedema. The small biopsy shows mainly Antoni A tissue, with striking Verocay body formation, which with the abundant pericellular reticulin content (d, left), could explain the relative T2 hypointensity (cord isointensity) of this lesion; note S100 positivity of Schwann cells (d, right)

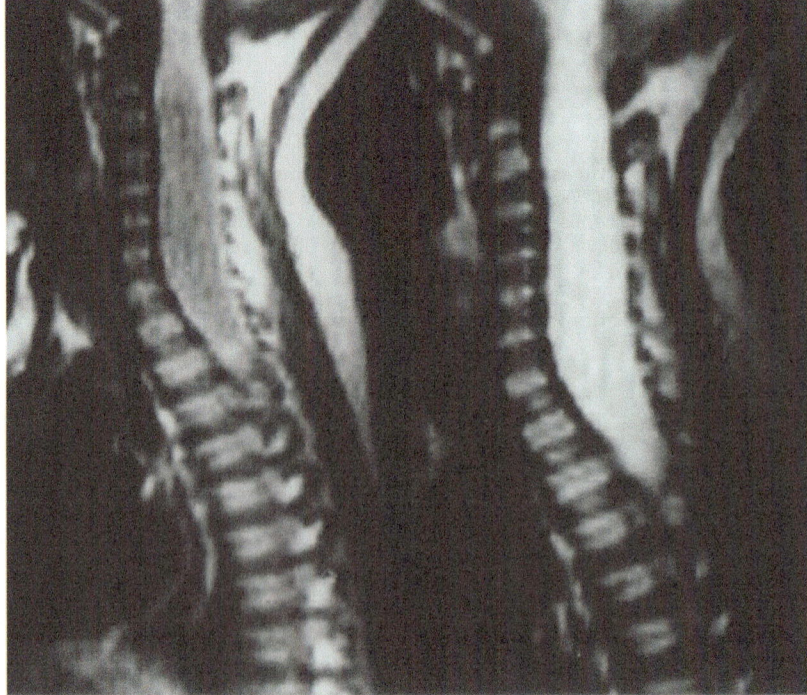

a   b   **Figure 7.51**   (*legend opposite*)

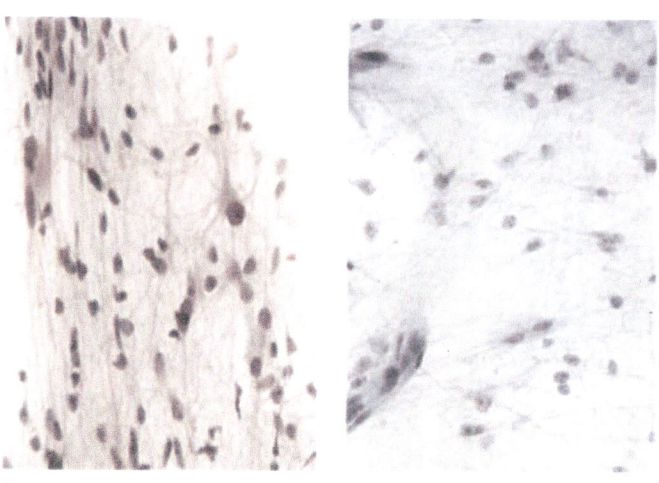

c

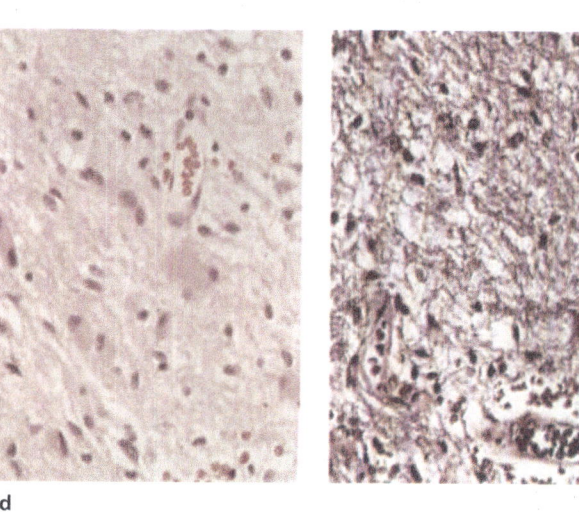

d

Figure 7.51 Astrocytoma, fibrillary, spinal cord: male, 2 years, fluctuating paraparesis and postural disturbance; (**a**) T1WI, (**b**) T2WI, (**c**) HE/Tol blue × 400, (**d**) HE/PTAH × 400; (non-enhancing), diffuse T1 hypointense (a), T2 hyperintense expansion of the cord (b); gross widening of the spinal canal is associated with pressure atrophy of the cervical vertebral bodies. Correlative imaging feature and pathomorphology (c,d) are pathognomonic, and are a faithful counterpart of the hemispheric fibrillary astrocytoma

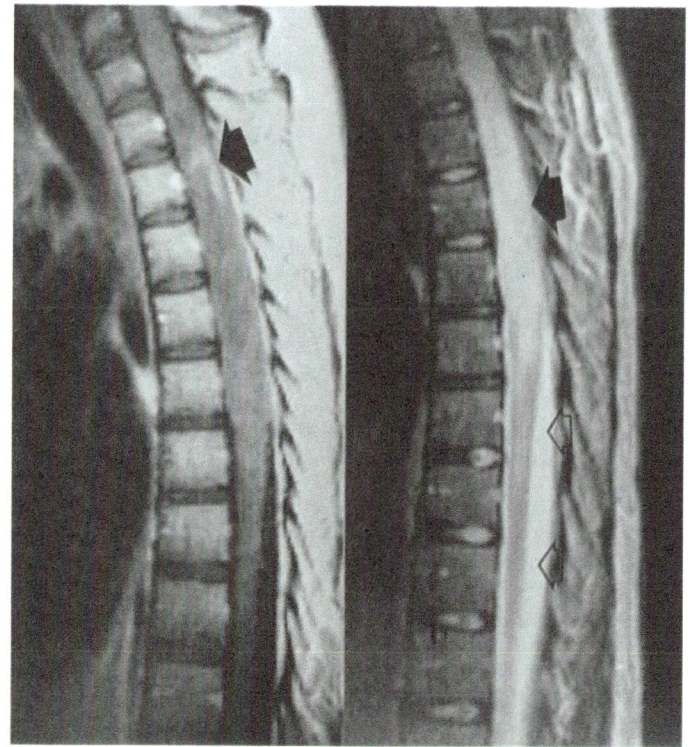

a   b

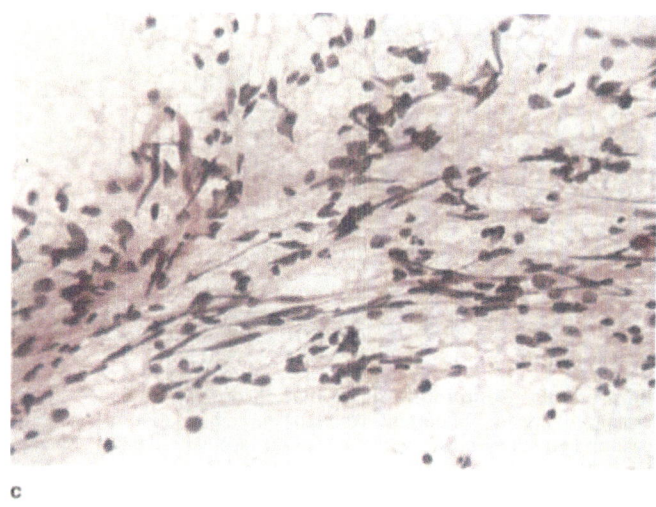

c

Figure 7.52 Astrocytoma, fibrillary, spinal cord: female, 14 years; (**a**) T1WI + C, (**b**) T2WI, (**c**) HE × 200, (**d**) GFAP/HE × 400/× 1000; extensive hypointense cord expansion, mainly non-enhancing except for a fragmentary linear focus (a, arrow); the lesion is weakly T2 hyperintense (b, arrow), compared with CSF (b, open arrows). At operation diffuse swelling of cord confirmed, and myelotomy did not disclose obviously abnormal tissue. Although biopsy specimen smear suffers from crush artefact, nuclei are clearly abnormal (c) and immunohistochemistry performed on cytological preparations confirms the astrocytic nature of the tumour cells (d). Morphology of enhancing focus is unknown, but may represent the more vascularized type of compact pilocytic astrocytoma (see **Figure 7.49**), or focal malignant change

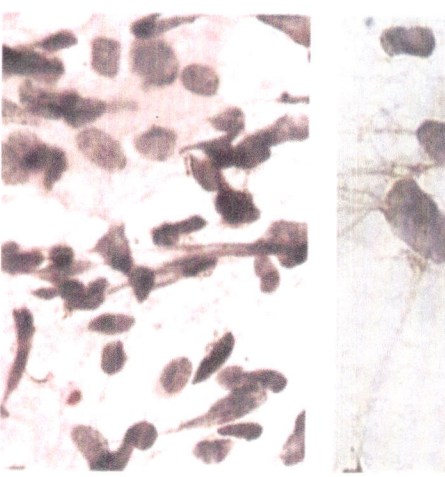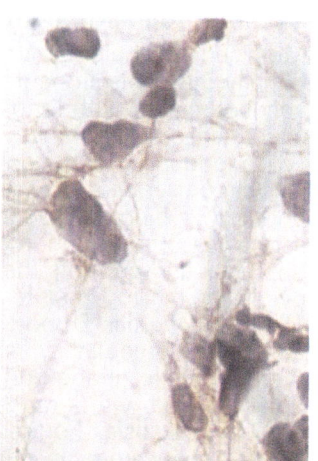

d

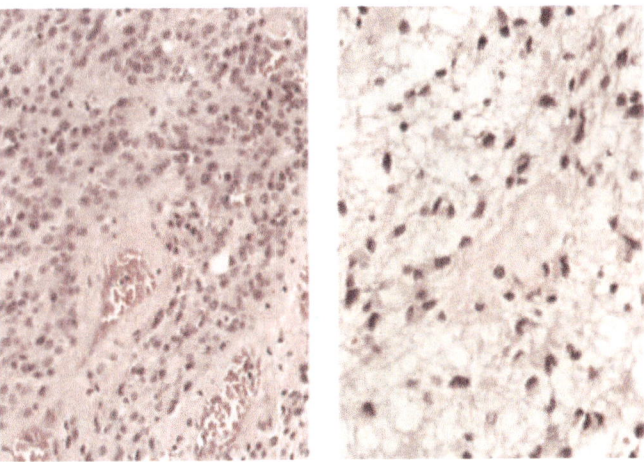

Figure 7.53 Ependymoastrocytoma, spinal cord: male, 47 years; typical ependymoma (left) and astrocytoma (right); note prominent vasculature of ependymomatous component compared with the relatively avascular astrocytoma; provided that these tissue types are sufficiently extensive, patchy or inhomogeneous enhancement may be expected. HE ×200

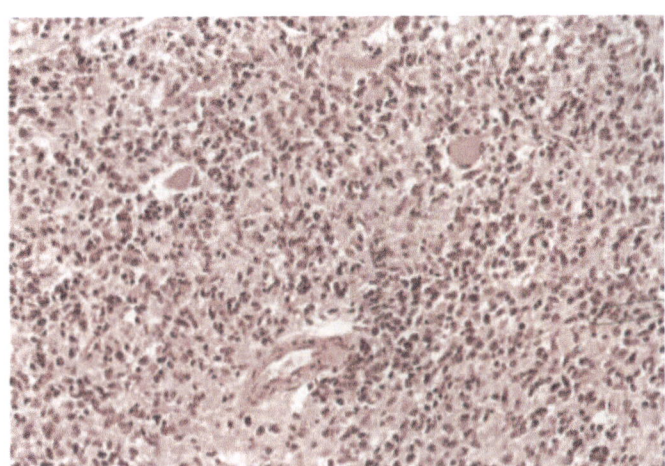

Figure 7.54 Glioma, NOS, spinal cord: male, 27 years; biopsy of extensive spinal tumour consisting of poorly differentiated glial cells, diffusely infiltrating cord parenchyma. HE ×200

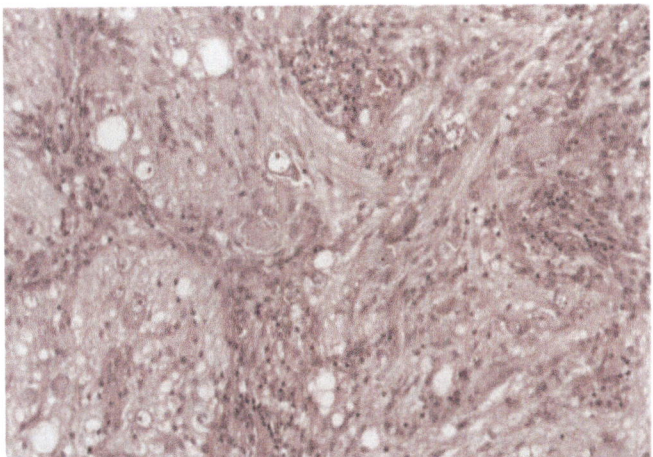

Figure 7.55 Ganglioglioma, spinal cord: male, 38 years; striking organized mixture of neuropil-like tissue containing abnormal ganglion cells and granular bodies, with interspersed vascularized glial trabeculae. HE ×200

ADDENDUM

Dysembryoplastic neuroepithelial tumour (DNT)

Most neuropathologists will have experience of an exceptionally indolent glioneuronal neoplasm which is invariably associated with longstanding epilepsy. The entity is characterized by its unchanging nature on serial images (CT hypodense, T1 hypo/T2 hyperintense, typically cortical, circumscribed and non-enhancing) and its histomorphology, which, although suggestive of protoplasmic astrocytes or oligodendroglia, is nevertheless somewhat untypical and prompts the notion of a hamartomatous or dysplastic mass. These features were first summarized in 1988 by Daumas-Duport, et al who also proposed the term dysembryoplastic neuroepithelial tumour[1]. Besides the diagnostic glioneuronal component, the lesion may be associated with a range of glial cell types and foci of cortical dysplasia. Furthermore, the imaging finding of strong enhancement in a number of otherwise microscopically characteristic tumours[2,3] has necessitated widening the concept to include two subtypes of DNT, namely simple (consisting solely of the specific glioneuronal element) and complex, with vascular arcades and hamartomatous vessels being present in the latter, and presumably accounting for contrast uptake.

Although since completing the text of this book we have identified two cases of complex DNT, we now think it probable that the tumour illustrated in Figure 4.22, as an example of protoplasmic astrocytoma, is in fact the simple form of DNT. This would be consistent with the recent suggestion[2] that histologically homogeneous protoplasmic tumours are properly simple DNTs.

We also draw attention to the importance of the possible imaging depiction of significant mass effect or peritumoural oedema, either as an initial event, or appearing in the scanning chronology. Such a finding, particularly if associated with focal enhancement, must denote new growth, and despite otherwise typical histology on biopsy, suggests an alternative diagnosis, or, if indeed a DNT, a more guarded prognosis seems appropriate.

References

1. Daumas-Duport C, Scheithauer BW, Chodkiewicz JP, et al. Dysembryoplastic neuroepithelial tumour: A surgically curable tumour of young patients with intractable partial seizures. Neurosurgery. 1988;23:545–6.
2. Daumas-Duport C. Dysembryoplastic neuroepithelial tumours. Brain Pathol. 1993;3:283–95.
3. Koeller KK, Dillon WP. Dysembryoplastic neuroepithelial tumors: MR appearance. AJNR. 1992;13:1319–25.

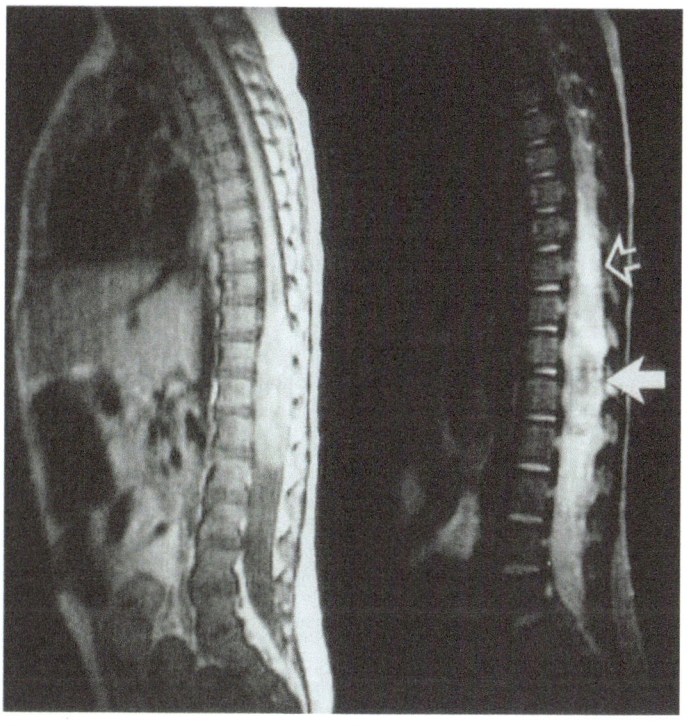

a   b

Figure 7.56 **Sarcoglioma, conus**: female, 1 year, paraplegia; (**a**) T1WI, (**b**) T2WI, (**c**) HE × 200/GFAP × 400, (**d**) HE × 200/ × 100, (**e**) HE/Retic × 400; smooth conus expansion is homogeneously cord T1 isointense (a), and mainly T2 isointense (b, closed arrow). Rostral parenchymal signal hyperintensity may be oedema (b, open arrow). Variable histological picture includes tumour composed of sarcomatous elements (c, left) with admixed neoplastic astrocytes (brown-staining cells on right – note mitosis (arrow); the tumour, which shows a sharp parenchymal interface (d, left), also contains sinusoidal vessels within myxomatous stroma (d, right) and abundant reticulin (e). (Histology reviewed by Prof LJ Rubinstein)

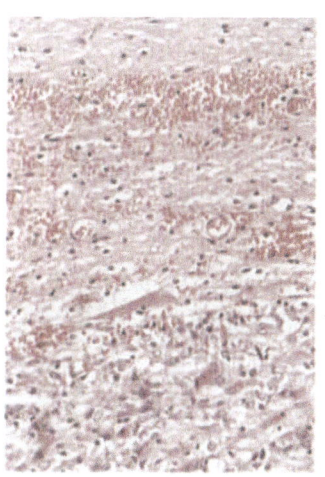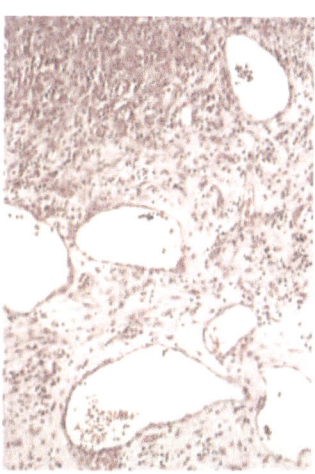

c   d

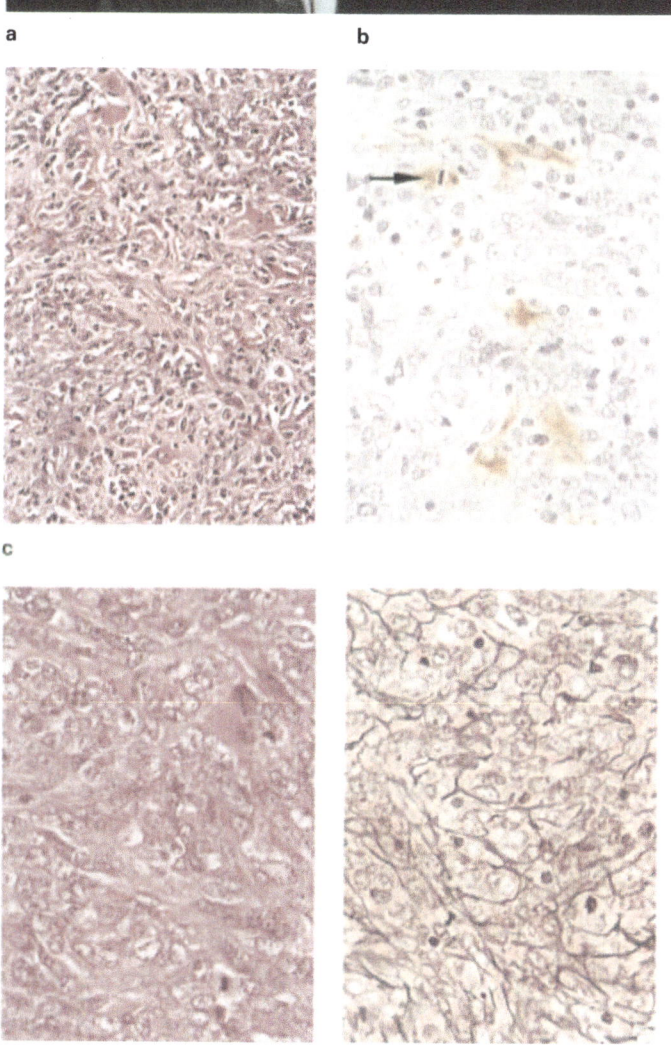

e

Index

The manufacturer's authorised representative in the EU is Springer
Nature Customer Service Centre GmbH, Europaplatz 3, 69115 Heidelberg,
Germany. If you have any concerns regarding our products, please
contact ProductSafety@springernature.com

Printed and bound by CPI Group (UK) Ltd, Croydon, CR0 4YY
27/04/2026
02097727-0001